Hematologic Malignancies

Series editor
Martin Dreyling
München, Germany

This series of professional books provides in-depth information on all aspects of the diagnosis and treatment of different hematologic cancers, including clinical evaluation, imaging diagnosis, staging, current treatment strategies, novel targeted approaches, and evaluation of treatment response. Readers will also find coverage of methodological and research issues and factors that influence treatment outcome. Each volume is designed to serve both as a quick reference and as a comprehensive source of knowledge that will be invaluable in improving management of the malignancy under consideration. The volume editors and authors have been selected for their international reputations and acknowledged expertise. The series will appeal to hematologists and oncologists in hospitals or private practices, residents, and others with an interest in the field.

More information about this series at http://www.springer.com/series/5416

Georg Lenz • Gilles Salles
Editors

Aggressive Lymphomas

Springer

Editors
Georg Lenz
Department of Translational Oncology
University-Hospital Münster
Münster
Germany

Gilles Salles
Department of Hematology
University Claude Bernard Lyon 1
Pierre-Benite cedex
France

ISSN 2197-9766 ISSN 2197-9774 (electronic)
Hematologic Malignancies
ISBN 978-3-030-00361-6 ISBN 978-3-030-00362-3 (eBook)
https://doi.org/10.1007/978-3-030-00362-3

Library of Congress Control Number: 2018964248

This Springer imprint is published by the registered company Springer Nature Switzerland AG
The registered company address is: Gewerbestrasse 11, 6330 Cham, Switzerland

Contents

Introduction

In the last several years, the understanding of the biology and the molecular pathogenesis of aggressive lymphomas has substantially improved. This significantly changed diagnostic and therapeutic algorithms. As a result, a variety of novel molecular lymphoma subtypes and patient risk groups have recently been identified, and various novel and very specific compounds as well as new immunologic approaches have shown impressive efficacy in clinical trials. These therapeutic improvements will soon translate into standard of care and will further improve the prognosis of affected patients.

Our textbook summarizes the current knowledge on the epidemiology, pathology, and biology of the major aggressive lymphoma subtypes. In the main section, we provide an up-to-date overview of the standard of care therapeutic approaches of patients affected by these diseases. In the last part, we describe how we believe that the field will develop and how future diagnostic and therapeutic strategies will look like. Thus, our textbook provides an up-to-date compendium on the recent developments in the field of aggressive lymphomas.

At last, we would like to thank all of the authors whose expertise and tremendous efforts made the completion of this textbook possible. Finally, we are very grateful to the Springer publisher and especially to Ejaz Ahmad, who continuously supported the development of this textbook.

September 2018
Münster, Germany — Georg Lenz
Pierre-Benite cedex, France — Gilles Salles

In the older version the spelling of book title was incorrect. Book title "Agressive Lymphomas" has been corrected to "Aggressive Lymphomas". https://doi.org/10.1007/978-3-030-00362-3

Part I

Epidemiology, Pathology and Molecular Pathogenesis

Epidemiology of Aggressive Lymphomas

1

James R. Cerhan

1.1 Introduction and Scope

Lymphomas are a heterogeneous group of nearly 100 variants of lymphoid malignancy that arise from lymphocytes and produce tumors in the lymph nodes, lymphatic organs, and extranodal lymphatic tissue (i.e., lymphoma), as well as the bone marrow (i.e., multiple myeloma) or peripheral blood (i.e., leukemia) [1]. Collectively, lymphoid neoplasms are the fourth most common cancers in the USA, with an estimated 136,960 cases in 2016 [2]. Lymphomas are considered to be clonal tumors of immature or mature B-cells, T-cells, or natural killer (NK) cells arrested at various stages of differentiation [3]. B-cell neoplasms appear to recapitulate the normal stages of B-cell differentiation, and many B-cell lymphomas can be linked to a presumed normal cell counterpart. The normal counterparts of T-cells and NK-cells are not as well characterized as B-cells, but they do share many immunophenotypic and functional properties and are currently grouped together. Based on this understanding, the current World Health Organization (WHO) classification system [4], which has been incorporated into the International Classification of Diseases for Oncology (ICD-O) [5], recognizes precursor lymphoid neoplasm (B- and T-cell), mature B-cell neoplasms, mature T/NK-cell neoplasms, Hodgkin lymphoma (HL), and histiocytic and dendritic cell neoplasms. Acute and chronic lymphocytic leukemia (ALL and CLL, respectively) and multiple myeloma (MM) are classified as a B-cell neoplasms [6]. The 2016 revision of the fourth edition of the WHO classification of lymphoid malignancies [1] was recently released, and although it did not allow for any new definitive entities, it incorporated new genetic/molecular and clinical data into current disease entities and added a limited number of new provisional entities.

While there are multiple B-cell [7, 8] and T-cell [9] subtypes that are considered to be aggressive lymphomas (with some entities changing or being added across editions of the WHO Classification in 2001 [6], 2008 [4], and 2016 [1]), in this chapter, the focus is on three broadly defined groups: diffuse large B-cell lymphoma (DLBCL), Burkitt lymphoma/leukemia (BL), and peripheral T-cell lymphoma (PTCL). Table 1.1 provides an overview of the major lymphoid malignancy subtypes by version of the WHO Classification, with more detail provided for the aggressive subtypes. Based on national US data, of the estimated 136,960 newly diagnosed lymphoid neoplasms in 2016, there were 8500 HL (6.2%), 117,470 B-cell lymphoid malignancies (85.8%), and 8380 T/NK-cell lymphoid malignancies (6.1%). In Table 1.1, we have

J. R. Cerhan (✉)
Department of Health Sciences Research, Mayo Clinic College of Medicine, Rochester, MN, USA
e-mail: Cerhan.james@mayo.edu

G. Lenz, G. Salles (eds.), *Aggressive Lymphomas*, Hematologic Malignancies,
https://doi.org/10.1007/978-3-030-00362-3_1

Table 1.1 Expected number of incident lymphoid neoplasms in 2016, USA, according to the WHO classification of lymphoid malignancies[a]

Subtype[b]	ICD-O-3 codes	WHO version			New cases, 2016	% of lymphoid neo-plasms
		2001	2008	2016		
Lymphoid neoplasms, total					136,960	100
1. Hodgkin lymphoma (HL)	9650–9655,9659,9661–9667	X	X	X	8500	6.2
2. Non-Hodgkin lymphoid neoplasms					125,850	91.9
2(a) Non-Hodgkin lymphoid neoplasms, B-cell					117,470	85.8
1. Precursor B-cell lymphoblastic leukemia/lymphoma	9727(B), 9728, 9811–9818, 9835(B), 9836	X	X	X	4930	3.6
1.1. Precursor B-cell lymphoblastic leukemia/ lymphoma, NOS	9727(B), 9728, 9811, 9835(B), 9836		X	X	4570	3.3
1.2. Precursor B-cell lymphoblastic leukemia/ lymphoma, with recurrent genetic abnormalities	9812–9818		X	X	360	0.3
2. Mature non-Hodgkin lymphoma, B-cell					105,190	76.8
2.1.1. Chronic lymphocytic leukemia/small lymphocytic leukemia (CLL/SLL)	9670, 9823	X	X	X	20,980	15.3
2.1.2. Prolymphocytic leukemia, B-cell	9832(B), 9833	X	X	X	120	0.1
2.1.3. Mantle cell lymphoma	9673	X	X	X	3320	2.4
2.2.1. Lymphoplasmacytic lymphoma	9671	X	X	X	1060	0.8
2.2.2. Waldenstrom macroglobulinemia	9761	X	X	X	1270	0.9
2.3. **Diffuse large B-cell lymphoma (DLBCL)**	**9678–9679, 9684(B), 9680, 9687–9688, 9712, 9735, 9737–9738**				**27,650**	**20.2**
2.3.1. **DLBCL-NOS**	**9684(B), 9680 (excluding C44.0–44.9, C49.9, C71.0–71.9)**	**X**	**X**	**X**	**25,380**	**18.5**
2.3.2. **Primary DLBCL of the CNS (PCNSL)**	**9680 (C71.0–71.9)**		**X**	**X**	**1100**	**0.8**
2.3.3. **Primary cutaneous DLBCL, leg type**	**9680 (C44.0–44.9)**		**X**	**X**	**400**	**0.3**
2.3.4. **T-cell/histiocyte-rich large B-cell lymphoma**	**9688**		**X**	**X**	**200**	**0.1**
2.3.5. **Intravascular large B-cell lymphoma**	**9712, 9680 (C49.9)**	**X**	**X**	**X**	**60**	**0.04**
2.3.6. **ALK positive large B-cell lymphoma**	**9737**		**X**	**X**	**<50**	**<0.04**
2.3.7. **Plasmablastic lymphoma**	**9735**		**X**	**X**	**180**	**0.1**

Table 1.1 (continued)

Subtype[b]	ICD-O-3 codes	WHO version			New cases, 2016	% of lymphoid neo-plasms
		2001	2008	2016		
2.3.8. **Large B-cell (plasmablastic) lymphoma arising from HHV-8 associated multicentric Castleman disease**	**9738**		**X**		**<50**	**<0.04**
2.3.9. **Primary effusion lymphoma (PEL)**	**9678**	**X**	**X**	**X**	**<50**	**<0.04**
2.3.10. **Primary mediastinal (thymic) large B-cell lymphoma (MLBCL)**	**9679**	**X**	**X**	**X**	**240**	**0.2**
EBV+ DLBCL of the elderly			X			
EBV+ DLBCL, NOS				X		
DLBCL associated with chronic inflammation			X	X		
Primary cutaneous DLBCL, leg type			X	X		
Lymphoid granulomatosis	9766	X	X	X		
Large B-cell lymphoma with IRF4 rearrangement				X		
EBV+ mucocutaneous ulcer				X		
HHV8+ DLBCL, NOS				X		
2.4. **Burkitt lymphoma/leukemia (BL)**	**9687, 9826**	**X**	**X**	**X**	**1480**	**1.1**
Burkitt-like lymphoma with chromosomal 11q aberrations				X		
High-grade B-cell lymphoma, with MYC and BCL2 and/or BCL6 rearrangements				X		
High-grade B-cell lymphoma, NOS				X		
B-cell lymphoma, classifiable, with feature intermediate between DLBCL and HL	9596		X	X		
2.5. Marginal zone lymphomas	9689, 9699	X	X	X	7460	5.4
2.6. Follicular lymphoma	9597,9690–9691,9695,9698	X	X	X	13,960	10.2
2.7. Hairy cell leukemia	9940	X	X	X	1100	0.8
2.8. Hairy cell leukemia variant	9591 (C42.1–42.2)		X	X	810	0.6
2.9. Plasma cell neoplasms	9731–9734	X	X	X	25,980	19.0
2.10. Heavy chain diseases	9762	X	X	X	<50	<0.04
3. B-cell lymphoid neoplasms, NOS	9590(B), 9591(B) (excluding C42.1–42.2), 9675(B), 9820(B)	X	X	X	7350	5.4

(continued)

Table 1.1 (continued)

Subtype[b]	ICD-O-3 codes	WHO version			New cases, 2016	% of lymphoid neo-plasms
		2001	2008	2016		
2(b) Non-Hodgkin lymphoid neoplasms, T/NK-cell					8380	6.1
1. Precursor T/NK-cell lymphoblastic leukemia/ lymphoma, NOS	9727(T, NK), 9729, 9835(T, NK), 9837	X	X	X	1070	0.8
2. Mature non-Hodgkin lymphoid neoplasms, T/NK-cell					7190	5.2
2.1. Mycosis fungoides/Sezary syndrome (MF/SS)	9700, 9701	X	X	X	1690	1.2
2.2. **Peripheral T-cell lymphomas (PTCL)**	**9675(T), 9702, 9705, 9708–9709, 9714, 9716–9717, 9724, 9726**				**3950**	**2.9**
2.2.1. **PTCL, NOS**	**9675(T, NK), 9702**	**X**	**X**	**X**	**1660**	**1.2**
2.2.2. **Angioimmunoblastic T-cell lymphoma (AITL)**	**9705**	**X**	**X**	**X**	**530**	**0.4**
2.2.3. **Subcutaneous panniculitis-like T-cell lymphoma (SPTCL)**	**9708**	**X**	**X**	**X**	**<50**	**<0.04**
2.2.4. **Anaplastic large cell lymphoma (ALCL) ALK-positive**	**9714**		**X**	**X**	**830**	**0.6**
2.2.5. **Hepatosplenic T-cell lymphoma (HSTL)**	**9716**	**X**	**X**	**X**	**<50**	**<0.04**
2.2.6. **Enteropathy-associated T-cell lymphoma (EATL)**	**9717**	**X**	**X**	**X**	**50**	**0.0**
2.2.7. **Primary cutaneous gamma-delta T-cell lymphoma**	**9726**		**X**	**X**	**<50**	**<0.04**
2.2.8. **Primary cutaneous T-cell lymphoma, NOS**	**9709**	**X**	**X**	**X**	**760**	**0.6**
2.2.9. **Systemic EBV-positive lymphoproliferative disease**	**9724**		**X**	**X**	**<50**	**<0.04**
Anaplastic large cell lymphoma ALK-negative				X		
Breast implant-associated anaplastic large-cell lymphoma				X		
Primary cutaneous CD8+ aggressive epidermotropic cytotoxic T-cell lymphoma				X		
Primary cutaneous CD4+ small/medium T-cell lymphoproliferative disorder				X		
Systemic EBV+ T-cell lymphoma of childhood				X		
Hydroa vacciniforme-like lymphoproliferative disorder				X		

Table 1.1 (continued)

Subtype[b]	ICD-O-3 codes	WHO version 2001	2008	2016	New cases, 2016	% of lymphoid neo-plasms
Follicular T-cell lymphoma				X		
Nodal peripheral T-cell lymphoma with TFH phenotype				X		
2.3. Adult T-cell leukemia/ lymphoma	9827	X	X	X	180	0.1
2.4. Extranodal NK/T-cell lymphoma, nasal type	9719	X	X	X	190	0.1
2.5. T-cell large granular lymphocytic leukemia	9831	X	X	X	670	0.5
2.6. T-cell prolymphocytic leukemia	9832(T, NK), 9834	X	X	X	160	0.1
2.7. Aggressive NK-cell leukemia	9948	X	X	X	<50	<0.04
2.8. Primary cutaneous CD30 + lymphoproliferative disorders (primary cutaneous anaplastic large cell lymphoma)	9718		X	X	310	0.2
Lymphomatoid papulosis				X		
Chronic lymphoproliferative disorder of NK cells				X		
Monomorphic epitheliotropic intestinal T-cell lymphoma				X		
Indolent T-cell lymphoproliferative disorder of the GI tract				X		
Primary cutaneous acral CD8+ T-cell lymphoma				X		
3. T/NK-cell, lymphoid neoplasms, NOS	9590–9591(T, NK), 9684(T, NK), 9820 (T, NK), 9970(T, NK)	X	X	X	120	0.1
3. B-cell lymphoma unclassifiable, with features intermediate between DLBCL and classical HL	9596				170	0.1
4. Lymphoid neoplasm, NOS	9590, 9727,9820, 9835 (excluding B, T, NK)	X	X	X	2440	1.8

[a]Adapted from Teras et al. [2]
[b]Subtypes defined using World Health Organization Classification of Tumours of Haematopoietic and Lymphoid Tissues and organized according to SEER Cancer Statistics Review (CSR), 1975–2012, and the InterLymph hierarchical classification of lymphoid neoplasms for epidemiologic research (2008)

bolded the specific WHO entities that are the focus of this chapter, and most of these entities were defined in the first WHO Classification in 2001 [6], which gives sufficient time to accrue cases into cancer registries to provide population-level data, as well as time for epidemiologic studies to be conducted to understand these entities. It should be kept in mind that registry data rely on routine pathology practice and concordance with expert review can vary by lymphoma subtype, as recently shown in a French study [10]. For major aggressive subtypes, concordance in the French study between referral and expert diagnosis was high for DLBCL not-otherwise-specific (NOS) (83.8%) and alkaline phosphatase (ALK)-positive anaplastic large cell lymphoma (ALCL)

(82.3%), followed by BL (76.0%), enteropathy-associated T-cell lymphoma (EATL) (74.2%), angioimmunoblastic T-cell lymphoma (AITL) (68.7%), PTCL-NOS (63.8%), and ALK-negative ALCL (47.2%).

1.2 Descriptive Epidemiology

Descriptive epidemiology evaluates the occurrence of disease and other health-related characteristics in human populations. Descriptive patterns are based on aggregate characteristics of disease frequency, person (age, sex, race, etc.), place (generally geographic region), and calendar time. Such data are critical for an initial basic understanding of a disease in the population and can also generate hypotheses regarding etiology.

1.2.1 Frequency

DLBCL is the most common lymphoid malignancy in the USA, with an estimated 27,650 new cases in 2016, which is 20.2% of all lymphoid malignancies. The vast majority of DLBCL is DLBCL-NOS (25,380 cases/year), with several rarer entities, including primary DLBCL of the central nervous system (PCNSL), with an estimated 1100 cases/years; intravascular large B-cell lymphoma (IVBCL), with 60 cases/year; primary effusion lymphoma (PEL), with <50 cases/year; and primary mediastinal (thymic) large B-cell lymphoma (MLBCL), with 240 cases/year.

BL, in contrast to DLBCL, is a rare subtype with an estimated 1480 cases/year or ~1% of all lymphoid malignancies in the USA [2]. It is commonly classified into the histologically indistinguishable subtypes of sporadic, endemic, and immunodeficiency-associated BL [11].

PTCL is also uncommon, with an estimated 3950 cases/year, representing approximately 3% of all lymphoid malignancies. There is great heterogeneity in this group, and it includes PTCL-NOS (1660 case/year), AITL (530 cases/year), subcutaneous panniculitis-like T-cell lymphoma (SPTCL, <50 cases/year), ALCL (830 cases/year), hepatosplenic T-cell lymphoma (HSTL, <50 cases/year), EATL (50 cases/year), primary cutaneous gamma-delta T-cell lymphoma (PCGD-TCL, <50 cases/year), and systemic EBV-positive lymphoproliferative disease (<50 cases/year). The entity "ALCL, T-cell or null-cell type," has evolved from the 2001 to the 2008 WHO classification to be classified as ALK-positive and ALK-negative ALCL, with the latter initially a provisional entity that is now classified as a definite entity [1]. Primary cutaneous T-cell lymphoma (CTCL, 760 cases/year), included in the 2001 and 2008 classification, now has two new provisional entities. This review does not include the less aggressive T-cell lymphomas, particularly mycosis fungoides/Sezary syndrome; most of the new provisional entities; precursor T/NK-cell lymphoblastic leukemia/lymphoma; or other rare NK and T-cell leukemias/lymphomas listed in Table 1.1.

Aggressive lymphomas, defined as DLBCL, BL, and PTCL (see Table 1.1), make up 24% of lymphoid malignancies overall. If non-Hodgkin lymphoma is defined using the traditional definition (i.e., after excluding HL, MM, and lymphoid malignancy NOS), then DLBCL accounts for 27.6% of cases, BL for 1.5%, and PTCL for 3.9% (1.7% for PTCL-NOS specifically). In the International Non-Hodgkin Lymphoma Classification Project of 4539 cases from 24 countries on five continents [12], 41% of NHLs from the USA and Europe were classified as aggressive (using the above definition) compared with 56.2% for all other world regions (i.e., non-US and European); a lower percentage distribution from the USA/Europe versus other regions was also observed individually for DLBCL (28.9% versus 42.5%), BL (0.8% versus 2.2%), and PTCL-NOS (2.6% versus 3.5%). Similar distributions from European [13, 14] and Asian [15–19] countries have also been reported, with a complementary decrease in the percentage of more indolent subtypes, particularly follicular lymphoma, in Asian studies.

1.2.2 Incidence

While frequency counts and distributions provide insight into the scope of cancer burden, these

Table 1.2 Incidence rates (age-adjusted per 100,000) and annual percent change (APC) for all lymphomas and selected aggressive subtypes, overall and by sex, USA, SEER 18, 2000–2014

			Sex specific				
	Overall		Males		Females		
Lymphoma subtype[a]	Rate	APC	Rate	APC	Rate	APC	IRR[c] (M:F)
All lymphomas	35.8	0.1	44.32	0.1	29.1	−0.1	1.5
DLBCL	6.95	0.5[b]	8.47	0.6[b]	5.72	0.2	1.5
DLBCL-NOS	6.88	0.4[b]	8.41	0.6[b]	5.65	0.1	1.5
IVBCL	0.0097	8.8[b]	0.01	[e]	0.0093	[e]	1.1
PEL	0.011	[e]	0.02	[e]	[d]	[e]	[e]
MLBCL	0.047	[e]	0.038	[e]	0.057	[e]	0.7
BL	0.40	0.2	0.60	0.3	0.21	−0.1	2.9
PTCL	1.15	0.5	1.48	0.4	0.88	0.7[b]	1.7
PTCL-NOS	0.41	1.2[b]	0.54	1.2	0.31	1.2	1.8
AITL	0.13	4.6[b]	0.16	4.9[b]	0.11	4.4[b]	1.4
SPTCL	0.014	3.5	0.0096	[e]	0.018	1.3	0.5
ALCL	0.24	−3.2[b]	0.31	−3.6[b]	0.17	−2.6[b]	1.8
HSTL	0.0091	7.1[b]	0.013	7.5[b]	0.0055	[e]	2.3
EATL	0.012	3.7	0.016	4.4	0.0094	[e]	1.7
CTCL	0.23	−0.3	0.30	−0.4	0.18	−0.3	1.6
PCALCL	0.095	0.5	0.12	0.4	0.075	0.4	1.6

[a]Subtypes: *DLBCL* diffuse large B-cell lymphoma, *NOS* not otherwise specified, *IVBCL* intravascular B-cell lymphoma, *PEL* primary effusion lymphoma, *MLBCL* mediastinal (thymic) large B-cell lymphoma, *BL* Burkitt lymphoma, *PTCL* peripheral T-cell lymphoma, *AITL* angioimmunoblastic T-cell lymphoma, *SPTCL* subcutaneous panniculitis-like T-cell lymphoma, *ALCL* anaplastic large cell lymphoma, *HSTL* hepatosplenic T-cell lymphoma, *EATL* enteropathy-associated T-cell lymphoma, *CTCL* cutaneous T-cell lymphoma, *PCALCL* primary cutaneous anaplastic large cell lymphoma
[b]$P < 0.05$
[c]*IRR* incidence rate ratio, male/female
[d]Unable to estimate (less than 25 cases)
[e]Statistic could not be calculated

measures do not take into account the size or age distribution of the underlying population that generates the case counts to provide rates for making comparisons. To do this, we use the incidence rate, which is defined as the number of newly diagnosed cancer cases in a defined population divided by the number of persons at risk from that population. Incidence rates are used to make comparisons across cancer types, geographic regions, calendar time, and in subgroups (e.g., defined by sex, race, ethnicity, etc.). The incidence rates for selected aggressive lymphomas in the USA are summarized in Tables 1.2 and 1.3 and are based on data from the 18 Surveillance, Epidemiology, and End Results (SEER) registries for 2000–2014 [20] using the WHO classification system as implemented with the InterLymph Classification [21, 22] and SEER*Stat [23]. Due to delays in implementing coding of new entities in population-based cancer registries, the subtypes are based on the 2001 WHO Classification (Table 1.1) [6]. Incidence rates were age-adjusted to the year 2000 US standard population. The annual percentage change (APC) was calculated using weighted least squares method, and the APC was evaluated on whether it was different from zero (no change), with statistical significance set at $P < 0.05$.

The age-adjusted incidence (per 100,000) was 35.8 for all lymphomas, 6.95 for DLBCL, 1.15 for PTCL, and 0.40 for BL. To put these rates in perspective to other lymphoma subtypes, the incidence of CLL/SLL is 5.87, MM is 5.86, follicular lymphoma is 3.57, classic HL is 2.57, and marginal zone lymphoma (MZL) is 1.89. Thus, DLBCL has the highest incidence rate, with both PTCL and BL being relatively uncommon.

Table 1.3 Incidence rates (age-adjusted per 100,000) and annual percent change (APC) for all lymphomas and selected aggressive subtypes by sex, race, and ethnicity, USA, SEER 18, 2000–2014

	Race specific								Hispanic ethnicity				
	White		Black			Asian or Pacific Islander			No		Yes		
Lymphoma subtype[a]	Rate	APC	Rate	APC	IRR[c] (B:W)	Rate	APC	IRR[c] (A:W)	Rate	APC	Rate	APC	IRR[c] (no/yes)
All lymphomas	37.1	0	34.9	0.4	0.9	21.5	−0.1	0.6	36.5	0.1	31.1	0	0.9
DLBCL	7.25	0.5[b]	4.84	0.7	0.7	5.96	0.6[b]	0.8	6.93	0.5[b]	7.30	0.5[b]	1.1
DLBCL-NOS	7.18	0.4[b]	4.77	0.6	0.7	5.89	0.4	0.8	6.86	0.3[b]	7.24	0.4	1.1
IVBCL	0.0092	7.3[b]	[d]	[e]	[e]	[d]	[e]	[e]	0.0096	8.5[b]	[d]	[e]	[e]
PEL	0.011	[e]	0.018	[e]	1.7	[d]	[e]	[e]	0.010	[e]	0.016	[e]	1.6
MLBCL	0.048	[e]	0.038	[e]	0.8	0.051	[e]	1.1	0.051	[e]	0.031	[e]	0.6
BL	0.42	0.3	0.32	0.3	0.8	0.34	−1.4	0.8	0.40	0.1	0.43	0.1	1.1
PTCL	1.11	0.3	1.47	0.7	1.3	0.92	0.6	0.8	1.19	0.7[b]	0.97	−0.2	0.8
PTCL-NOS	0.38	0.9	0.66	1.7	1.7	0.39	1.1	1.0	0.42	1.5[b]	0.36	−0.6	0.8
AITL	0.13	5.1[b]	0.092	1.8	0.7	0.19	3	1.4	0.13	4.6[b]	0.15	4.7[b]	1.1
SPTCL	0.011	2.9	0.025	−2.3	2.4	0.020	[e]	1.9	0.014	3.3	0.013	[e]	0.9
ALCL	0.24	−2.9[b]	0.28	−3.9[b]	1.2	0.16	−4.4[b]	0.7	0.24	−2.8[b]	0.23	−4.5[b]	0.9
HSTL	0.0071	[e]	0.021	[e]	2.9	[d]	[e]	[e]	0.011	8.3[b]	[d]	[e]	[e]
EATL	0.012	5.4[b]	[d]	[e]	[e]	[d]	[e]	[e]	0.012	3.1	[d]	[e]	[e]
CTCL	0.23	−1.1[b]	0.31	1.8	1.3	0.092	0	0.4	0.25	−0.3	0.14	1.2	0.6
PCALCL	0.096	0.2	0.0881	1.1	0.9	0.046	−3	0.5	0.10	0.4	0.063	1.6	0.6

[a]Subtypes: *DLBCL* diffuse large B-cell lymphoma, *NOS* not otherwise specified, *IVBCL* intravascular B-cell lymphoma, *PEL* primary effusion lymphoma, *MLBCL* mediastinal (thymic) large B-cell lymphoma, *BL* Burkitt lymphoma, *PTCL* peripheral T-cell lymphoma, *AITL* angioimmunoblastic T-cell lymphoma, *SPTCL* subcutaneous panniculitis-like T-cell lymphoma, *ALCL* anaplastic large cell lymphoma, *HSTL* hepatosplenic T-cell lymphoma, *EATL* enteropathy-associated T-cell lymphoma, *CTCL* cutaneous T-cell lymphoma, *PCALCL* primary cutaneous anaplastic large cell lymphoma

[b]$P < 0.05$

[c]*IRR* incidence rate ratio

[d]Unable to estimate (less than 25 cases)

[e]Statistic could not be calculated

1.2.2.1 DLBCL

For DLBCL, the age-adjusted incidence rates per 100,000 were 1.5 times greater in men (8.47) compared to women (5.72), were higher in whites (7.25) compared to blacks (4.84) and Asian/Pacific Islanders (5.96), and were similar in Hispanic (7.30) compared to non-Hispanic (6.93) ethnicity. From 2000 to 2014, the incidence of DLBCL increased at an annual rate of 0.5% per year ($P < 0.05$), and this rate of increase was similar across race groups and Hispanic ethnicity. There was heterogeneity by gender, however, with the APC greater for men (0.8% per year, $P < 0.05$) than for women (0.2% per year, $P > 0.05$). The time trends by sex and race of DLBCL are shown in Fig. 1.1.

Within the DLBCL category, DLBCL-NOS had by far the highest incidence (6.88), while the incidence of IVBCL (0.0097), PEL (0.011), and MLBCL (0.047) was much lower. Indeed, the rarity of the latter subtypes largely precluded any detailed comparison by gender, race/ethnicity, or time trends. Of note, the APC of IVBCL has been increasing at 8.8% per year ($P < 0.05$), and unlike the other DLBCL subtypes, the incidence of MLBCL was higher in women (0.057) than men (0.038). The age-incidence curve for DLBCL-NOS (Fig. 1.2) showed a logarithmic increase with age, similar to other common cancers like colorectal cancer, and suggests a similar impact of cumulative risk with age. In contrast, the age-incidence curve for MLBCL rapidly increased in the late teens, peaked in the 20s, and then declined until the 60s, when it slowly increased again with age. This pattern has led to hypotheses regarding reproductive factors in the etiology of MLBCL. PEL incidence increased to age 40 years and then stabilized, while IVBCL was not observed in those <35 years but then rapidly increased with age.

Comparison of incidence rates globally is more difficult for the hematologic malignancies

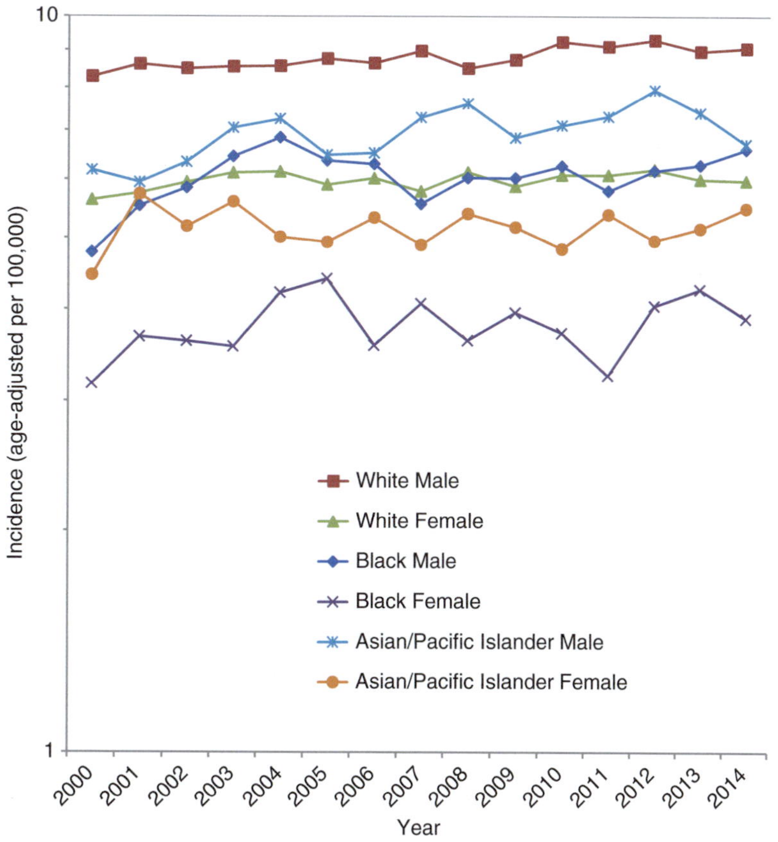

Fig. 1.1 Time trends in the age-adjusted incidence for DLBCL by race and sex groups, USA, SEER 18, 2000–2014

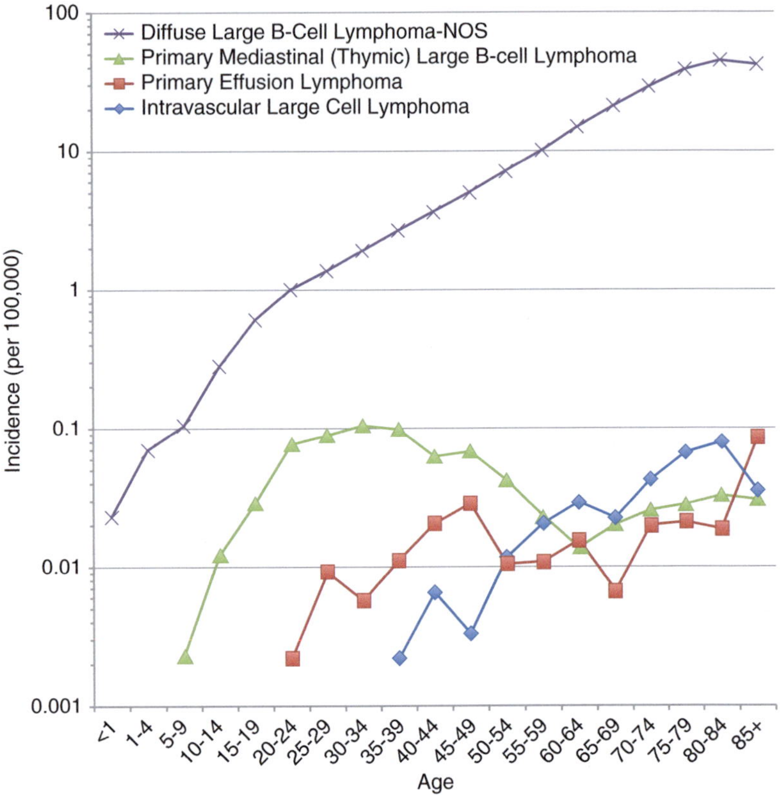

Fig. 1.2 Age-incidence curves for DLBCL subtypes, USA, SEER 18, 2000–2014

due to differences in pathology practice, level of abstraction, coding systems, and use of population standards (e.g., US 2000 standard has an older age distribution than the world standard, leading to higher rates). Nevertheless, broad comparisons are possible. For example, the age-standardized incidence rates, male/female ratios, and age-incidence curves for DLBCL in Europe for 2000–2002 [13], Australia for 1997–2006 [24], and the UK for 2004–2012 [14] were all similar to those reported here, although rates were somewhat lower for Australia as well as Europe combined, noting that there was a relatively wide range among individual European countries. In the UK, age-standardized incidence rates for DLBCL were highest for whites, intermediate for South Asian and blacks, and lowest for Chinese [25]. Compared to the USA, age-adjusted rates of DLBCL were lower in Singapore [19] and Japan [18], although they have been rapidly rising since the 1990s in both Asian countries.

1.2.2.2 BL

BL is one of the most male predominant lymphoma subtypes and had approximately threefold higher age-adjusted incidence per 100,000 for men (0.60) compared to women (0.21) in the USA for 2000–2014 (Table 1.2). BL also had a higher incidence in whites (0.42) compared to blacks (0.32) and Asian/Pacific Islanders (0.34), while there was little difference in incidence rates between Hispanic (0.43) and non-Hispanic (0.40) ethnicity (Table 1.3). Over the time frame 2000–2014, there were no statistically significant changes observed for BL incidence overall, or in any subgroup defined by gender, race, or ethnicity. The age-standardized incidence rates, male/female ratios, and age-incidence curves for BL in Europe for 2000–2002 [13], Australia for 1997–2006 [24], and the UK for 2004–2012 [14] were all similar to those reported here. Compared to the USA, BL rates in Singapore for 2003–2012 [19] were only slightly lower, while rates were fourfold lower in Japan for 2008 [18].

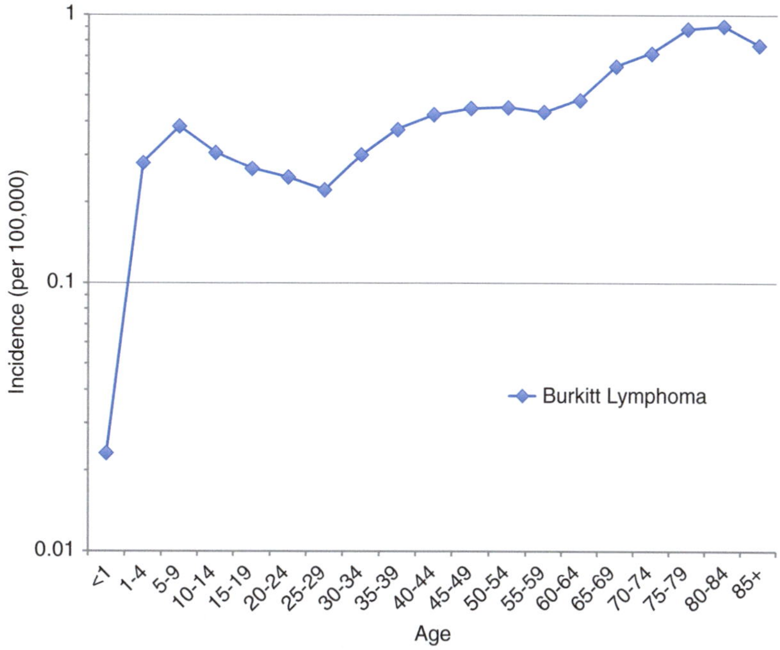

Fig. 1.3 Age-incidence curve for Burkitt lymphoma, USA, SEER 18, 2000–2014

The age-incidence pattern for BL is unique, with a peak in childhood (age 5–9 years), which then slowly declines to approximately age 30 years, followed by a second peak around age 50 years, and then an increase into old age (Fig. 1.3). This age-incidence pattern has been previously reported in the SEER data for 1973–2005, where there were two separate peaks in both males and females near ages 10 and 75 years and a third peak around age 40 years in males [26]. The latter peak attenuated with the exclusion of registries enriched for HIV/AIDs cases, and age-period-cohort models further supported a role for HIV/AIDs in the middle age peak in the age-incidence curve. This pattern was confirmed using data from cancer registries from four continents (excluding Africa) for 1963–2002, with age-specific peaks at age 10 and 70 years in all regions and time periods and a third peak around 40 years that only emerged in the mid-1990s and more strikingly in men [27]. Because BL is one of the most rapidly growing tumors known (with cell mass doubling every 1–2 days) [28], the interval from initiation to diagnosis is likely to be relatively short and, together with the distinctive age-incidence pattern, suggests potentially unique etiology, biology, and risk factors for the different age peaks.

1.2.2.3 PTCL

For PTCL overall, the age-adjusted incidence rates per 100,000 were 1.7 times greater in men (1.48) compared to women (0.88). Unlike most other NHL subtypes, they were higher in blacks (1.47) compared to whites (1.11) and lowest in Asian/Pacific Islanders (0.92); they were also somewhat higher in non-Hispanic (1.19) compared to Hispanic (0.97) ethnicity.

Data on eight of the PTCL entities are provided in Table 1.2 and show the heterogeneity of PTCL. The highest incidence was observed for PTCL-NOS (0.41), followed by ALCL (0.24) and CTCL (0.23). By gender, all of the subtypes showed higher incidence in men compared to women (IRRs 1.4–2.3) except for SPTCL, which had a higher incidence in women (0.018) compared to men (0.0096). Compared to whites, blacks had a higher incidence for all of the PTCL subtypes except AITL and PCALCL, while patterns were more mixed (and less stable due to small numbers) for Asian/Pacific Islander (Table 1.3). For most PTCL subtypes, incidence rates were

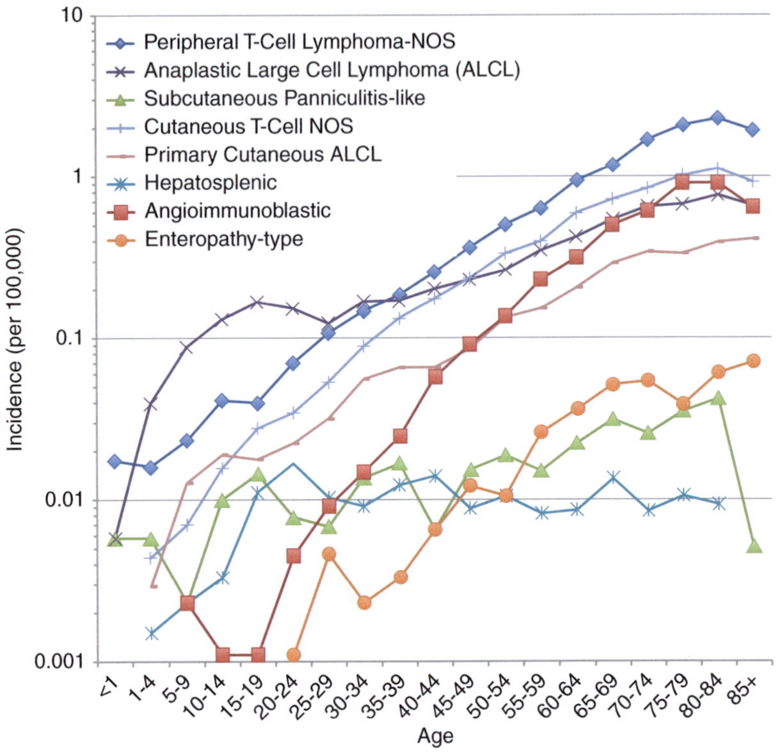

Fig. 1.4 Age-incidence curves for PTCL subtypes, USA, SEER 18, 2000–2014

generally higher in people of non-Hispanic ethnicity. The age-incidence curves for PTCL subtypes are shown in Fig. 1.4. PTCL-NOS, CTCL, PCALCL, and AITL all showed strong increases in incidence with age and, except for its rarity in those <20 years, so did EATL. ALCL showed a very rapid increase to age 15–19 years and then a decrease to age 30 years, followed by an increase into older age. HSTL showed an increase to age 20–24 years and then no change in incidence with age, while SPTCL showed a weakly positive overall trend in incidence with age.

While there was no evidence for changes in incidence of PTCL over the 2000–2014 timeframe, there were statistically significant ($P < 0.05$) increases in the APC for PTCL in women (0.7% per year) and in people of non-Hispanic ethnicity (0.7% per year). The time trends by sex and race for PTCL are shown in Fig. 1.5. By PTCL subtype, statistically significant increases in incidence were observed for PTCL-NOS (1.2% per year), AITL (4.6% per year), and HSTL (7.1% per year). For PTCL-NOS, the increase in APC was also statistically significant for non-Hispanics. For AITL the increase in APC was statistically significant in whites, both genders, and both Hispanic and non-Hispanic ethnicity. For HSTL, the increase was statistically significant in men and non-Hispanic ethnicity. The only PTCL subtype to show a statistically significant decline was for ALCL (−3.2% per year), and this decline was observed in both genders and all racial and ethnic subgroups.

Compared to the USA, the age-standardized incidence rates for PTCL-NOS were slightly lower in Australia for 1997–2006 [24] and the UK for 2004–2012 [14], although male/female ratios were similar. In 2008, age-standardized rates for PTCL-NOS in Japan were virtually the same as in the USA [18]. Fewer data are available for comparisons with other T-cell subtypes, but in a direct comparison between the USA versus Japan for 2008 using incidence rate ratios (IRR), CTCL (IRR = 6.42) and ALCL (IRR = 1.78) were more common in the USA, while AITL was less common (IRR = 0.80) [18]. In that study,

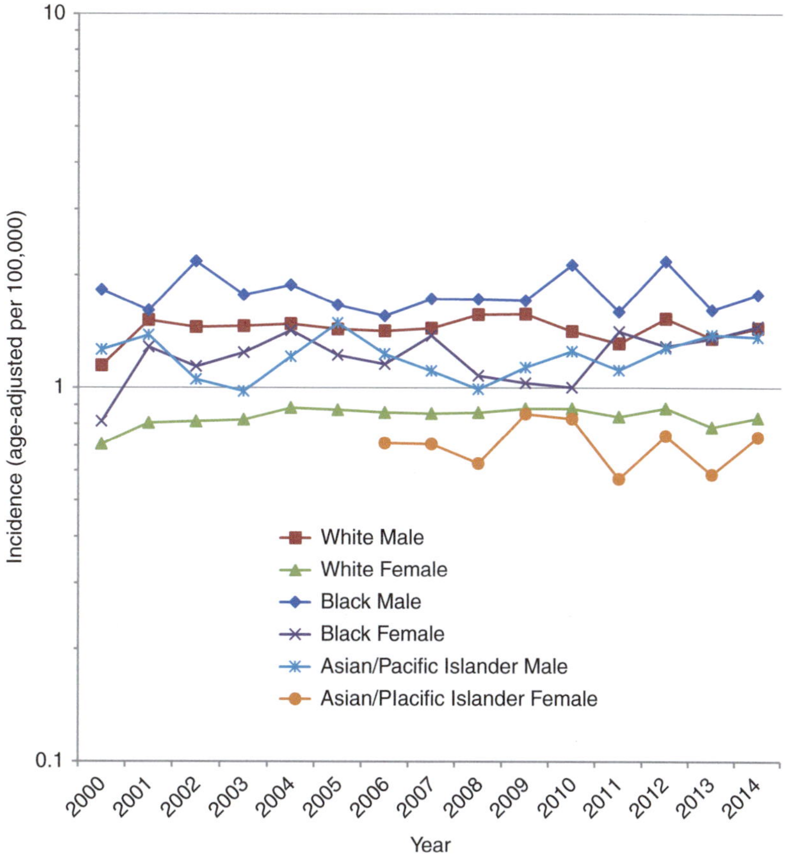

Fig. 1.5 Time trends in the age-adjusted incidence for PTCL by race and sex groups, USA, SEER 18, 2000–2014

besides AITL, only NK/T-cell lymphoma nasal type and adult T-cell leukemia/lymphoma had higher incidence rates in Japan compared to the USA, while all other T-cell and B-cell subtypes had higher incidence rates in the USA, showing that while the proportion of T- versus B-cell lymphomas were greater in Japan, this is due to lower incidence of B-cell malignancies and not a higher incidence of T-cell malignancies.

1.2.3 Survival

Survival is another important parameter in understanding the descriptive epidemiology of a cancer. Observed survival is the proportion of patients surviving for a specified length of time after diagnosis and is obtained using standard life table procedures. However, from a population perspective, we would like to account for competing causes of mortality in comparing survival rates, and for this we can use relative survival, which is essentially the observed survival rate adjusted for expected mortality. This tells us whether the specific disease (here, lymphoma) shortens life.

The 5-year relative survival rates for selected aggressive lymphomas are summarized in Table 1.4, which is based on data from the 18 SEER registries for 2000–2010 [20] using the WHO classification system as implemented with the InterLymph classification [21, 22] and SEER*Stat [23]. Expected survival was derived from US data for 1970–2012.

1.2.3.1 DLBCL

Five-year relative survival for DLBCL as a group for cases diagnosed 2000–2010 in the US SEER 18 registries was 59.6%, but there was significant heterogeneity for the DLBCL subtypes of MLBCL (84.0%), DLBCL-NOS (59.5%), IVBCL (53.6%), and PEL (24.8%). For DLBCL-NOS, relative

Table 1.4 Five-year relative survival rates (percent) for selected aggressive lymphoma subtypes, USA, SEER 18, 2000–2010

Lymphoma subtype[a]	All (%)	Sex specific: Male (%)	Sex specific: Female (%)	Race specific: White (%)	Race specific: Black (%)	Race specific: Asian or Pacific Islander (%)	Hispanic ethnicity: No (%)	Hispanic ethnicity: Yes (%)
All lymphomas	67.5	66.9	68.2	68.5	58.6	63.3	67.7	65.6
DLBCL	59.6	59.3	60.0	60.2	54.6	57.0	59.7	58.8
DLBCL-NOS	59.5	59.3	59.8	60.1	54.5[b]	56.9	59.6	58.8
IVBCL	53.6[b]	[c]	56.9[b]	57.5[b]	[c]	[c]	54.6[b]	[c]
PEL	24.8[b]	22.5[b]	[c]	22.5[b]	[c]	[c]	23.6[b]	[c]
MLBCL	84.0	83.0	84.1[b]	86.3[b]	79.9	67.0[b]	84.8	77.8[b]
BL	56.4	57.6	53.1[b]	57.6[b]	45.9[b]	58.2	56.2	57.4[b]
PTCL	56.0	54.6	58.0	57.9	45.9	46.3	56.6	51.6
PTCL-NOS	37.5	37.3	37.7	39.0	32.4	30.3[b]	37.8	34.5
AITL	42.5	38.4	46.8[b]	44.0[b]	32.5[b]	39.2	41.1	52.3[b]
SPTCL	67.0[b]	66.1[b]	67.5[b]	57.7[b]	[c]	[c]	64.2[b]	[c]
ALCL	56.1	54.8	58.4	57.9	42.8	55.9[b]	57.3	49.8
HSTL	21.9[b]	17.8[b]	[c]	15.4[b]	[c]	[c]	23.3[b]	[c]
EATL	14.2[b]	10.4[b]	19.9[b]	18.6[b]	[c]	[c]	14.5[b]	[c]
CTCL	82.1[b]	81.4[b]	83.1[b]	83.3[b]	72.2[b]	72.4[b]	82.2[b]	81.2[b]
PCALCL	89.3[b]	87.6[b]	91.2	89.7[b]	76.6	94.2[b]	89.3[b]	86.0[b]

[a]Subtypes: *DLBCL* diffuse large B-cell lymphoma, *NOS* not otherwise specified, *IVBCL* intravascular B-cell lymphoma, *PEL* primary effusion lymphoma, *MLBCL* mediastinal (thymic) large B-cell lymphoma, *BL* Burkitt lymphoma, *PTCL* peripheral T-cell lymphoma, *AITL* angioimmunoblastic T-cell lymphoma, *SPTCL* subcutaneous panniculitis-like T-cell lymphoma, *ALCL* anaplastic large cell lymphoma, *HSTL* hepatosplenic T-cell lymphoma, *EATL* enteropathy-associated T-cell lymphoma, *CTCL* cutaneous T-cell lymphoma, *PCALCL* primary cutaneous anaplastic large cell lymphoma
[b]The relative cumulative survival increased from a prior interval and has been adjusted
[c]Unable to estimate (less than 25 cases)

survival rates were similar by sex and Hispanic ethnicity but were slightly higher in whites (60.1%) compared to Asian/Pacific Islanders (56.9%) and blacks (54.5%). Comparison of relative survival rates by sex, race, and ethnicity was not possible for the other three rarer subtypes due to small numbers.

Five-year relative survival for DLBCL in the EUROCARE-5 study [29] increased from 2000–2002 (44.8%) to 2003–2005 (50.9%) to 2006–2008 (55.4%), while in the UK [14], it was 54.8% for cases diagnosed 2004–2012. In Singapore, 5-year age-standardized relative survival for DLBCL increased from 1998–2002 (34.7%) to 2003–2007 (46.5%) to 2008–2012 (49.2%) [19]. Increasing overall survival in DLBCL, which leads to increasing relative survival and decreasing mortality rates since 2000 at the population level, has been largely attributed to the widespread adoption of immunochemotherapy [30]. Racial disparities in the early adoption of immunochemotherapy for DLBCL appear to account for some of the difference by race in the USA [31].

1.2.3.2 BL

Five-year relative survival for BL overall for cases diagnosed 2000–2010 in the US SEER 18 registries was 56.4% and was slightly higher for males (57.6%) compared to females (53.1%); was similar for whites and Asian/Pacific Islander (~58%) but much lower for blacks (45.9%); and was similar by Hispanic ethnicity. A prior analysis of SEER data for 1973–2005 reported that 5-year death rates due to BL (Kaplan-Meier; not accounting for competing causes of death) were ~25% for pediatric BL (<20 years at diagnosis), ~50% for adult BL (20–59 years), and ~70% for geriatric BL (60+ years), with similar rates for males and females except for adult BL, where rates were slightly higher in males [26]. Five-year relative survival for BL in the UK for cases diagnosed 2004–2012 was 52.9% and was higher for males (57.7%) than females (39.9%) [14].

1.2.3.3 PTCL

The 5-year relative survival for PTCL for cases diagnosed 2000–2010 in the US SEER 18 registries as a group was 56.0%, but within this group, there was substantial heterogeneity, ranging from 89.3% for PCALCL to 14.2% for EATL (Table 1.4). There were no strong sex differences for most of the subtypes, and in general whites had somewhat higher survival rates, although for many of the rarest subtypes, comparisons were unstable due to small numbers. Compared to the USA, 5-year relative survival for selected T-cell subtypes diagnosed from 2004 to 2012 was lower in the UK for PTCL-NOS (37.5% versus 19.7%) and AITL (42.5% versus 26.2%), similar for ALCL (56.1% versus 50.8%) and higher for EATL (14.2% versus 28.0%); similar to the USA, there were no statistically significant difference in relative survival by gender in the UK [14].

1.2.4 Other Measures

1.2.4.1 Mortality Rate

The cancer mortality rate is defined as the number of cancer deaths in a given year divided by the number of persons in the population. This is a function of both incidence and survival and is generally based on death certificate data [32]. While less useful for understanding etiology, cancer mortality rates are considered the best basis for judging progress against cancer by Extramural Committee to Assess Measures of Progress Against Cancer [33].

While there have been recent substantial declines in NHL mortality overall in the USA and other Western countries [14, 24, 34, 35], it has been difficult to parse the contribution of NHL subtypes to these changes as subtype information is generally not recorded on death certificates. Using SEER and other population data, Howlader et al. [36] showed that overall NHL mortality rates increased from 1975 to 1997 and then decreased from 1998 to 2011 and that incidence-based mortality rates (an approach to link subtype-specific incidence data with mortality data) for DLBCL began to decline 3% per year after 1998, while PTCL (which had more limited data) showed no clear trend over 2006–2011. In 2011, an estimated 33% of NHL deaths were due to DLBCL, and 7% of NHL deaths were due to PTCL.

1.2.4.2 Event-Free Status at 24 Months (EFS24)

In an observational cohort of newly diagnosed DLBCL patients treated with immunochemotherapy for curative intent, approximately 70% of DLBCL patients did not have progression or relapse, retreatment, or death within 24 months of diagnosis (termed event-free survival or EFS24). These patients had an 8% absolute risk of DLBCL relapse in the next 5 years (95% CI 5–12%) and a subsequent overall survival equivalent to that of the age- and sex-matched general population (standardized mortality ratio [SMR] = 1.18, 95% CI 0.89–1.57) (Fig. 1.6); this finding was replicated in French clinical and registry-based data [37]. The 30% of DLBCL patients who did not achieve EFS24 had a very poor outcome, with a median survival of 13 months (95% CI 10–16 months) after a relapse or retreatment event and much higher mortality compared to the age- and sex-matched population (SMR = 16.9, 95 CI% 14.0–20.2). DLBCL relapses after 24 months also appeared to be less aggressive than early relapses, with a median OS of 36 months (95% CI 29–55 months). Similar results have been reported in the Danish population [38]. These findings have implications for patient counseling [39], patient surveillance after 24 months [40], study design to identify the biology of aggressive DLBCL [41], and use as a surrogate end point in clinical trials (as early failures are largely driven by DLBCL compared to later EFS events, which are more likely to be from unrelated competing mortality in patients in remission) [37].

In a similar analysis of cohorts from the USA, Sweden, and British Columbia, 36% of patient with PTCL treated with anthracycline-based chemotherapy regimens achieved EFS24, and the median survival after this landmark was not reached, and the 5-year OS was 78% (95% CI 73–84%). Expected 5-year survival based on age-, sex-, and country-matched population was

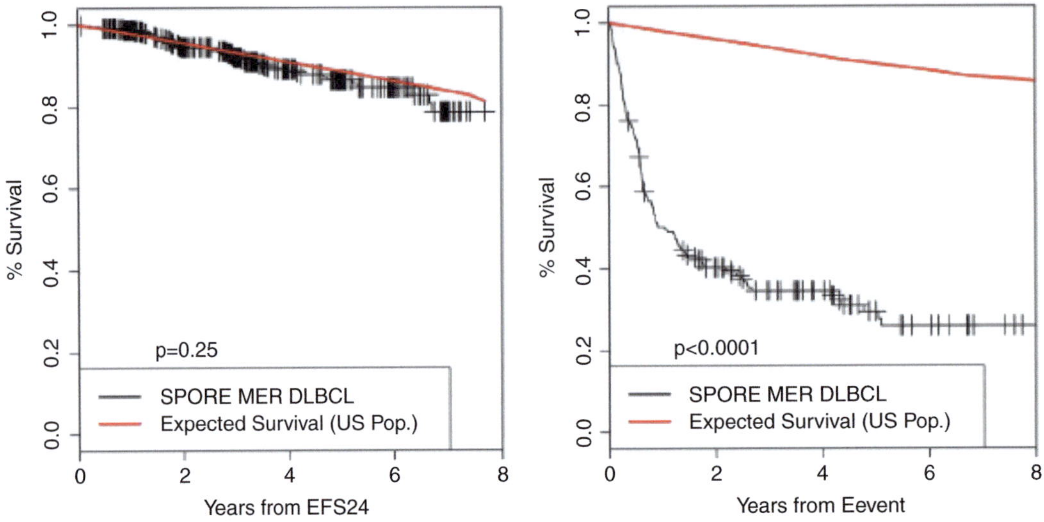

Fig. 1.6 Subsequent overall survival in the SPORE Molecular Epidemiology Resource (MER) versus expected survival (US population) for R-CHOP-treated DLBCL patients achieving EFS24 (left) or failing to achieve EFS24 (right)

92% (SMR = 3.16, 95% CI 2.48–3.98). In contrast, the 64% of patients with PTCL who progressed in the first 24 months had a subsequent median survival of 4.9 months (95% CI 3.8–5.9 months), a 5-year OS of 11%, and an SMR of 46.4 (95% CI 41.9–51.3) [42]. Similar to DLBCL, EFS24 can be used in this setting to help inform patient counseling, biomarker discovery, and clinical trial design for PTCL.

1.3 Analytic Epidemiology of Aggressive Lymphomas

1.3.1 General Considerations

In contrast to descriptive epidemiology, analytic epidemiology tests hypotheses about associations of exposure with disease risk. While intervention studies, including randomized controlled clinical trials, are the gold standard for evaluating causal associations, this approach is not practical for many if not most exposures and is not ethical to evaluate exposures that cause harm. Thus, most epidemiology studies are observational, in that exposure is not manipulated but rather is observed (measured) as it occurs in the population. The most common study designs utilized to study cancer etiology are case-control and cohort studies, with the latter considered a stronger form of evidence. However, all observational studies are subject to various types of bias (most prominently selection and recall bias), confounding (a factor that creates a spurious association due to its association with both exposure and outcome), and chance (random error). Thus, observational studies must be carefully designed to minimize bias and address potential confounding, although bias can rarely be completely eliminated and there always remains the possibility of confounding by unknown/unmeasured exposures. Chance findings (false positives) are addressed with stringent statistical evaluation and replication in independent studies, while false negatives are addressed by ensuring sufficient study power. Analytic studies also incorporate biomarkers to help infer disease mechanisms. A framework to evaluate causality incorporates these issues, and while intervention data provide the strongest evidence for causality, observational data, particularly from pooled and meta-analyses and in the context of biologic evidence, can provide sufficiently robust data to make a causal claim.

1.3.2 Specific Considerations

There have been several recent reviews of the epidemiology of NHL in general [43–45], which is not repeated here. Rather, the goal of this chapter is to highlight what is known about the epidemiology of the three most common aggressive NHL subtypes of DLBCL, BL, and PTCL. This leads to several specific issues unique to this task. Most studies have historically analyzed all NHL, with subtypes either not addressed or a secondary objective. This leads to inconsistent reporting of results for subtypes, if at all. Also, rare subtypes, like BL and PTCL usually did not have a sufficient number of cases in a given study to even present any associations. Further, most studies were not designed with sufficient power to address subtype-specific associations or to formally test for heterogeneity of risk factor associations across the major NHL subtypes ("etiologic heterogeneity"). This issue has been addressed in part through meta-analysis of published studies and pooling of studies through consortium efforts such as InterLymph [46]. The InterLymph Consortium was launched in 2001 to specifically create a structure and venue for pooling of individual-level study data from case-control studies in order to increase statistical power to address rare exposures; lymphoma subtypes; interactions between risk factors, both environmental and genetic; and provide definitive results on inconsistent findings identified in individual studies [46]. There are many advantages to pooled analysis of primary data, including more in-depth analyses based on detailed and harmonized exposure data, adjustment for potential confounding factors, evaluation of interactions and subgroup associations, systematic and comprehensive evaluation of NHL subtypes, and more robust statistical inferences relative to meta-analysis [47].

Another major issue is the classification of NHL subtypes. Prior to the adoption of the Working Formulation in 1982, there was no consensus approach for defining NHL subtypes which hampered analytic epidemiology studies [48]. However, that system only translated across different systems. The first true consensus classification for clinical and pathologic use was developed in 1994 as the Revised European-American Lymphoma (REAL) classification [49], which was incorporated in 2001 in the WHO Classification of Tumours of the Haematopoietic and Lymphoid Tissues [6]. This system was adopted worldwide, including incorporation into the *International Classification of Diseases for Oncology*, third Edition (ICD-O-3) [5]. In 2007, the InterLymph Consortium Pathology Working Group developed a nested classification system based on the WHO system and ICD-O-3 to group subtypes and to provide a translation from classifications before 2001 [21]. This system greatly facilitated analysis of lymphoid malignancies in epidemiologic studies and was able to incorporate updates [22], such as with the third edition of the WHO Classification [4].

These issues have been taken into consideration for this review. The initial focus is on results for each subtype from meta-analysis, pooled analysis, or large cohort studies. This approach will tend to overly emphasize positive results, as null results (no association) are less well reported due to publication bias. The InterLymph pooling projects partially overcomes this limitation, as there has been a more systemic evaluation that includes publication of null results. Many of the InterLymph pooling projects focused on specific exposures and ensured consistent harmonization of selected exposures. Subsequently, the InterLymph Subtypes Project was launched to examine a range of risk factors for each NHL subtype and to systematically assess commonalities and differences in risk factor associations across the common NHL subtypes [50].

1.3.3 DLBCL

1.3.3.1 Family History and Genetics

In the InterLymph Subtypes Project, a family history of NHL was associated with 1.84-fold increased risk of DLBCL (95% CI 1.46–2.33), and this association slightly strengthened after adjustment for DLBCL-specific risk factors (OR = 1.95, 95% CI 1.54–2.47) [51]. This risk estimate is in agreement with data from a pooled analysis of Scandinavian registries (SIR = 1.9; 95% CI 1.6–2.2) [52]. Risk of DLBCL was also elevated for persons with a first-degree relative with DLBCL (SIR = 1.9, 95% CI 1.4–2.6), FL (SIR = 2.6, 95% CI 1.7–3.6), LPL/WM (SIR = 3.5, 95% CI 1.3–7.5), MCL (SIR = 1.9, 95% CI 0.5–4.8), or mature T-cell lymphoma (SIR = 2.1, 95% CI 0.4–6.2), although the latter two associations were not statistically significant [52]. Risk of DLBCL was also elevated ~2-fold for a family history of HL [51, 53], but there was no association for CLL [51, 54] or MM [51]. Familial aggregation represents both shared genetics and environmental factors, and the findings summarized above suggest that familial risk is not strongly confounded by nongenetic risk factors and that there may be shared factors among lymphoma subtypes, perhaps exclusive of CLL and MM. Interestingly, results for familial aggregation of other lymphoma subtypes tend to show that a family history of a specific lymphoma subtype is most strongly associated with risk for that specific lymphoma [55], suggesting that there may also be genetic factors unique to a subtype.

While studies of familial aggregation are consistent with an important role for genetics in lymphoma development, only genetic studies can definitively identify risk loci. Prior to the advent of genome-wide association studies (GWAS), there were a large number of candidate gene studies in lymphoma (reviewed in [56–61], but for a variety of reasons, including biased study design, small sample size (low power), uncontrolled multiple testing (leading to false positive associations), lumping together of all subtypes, and unrealistic expectations in our ability to choose variants and genes, these studies have largely failed to replicate. However, one of the most robust candidate gene findings in lymphoma has been for an *LTA-TNF* haplotype with DLBCL risk ($P = 2.93 \times 10^{-8}$) [62, 63].

In contrast to candidate gene/pathway studies, GWA studies have definitively identified several susceptibility loci for DLBCL. In a large GWAS of European ancestry [64], novel loci identified included 6p25.3 (*EXOC2*), 6p21.33 (*HLA-B*), 2p23.3 (*NCOA1*), and 8q24.21 (near *PVT1* and *MYC*). The strongest finding after imputing HLA alleles and amino acids was with *HLA-B*08:01* although this could not be statistically distinguished from the *HLA-B* SNP due to high linkage disequilibrium. Based on the GWAS data, common SNPs including but not limited to the GWAS-discovered loci were estimated to explain approximately 16% of the variance in DLBCL risk overall [64]. Three of the five GWAS-discovered SNPs for DLBCL in Europeans were significantly associated with DLBCL in an East Asian population [65], including *EXOC2* (OR = 2.04, $P = 3.9 \times 10^{-10}$), *PVT1* (OR = 1.34, $P = 2.1 \times 10^{-6}$), and *HLA-B* (OR = 3.05, $P = 0.009$). Overall, MAFs were similar or only modestly lower in the East Asian population for all SNPs except for one of the 8q24 SNPs, which was much rarer. In a GWAS conducted in an East Asian population, a locus at 3q27 (near *BCL6* and *LPP*) was identified [66], although this could not be replicated in independent studies of East Asian [65] or European ancestry [64]. The GWAS results strongly support a role for immunologic pathways in the etiology of DLBCL, but more studies are needed to identify additional loci, particularly for DLBCL subtypes defined by cell of origin and in populations of contrasting risk.

1.3.3.2 Immune Biomarkers

Biomarkers of immune function, most prominently circulating cytokines and chemokines, allow epidemiologists to link subclinical immunologic alterations in otherwise normal people to future lymphoma risk using banked samples from large cohort studies. While most studies have reported only overall NHL associations, a meta-analysis of four studies found a strong and consistent positive association of soluble CD30 (OR = 2.07, 95% CI 1.41–3.03) and to a somewhat lesser extent soluble CD27 (OR = 1.86, 95% CI 0.92–3.78) with DLBCL risk [67]. Several studies have also reported a positive association of soluble CD23 with DLBCL risk [68, 69]. These findings taken together imply a role for B-cell activation markers as predictors of future DLBCL risk. There are also suggestive data for a positive association of soluble B-cell attracting chemokine (BCA-1, or CXCL3) with DLBCL risk [68, 70], suggesting a role for chemotaxis in DLBCL pathogenesis.

1.3.3.3 Infectious Agents

There are strong data linking several types of infections to DLBCL risk. DLBCL, including PCNSL, are both AIDS-defining cancers [71], and recent estimates from the USA for 1996–2010 show that HIV infection or AIDS increased risk of DLBCL 17.6-fold (95% CI 16.7–18.6) and PCNSL 47.7-fold (95% CI 43.4–52.2) [72]. Risk of DLBCL and PCNSL has declined with the advent of highly active antiretroviral therapy (HAART) in 1996, although risks continue to be substantially elevated for these subtypes [73, 74]. The International Agency for Research on Cancer (IARC) has listed Kaposi sarcoma-associated herpesvirus 8 (HHV8) as an established cause of PEL [75]. PEL is primarily observed in people with immunodeficiency, and the majority of patients are EBV positive [76]. Hepatitis C virus (HCV) is also an established cause of NHL [75], and HCV has been positively associated with DLBCL risk in an InterLymph pooled analysis (OR = 2.24, 95% CI 1.68–2.99) [77], including after adjusting for other risk factors (OR = 2.02, 95% CI 1.47–2.76) [51], as well as in a large SEER-Medicare analysis (OR = 1.52, 95% CI 1.05–2.18) [78]. While hepatitis B virus (HBV) is considered to only have limited evidence to cause NHL in the 2009 IARC review, a recent meta-analysis of 17 case-control and five cohort studies (with over 40,000 cases) found a positive association with DLBCL (OR = 1.84, 95% CI 1.13–3.01), which was restricted to high (OR = 2.73, 95% CI 1.62–4.59) but not low (OR = 1.11, 95% CI 0.73–1.69) HBV prevalence countries [79]. Human pegivirus (HPgV), previously known as GB virus C (GBV-C) [80], viremia has been associated with DLBCL risk in a population-based case-control study (OR = 5.18, 95% CI 2.06–13.7) [81] and a nested case-control study with prediagnostic samples (OR = 5.31, 95% CI 1.54–18.4) [82] independent of HBV and HCV. HPgV is a single-stranded RNA virus from *Flaviviridae* that is closely related to HCV but is lymphotropic and could impact lymphoma risk by causing chronic immune stimulation or impaired immunosurveillance.

1.3.3.4 Medical History

Solid organ transplantation is associated with an increased risk of DLBCL, most recently estimated at a 13.5-fold increased risk (95% CI 12.7–14.4) based on data from a US population-based study of transplant recipients from 1987 to 2008 [83], which is consistent with other recent studies [84, 85]. In the former study, DLBCL made up over 50% of the NHLs, which is much greater than the 25–30% observed at the population level. Other aggressive lymphomas (BL, PTCL) were also overrepresented in this setting [83]. Risk of DLBCL was particularly elevated for transplants given before age 20 years (SIR = 379, 95% CI 318–447) and for pancreas or pancreas/kidney transplants (SIR = 32.6, 95% CI 24.6–42.5). There was also evidence for a U-shaped curve, with risk highest in the first year after transplantation and then after 5 years [83], consistent with patterns seen for NHL overall in this setting [86, 87]. Mechanistically, these findings suggest important roles for immunosuppression (specifically in the early, intense induction phase as well as in the later long-term maintenance phase), chronic immune activation (due to the presence of donor organ), or the combined effects of these, resulting in long-term, chronic immune dysfunction.

History of blood transfusion was not associated with DLBCL risk in a meta-analysis of case-control and cohort studies [88]. In the InterLymph Subtypes Project, there was an unexpected inverse association of blood transfusion with DLBCL risk (OR = 0.81, 95% CI 0.72–0.91) after adjusting for other DLBCL risk factors; in sex-specific models, transfusion history only remained significantly associated with DLBCL risk among men [51].

In the InterLymph autoimmune pooling project [89], DLBCL risk was associated with systemic lupus erythematosus (SLE, OR = 2.74, 95% CI 1.47–5.11) and Sjogren syndrome (OR = 8.92, 95% CI 3.83–20.7), consistent with other studies [90–92]. There were also associations with hemolytic anemia (OR = 3.22, 95% CI 1.31–7.89) and a suggestive association with celiac disease (OR = 1.83, 95% CI, 0.89–3.74), with the latter finding more definitively confirmed in a recent meta-analysis (OR = 2.25, 95% 1.32–3.85) [93]. In the InterLymph Subtypes Project, a history of B-cell-activating (OR = 2.36, 95% CI 1.80–3.09) or both B-cell- and T-cell-activating (OR = 4.86, 95% CI 2.31–10.3) but not T-cell-activating (OR = 1.03, 95% CI 0.86–1.24) autoimmune diseases was associated with DLBCL risk after adjusting for other DLBCL-specific risk factors [51]. These results were similar for men and women and held for DLBCL of the GI tract, testis, mediastinum, and skin, but not of the CNS [51]. The overall association with autoimmune disease was mainly driven by individual associations with multiple B-cell-activating autoimmune diseases (Sjogren syndrome, SLE, hemolytic anemia, and RA) but only one T-cell-activating autoimmune disease (celiac), suggesting a more prominent role for the former mechanism in DLBCL etiology. While it has been challenging to disentangle autoimmune disease, treatment (i.e., confounding by indication), and shared genetics or other host factors in understanding these associations, they do support the role of chronic inflammation, antigenic stimulation, and overall immune dysregulation in DLBCL pathogenesis [94].

History of an atopic condition was inversely associated with DLBCL risk after accounting for other DLBCL-specific risk factors (OR = 0.82; 95% CI 0.76–0.89) in the InterLymph Subtypes Project; specific inverse associations included allergies, asthma, and hay fever [51]. The atopy association was particularly strong for PCNSL. However, the association of allergies with DLBCL was null in a large cohort study [95], raising concerns about reverse causality from case-control studies that needs further evaluation. In the InterLymph Subtypes Project for DLBCL, the autoimmune and HCV risk associations and the atopy protective association remained statistically significant in a multivariate model, suggesting a complex interplay of immune stimulation (autoimmunity and HCV infection) and hypersensitivity (atopy) in DLBCL pathogenesis that requires further understanding [96].

In a meta-analysis of type 2 diabetes and lymphoma risk, there was no overall increased risk for DLBCL (OR = 1.16, 95% CI 0.92–1.48), although there was increased risk in European (OR = 1.48, 95% CI 1.10–2.01) but not US populations [97].

1.3.3.5 Hormonal and Reproductive Factors

In the InterLymph reproductive factors pooling project [98, 99], there were no associations of menstrual (including age at menarche or age at menopause), reproductive (including parity/number of children and age at first and last child), or hormonal contraception history with DLBCL risk. In contrast, there was an inverse association for use of postmenopausal hormone therapy (OR = 0.66, 95% CI 0.54–0.80), although there was no trend with years of use. In the InterLymph Subtypes Project, both OC use prior to 1970 (OR = 0.78 compared to no OC use, 95% CI 0.62–1.00) and hormone therapy use initiated at age 50 years or older (OR = 0.68 compared to never use, 95% CI 0.52–0.88) were inversely associated with DLBCL risk in the final multivariable model that also adjusted for other DLBCL risk factors [51]. However, cohort studies evaluating these factors for DLBCL risk have not been consistent nor supportive of these associations [100–103].

1.3.3.6 Occupations and Environmental Factors

In the InterLymph occupational pooling project of ten case-control studies [104], DLBCL risk was positively associated with the occupational groups hairdresser (OR = 1.47, 95% CI 1.08–2.00) and textile worker (OR = 1.19, 95% CI 1.01–1.41), as well as the specific occupations of charworkers, cleaners, and related workers (OR = 1.27, 95% CI 1.03–1.58); field crop and vegetable farm workers (OR = 1.50, 95% CI 1.15–1.97); metal melters and reheaters (OR = 2.31, 95% CI 1.01–5.26); and special education teachers (OR = 1.94, 95% CI 1.01–3.71). In the InterLymph Subtypes Project, field crop and vegetable farmer (OR = 1.49, 95% CI 1.14–1.95), sewer and embroiderer (OR = 1.43, 95% CI 1.10–1.87), women's hairdresser (OR = 1.61, 95% CI 1.13–2.31), and driver/material handling equipment operator (OR = 1.47, 95% CI 0.97–2.25) were all associated with DLBCL risk after adjustment for other DLBCL-specific risk factors [51]. In sex-specific models, the former three occupations were retained for women, and the latter occupation was retained for men. In a meta-analysis of occupational exposures to agricultural pesticide groups [105], DLBCL was associated with phenoxy herbicide exposure (OR = 2.0, 95% CI 1.1–3.7) and weakly associated with DDT exposure (OR = 1.2, 95% CI 0.9–1.7). In the Agricultural Health Study cohort [106], there were no statistically significant associations of DLBCL with any of 26 insecticides, fungicides, and fumigants evaluated, including DDT. In the Agricultural Health Study, a recent report found no association of 2,4-D with NHL overall, consistent with prior and an updated meta-analysis of this association [107]; no data for DLBCL were available.

1.3.3.7 Hair Dye

In the InterLymph hair dye pooling project, there was an increased risk of NHL among women who started using hair dyes before 1980 (OR = 1.3, 95% 1.1–1.4), but there was no association with DLBCL (OR = 1.1, 95% CI 0.9–1.3) [108]. In the InterLymph Subtypes Project, hair dye use was not associated with DLBCL, but duration of hair dye use was positively associated with MLBCL risk (OR = 4.97 for 20+ years of use versus never use, *P*-trend < 0.001) [51]. While the latter finding was based on a small number of cases and thus requires replication, it is somewhat provocative given the distinct descriptive epidemiology of this lymphoma subtype, including excess female incidence and peak incidence around age 30 years.

1.3.3.8 Anthropometrics and Physical Activity

Body mass index (BMI) was positively associated with NHL (OR = 1.07 per 5 kg/m^2, 95% CI 1.04–1.10) in a meta-analysis of prospective cohort studies, and the association was specifically observed for DLBCL (OR = 1.13 per 5 kg/m^2, 95% CI 1.02–1.26) and not for FL or CLL/SLL [109]. In a meta-analysis of six case-control and ten cohort studies specifically focused on DLBCL, overweight (25–29.9 kg/m^2, OR = 1.14, 95% CI 1.04–1.24) and obesity (30+ kg/m^2, OR = 1.29, 95% CI 1.16–1.43) were associated with increased risk. Estimates were similar by study design (case-control versus cohort) and gender but stronger in American and Asian relative to European populations [110]. The latter study suggested a linear association for BMI and DLBCL, such that each 10 kg/m^2 increase in BMI was associated with a 14% increase in DLBCL risk. In the InterLymph Subtypes Project, usual adult BMI ($P = 0.002$) and BMI as a young adult ($P < 0.001$) both showed positive, monotonic associations with DLBCL risk in models adjusted for age, sex, race/ethnicity, and study [51]. When both variables were simultaneously included in a multivariable model that also included other DLBCL-specific risk factors (including socioeconomic status), the association for usual adult BMI greatly attenuated and only showed an association for underweight (OR = 0.58 for 15–18.4 versus 18.5–22.4 kg/m^2, 95% CI 0.39–0.85), while young adult BMI only slightly attenuated and continued to show a monotonic association with DLBCL risk (OR = 1.58 for 30–50 versus 18.5–22.4 kg/m^2, 95% CI 1.12–2.23). The association of young adult BMI with DLBCL risk is supported by cohort studies [111–113], including after adjustment for adult BMI [114]. While specific mechanisms linking BMI and DLBCL risk are not known, immune (including chronic inflammation) or hormonal mechanisms have been postulated [115].

Greater physical activity showed a weak inverse association with NHL risk in a meta-analysis of eight case-control and 15 cohort studies (RR = 0.91, 95% CI 0.82–1.00), but there was no association for DLBCL (RR = 0.95, 95% CI 0.80–1.14) [116]. In the InterLymph Subtypes Project, leisure time physical activity was not associated with DLBCL risk (OR = 0.85 for vigorous versus low activity, *P*-trend = 0.23). Leisure-time sitting (hours/day) was positively associated with NHL risk (HR = 2.18 for 6+ versus <3 h/day, *P*-trend = 0.008) in a large cohort study, but there was no association with DLBCL risk (*P*-trend = 0.98) [117]. The positive association of BMI with DLBCL risk, but lack of association with physical activity, will require further investigation.

1.3.3.9 Smoking and Alcohol Consumption

Cigarette smoking history was not associated with DLBCL risk in a large meta-analyses [118, 119] nor in the InterLymph pooling projects [51, 120]. However, in the InterLymph Subtypes Project, there were positive associations of smoking (>35 years versus nonsmoker) with risk of PCNSL (OR = 1.52, *P*-trend = 0.024), testicular DLBCL (OR = 2.72, *P*-trend = 0.091), and cutaneous DLBCL (OR = 1.88, *P*-trend = 0.015). A positive association of smoking with PCNSL has been previously reported [121], while the other associations require replication.

Alcohol drinkers had a lower risk of DLBCL (OR = 0.79, 95% CI 0.68–0.91) in recent meta-analysis of 21 case-control and eight cohort studies, which was also observed for NHL overall (OR = 0.85, 95% CI 0.79–0.91) and for most major NHL subtypes except CLL/SLL [122]. In the InterLymph Subtypes Project, greater lifetime consumption of alcohol was inversely associated with DLBCL risk after adjusting for DLBCL-specific risk factors including socioeconomic status and body mass index (OR = 0.64 for >400 kg versus nondrinker, 95% CI 0.51–0.79, *P*-trend < 0.001) [51]. Inverse associations were observed for multiple alcohol variables defined by type, intensity, and duration of use, and the inverse associations were stronger in men. The mechanistic underpinning of this association is unknown, but both the impact of alcohol use on general immune function [123] and specific effects on cell signaling pathways related to lymphomagenesis [124] have been suggested.

1.3.3.10 Diet

While several associations had been suggested between diet and cancers of the lymphoid and hematopoietic system, including milk and dairy, meat, fat, fish, and fruit and vegetables [125], the Panel for the 2007 *Food, Nutrition, Physical Activity, and the Prevention of Cancer* [126] report concluded that more work was needed into mechanisms that underlie putative dietary associations as well as the need to better investigate lymphoma subtypes, for which there were only limited data. Our knowledge state has not increased much since that report [43]. The strongest and most consistent data have been for vegetable intake. In a meta-analysis of nine case-control studies and five cohort studies, vegetable intake was inversely associated with NHL risk (RR = 0.81 for low versus high intake, 95% CI 0.71–0.92), and this was also observed for DLBCL risk (RR = 0.70, 95% CI 0.54–0.91) [127]. Vegetables are a rich source of phytochemicals, vitamins, and antioxidants, which have chemopreventive properties and can enhance immune function, both mechanisms relevant to lymphomagenesis.

In the California Teacher's Cohort, an antioxidant index measuring hydroxyl radical absorbance capacity showed a suggestive inverse association with DLBCL risk (RR = 0.68 for highest versus lowest quartile, *P*-trend = 0.08) [128], which was replicated and expanded in a case-control study using an updated and more comprehensive measure of hydroxyl radical absorbance (OR = 0.43 for highest versus lowest quartile, *P*-trend = 0.026) [129]. In support of these latter findings, inverse associations for DLBCL from large cohort studies have been reported for dietary and supplemental intake of vitamin C (RR = 0.69 for highest versus lowest quartile, *P*-trend = 0.030) [130]; serum levels of total carotenoids (OR = 0.46 for highest versus lowest tertile, *P*-trend < 0.01), β-carotene (OR = 0.38, *P*-trend < 0.01), lycopene (OR = 0.51, *P*-trend < 0.01), and α-cryptoxanthin (OR = 0.35, *P*-trend = 0.02) [131]; and α-tocopherol in a nonlinear (U-shaped) manner [132]. While suggestive, a specific antioxidant mechanism vrelated to DLBCL pathogenesis has yet to be identified.

1.3.3.11 Sun Exposure

In the InterLymph sun exposure pooling project, higher composite recreational sun exposure was inversely associated with NHL risk (OR = 0.76 for highest versus lowest quartile, *P*-trend = 0.005) as well as for DLBCL risk (OR = 0.69, *P*-trend < 0.001), while there was no association with occupational sun exposure [133]. In the InterLymph Subtypes Project, recreational sun exposure was inversely associated with DLBCL risk (OR = 0.78 for highest versus lowest quartile, *P*-trend < 0.001) after adjusting for DLBCL-specific risk factors [51]. In the California Teachers Study cohort, residential UVR levels within a 20-km radius were associated with reduced risk of DLBCL (RR = 0.36 for highest versus lowest statewide quartile of minimum UV, 95% CI, 0.17–0.78; *P*-trend = 0.07) [134], and this association was not modified by skin sensitivity to sunlight, race/ethnicity, body mass index, or neighborhood socioeconomic status. In the Nurses' Health Study, multiple measures of higher average annual UV-B flux, most prominently at age 15 (RR = 0.67, *P*-trend = 0.37) and as a lifetime cumulative average (RR = 0.84, *P*-trend = 0.68), showed weak and not statistically significant but nevertheless inverse associations with DLBCL risk [135]. In an ecologic study from Australia [136], higher latitude (a surrogate for lower residential ambient UVR exposure) was correlated with higher DLBCL incidence rates (IRR = 1.37, 95% CI 1.16–1.61), and in an ecologic study in the USA [137], greater ambient UV radiation based on satellite estimates was inversely associated with DLBCL incidence rates (IRR = 0.84, 95% CI 0.76–0.94). The latter study also reported that the elevated IRRs for DLBCL were similar for whites, blacks, and Hispanics.

The underlying biological mechanism for any putative inverse association with DLBCL risk is not known, but dietary vitamin D intake is not a likely mechanism as a meta-analysis found no association for DLBCL (OR = 1.05 for highest versus lowest category, 95% CI 0.73–1.52) [138], and in the California Teachers Cohort, neither dietary nor supplemental vitamin D intake was associated with DLBCL risk [134]. A pooled nested case-control analysis of ten cohort studies found no association of circulating 25-hydroxyvitamin D with DLBCL risk (*P*-trend = 0.40), although the highest category showed a protective effect (OR = 0.74 for >100 versus 50 to <75 nmol/L, 95%CI 0.39–1.42) and the lowest category showed a slightly elevated risk (OR = 1.27 for <25 versus 50 to <75 nmol/L, 95%CI 0.76–2.12) [139]. These and other results suggest that long-term and cumulative UV exposure, relative to intermittent intense exposure, are more relevant, which would impact the ability of one-time sampling of circulating vitamin D levels to detect an association. Alternatively, immunologic effects of UV radiation and impacts on circadian rhythm have been suggested as alternative mechanisms [138].

1.3.4 Burkitt Lymphoma

The analytic epidemiology of BL is strongly linked to the main clinical variants of endemic, immunodeficiency-associated, and sporadic BL. The translocation involving *MYC* is highly characteristic but not specific [140].

1.3.4.1 Endemic BL

Endemic BL occurs predominately in equatorial Africa and Papua New Guinea, where it is the most common childhood cancer [11]. It most commonly presents as a clinically striking extranodal jaw or orbital mass, but histologically it cannot be distinguished from other variants of BL. The incidence of endemic BL is closely linked to areas with high rates of *Plasmodium falciparum* infection and early infection with EBV. Rates of BL also correlate with intensity and changes of malaria transmission related to malaria control efforts [141, 142]. Both malaria and EBV induce B-cell hyperplasia, and while the exact mechanism is not definitive, malaria can directly influence lymphomagenesis through induction of activation-induced cytidine deaminase (AID), leading to the creation of a *MYC* translocation with immunoglobulin genes and ectopic *MYC* expression [11]. This, coupled with EBV's ability to block apoptosis of genetically altered cells as they go through the germinal-center reaction, is thought to underlie BL pathogenesis [11].

1.3.4.2 Immunodeficiency-Associated BL

In 1982, HIV infection was linked to an increased risk of BL [143, 144], and ultimately BL became an AIDS-defining condition [71] and was included as a BL variant in 2008 WHO Classification of Hematopoietic Tumors [4]. HIV/AIDS has been hypothesized to explain the third peak in the age-incidence curve that was discussed above. In contrast to DLBCL, risk of BL did not decline as much after the introduction of HAART in 1996 [73, 74]. Based on SEER data, Mbulaiteye et al. have estimated that in the USA, 71% of adult BL was AIDS related and 29% was non-AIDS related [26]. Mechanistically, HIV may play a similar role as malaria, as high expression of AID in peripheral blood mononuclear cells has been shown to be associated with later risk of BL in HIV-infected patients [145], which is consistent with AID-mediated *MYC*/Ig translocations characteristic of BL.

Solid organ transplantation is associated with an increased risk of BL, most recently estimated at 24.5-fold excess risk (95% CI 19.7–30.2) based on data from a US population-based study of transplant recipients from 1987 to 2008 [83]. Risk was particularly elevated for transplants given before age 20 years (SIR = 123, 95% CI 79–183) and for liver transplants (SIR = 47.1, 95% CI 33.3–64.6). In contrast to DLBCL, BL risk was not elevated in the first year after transplantation but rather increased with time since transplant. While EBV appears to drive most of the excess risk of DLBCL in children under age 20 and in the first year of transplantation (noting that DLBCL comprises a larger fraction of posttransplant lymphoproliferative disorders), this is probably heterogeneous in immunodeficiency-associated BL, where only ~50% of HIV-associated BL is EBV positive [146].

1.3.4.3 Sporadic BL

Sporadic BL is observed globally, although it is more common in developed countries [11]. EBV is detected in approximately 30% of sporadic BL cases, and EBV+ sporadic BL is associated with lower socioeconomic status and early EBV infection [11]. There have been relatively few epidemiologic studies of this entity due to its overall rarity.

For adult BL, the largest study to date is the InterLymph Subtypes Project, which published risk factors for sporadic BL based on a pooled dataset of 295 cases and 21,818 controls from 18 case-control studies [147]. The study included typical BL and Burkitt-like lymphomas and excluded cases with HIV infection or history of solid organ transplantation. Because of the unique descriptive epidemiology of sporadic BL, analyses were stratified on younger (<50 years) and older (50+ years) age at diagnosis. In the final multivariable model, BL in younger participants was inversely associated with a history of allergy (OR = 0.58, 95% CI 0.32–1.05) and positively associated with a history of eczema among individuals without other atopic conditions (OR = 2.54, 95% CI 1.20–5.40), taller height (OR = 2.17 for highest versus lowest quartile, 95% CI 1.08–4.36), use of light color hair dye (OR = 2.89 versus never used hair dye, 95% CI 0.84–9.94), and employment as a charworker cleaner (OR = 3.49, 95% CI 1.13–10.7). BL in older individuals was positively associated with a history of HCV seropositivity (OR = 4.19, 95% CI 1.05–16.6) and inversely associated with usual adult BMI (OR = 0.16 for 35–50 versus <18.5 kg/m^2, 95% CI 0.02–1.05) and use of alcohol (OR = 0.63 at least one drink per month versus nondrinker, 95% CI 0.40–0.98). These associations were largely age-specific, although there was a suggestive inverse association with alcohol use among younger individuals and a suggestive positive association with height among older individuals.

One notable finding was a lack of an association of a family history of any hematologic malignancy with risk of BL (OR = 0.81, 95% CI 0.41–1.62), and this was the only subtype (of 11 subtypes evaluated) besides mycosis fungoides/

Sezary syndrome to not have an association with family history [148]. Similarly, in the Scandinavian registries, there was no association of any family history of NHL with BL risk (SIR = 0.9, 95% CI 0.3–1.9) [52]. It is not clear if the lack of association is real (and perhaps suggesting a smaller role for genetic susceptibility) or that these studies have been underpowered due to the rarity of BL.

The association of hepatitis viruses with BL remains unclear. In an Australian cohort of over 110,000 HBV and HCV patients identified from 1990 to 2002 and linked to a population-based cancer registry, there was excess risk of BL in HBV (SIR = 12.9, 95% CI 5.4–30.9) but not HCV patients [149]. In contrast, in the SEER-Medicare study of individuals aged 65+ years, there was a positive association of BL with HCV (OR = 5.21, 95% CI 1.62–16.8) but not HBV [78].

1.3.5 PTCL

1.3.5.1 Family History and Genetics

In the InterLymph Subtypes Project [150], a first-degree family history of a hematologic malignancy was associated with 1.92-fold increased risk of PTCL (95% CI 1.30–2.84) after adjusting for PTCL-specific risk factors. This association was observed for PTCL-NOS (OR = 1.92, 95% CI 1.05–3.49) and AITL (OR = 2.55, 95% CI 1.10–5.89) but was much weaker and not statistically significant for ALCL (OR = 1.36, 95% CI 0.54–3.44). In registry-based studies from Scandinavia, first-degree relatives of patients with HL, CLL, DLBCL, or FL specifically were not at elevated risk of T-cell lymphoma [53, 54]. There was increased risk of mature T-cell lymphoma for a first-degree relative with any NHL (SIR = 1.7, 95% CI 0.9–3.0), LPL/WM (SIR = 17, 95% CI 2.0–60), or mature T-cell lymphoma (SIR = 8.2, 95% CI 0.2–46), although only the LPL/WM was statistically significant and the mature T-cell lymphoma SIR was based on only one exposed case [52]. The only GWAS conducted in T-cell lymphoma was for extranodal natural killer T-cell lymphoma (NKTCL) in Asians, which identified a locus at 6p21.32 (*HLA-DPB1* in HLA class II) [151]. Imputation-based fine-mapping implicated four AA residues (Gly84-Gly85-Pro86-Met87) at the edge of the HLA-DPB1 peptide-binding groove as accounting for most the association of the top SNP in this region.

1.3.5.2 Infections

Although not an AIDS-defining cancer, AIDS was associated with a 24.3-fold increased risk of PTCL (95% CI 11.7–44.8) in the pre-HAART era [152], and US data from 1996 to 2010 showed that HIV infection or AIDS was still associated with an increased, albeit weaker, risk of PTCL (RR = 3.6, 95% CI 2.6–4.9) [72], supporting a role for immunosuppression or other immune dysregulation in this subtype. ALCL and NKTCL were also elevated in HIV/AIDS patients [72]. In an InterLymph pooled analysis of 17 case-control studies, a self-reported history of infectious mononucleosis was associated with an increased risk of PTCL (OR = 1.72, 95% CI 1.14–2.59) [153].

While HCV does not appear to be linked to PTCL, there is some suggestive evidence for an association of HBV with T-cell malignancies, as a recent meta-analysis of 17 case-control and five cohort studies (with over 40,000 cases) found a positive association with T-cell lymphoma (OR = 1.44, 95% CI 1.08–1.91); specific results for PTCL were not available [79].

1.3.5.3 Medical History

Solid organ transplantation was associated with an increased risk of PTCL, most recently estimated at a 3.9-fold excess risk (95% CI 2.7–5.6) based on data from a US population-based study of transplant recipients from 1987 to 2008 [83]. Risk was particularly elevated for transplants given before age 20 years (SIR = 172, 95% CI 69–354) and with time since transplantation, but it did not vary by type of transplanted organ. Risks were also elevated for ALCL (SIR = 12.8, 95% CI 9.0–17.7), PCALCL (SIR = 13.5, 95% CI 6.2–25.5), and HSTL (SIR = 100, 95% CI 33–234).

Celiac disease was associated with T-cell lymphoma overall in the InterLymph autoimmune pooling project (OR = 6.21, 95% CI 2.82–13.6) [89], in the SEER-Medicare study (OR = 5.9, 95% CI 2.4–14) [92], and in a recent comprehensive meta-analysis (OR = 15.8, 95% CI 7.85–31.9) [93]. The InterLymph analysis also found an association with psoriasis (OR = 1.63, 95% CI 1.03–2.57) [89]. In the InterLymph Subtypes Project, both celiac (OR = 17.8, 95% CI 8.61–36.8) and psoriasis (OR = 1.97, 95% CI 1.17–3.32) were associated with PTCL in a multivariable model that adjusted for a variety of PTCL risk factors [150]. The association with celiac disease was also significant for PTCL-NOS (OR = 8.66, 95% CI 1.97–38.1), ALCL (OR = 16.6, 95% CI 3.27–84.3), and EATL (OR = 215, 95% CI 44–1041). While inflammatory bowel disease per se has not been clearly linked to lymphoma risk, thiopurine use appears to increase risk, particularly risk of HSTL, with or without TNF-α inhibitors [154, 155].

A history of allergies was inversely associated with PTCL risk (OR = 0.69, 95% CI 0.54–0.87), while a history of eczema (OR = 1.41, 95% CI 1.07–1.85) was positively associated with risk after simultaneous adjustment for each other and other PTCL-specific risk factors in the InterLymph Subtypes Project.

In a meta-analysis of type 2 diabetes and lymphoma risk, there was an overall increased risk for PTCL (OR = 2.42, 95% CI 1.24–4.72), and this was most pronounced for Asian studies [97]. There is evidence of intrinsic T-cell dysfunction in patients with type 2 diabetes [156], and given the PTCL associations with the T-cell-activating autoimmune diseases of celiac disease and psoriasis, it suggests potential shared mechanisms, but further research is needed, particularly with respect to potential confounding factors.

The association of breast implants and ALCL was first describe in 1997 [157], and to date two population-based studies from the Netherlands (OR = 18.2, 95% CI 2.1–157) [158] and California (HR = 10.9, 95% CI 2.18–54.0) [159] have shown increased risk at the population level. Additional evidence strongly supports this association, and although causation has not been fully established [160], a provisional entity called breast implant-associated ALCL, to be distinguished from other ALK-ALCL, has been proposed in the 2016 WHO update [1].

1.3.5.4 Occupations and Environmental Factors

In the InterLymph occupational pooling project [104], PTCL risk was positively associated with ever employment as a painter (OR = 1.80, 95% CI 1.14–2.84), textile worker (OR = 1.60, 95% CI 1.18–2.17), wood worker (OR = 1.54, 95% CI 1.04–2.27), or electrical fitter (OR = 2.02, 95% CI 1.03–3.97). In the InterLymph Subtypes Project, PTCL risk was positively associated with ever employment as a textile worker (OR = 1.58, 95% CI 1.05–2.83) or electrical fitter (OR = 2.89, 95% CI 1.41–5.95) and was inversely associated with having ever lived or worked on a farm (OR = 0.72, 95% CI 0.55–0.95) after adjusting for other PTCL-specific risk factors [150]. In exploratory analyses, there was suggestive evidence that employment as a textile worker was associated with increased risk of ALCL and as an electrical fitter was associated with increased risk of ALCL and AITL.

1.3.5.5 Anthropometrics

In the InterLymph Subtypes Project, there was no association of body mass index or height with risk of PTCL, or specifically PTCL-NOS, ALCL, or AITL [150].

1.3.5.6 Smoking and Alcohol Use

Ever cigarette smoking was associated with T-cell lymphoma (OR = 1.23, 95% CI 1.09–1.38) in a meta-analysis of 41 case-control and nine cohort studies [119]. In the InterLymph Subtypes Project, cigarette smoking was a strong, independent risk factor for PTCL, with a clear dose response with duration of smoking (*P* trend <0.001): 40+ year smokers had a 1.92-fold higher risk of PTCL compared to nonsmokers (95% CI 1.41–2.62) [150]. In exploratory analyses, the smoking association was strongest for ALCL and PTCL-NOS. In a separate analysis of mycosis fungoides/Sezary syndrome, cigarette smoking was also associated with increased risk (OR = 1.55 for 40+ years versus nonsmoker, 95% CI 1.04–2.31) [161], supporting a broad T-cell lymphoma association observed in meta-analysis and pooled analysis. While this does not establish a causal association, there are accumulating data that T lymphocytes may be particularly susceptible smoking [119].

Alcohol drinkers compared to nondrinkers had a lower risk of T-cell lymphoma (OR = 0.78, 95% CI 0.58–1.05) in a recent meta-analysis of 21 case-control and eight cohort studies [122]. In the InterLymph Subtypes Project, consumption of at least one alcoholic drink per month was inversely associated with PTCL risk (OR = 0.64, 95% CI 0.49–0.82) after adjusting for other PTCL-specific risk factors including cigarette smoking [150]. In exploratory analyses, alcohol use was inversely associated with PTCL-NOS but not ALCL or AITL.

1.3.5.7 Sun Exposure

In the InterLymph sun exposure pooling project, recreational sun exposure was not associated with PTCL risk (*P*-trend = 0.67), although there was an inverse association for the highest level of exposure (OR = 0.83 for highest versus lowest quartile, 95% CI 0.46–1.49) [133]. In the InterLymph Subtypes Project, recreational sun exposure showed a suggestive inverse association with PTCL risk (OR = 0.79 for highest versus lowest quartile, *P*-trend = 0.1), but the association attenuated after adjusting for other PTCL risk factors, and it was not included in the final multivariable model [150]. In exploratory analyses, recreational sun exposure was inversely associated with ALCL, but not PTCL-NOS or AITL. Of some interest, ecologic data from both Australia and the USA support an inverse association of PTCL-NOS and ambient UV radiation [136, 137], and for the latter study, associations were strongest among blacks.

1.3.6 Cross-Subtype Patterns

As discussed above, we have focused on risk factor associations for the three major aggressive subtypes, which are summarized in Table 1.5. However, this approach does not put these risk factor associations in the context of each other or relative to the common indolent subtypes, which is needed to gain a more systematic insight into the etiologic heterogeneity of NHL. To achieve such a goal, there needs to be a sufficient sample size for at least the more common subtypes, harmonized risk factor data, and formal statistical testing approaches to evaluate heterogeneity and clustering. One of the largest and most comprehensive analyses to date has been the InterLymph Subtypes Project [50], which has already been highlighted above for the individual subtypes of DLBCL [51], BL [147], and PTCL [150], but which also conducted a formal cross-subtype evaluation [148] for 11 subtypes that included 4667 DLBCL, 3530 FL, 2440 CLL/SLL, 1052 MZL, 584 PTCL, 557 MCL, 374 LPL/WM, 324 MF/SS, 295 BL, 154 hairy cell leukemia, 152 ALL, and 23,096 controls. Risk factor data were centrally harmonized and included data on medical history, family history of hematologic malignancies, lifestyle factors, and occupation.

With respect to etiologic heterogeneity, Table 1.6 summarizes risk factors that were associated with 1 or more NHL subtypes ($P < 0.01$ based on the ASSET test [162], a subset-based statistical approach that was used to test whether an exposure was associated with at least 1 of the 11 subtypes [148]). For example, family history of NHL was strongly associated with 1 or more of the NHL subtypes ($P_{ASSET} = 1.7 \times 10^{-13}$), and there was no evidence for subtype heterogeneity across subtypes ($P = 0.52$) based on a test of homogeneity of ORs among NHL subtypes from the random effects meta-analysis *Q* statistic [163]; eight of the 11 subtypes showed a positive association with risk (OR > 1.6), 5 at $P < 0.05$. Notably, while both DLBCL and PTCL were associated with family history of NHL, BL (along with MF/SS and LPL/WM) did not.

Overall, there was evidence for heterogeneity (i.e., risk factors differed among NHL subtypes) based on the *Q* statistic ($P < 0.05$) for most autoimmune diseases, eczema, HCV, blood transfusion, height, cigarette smoking, and teaching occupation, whereas generally homogeneous risks were observed for a family history of NHL, alcohol

Table 1.5 Summary of risk factor associations for the major aggressive subtypes of DLBCL, BL, and PTCL

Risk factor	DLBCL	BL	PTCL	Comments
Family history of NHL	↑	Ø	↑	
Genetic loci				
TNF-LTA Haplotype	↑			
6p25.3	↑			Near *EXOC2*
6p21.33	↑			*HLA-B*08:01* implicated through HLA imputation
2p23.3	↑			Near *NCOA1*
8q24.21	↑			2 independent SNPs at this locus; near *PVT1* and *MYC*
Immune biomarkers				
Soluble CD30	↑			
Infections				
HIV/AIDS	↑	↑	↑	Both DLBCL and BL are AIDS-defining conditions
HHV8	↑			Considered causal for PEL
EBV		↑		
Malaria		↑		
HCV	↑		Ø	Established carcinogen for NHL; mixed data for BL
HBV	↑			
Solid organ transplantation	↑	↑	↑	Particularly strong in pediatric population
Breast implants			↑	ALCL
Autoimmune disorders				
System lupus erythematosus	↑			
Sjogren syndrome	↑			
Celiac disease	↑		↑	Data are strongest for PTCL
Psoriasis			↑	
Allergies (including hay fever)	↓	↓	↓	Few data from cohort studies (? reverse causality)
Eczema		↑	↑	
Type 2 diabetes	Ø		↑	↑ for DLBCL in Europe; ↑ for PTCL in Asia
Body mass index	↑	↓	Ø	
Cigarette smoking	Ø		↑	↑ for PCNSL
Alcohol consumption	↓	↓	↓	For DLBCL, stronger in males
Vegetable consumption	↓			
Recreational sun exposure	↓	Ø	Ø	

DLBCL diffuse large B-cell lymphoma, *BL* Burkitt lymphoma, *PTCL* peripheral T-cell lymphoma, *ALCL* anaplastic large cell lymphoma, *PCNSL* primary central nervous system lymphoma
Key: ↑ = increases risk; ↓ = decreases risk; Ø = no association

consumption, recreational sun exposure, allergy, hay fever, young adult BMI, socioeconomic status, and the occupations of general farm worker and painter. However, from inspection of Tables 1.5 and 1.6, no unique risk factor patterns for the three main aggressive subtypes were evident.

A second approach used in the InterLymph Subtypes Initiative was to evaluate clustering of subtypes based on their shared risk factor profiles when all available risk factors were taken into account simultaneously. Statistically significant clustering among subtypes based on risk factor profiles was identified and is summarized

Table 1.6 Heterogeneity of risk factor associations for aggressive subtypes (DLBCL, BL, and PTCL) and other indolent subtypes, InterLymph subtypes project

Risk factor	*P* ASSET[a]	NHL OR[b] (95% CI)	DLBCL OR[b] (95% CI)	BL OR[b] (95% CI)	PTCL OR[b] (95% CI)	*P* homogeneity[c]	Other statistically significant subtypes (direction of OR)
Family history of NHL	1.7×10^{-13}	1.79 (1.51–2.13)	1.57 (1.34–1.83)	0.75 (0.23–2.43)	1.69 (0.92–3.12)	0.52	MZL(↑),CLL/SLL(↑), FL(↑), MCL(↑)
B-cell-activating autoimmune disease	3.8×10^{-22}	1.96 (1.60–2.40)	2.45 (1.91–3.16)	1.22 (0.29–5.04)	1.81 (0.87–3.79)	9.8×10^{-10}	MZL(↑), LPL/WM(↑)
– Systemic lupus erythematosus	1.9×10^{-8}	2.83 (1.82–4.41)	2.49 (1.42–4.37)	~	3.90 (1.24–12.3)	0.18	MF/SS(↑), MZL(↑), LPL/WM(↑)
– Sjogren syndrome	6.3×10^{-18}	7.52 (3.68–15.4)	8.77 (3.94–19.5)	~	3.68 (0.48–31.0)	7.3×10^{-9}	FL(↑)
T-cell-activating autoimmune disease	0.0053	1.07 (0.95–1.21)	1.08 (0.91–1.28)	0.57 (0.25–1.32)	1.95 (1.37–2.77)	0.012	MF/SS (↑)
– Celiac disease	5.2×10^{-11}	1.77 (1.05–2.99)	2.09 (1.04–4.18)	~	14.8 (7.27–30.2)	5.1×10^{-8}	
– Systemic sclerosis/scleroderma	0.0051	1.03 (0.41–2.58)	0.71 (0.16–3.24)	20.2 (2.44–166)	~	0.065	MF/SS(↑), HCL(↑)
Allergy	5.9×10^{-8}	0.86 (0.81–0.92)	0.82 (0.74–0.90)	0.75 (0.51–1.10)	0.75 (0.60–0.94)	0.24	CLL/SLL(↓), FL(↓), MCL(↓)
Hay fever	9.1×10^{-9}	0.82 (0.77–0.88)	0.78 (0.70–0.86)	0.64 (0.44–0.95)	0.95 (0.74–1.21)	0.12	LPL/WM(↓), FL(↓), MCL(↓)
Eczema	5.0×10^{-5}	1.01 (0.93–1.10)	0.91 (0.80–1.03)	1.03 (0.64–1.66)	1.27 (0.97–1.65)	2.6×10^{-5}	MF/SS(↑)
HCV	2.3×10^{-8}	1.81 (1.39–2.37)	2.33 (1.71–3.19)	3.05 (0.90–10.3)	1.88 (0.66–5.33)	0.0021	MZL(↑), LPL/WM(↑), CLL/SLL(↑)
Blood transfusion (before 1990)	8.8×10^{-5}	0.83 (0.77–0.91)	0.84 (0.75–0.95)	0.81 (0.49–1.34)	0.78 (0.54–1.12)	0.050	CLL/SLL(↓), FL(↓), HCL(↓)
Young adult BMI	4.2×10^{-9}	1.95 (1.51–2.53)	3.02 (2.13–4.27)	1.67 (0.57–4.87)	1.14 (0.49–2.62)	0.28	FL(↑)
Height	0.0017	1.20 (1.08–1.32)	1.16 (1.01–1.33)	2.43 (1.37–4.31)	1.26 (0.89–1.79)	0.024	CLL/SLL(↑), FL(↑), HCL(↑)
Alcohol consumption (any)	8.9×10^{-8}	0.87 (0.81–0.93)	0.81 (0.73–0.89)	0.64 (0.48–0.87)	0.68 (0.53–0.87)	0.062	MZL(↓), FL(↓)
Smoking (duration)	2.2×10^{-5}	1.06 (0.99–1.14)	1.02 (0.92–1.12)	0.77 (0.51–1.17)	1.75 (1.33–2.30)	3.2×10^{-9}	MZL(↑), LPL/WM(↑), CLL/SLL(↓), FL(↑)

(continued)

Table 1.6 (continued)

Risk factor	*P* ASSET[a]	NHL OR[b] (95% CI)	DLBCL OR[b] (95% CI)	BL OR[b] (95% CI)	PTCL OR[b] (95% CI)	*P* homogeneity[c]	Other statistically significant subtypes (direction of OR)
Recreational sun exposure	2.7×10^{-9}	0.74 (0.66–0.83)	0.75 (0.64–0.88)	0.72 (0.33–1.59)	0.67 (0.46–1.00)	0.79	MZL(↓), CLL/SLL(↓), FL(↓)
Socioeconomic status	3.4×10^{-5}	0.88 (0.83–0.93)	0.82 (0.76–0.90)	0.65 (0.48–0.90)	0.84 (0.67–1.05)	0.061	HCL(↑)
General farm worker	0.0082	1.28 (1.10–1.50)	1.09 (0.87–1.37)	1.49 (0.59–3.78)	0.79 (0.40–1.56)	0.34	MF/SS(↑), CLL/SLL(↑),
Painter	0.0048	1.22 (0.99–1.51)	1.02 (0.76–1.37)	2.28 (0.97–5.33)	1.45 (0.73–2.88)	0.085	MF/SS(↑)
Teacher	5.6×10^{-5}	0.86 (0.77–0.95)	0.87 (0.75–1.00)	0.27 (0.09–0.87)	0.79 (0.51–1.22)	0.0062	MZL(↓)

NHL non-Hodgkin lymphoma, *DLBCL* diffuse large B-cell lymphoma, *BL* Burkitt lymphoma, *PTCL* peripheral T-cell lymphoma, *MZL* marginal zone lymphoma, *CLL/SLL* chronic lymphocytic leukemia/small lymphocytic lymphoma, *FL* follicular lymphoma, *MCL* mantle cell lymphoma, *LPL/WM* lymphoplasmacytic lymphoma/Waldenstrom macroglobulinemia, *MF/SS* mycosis fungoides/Sezary syndrome, *HCL* hairy cell leukemia

[a]*P*-ASSET is the *P*-value for overall association of the risk factor with one or more NHL subtypes

[b]*OR* Odds ratio and 95% *CI* confidence intervals, adjusted for age, sex, race/ethnicity, and study. OR represents risk per increasing category of an ordinal variable for body mass index as a young adult (<18.5, 18.5–22.4, 22.5–24.9, 25.0–29.9, ≥30 kg/m^2), height (sex-specific quartiles, males, <172.0, 172.0–177.7, 177.8–181.9, ≥182.0 cm; females, <159.0, 159.0–162.9, 163.0–167.9, ≥168.0 cm), weight (sex-specific quartiles, males, <72.57, 72.57–79.99, 80.00–88.99, ≥89.00 kg; females, <58.05, 58.06–64.99, 65.00–74.83, ≥74.84 kg), duration of cigarette smoking (0, 1–19, 20–29, 30–39, ≥40 years), recreational sun exposure (hours/week, study-specific quartiles), and socioeconomic status (low, medium, high; measured by years of education for studies in North America or by dividing measures of education or socioeconomic status into tertiles for studies in Europe or Australia)

[c]$P_{homogeneity}$ derived from the random effects meta-analysis *Q* statistic

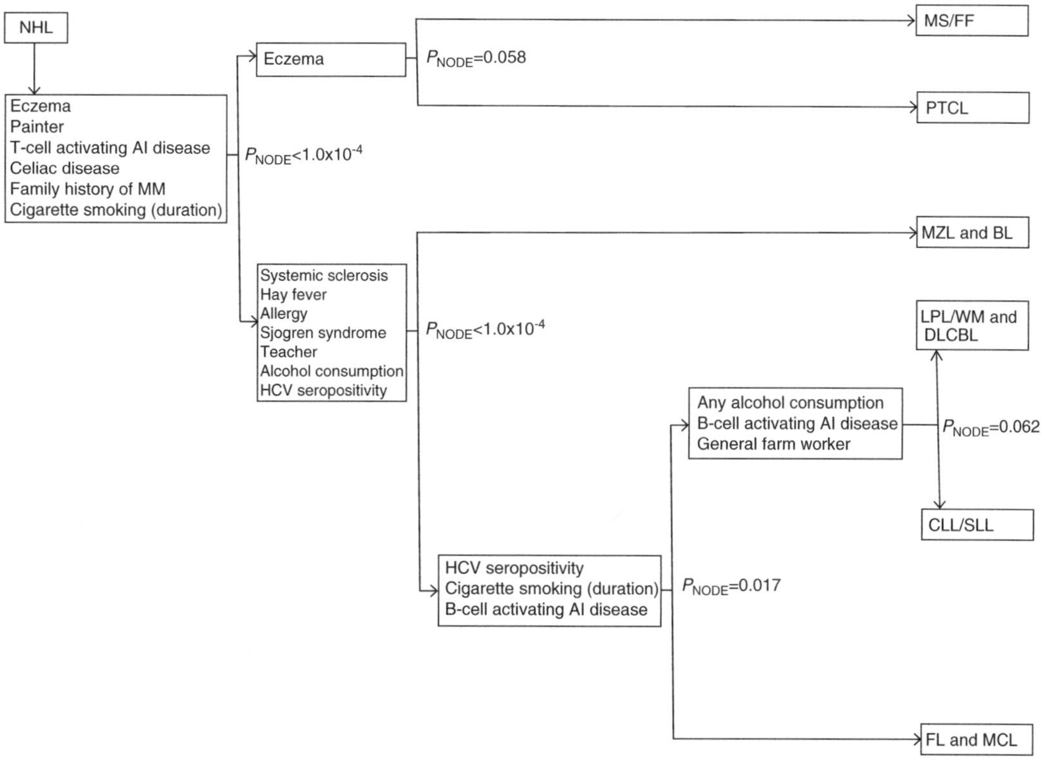

Fig. 1.7 Top-down hierarchical clustering of risk factors for groups of NHL subtypes, InterLymph Subtypes Project (Adapted from Morton et al. J Natl Cancer Inst Monogr 2014;48:130–144). P_{NODE} is the *P*-value for creation of a node in the tree during hierarchical clustering. *AI* autoimmune disease, *NHL* non-Hodgkin lymphoma, *DLBCL* diffuse large B-cell lymphoma, *BL* Burkitt lymphoma, *PTCL* peripheral T-cell lymphoma, *MZL* marginal zone lymphoma, *CLL/SLL* chronic lymphocytic leukemia/small lymphocytic lymphoma, *FL* follicular lymphoma, *MCL* mantle cell lymphoma, *LPL/WM* lymphoplasmacytic lymphoma/Waldenstrom macroglobulinemia, *MF/SS* mycosis fungoides/Sezary syndrome

in Fig. 1.7 [148]. The greatest difference in risk factor patterns was between B-cell and T-cell lymphomas ($P < 0.0001$, which is the *P*-value for creation of a node in the tree during hierarchical clustering), with eczema, occupation as a painter, T-cell-activating autoimmune diseases, family history of MM, and cigarette smoking more strongly (although not necessarily exclusively) associated with risk of T-cell compared to B-cell lymphomas. For the T-cell lymphoma arm of the tree, there was a second suggestive split separating PTCL from MF/SS ($P = 0.058$) mainly based on the strong association of eczema with MF/SS. For the B-cell arm, there remained additional substantial heterogeneity, with the tree first separating MZL and BL into a cluster ($P < 0.0001$), then FL and MCL into a cluster ($P = 0.017$), then DLBCL and LPL/WM into a cluster, and then a final suggestive separation of CLL/SLL (P = 0.062); key differentiating risk factors are shown in Fig. 1.7. The three aggressive subtypes of DLBCL, BL, and PTCL all ended up in separate final nodes, further suggesting that there is unlikely to be a common set of risk factors that lead to aggressive lymphoma.

Another approach to identify risk factor profiles for NHL subtypes has been termed as "MedWAS" (medical condition-wide association study), which used SEER-Medicare data to agnostically (like GWAS) and comprehensively evaluate 5296 medical conditions in claims data for 52,691 cases of five subtypes (CLL/SLL, DLBCL, FL, MZL, and T-cell lymphoma) and 200,000 controls, all with no history of cancer (except for nonmelanoma skin cancer) [164]. After accounting for multiple testing, 55 unique conditions were associated with 1 or more of the 5 NHL subtypes, of which 49 (89%) varied significantly in the association across subtype ($P_{heterogeneity} < 0.05$). Only history of nonmelanoma skin cancer (ORs 1.19–1.55), actinic keratosis (ORs 1.12–1.25), and hemolytic anemia (ORs 1.64–4.07) was associated with increased risk of all five subtypes. Several well-established subtype-specific risk factor associations were observed, including HIV/AIDs and DLBCL (OR = 3.83, 95% CI 2.28–6.43); solid organ transplantation and DLBCL (OR = 4.27; 95% CI 3.23–5.64) and TCL (OR = 3.58, 95% CI 1.82–7.03); HCV and DLBCL (OR = 1.74; 95% CI 1.37–2.22); SLE and DLBCL (OR = 1.74, 95% CI 1.39–2.17) and MZL (OR = 2.57, 95% CI 1.84–3.58); Sjogren syndrome and DLBCL (OR = 2.10, 95% CI 1.77–2.49) and MZL (OR = 4.74, 95% CI 3.81–5.89); and celiac and T-cell lymphoma (OR = 8.09, 95% CI 4.36–15.0). Nine skin diseases (e.g., atopic dermatitis, psoriasis) were specifically associated with T-cell lymphoma, likely related to the fact that 48% of T-cell lymphomas in the study were cutaneous, particularly MF/SS.

1.4 Conclusions and Future Directions

With the maturation of the WHO classification system and its incorporation into population-based cancer registries, the descriptive epidemiology of DLBCL, BL, and PTCL has become better defined, acknowledging the challenges of changing entities within the WHO classification and the likely substantial heterogeneity for PTCL in particular. The analytic epidemiology of these subtypes has only recently been systematically addressed through use of standardized definitions (e.g., InterLymph classification) and the use of pooled and meta-analysis approaches to increase study power and assess consistency across multiple studies and populations. The analytic epidemiology suggests that some risk factors are associated with all three of these aggressive subtypes but that they are not specific to aggressive lymphoma as a group. Furthermore, both the descriptive and analytic epidemiology suggests that these three entities are likely to be largely unique in their risk factor profile and hence etiology, which has clear implications for understanding pathogenesis and primary prevention. International comparisons suggest that the overrepresentation of aggressive subtypes relative to North America and Europe, particularly T-cell lymphomas, is due to underrepresentation of indolent subtypes as incidence rates for DLBCL, sporadic BL, and most T-cell subtypes are lower in Asian compared to Western countries.

While we are increasing our understanding of these entities, much more research is needed to identify environment and genetic risk factors and understand differences by race/ethnicity and geography. In particular, a better understanding between populations of European and non-European ancestry may lead to novel biologic insights. Our current knowledge base is largely from pooling of case-control studies, which are susceptible to survival, recall, and selection biases, and thus more cohort studies are needed. However, given the rarity of many of these entities, this will be challenging, and pooling of cohorts will also be needed through consortial efforts. There will also be continued value in clinical series and careful biologic studies as a companion to large epidemiologic studies.

Rapidly evolving knowledge about the molecular heterogeneity of DLBCL, BL, and PTCL will also need to be incorporated into epidemiologic studies. For example, DLBCL is classified into germinal center B-cell type (GCB) and activated B-cell type (ABC) in the 2016 update of the WHO Classification [1]. PTCL is even more challenging, given our evolving knowledge of the heterogeneity of the more well-defined PTCL subtypes as well as the yet to be defined heterogeneity underling PTCL-NOS [1, 9]. This will be challenging for epidemiology studies due to the need to incorporate these entities into cancer registries and new studies, as well as the challenges of achieving sufficiently powered studies. Sequencing studies of the somatic (tumor) genome will also provide new biologic insights that can be incorporated into epidemiology studies, for example, by defining sub-entities, identifying pathways that cross subtypes, as well as linking environmental exposures to somatic alterations. While there has been much progress identifying and understanding precursor conditions to CLL/SLL and MM, there is little understanding for DLBCL, BL, and PTCL.

In conclusion, there has been a dramatic increase in our understanding of both the descriptive and analytic epidemiology of DLBCL, BL, and PTCL over the past 20 years, and in parallel, it has also become clear of the need for much more additional work to fully understand and better prevent these aggressive cancers.

References

1. Swerdlow SH, Campo E, Pileri SA, et al. The 2016 revision of the World Health Organization classification of lymphoid neoplasms. Blood. 2016;127(20):2375–90.
2. Teras LR, DeSantis CE, Cerhan JR, et al. 2016 US lymphoid malignancy statistics by World Health Organization subtypes. CA Cancer J Clin. 2016;66(6):443–59.
3. Jaffe ES, Harris NHL, Stein H, et al. Introduction and overview of the classification of lymphoid neoplasms. In: Swerdlow SH, Campo E, Harris NL, et al., editors. WHO classification of tumours of the haematopoietic and lymphoid tissues. Lyon: IARC; 2008.
4. Swerdlow SH, Campo E, Harris NL, et al. WHO classification of tumours of the haematopoietic and lymphoid tissues. In: Bosman FT, Jaffe ES, Lakhani SR, et al., editors. World Health Organization classification of tumours. Lyon: IARC Press; 2008.
5. Fritz A, Percy C, Jack A, et al. International classification of diseases for oncology. 3rd ed. Geneva: World Health Organization; 2000.
6. Jaffe ES, Harris NL, Stein H, et al. World Health Organization classification of tumours: pathology and genetics of tumours of haematopoietic and lymphoid tissues. Lyon: IARC Press; 2001.
7. Jaffe ES, Pittaluga S. Aggressive B-cell lymphomas: a review of new and old entities in the WHO classification. Hematology Am Soc Hematol Educ Program. 2011;2011:506–14.
8. Ott G. Aggressive B-cell lymphomas in the update of the 4th edition of the World Health Organization classification of haematopoietic and lymphatic tissues: refinements of the classification, new entities and genetic findings. Br J Haematol. 2017;178(6):871–87.
9. Armitage JO. The aggressive peripheral T-cell lymphomas: 2017. Am J Hematol. 2017;92(7):706–15.
10. Laurent C, Baron M, Amara N, et al. Impact of expert pathologic review of lymphoma diagnosis: study of patients from the French Lymphopath Network. J Clin Oncol. 2017;35(18):2008–17.
11. Magrath I. Epidemiology: clues to the pathogenesis of Burkitt lymphoma. Br J Haematol. 2012;156(6):744–56.
12. Perry AM, Diebold J, Nathwani BN, et al. Non-Hodgkin lymphoma in the developing world: review of 4539 cases from the International Non-Hodgkin Lymphoma Classification Project. Haematologica. 2016;101(10):1244–50.
13. Sant M, Allemani C, Tereanu C, et al. Incidence of hematologic malignancies in Europe by morphologic subtype: results of the HAEMACARE project. Blood. 2010;116(19):3724–34.
14. Smith A, Crouch S, Lax S, et al. Lymphoma incidence, survival and prevalence 2004-2014: sub-type analyses from the UK's Haematological Malignancy Research Network. Br J Cancer. 2015;112(9):1575–84.
15. Yoon SO, Suh C, Lee DH, et al. Distribution of lymphoid neoplasms in the Republic of Korea: analysis of 5318 cases according to the World Health Organization classification. Am J Hematol. 2010;85(10):760–4.
16. Sun J, Yang Q, Lu Z, et al. Distribution of lymphoid neoplasms in China: analysis of 4,638 cases according to the World Health Organization classification. Am J Clin Pathol. 2012;138(3):429–34.
17. Arora N, Manipadam MT, Nair S. Frequency and distribution of lymphoma types in a tertiary care hospital in South India: analysis of 5115 cases using the World Health Organization 2008 classification and comparison with world literature. Leuk Lymphoma. 2013;54(5):1004–11.
18. Chihara D, Ito H, Matsuda T, et al. Differences in incidence and trends of haematological malignancies in Japan and the United States. Br J Haematol. 2014;164(4):536–45.
19. Lim RB, Loy EY, Lim GH, et al. Gender and ethnic differences in incidence and survival of lymphoid neoplasm subtypes in an Asian population: secular trends of a population-based cancer registry from 1998 to 2012. Int J Cancer. 2015;137(11):2674–87.
20. National Cancer Institute. Surveillance, epidemiology, and end results (SEER) program. www.seer.cancer.gov. SEER*stat database: incidence—SEER 18 regs research data + hurricane katrina impacted. Accessed 29 April 2017.
21. Morton LM, Turner JJ, Cerhan JR, et al. Proposed classification of lymphoid neoplasms for epidemiologic research from the Pathology Working Group of the International Lymphoma Epidemiology Consortium (InterLymph). Blood. 2007;110(2):695–708.
22. Turner JJ, Morton LM, Linet MS, et al. InterLymph hierarchical classification of lymphoid neoplasms for epidemiologic research based on the WHO

classification (2008): update and future directions. Blood. 2010;116(20):e90–8.
23. National Cancer Institute. Surveillance research program, National Cancer Institute SEER*stat software version 8.3.4. www.seer.cancer.gov/seerstat.
24. van Leeuwen MT, Turner JJ, Joske DJ, et al. Lymphoid neoplasm incidence by WHO subtype in Australia 1982-2006. Int J Cancer. 2014;135(9):2146–56.
25. Shirley MH, Sayeed S, Barnes I, et al. Incidence of haematological malignancies by ethnic group in England, 2001-7. Br J Haematol. 2013;163(4):465–77.
26. Mbulaiteye SM, Anderson WF, Bhatia K, et al. Trimodal age-specific incidence patterns for Burkitt lymphoma in the United States, 1973-2005. Int J Cancer. 2010;126(7):1732–9.
27. Mbulaiteye SM, Anderson WF, Ferlay J, et al. Pediatric, elderly, and emerging adult-onset peaks in Burkitt's lymphoma incidence diagnosed in four continents, excluding Africa. Am J Hematol. 2012;87(6):573–8.
28. Iversen U, Iversen OH, Bluming AZ, et al. Cell kinetics of African cases of Burkitt lymphoma. A preliminary report. Eur J Cancer. 1972;8(3):305–8.
29. Sant M, Minicozzi P, Mounier M, et al. Survival for haematological malignancies in Europe between 1997 and 2008 by region and age: results of EUROCARE-5, a population-based study. Lancet Oncol. 2014;15(9):931–42.
30. Sehn LH, Donaldson J, Chhanabhai M, et al. Introduction of combined CHOP plus rituximab therapy dramatically improved outcome of diffuse large B-cell lymphoma in British Columbia. J Clin Oncol. 2005;23(22):5027–33.
31. Flowers CR, Fedewa SA, Chen AY, et al. Disparities in the early adoption of chemoimmunotherapy for diffuse large B-cell lymphoma in the United States. Cancer Epidemiol Biomark Prev. 2012;21(9):1520–30.
32. Boyle P. Relative value of incidence and mortality data in cancer research. Recent Results Cancer Res. 1989;114(4):41–63.
33. Measurement of progress against cancer. Extramural Committee to Assess Measures of Progress Against Cancer. J Natl Cancer Inst. 1990;82(10):825–35.
34. Clarke CA, Glaser SL. Changing incidence of non-Hodgkin lymphomas in the United States. Cancer. 2002;94(7):2015–23.
35. Bosetti C, Levi F, Ferlay J, et al. Incidence and mortality from non-Hodgkin lymphoma in Europe: the end of an epidemic? Int J Cancer. 2008;123(8):1917–23.
36. Howlader N, Morton LM, Feuer EJ, et al. Contributions of subtypes of non-Hodgkin lymphoma to mortality trends. Cancer Epidemiol Biomark Prev. 2016;25(1):174–9.
37. Maurer MJ, Ghesquieres H, Jais JP, et al. Event-free survival at 24 months is a robust end point for disease-related outcome in diffuse large B-cell lymphoma treated with immunochemotherapy. J Clin Oncol. 2014;32(10):1066–73.
38. Jakobsen LH, Bogsted M, Brown PN, et al. Minimal loss of lifetime for patients with diffuse large B-cell lymphoma in remission and event free 24 months after treatment: a Danish population-based study. J Clin Oncol. 2017;35(7):778–84.
39. Maurer MJ, Jais JP, Ghesquieres H, et al. Personalized risk prediction for event-free survival at 24 months in patients with diffuse large B-cell lymphoma. Am J Hematol. 2016;91(2):179–84.
40. Thompson CA, Ghesquieres H, Maurer MJ, et al. Utility of routine post-therapy surveillance scans in diffuse large B-cell lymphoma. J Clin Oncol. 2014;32(31):3506–12.
41. Novak AJ, Asmann YW, Maurer MJ, et al. Whole-exome analysis reveals novel somatic genomic alterations associated with outcome in immunochemotherapy-treated diffuse large B-cell lymphoma. Blood Cancer J. 2015;5:e346.
42. Maurer MJ, Ellin F, Srour L, et al. An international assessment of event-free survival at 24 months (EFS24) and subsequent survival in peripheral T-cell lymphoma. J Clin Oncol. 2017;35(36):4019–26.
43. Bassig BA, Lan Q, Rothman N, et al. Current understanding of lifestyle and environmental factors and risk of non-hodgkin lymphoma: an epidemiological update. J Cancer Epidemiol. 2012;2012:978930.
44. Boffetta P. I. Epidemiology of adult non-Hodgkin lymphoma. Ann Oncol. 2011;22(4):iv27–31.
45. Cerhan JR, Vajdic CM, Spinelli JJ. Non-Hodgkin lymphoma. In: Schottenfeld D, Fraumeni JF, editors. Cancer epidemiology and prevention. New York: Oxford University Press; 2017. in press.
46. Boffetta P, Armstrong B, Linet M, et al. Consortia in cancer epidemiology: lessons from InterLymph. Cancer Epidemiol Biomark Prev. 2007;16(2):197–9.
47. Blettner M, Sauerbrei W, Schlehofer B, et al. Traditional reviews, meta-analyses and pooled analyses in epidemiology. Int J Epidemiol. 1999;28(1):1–9.
48. Weisenburger DD. Pathological classification of non-Hodgkin's lymphoma for epidemiological studies. Cancer Res. 1992;52(Suppl 19):5456s–62s; discussion 5462s–5464s.
49. Harris NL, Jaffe ES, Stein H, et al. A revised European-American classification of lymphoid neoplasms: a proposal from the International Lymphoma Study Group. Blood. 1994;84(5):1361–92.
50. Morton LM, Sampson JN, Cerhan JR, et al. Rationale and design of the International Lymphoma Epidemiology Consortium (InterLymph) non-Hodgkin Lymphoma Subtypes Project. J Natl Cancer Inst Monogr. 2014;2014(48):1–14.
51. Cerhan JR, Kricker A, Paltiel O, et al. Medical history, lifestyle, family history, and occupational risk factors for diffuse large B-cell lymphoma: the InterLymph Non-Hodgkin Lymphoma Subtypes Project. J Natl Cancer Inst Monogr. 2014;2014(48):15–25.
52. Fallah M, Kharazmi E, Pukkala E, et al. Familial risk of non-Hodgkin lymphoma by sex, relationship, age

at diagnosis and histology: a joint study from five Nordic countries. Leukemia. 2016;30(2):373–8.
53. Goldin LR, Bjorkholm M, Kristinsson SY, et al. Highly increased familial risks for specific lymphoma subtypes. Br J Haematol. 2009;146(1):91–4.
54. Goldin LR, Bjorkholm M, Kristinsson SY, et al. Elevated risk of chronic lymphocytic leukemia and other indolent non-Hodgkin's lymphomas among relatives of patients with chronic lymphocytic leukemia. Haematologica. 2009;94(5): 647–53.
55. Cerhan JR, Slager SL. Familial predisposition and genetic risk factors for lymphoma. Blood. 2015;126:2265–73.
56. Skibola CF, Curry JD, Nieters A. Genetic susceptibility to lymphoma. Haematologica. 2007;92(7):960–9.
57. Cerhan JR. Host genetics in follicular lymphoma. Best Pract Res Clin Haematol. 2011;24(2): 121–34.
58. Slager SL, Caporaso NE, de Sanjose S, et al. Genetic susceptibility to chronic lymphocytic leukemia. Semin Hematol. 2013;50(4):296–302.
59. Sud A, Hemminki K, Houlston RS. Candidate gene association studies and risk of Hodgkin lymphoma: a systematic review and meta-analysis. Hematol Oncol. 2017;35(1):34–50.
60. Kushekhar K, van den Berg A, Nolte I, et al. Genetic associations in classical hodgkin lymphoma: a systematic review and insights into susceptibility mechanisms. Cancer Epidemiol Biomark Prev. 2014;23(12):2737–47.
61. McAulay KA, Jarrett RF. Human leukocyte antigens and genetic susceptibility to lymphoma. Tissue Antigens. 2015;86(2):98–113.
62. Skibola CF, Bracci PM, Nieters A, et al. Tumor necrosis factor (TNF) and lymphotoxin-alpha (LTA) polymorphisms and risk of non-Hodgkin lymphoma in the InterLymph Consortium. Am J Epidemiol. 2010;171(3):267–76.
63. Rothman N, Skibola CF, Wang SS, et al. Genetic variation in TNF and IL10 and risk of non-Hodgkin lymphoma: a report from the InterLymph Consortium. Lancet Oncol. 2006;7(1):27–38.
64. Cerhan JR, Berndt SI, Vijai J, et al. Genome-wide association study identifies multiple susceptibility loci for diffuse large B cell lymphoma. Nat Genet. 2014;46(11):1233–8.
65. Bassig BA, Cerhan JR, Au W-Y, et al. Genetic susceptibility to diffuse large B-cell lymphoma in a pooled study of three Eastern Asian populations. Eur J Haematol. 2015;95(5):442–8.
66. Tan DE, Foo JN, Bei JX, et al. Genome-wide association study of B cell non-Hodgkin lymphoma identifies 3q27 as a susceptibility locus in the Chinese population. Nat Genet. 2013;45(7):804–7.
67. Hosnijeh FS, Portengen L, Spath F, et al. Soluble B-cell activation marker of sCD27 and sCD30 and future risk of B-cell lymphomas: a nested case-control study and meta-analyses. Int J Cancer. 2016;138(10):2357–67.
68. De Roos AJ, Mirick DK, Edlefsen KL, et al. Markers of B-cell activation in relation to risk of non-Hodgkin lymphoma. Cancer Res. 2012;72(18):4733–43.
69. Purdue MP, Lan Q, Kemp TJ, et al. Elevated serum sCD23 and sCD30 up to two decades prior to diagnosis associated with increased risk of non-Hodgkin lymphoma. Leukemia. 2015;29(6):1429–31.
70. Purdue MP, Hofmann JN, Kemp TJ, et al. A prospective study of 67 serum immune and inflammation markers and risk of non-Hodgkin lymphoma. Blood. 2013;122(6):951–7.
71. Centers for Disease Control (CDC). Revision of the CDC surveillance case definition for acquired immunodeficiency syndrome. Council of State and Territorial Epidemiologists; AIDS Program, Center for Infectious Diseases. MMWR Suppl. 1987;36(1):1S–15S.
72. Gibson TM, Morton LM, Shiels MS, et al. Risk of non-Hodgkin lymphoma subtypes in HIV-infected people during the HAART era: a population-based study. AIDS. 2014;28(15):2313–8.
73. van Leeuwen MT, Vajdic CM, Middleton MG, et al. Continuing declines in some but not all HIV-associated cancers in Australia after widespread use of antiretroviral therapy. AIDS. 2009;23(16):2183–90.
74. Simard EP, Pfeiffer RM, Engels EA. Spectrum of cancer risk late after AIDS onset in the United States. Arch Intern Med. 2010;170(15):1337–45.
75. Bouvard V, Baan R, Straif K, et al. A review of human carcinogens—part B: biological agents. Lancet Oncol. 2009;10(4):321–2.
76. Pinzone MR, Berretta M, Cacopardo B, et al. Epstein-barr virus- and Kaposi sarcoma-associated herpesvirus-related malignancies in the setting of human immunodeficiency virus infection. Semin Oncol. 2015;42(2):258–71.
77. de Sanjose S, Benavente Y, Vajdic CM, et al. Hepatitis C and non-Hodgkin lymphoma among 4784 cases and 6269 controls from the International Lymphoma Epidemiology Consortium. Clin Gastroenterol Hepatol. 2008;6(4):451–8.
78. Anderson LA, Pfeiffer R, Warren JL, et al. Hematopoietic malignancies associated with viral and alcoholic hepatitis. Cancer Epidemiol Biomark Prev. 2008;17(11):3069–75.
79. Dalia S, Chavez J, Castillo JJ, et al. Hepatitis B infection increases the risk of non-Hodgkin lymphoma: a meta-analysis of observational studies. Leuk Res. 2013;37(9):1107–15.
80. Stapleton JT, Xiang J, McLinden JH, et al. A novel T cell evasion mechanism in persistent RNA virus infection. Trans Am Clin Climatol Assoc. 2014;125:14–24; discussion 24–6.
81. Krajden M, Yu A, Braybrook H, et al. GBV-C/hepatitis G virus infection and non-Hodgkin lymphoma: a case control study. Int J Cancer. 2010;126(12):2885–92.
82. Chang CM, Stapleton JT, Klinzman D, et al. GBV-C infection and risk of NHL among U.S. adults. Cancer Res. 2014;74(19):5553–60.

83. Clarke CA, Morton LM, Lynch C, et al. Risk of lymphoma subtypes after solid organ transplantation in the United States. Br J Cancer. 2013;109(1):280–8.
84. Vajdic CM, van Leeuwen MT, Turner JJ, et al. No excess risk of follicular lymphoma in kidney transplant and HIV-related immunodeficiency. Int J Cancer. 2010;127(11):2732–5.
85. Quinlan SC, Morton LM, Pfeiffer RM, et al. Increased risk for lymphoid and myeloid neoplasms in elderly solid-organ transplant recipients. Cancer Epidemiol Biomark Prev. 2010;19(5):1229–37.
86. van Leeuwen MT, Grulich AE, Webster AC, et al. Immunosuppression and other risk factors for early and late non-Hodgkin lymphoma after kidney transplantation. Blood. 2009;114(3):630–7.
87. Quinlan SC, Pfeiffer RM, Morton LM, et al. Risk factors for early-onset and late-onset post-transplant lymphoproliferative disorder in kidney recipients in the United States. Am J Hematol. 2011;86(2):206–9.
88. Castillo JJ, Dalia S, Pascual SK. Association between red blood cell transfusions and development of non-Hodgkin lymphoma: a meta-analysis of observational studies. Blood. 2010;116(16):2897–907.
89. Ekstrom Smedby K, Vajdic CM, Falster M, et al. Autoimmune disorders and risk of non-Hodgkin lymphoma subtypes: a pooled analysis within the InterLymph Consortium. Blood. 2008;111(8):4029–38.
90. Apor E, O'Brien J, Stephen M, et al. Systemic lupus erythematosus is associated with increased incidence of hematologic malignancies: a meta-analysis of prospective cohort studies. Leuk Res. 2014;38(9):1067–71.
91. Theander E, Henriksson G, Ljungberg O, et al. Lymphoma and other malignancies in primary Sjogren's syndrome: a cohort study on cancer incidence and lymphoma predictors. Ann Rheum Dis. 2006;65(6):796–803.
92. Anderson LA, Gadalla S, Morton LM, et al. Population-based study of autoimmune conditions and the risk of specific lymphoid malignancies. Int J Cancer. 2009;125(2):398–405.
93. Tio M, Cox MR, Eslick GD. Meta-analysis: coeliac disease and the risk of all-cause mortality, any malignancy and lymphoid malignancy. Aliment Pharmacol Ther. 2012;35(5):540–51.
94. Baecklund E, Smedby KE, Sutton LA, et al. Lymphoma development in patients with autoimmune and inflammatory disorders—what are the driving forces? Semin Cancer Biol. 2014;24:61–70.
95. Erber E, Lim U, Maskarinec G, et al. Common immune-related risk factors and incident non-Hodgkin lymphoma: the multiethnic cohort. Int J Cancer. 2009;125(6):1440–5.
96. Musolino C, Allegra A, Minciullo PL, et al. Allergy and risk of hematologic malignancies: associations and mechanisms. Leuk Res. 2014;38(10):1137–44.
97. Castillo JJ, Mull N, Reagan JL, et al. Increased incidence of non-Hodgkin lymphoma, leukemia, and myeloma in patients with diabetes mellitus type 2: a meta-analysis of observational studies. Blood. 2012;119(21):4845–50.
98. Kane EV, Roman E, Becker N, et al. Menstrual and reproductive factors, and hormonal contraception use: associations with non-Hodgkin lymphoma in a pooled analysis of InterLymph case-control studies. Ann Oncol. 2012;23(9):2362–74.
99. Kane EV, Bernstein L, Bracci PM, et al. Postmenopausal hormone therapy and non-Hodgkin lymphoma: a pooled analysis of InterLymph case-control studies. Ann Oncol. 2013;24(2):433–41.
100. Cerhan JR, Vachon CM, Habermann TM, et al. Hormone replacement therapy and risk of non-Hodgkin lymphoma and chronic lymphocytic leukemia. Cancer Epidemiol Biomark Prev. 2002;11:1466–71.
101. Lu Y, Wang SS, Sullivan-Halley J, et al. Oral contraceptives, menopausal hormone therapy use and risk of B-cell non-Hodgkin lymphoma in the California Teachers Study. Int J Cancer. 2011;129(4):974–82.
102. Morton LM, Wang SS, Richesson DA, et al. Reproductive factors, exogenous hormone use and risk of lymphoid neoplasms among women in the National Institutes of Health-AARP Diet and Health Study Cohort. Int J Cancer. 2009;124(11):2737–43.
103. Kato I, Chlebowski RT, Hou L, et al. Menopausal estrogen therapy and non-Hodgkin's lymphoma: a post-hoc analysis of women's health initiative randomized clinical trial. Int J Cancer. 2016;138(3):604–11.
104. t Mannetje A, De Roos AJ, Boffetta P, et al. Occupation and risk of non-Hodgkin lymphoma and its subtypes: a pooled analysis from the InterLymph consortium. Environ Health Perspect. 2016;124(4):396–405.
105. Schinasi L, Leon ME. Non-Hodgkin lymphoma and occupational exposure to agricultural pesticide chemical groups and active ingredients: a systematic review and meta-analysis. Int J Environ Res Public Health. 2014;11(4):4449–527.
106. Alavanja MC, Hofmann JN, Lynch CF, et al. Non-hodgkin lymphoma risk and insecticide, fungicide and fumigant use in the agricultural health study. PLoS One. 2014;9(10):e109332.
107. Goodman JE, Loftus CT, Zu K. 2,4-Dichlorophenoxyacetic acid and non-Hodgkin's lymphoma: results from the Agricultural Health Study and an updated meta-analysis. Ann Epidemiol. 2017;27(4):290–292 e5.
108. Zhang Y, Sanjose SD, Bracci PM, et al. Personal use of hair dye and the risk of certain subtypes of non-Hodgkin lymphoma. Am J Epidemiol. 2008;167(11):1321–31.
109. Larsson SC, Wolk A. Body mass index and risk of non-Hodgkin's and Hodgkin's lymphoma: a meta-analysis of prospective studies. Eur J Cancer. 2011;47(16):2422–30.
110. Castillo JJ, Ingham RR, Reagan JL, et al. Obesity is associated with increased relative risk of diffuse large B-cell lymphoma: a meta-analysis of

observational studies. Clin Lymphoma Myeloma Leuk. 2014;14(2):122–30.
111. Cerhan JR, Janney CA, Vachon CM, et al. Anthropometric characteristics, physical activity, and risk of non-Hodgkin's lymphoma subtypes and B-cell chronic lymphocytic leukemia: a prospective study. Am J Epidemiol. 2002;156(6):527–35.
112. Bertrand KA, Giovannucci E, Zhang SM, et al. A prospective analysis of body size during childhood, adolescence, and adulthood and risk of non-Hodgkin lymphoma. Cancer Prev Res (Phila). 2013;6(8):864–73.
113. Pylypchuk RD, Schouten LJ, Goldbohm RA, et al. Body mass index, height, and risk of lymphatic malignancies: a prospective cohort study. Am J Epidemiol. 2009;170(3):297–307.
114. Yang TO, Cairns BJ, Kroll ME, et al. Body size in early life and risk of lymphoid malignancies and histological subtypes in adulthood. Int J Cancer. 2016;139(1):42–9.
115. Roberts DL, Dive C, Renehan AG. Biological mechanisms linking obesity and cancer risk: new perspectives. Annu Rev Med. 2010;61:301–16.
116. Jochem C, Leitzmann MF, Keimling M, et al. Physical activity in relation to risk of hematologic cancers: a systematic review and meta-analysis. Cancer Epidemiol Biomark Prev. 2014;23(5):833–46.
117. Teras LR, Gapstur SM, Diver WR, et al. Recreational physical activity, leisure sitting time and risk of non-Hodgkin lymphoid neoplasms in the American Cancer Society Cancer Prevention Study II Cohort. Int J Cancer. 2012;131(8):1912–20.
118. Castillo JJ, Dalia S. Cigarette smoking is associated with a small increase in the incidence of non-Hodgkin lymphoma: a meta-analysis of 24 observational studies. Leuk Lymphoma. 2012;53(10):1911–9.
119. Sergentanis TN, Kanavidis P, Michelakos T, et al. Cigarette smoking and risk of lymphoma in adults: a comprehensive meta-analysis on Hodgkin and non-Hodgkin disease. Eur J Cancer Prev. 2013;22(2):131–50.
120. Morton LM, Hartge P, Holford TR, et al. Cigarette smoking and risk of non-Hodgkin lymphoma: a pooled analysis from the International Lymphoma Epidemiology Consortium (interlymph). Cancer Epidemiol Biomark Prev. 2005;14(4):925–33.
121. Schiff D, Suman VJ, Yang P, et al. Risk factors for primary central nervous system lymphoma: a case-control study. Cancer. 1998;82(5):975–82.
122. Tramacere I, Pelucchi C, Bonifazi M, et al. Alcohol drinking and non-Hodgkin lymphoma risk: a systematic review and a meta-analysis. Ann Oncol. 2012;23(11):2791–8.
123. Romeo J, Warnberg J, Nova E, et al. Moderate alcohol consumption and the immune system: a review. Br J Nutr. 2007;98(Suppl 1):S111–5.
124. Hagner PR, Mazan-Mamczarz K, Dai B, et al. Alcohol consumption and decreased risk of non-Hodgkin lymphoma: role of mTOR dysfunction. Blood. 2009;113(22):5526–35.
125. Cross AJ, Lim U. The role of dietary factors in the epidemiology of non-Hodgkin's lymphoma. Leuk Lymphoma. 2006;47(12):2477–87.
126. World Cancer Research Fund and American Institute for Cancer Research. Food, nutrition, physical activity, and the prevention of cancer: a global perspective. Washington, DC: AICR; 2007.
127. Chen GC, Lv DB, Pang Z, et al. Fruits and vegetables consumption and risk of non-Hodgkin's lymphoma: a meta-analysis of observational studies. Int J Cancer. 2013;133(1):190–200.
128. Chang ET, Canchola AJ, Clarke CA, et al. Dietary phytocompounds and risk of lymphoid malignancies in the California Teachers Study cohort. Cancer Causes Control. 2011;22(2):237–49.
129. Holtan SG, O'Connor HM, Fredericksen ZS, et al. Food-frequency questionnaire-based estimates of total antioxidant capacity and risk of non-Hodgkin lymphoma. Int J Cancer. 2012;131(5):1158–68.
130. Kabat GC, Kim MY, Wactawski-Wende J, et al. Intake of antioxidant nutrients and risk of non-Hodgkin's Lymphoma in the Women's Health Initiative. Nutr Cancer. 2012;64(2):245–54.
131. Ollberding NJ, Maskarinec G, Conroy SM, et al. Prediagnostic circulating carotenoid levels and the risk of non-Hodgkin lymphoma: the Multiethnic Cohort. Blood. 2012;119(24):5817–23.
132. Morimoto Y, Ollberding NJ, Cooney RV, et al. Prediagnostic serum tocopherol levels and the risk of non-hodgkin lymphoma: the multiethnic cohort. Cancer Epidemiol Biomark Prev. 2013;22(11):2075–83.
133. Kricker A, Armstrong BK, Hughes AM, et al. Personal sun exposure and risk of non Hodgkin lymphoma: a pooled analysis from the Interlymph Consortium. Int J Cancer. 2008;122(1):144–54.
134. Chang ET, Canchola AJ, Cockburn M, et al. Adulthood residential ultraviolet radiation, sun sensitivity, dietary vitamin D, and risk of lymphoid malignancies in the California Teachers Study. Blood. 2011;118(6):1591–9.
135. Bertrand KA, Chang ET, Abel GA, et al. Sunlight exposure, vitamin D, and risk of non-Hodgkin lymphoma in the Nurses' Health Study. Cancer Causes Control. 2011;22(12):1731–41.
136. van Leeuwen MT, Turner JJ, Falster MO, et al. Latitude gradients for lymphoid neoplasm subtypes in Australia support an association with ultraviolet radiation exposure. Int J Cancer. 2013;133(4):944–51.
137. Cahoon EK, Pfeiffer RM, Wheeler DC, et al. Relationship between ambient ultraviolet radiation and non-Hodgkin lymphoma subtypes: a U.S. population-based study of racial and ethnic groups. Int J Cancer. 2015;136(5):E432–41.
138. Lu D, Chen J, Jin J. Vitamin D status and risk of non-Hodgkin lymphoma: a meta-analysis. Cancer Causes Control. 2014;25(11):1553–63.
139. Purdue MP, Freedman DM, Gapstur SM, et al. Circulating 25-hydroxyvitamin D and risk of

non-hodgkin lymphoma: cohort consortium vitamin D pooling project of rarer cancers. Am J Epidemiol. 2010;172(1):58–69.
140. Leoncini L, Raphael M, Stein H, et al. Burkitt lymphoma. In: Swerdlow SH, Campo E, Harris NL, et al., editors. WHO classification of tumours of the haematopoietic and lymphoid tissues. Lyon: IARC; 2008. p. 262–4.
141. Morrow RH Jr. Epidemiological evidence for the role of falciparum malaria in the pathogenesis of Burkitt's lymphoma. IARC Sci Publ. 1985;60: 177–86.
142. Rainey JJ, Mwanda WO, Wairiumu P, et al. Spatial distribution of Burkitt's lymphoma in Kenya and association with malaria risk. Tropical Med Int Health. 2007;12(8):936–43.
143. Doll DC, List AF. Burkitt's lymphoma in a homosexual. Lancet. 1982;1(8279):1026–7.
144. Ziegler JL, Drew WL, Miner RC, et al. Outbreak of Burkitt's-like lymphoma in homosexual men. Lancet. 1982;2(8299):631–3.
145. Epeldegui M, Breen EC, Hung YP, et al. Elevated expression of activation induced cytidine deaminase in peripheral blood mononuclear cells precedes AIDS-NHL diagnosis. AIDS. 2007;21(17): 2265–70.
146. Carbone A, Cesarman E, Spina M, et al. HIV-associated lymphomas and gamma-herpesviruses. Blood. 2009;113(6):1213–24.
147. Mbulaiteye SM, Morton LM, Sampson JN, et al. Medical history, lifestyle, family history, and occupational risk factors for sporadic Burkitt lymphoma/leukemia: the Interlymph Non-Hodgkin Lymphoma Subtypes Project. J Natl Cancer Inst Monogr. 2014;2014(48):106–14.
148. Morton LM, Slager SL, Cerhan JR, et al. Etiologic heterogeneity among non-Hodgkin lymphoma subtypes: the InterLymph non-Hodgkin lymphoma subtypes project. J Natl Cancer Inst Monogr. 2014;2014(48):130–44.
149. Amin J, Dore GJ, O'Connell DL, et al. Cancer incidence in people with hepatitis B or C infection: a large community-based linkage study. J Hepatol. 2006;45(2):197–203.
150. Wang SS, Flowers CR, Kadin ME, et al. Medical history, lifestyle, family history, and occupational risk factors for peripheral T-cell lymphomas: the InterLymph non-Hodgkin lymphoma subtypes project. J Natl Cancer Inst Monogr. 2014;2014(48):66–75.
151. Li Z, Xia Y, Feng LN, et al. Genetic risk of extranodal natural killer T-cell lymphoma: a genome-wide association study. Lancet Oncol. 2016;17(9): 1240–7.
152. Biggar RJ, Engels EA, Frisch M, et al. Risk of T-cell lymphomas in persons with AIDS. J Acquir Immune Defic Syndr. 2001;26(4):371–6.
153. Becker N, Falster MO, Vajdic CM, et al. Self-reported history of infections and the risk of non-Hodgkin lymphoma: an InterLymph pooled analysis. Int J Cancer. 2012;131(10):2342–8.
154. Kotlyar DS, Lewis JD, Beaugerie L, et al. Risk of lymphoma in patients with inflammatory bowel disease treated with azathioprine and 6-mercaptopurine: a meta-analysis. Clin Gastroenterol Hepatol. 2015;13(5):847–58.e4; quiz e48–50.
155. Deepak P, Sifuentes H, Sherid M, et al. T-cell non-Hodgkin's lymphomas reported to the FDA AERS with tumor necrosis factor-alpha (TNF-alpha) inhibitors: results of the REFURBISH study. Am J Gastroenterol. 2013;108(1):99–105.
156. Jagannathan-Bogdan M, McDonnell ME, Shin H, et al. Elevated proinflammatory cytokine production by a skewed T cell compartment requires monocytes and promotes inflammation in type 2 diabetes. J Immunol. 2011;186(2):1162–72.
157. Keech JA Jr, Creech BJ. Anaplastic T-cell lymphoma in proximity to a saline-filled breast implant. Plast Reconstr Surg. 1997;100(2):554–5.
158. de Jong D, Vasmel WL, de Boer JP, et al. Anaplastic large-cell lymphoma in women with breast implants. JAMA. 2008;300(17):2030–5.
159. Wang SS, Deapen D, Voutsinas J, et al. Breast implants and anaplastic large cell lymphomas among females in the California Teachers Study cohort. Br J Haematol. 2016;174(3):480–3.
160. Kim B, Roth C, Chung KC, et al. Anaplastic large cell lymphoma and breast implants: a systematic review. Plast Reconstr Surg. 2011;127(6):2141–50.
161. Aschebrook-Kilfoy B, Cocco P, La Vecchia C, et al. Medical history, lifestyle, family history, and occupational risk factors for mycosis fungoides and Sezary syndrome: the InterLymph non-Hodgkin lymphoma subtypes project. J Natl Cancer Inst Monogr. 2014;2014(48):98–105.
162. Bhattacharjee S, Rajaraman P, Jacobs KB, et al. A subset-based approach improves power and interpretation for the combined analysis of genetic association studies of heterogeneous traits. Am J Hum Genet. 2012;90(5):821–35.
163. Higgins JP, Thompson SG. Quantifying heterogeneity in a meta-analysis. Stat Med. 2002;21(11): 1539–58.
164. Engels EA, Parsons R, Besson C, et al. Comprehensive evaluation of medical conditions associated with risk of non-Hodgkin lymphoma using Medicare claims ("MedWAS"). Cancer Epidemiol Biomark Prev. 2016;25(7):1105–13.

Pathology and Molecular Pathogenesis of DLBCL and Related Entities

2

Laura Pasqualucci and German Ott

2.1 Introduction

Diffuse large B-cell lymphoma (DLBCL) represents a heterogeneous group of aggressive lymphoid neoplasms that originate, in most cases, from the malignant transformation of B cells within the germinal center (GC) and feature distinct genetic, phenotypic, and clinical behavior. The 2017 update of the fourth edition of the WHO classification of lymphoid, histiocytic, and dendritic cell neoplasms reflects this heterogeneity by recognizing over ten large B-cell lymphoma entities, including, among others, the most common DLBCL not otherwise specified (NOS), primary mediastinal large B-cell lymphoma (PMBCL), intravascular large B-cell lymphoma, and a few new categories or provisional entities (Table 2.1) [1, 2]. Of importance, the revised classification requires the distinction of DLBCL-NOS into two "cell-of-origin" molecular subtypes, i.e., germinal center B-cell-like (GCB) and activated B-cell-like (ABC) DLBCL, incorporating the notion that these tumors are addicted to distinct oncogenic pathways and differ in clinical outcome. Moreover, a separate category has been introduced for DLBCL harboring chromosomal translocations of both *MYC* and *BCL2* and/or *BCL6* (the so-called double-hit or triple-hit lymphomas).

Table 2.1 Lymphomas of large B cells in the updated WHO classification

DLBCL, NOS
T-cell/histiocyte-rich large B-cell lymphoma
Intravascular large B-cell lymphoma
Plasmablastic lymphoma
ALK-positive large B-cell lymphoma
EBV-positive DLBCL, NOS
HHV8-positive DLBCL
Primary DLBCL of the CNS
Primary cutaneous DLBCL, leg type
Large B-cell lymphoma with *IRF4* rearrangements
Primary mediastinal (thymic) large B-cell lymphoma
DLBCL associated with chronic inflammation
Primary effusion lymphoma
High-grade B-cell lymphoma
– *High-grade B-cell lymphoma, with MYC and BCL2 and/or BCL6 rearrangements*
– *High-grade B-cell lymphoma, NOS*
B-cell lymphoma, unclassifiable, with features intermediate between DLBCL and classical Hodgkin lymphoma

From a genetic standpoint, fundamental new insights have been gained over the past decade, particularly regarding the mutational landscape of DLBCL-NOS and PMBCL. These studies led to the identification of multiple genes and pathways that are recurrently disrupted by genetic

L. Pasqualucci (✉)
Institute for Cancer Genetics, Columbia University, New York, NY, USA
e-mail: lp171@columbia.edu

G. Ott
Department of Clinical Pathology, Robert-Bosch-Krankenhaus, Stuttgart, Germany
e-mail: german.ott@rbk.de

G. Lenz, G. Salles (eds.), *Aggressive Lymphomas*, Hematologic Malignancies,
https://doi.org/10.1007/978-3-030-00362-3_2

lesions in these tumors and likely play significant roles in their pathogenesis. Of note, a number of the affected genes represent potentially actionable targets that could be exploited for precision medicine approaches.

This chapter will cover the pathology and genetics of DLBCL and related entities, according to the definition of the updated 2017 WHO classification, with special emphasis on the most common and molecularly better characterized DLBCL-NOS and PMBCL.

2.2 Diffuse Large B-Cell Lymphoma, NOS

DLBCL not otherwise specified (NOS) constitutes the most common type of B-cell lymphoma in adults, accounting for approximately 30% of all diagnoses, and includes cases that cannot be assigned to any other specific subtype or disease entity. Morphologically, these tumors consist of large lymphoid cells with basophilic cytoplasm and vesicular nuclei that are at least twice the size of normal lymphocytes and exhibit a diffuse growth pattern in the large majority of cases. DLBCLs are mainly nodal lymphomas, although roughly 40% of cases are considered primary extranodal in origin [3]. Among them, the most common extranodal site is the gastrointestinal tract; however, DLBCL can involve virtually every lymphoid and nonlymphoid organ, including the Waldeyer's ring, spleen, bones, gonads, thyroid, liver, and kidneys. DLBCL cases localized to some of these sites are considered separate entities, as it is the case for primary DLBCL of the central nervous system (PCNSL) and primary mediastinal (thymic) large B-cell lymphoma (PMBCL). Leukemic spread is rare in DLBCL.

The etiology of DLBCL remains largely unknown; however, a few specific risk factors have been recognized, such as immunodeficiency and chronic inflammation. In particular, DLBCL NOS arising in the setting of immunodeficiency is associated with infection by the Epstein-Barr virus (EBV) in a large number of cases, a finding that is relatively uncommon in sporadic DLBCL. While most DLBCL cases arise de novo, they can also be seen in the setting of transformation from preexisting low-grade lymphoid tumors, including chronic lymphocytic leukemia (so-called Richter's syndrome) and follicular lymphoma.

Patients with DLBCL can be asymptomatic or present with systemic symptoms such as fatigue, fever, and night sweats. Often, a rapidly growing mass is found at the site of involvement, and after appropriate clinical staging, only 25–30% of patients show localized (stage I or II) disease. In many cases, specific symptoms are related to the site of origin and/or the site of the predominantly manifesting tumor mass [4].

2.2.1 Pathology

In *lymph nodes*, tumor infiltrates may totally efface the underlying architecture of the parenchyma, while partial infiltration is found more rarely. The perinodal soft tissues are often affected as well. In *extranodal* localizations, the pattern of infiltration is generally related to the specific site involved, e.g., a diffuse infiltration of the lung parenchyma by PMBCL or the confinement of the infiltrate to the luminal parts of the bowel wall in primary intestinal lymphoma. Common morphological variants of DLBCL include the centroblastic, immunoblastic, and anaplastic variants (Fig. 2.1). Of these, the most common one is represented by *centroblastic* DLBCL, which consists of medium- to large-sized cells with scant to slightly basophilic cytoplasm, an open vesicular chromatin structure, and several small membrane-bound nucleoli (Fig. 2.1a). This classical tumor cell type (referred to as the monomorphic variant) may be admixed with immunoblasts (the so-called polymorphic variant of DLBCL-centroblastic), and nuclei with a conspicuously multilobated shape may be observed. Roughly 60–70% of centroblastic-type DLBCL cases show a germinal center B-cell-like gene expression profile (GEP) (see next paragraph). *Immunoblastic* DLBCLs are composed of large cells with broad basophilic cytoplasm and large vesicular nuclei showing a single central nucleolus (Fig. 2.1b).

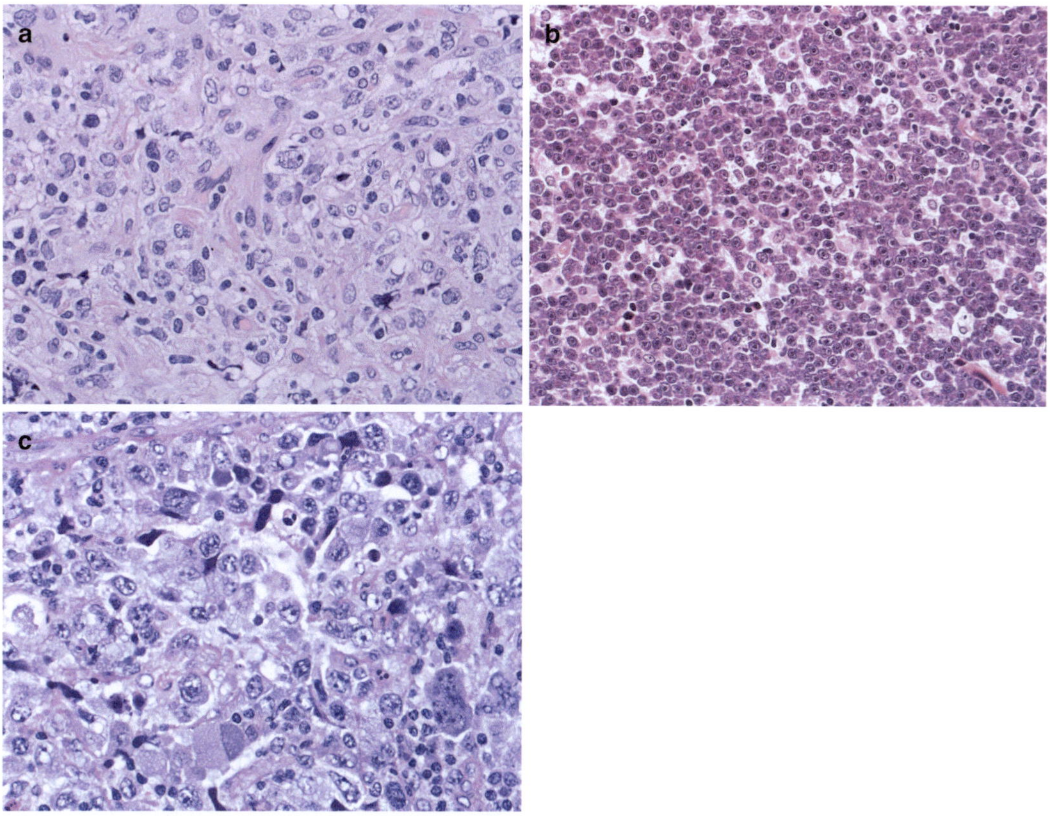

Fig. 2.1 Morphological variants of DLBCL, NOS. (**a**) Centroblastic variant of DLBCL, characterized by medium-sized to large cells with a narrow, slightly basophilic cytoplasm and round to oval, or lobulated, nuclei with vesicular chromatin and several membrane-bound nucleoli. (**b**) Immunoblastic lymphoma, displaying a broader, basophilic cytoplasm and round nuclei with loose chromatin and a single, prominent nucleolus. (**c**) Anaplastic variant of DLBCL, characterized by large and at times very pleomorphic cells with large, irregular nuclei and bizarre or multinucleated giant cells

In this variant, partial plasmablastic differentiation may be observed, and most cases show an activated B-cell-like GEP [5]. The *anaplastic* DLBCL variant is characterized by large to very large cells with equally large and pleomorphic, sometimes bizarre nuclei resembling Hodgkin or Reed-Sternberg-like cells, and a cohesive growth pattern with occasional intrasinusoidal spread (Fig. 2.1c). CD30 expression is frequently observed. In many cases, immunohistochemistry is needed in order to differentiate this variant from anaplastic large cell lymphoma of T-/null-cell linage [6–8]. Often, however, DLBCL shows a mixed composition of these cell types, and no specific variant can be diagnosed. In addition, a varying number of accompanying interspersed T cells and histiocytes can be seen in the background, reflecting different interactions of the tumor cells with the surrounding microenvironment.

2.2.2 Immunophenotype

The tumor cells of DLBCL express by definition pan B-cell markers such as CD19, CD20, or CD22. A number of other antigens may also be expressed on the membrane, in the cytoplasm, or in the nuclei of the tumor cells, including CD5 (5–10% of cases), CD10 (30%), or CD30 (10–20%). Reactivity for CD5 or CD10 does not necessarily indicate transformation from indolent lymphomas, and the vast majority of CD5- and/or CD10-positive DLBCL are de novo diagnoses.

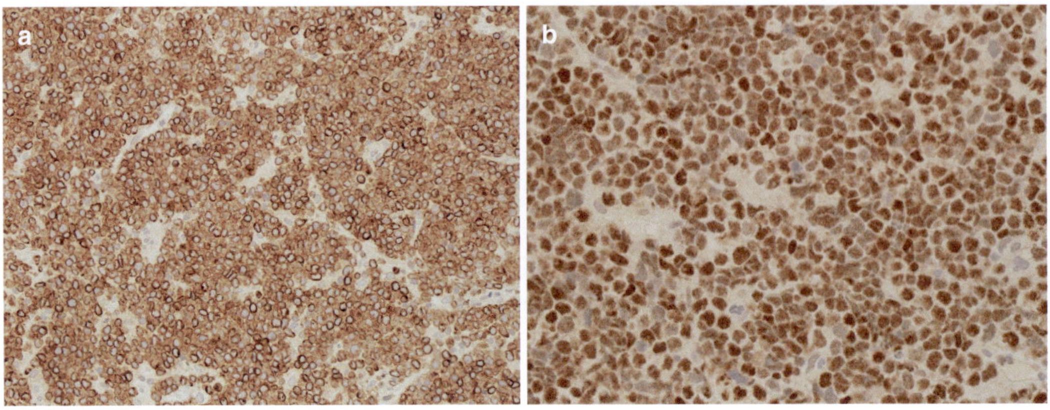

Fig. 2.2 Double expressor lymphoma. (**a**) Immunohistochemical analysis of BCL2 expression, showing positivity in the cytoplasm of virtually all tumor cells. (**b**) The vast majority of the cells also express nuclear MYC protein

Additional markers include CD38, CD138, immunoglobulin (cytoplasmic), IRF4/MUM1, the GC-associated protein BCL6, and BCL2 [2]. Apart from correctly identifying the B-cell derivation of the tumor cells and rendering predictive information on CD20 expression (the target of anti-CD20 immunotherapy), various immunohistochemical algorithms have been constructed to assign DLBCL samples to the two main molecular classes identified by GEP analysis (discussed in the next section). The Ki67 proliferation index is generally high, and nuclear reactivity is often seen in 60–90% of tumor cells.

Of particular relevance is the immunohistochemical analysis of MYC and BCL2, because the simultaneous expression of these two proteins, either due to concurrent chromosomal translocations (double-hit lymphomas, 5–8% of cases) or independently of genetic lesions (so-called double-expressor lymphomas, accounting for 20–30% of cases), has been associated with inferior prognosis, although more recent prospective studies are starting to reveal comparable overall survival [9–13]. In the WHO update, "double-hit" or "triple-hit" lymphomas are included in the new category of high-grade B-cell lymphoma (see corresponding section for a detailed description), while dual expression of BCL2 and MYC without *MYC/BCL2* chromosomal alterations is recognized as a negative prognostic indicator within DLBCL, NOS, but not as a separate category. The recommended cutoffs to define double-expressor DLBCLs are >40% for MYC expression and >50% for BCL2 expression (Fig. 2.2a, b) [1].

2.2.3 Cell of Origin and Gene Expression Profiling

The normal counterpart of DLBCL is a peripheral mature B-cell that has experienced the GC reaction, as demonstrated by the presence in these tumors of clonally rearranged, somatically hypermutated immunoglobulin genes [14]. Seminal studies utilizing genome-wide transcriptional profiling approaches allowed the identification of at least two molecular subtypes of DLBCL, NOS, with an intermediate group that remains unclassifiable [5, 15]. The *germinal center B-cell-like* (GCB) DLBCL is characterized by a gene expression pattern that is more similar to that of a light zone (LZ) B cell, possibly recirculating toward the dark zone [15, 16]. Conversely, the *activated B-cell-like* (ABC) DLBCL is characterized by the expression of genes that are typically upregulated in a subset of GC LZ B cells poised to differentiate into plasma cells [15, 16]. Besides indicating the putative cell of origin (COO) of the disease, this classification identifies tumors with fundamentally different biological and genetic features, as well as clinical outcome, with ABC-DLBCL being generally less curable [5, 17, 18]. In the upcoming area of targeted therapies [19], the COO classification is, therefore, of important predictive impact in the management of DLBCL. Moreover, some association has been reported between COO subtype and cytomorphology, site of origin, and age at diagnosis [2, 5]. Particularly, centroblastic lymphomas are more often of GCB type, whereas immunoblastic tumors more often display an ABC-like GEP [5]. The tumor cells in specific entities such as PCNSL or DLBCL of the leg are more often of the ABC-type [20]. Finally, the prevalence of ABC-type tumors appears to rise with age [21].

The distinction in ABC- and GCB-DLBCL has now been officially incorporated into the updated WHO classification and is strongly recommended in the clinical practice [1]. Because genome-wide molecular profiling is not available in all laboratories, a number of immunohistochemical algorithms have been developed over the past decades in order to predict DLBCL molecular subtype on routine formalin-fixed paraffin-embedded (FFPE) material. Among these classifiers, the most widely used is the so-called Hans algorithm [22] that utilizes expression of CD10, BCL6, and IRF4/MUM1 to distinguish GC and non-GC DLBCL. However, other algorithms have been proposed, which employ additional markers such as GCET1, FOXP1, and LMO2 [23]. While the use of immunohistochemical algorithms is considered acceptable in the revised WHO classification, two major caveats have to be kept in mind: (1) these classifiers do not—at least formally—define an "unclassified" variant; (2) lack of reproducibility in the staining pattern and intensity has been frequently observed across different laboratories and institutions [24]. Indeed, the individual immunohistochemistry-based algorithms are far from yielding identical results, even when applied on the same case series [25]. In order to overcome these limits, several low-density GEP platforms have been recently developed, which can be applied to FFPE material and provided reproducible results comparable to conventional microarray-based GEP, thus showing promise as a routine diagnostic tool [26, 27].

2.2.4 Molecular Pathogenesis

Over the past decade, the rapid expansion of next-generation sequencing technologies has significantly advanced our understanding of the molecular pathogenesis of DLBCL. These studies revealed a remarkable complexity in the DLBCL coding genome, which harbors between 30 and >100 lesions/case [28–31] and features approximately 150 candidate driver genes, as predicted in a recent study of over 500 cases [32]. Even greater complexity is expected to emerge as we start interrogating the noncoding portion of the DLBCL genome, including long noncoding RNAs, microRNAs, and promoter/enhancer elements that could be targeted by ASHM. Consistently, recent whole-genome sequencing studies uncovered clusters of mutations at enhancers, which may reflect the activity of the AID cytidine deaminase [33, 34]. While only a subset of the identified lesions has undergone detailed functional characterization to date, these studies revolutionized our knowledge of DLBCL biology, leading to the discovery of several potential targets for therapy. Here we will focus on selected genetic alterations that are more frequently observed and have been functionally dissected (Fig. 2.3).

2.2.4.1 Genetic Lesions Found in Both GCB-DLBCL and ABC-DLBCL

Histone/chromatin modifier genes. A consistent theme in recent DLBCL sequencing studies has been the discovery of recurrent mutations in genes encoding for histone/chromatin modifiers, including methyltransferases, acetyltransferases, and linker histones [28–30]. Mutations of epigenetic modifiers (particularly, *CREBBP* and *KMT2D*) were shown to represent early events that are acquired by a common ancestral clone before final clonal expansion and, in the context of FL transformation, divergent evolution to FL or tFL [35–38], suggesting that these lesions contribute to the initial phases of lymphomagenesis.

Overall, ~30% of all DLBCL samples, with some enrichment for GCB-DLBCL, carry mutations and/or deletions inactivating the

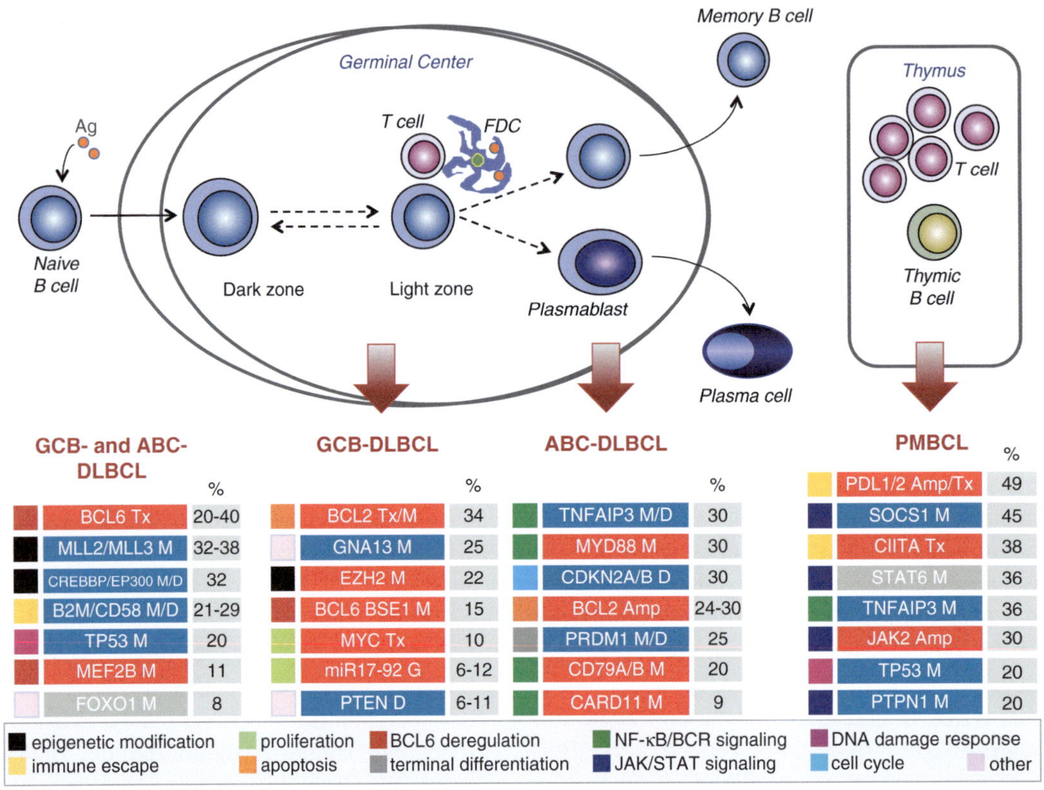

Fig. 2.3 Most common genetic lesions in DLBCL, NOS and PMBCL. Postulated cell of origin for germinal center B-cell-like (GCB) DLBCL, activated B-cell-like (ABC) DLBCL, and primary mediastinal B-cell lymphoma (PMBCL). The most common genetic alterations associated with these diseases (including those shared across different subtypes and those subtype-specific) are shown, with color codes indicating the subverted biological pathway. Blue textbox, loss-of-function; red, gain-of-function (Modified from Pasqualucci and Dalla-Favera, Semin Hematol, 2015) [18]

acetyltransferase genes *CREBBP* (25%) and *EP300 (5%)* [39]. These two highly conserved and ubiquitously expressed enzymes catalyze the addition of acetyl groups to the lysine residues of multiple histone and nonhistone proteins implicated in diverse signaling and developmental pathways [40]. Mutations include prototypical loss-of-function events that truncate the CREBBP/EP300 polypeptide, abolishing the histone acetyltransferase (HAT) domain, as well as amino acid changes that target the HAT domain, leading to diminished affinity for Acetyl-CoA and thus impaired enzymatic activity [39]. Of note, most of these events are heterozygous, and the residual wild-type allele is expressed, implicating a haploinsufficient tumor suppressor role. Indeed, reduced dosage of CREBBP/EP300 in mouse GC B cells was shown to cooperate with BCL2 deregulation to facilitate the development of FL [41]. Recent studies have started to unveil the mechanism by which these mutations contribute to neoplastic transformation. This involves in part the reduced ability of CREBBP to acetylate the oncoprotein BCL6, where acetylation serves as a negative modulator [42], and the tumor suppressor TP53, which, conversely, requires acetylation for its transcriptional activation [43, 44]. The balanced activity of these two proteins is fundamental for GC physiology and pathology and particularly for the regulation of DNA damage checkpoints during *IG* remodeling processes [45]; thus, one consequence of BCL6 activity overriding p53 would be an increased tolerance for DNA damage in the absence of proper apoptotic responses. CREBBP opposes the activity of BCL6 also by acetylating H3K27 residues at the promoter/enhancer sequences of most of its target genes, facilitating their transcription. This is particularly important for the commissioning of enhancers that need to be activated during the transition between GC and post-GC stages, when cells receive signals to down-regulate BCL6 and become plasma cells [41]. Reduced CREBBP acetyltransferase activity will impact on multiple biological programs that are critical to the normal GC reaction, with genes involved in GC exit being especially susceptible. The discovery of mutations in *CREBBP* and *EP300* has clinical implications in view of available drugs (i.e., histone deacetylase inhibitors) that could provide therapeutic benefits by re-establishing physiologic acetylation levels in tumors carrying these alterations.

Inactivating mutations *of KMT2D* (also known as *MLL2*) are found in approximately one third of DLBCL cases and >80% of FL cases, representing one of the most frequent genetic aberrations associated with GC-derived malignancies [28, 29]. KMT2D is a member of the SET1 family of histone methyltransferases and controls epigenetic transcriptional regulation mostly by mono- and dimethylating the lysine 4 position of histone H3 (H3K4), a mark associated with active chromatin conformation [46]. In GC B cells, KMT2D occupies chromatin domains at enhancer and less frequently at promoter regions of genes that have established roles in B-cell physiology, including immune regulators and components of BCR and CD40 receptor-mediated signaling responses [47, 48].

KMT2D mutations impair the protein methyltransferase activity by either removing the C-terminal cluster of conserved domains, including the SET module (truncating mutations) [28, 39], or by introducing disruptive amino acid changes in the same portion of the protein (missense mutations) [48]. In analogy to the human data, conditional B-cell-specific deletion of *KMT2D* before GC formation leads to a significant increase in the GC B-cell population and to the establishment of a distinct transcriptional program enriched in anti-apoptotic and cell cycle regulatory genes [48]. While loss of *KMT2D* is insufficient to drive tumor formation, combined *KMT2D* deletion and BCL2 deregulation led to a significant increase in the development of lymphomas recapitulating the spectrum of phenotypes observed during human FL to DLBCL transition [48].

Collectively, the findings accumulated to date suggest that alterations in epigenetic modifiers may act differently from classical tumor suppressor genes and facilitate the initial stages of transformation by creating a permissive environment for the proliferation and survival of the cancer clone, in cooperation with other genetic lesions (e.g., BCL2 translocations).

Deregulation of BCL6 activity. BCL6 is a master regulator of the GC reaction [49, 50], and deregulation of its activity constitutes a major oncogenic mechanism exploited by DLBCL cells. The function of BCL6 is required in normal GC B cells to negatively modulate multiple biological programs that are critical for allowing the selection of cells with high-affinity antigen receptors and include the establishment of a proliferative phenotype, the attenuation of DNA damage sensing and replication checkpoints [45, 51–53], the protection from programed cell death [54, 55], and the block of terminal differentiation [56]. These programs are hijacked by DLBCL cells through multiple genetic aberrations that dysregulate BCL6 function either directly or indirectly (Fig. 2.4). Approximately 30% of cases—with a preference for ABC-DLBCL [57]—carry chromosomal translocations that juxtapose the intact coding domains of *BCL6* to heterologous sequences derived from over 20 chromosomal partners (the *IG* heavy and light chain loci being most commonly involved) [58–61]. In an additional ~6% of cases, translocations cluster at an alternative breakpoint region and link BCL6 to distantly acting transcriptional regulatory elements [62]. The common feature of these promoters is a broader activity that extends past the GC stage [63], thus preventing the down-regulation of BCL6 transcription necessary for differentiation into post-GC B cells.

BCL6 is also altered by multiple somatically acquired mutations that are distributed within a ~2 kb region downstream to its TSS, encompassing the first noncoding exon (~75% of cases). While most of these events reflect the physiologic activity of the SHM process [64, 65],

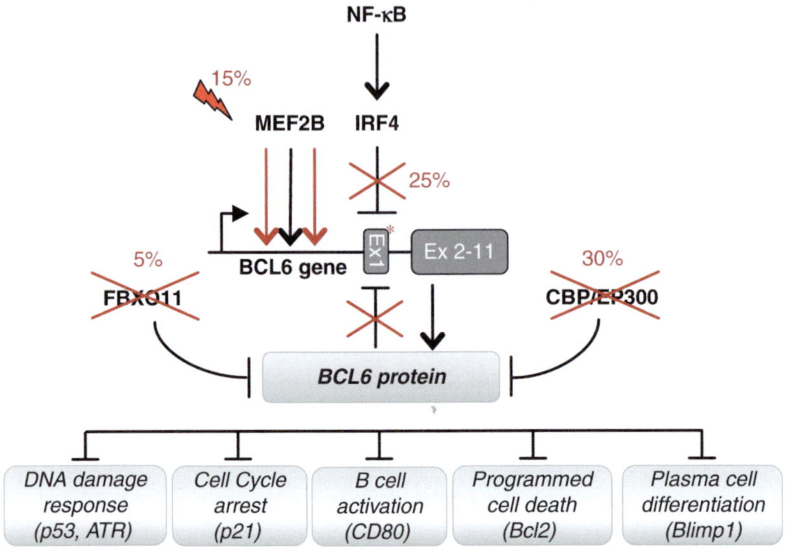

Fig. 2.4 Deregulation of BCL6 activity by genetic lesions in DLBCL. Recurrent genetic alterations deregulating the function of BCL6 in DLBCL, either directly or indirectly. Representative biological programs modulated by BCL6 in the GC and disrupted as a consequence of these lesions are shown at the bottom. Symbols depict loss-of-function and gain-of-function genetic alterations (Modified from Pasqualucci and Dalla-Favera, Semin Hematol, 2015) [18]

selected nucleotide changes within its untranslated first exon appear to be restricted to lymphoma cells, where they abrogate a negative autoregulatory feedback loop (10% of GCB-DLBCL cases) [66, 67] or prevent the IRF4-mediated BCL6 transcriptional repression induced by CD40 signaling in the GC LZ [68].

Besides genetic lesions directly affecting the BCL6 locus, several indirect mechanisms lead to deregulated BCL6 activity in DLBCL (Fig. 2.4). These include (1) inactivating mutations of *CREBBP/EP300* (discussed above) [41, 42, 69]; (2) somatic mutations in the GC-specific transcription factor *MEF2B* [28, 70], which enhances BCL6 expression in ~15% of cases, by abrogating the binding to the corepressor CABIN1 (missense mutations in the N-terminal MEF/MAD domain) or by generating truncated proteins that lack phosphorylation- and sumoylation-mediated negative regulatory motifs located in the C-terminal portion of the protein (truncating mutations) [70, 71]; and (3) loss-of-function mutations and/or deletions of the ubiquitin adaptor protein *FBXO11* (~5% of cases), leading to increased BCL6 protein stability [72]. In line with the genetic data, mouse models recapitulating these lesions develop clonal lymphoproliferative disorders mimicking various stages of the human disease [41, 73, 74]. Collectively, these data highlight BCL6 as an attractive therapeutic target for DLBCL, with several in vitro and preclinical studies showing promising results upon the use of small peptide inhibitors [75, 76].

Escape from immune surveillance. DLBCL cells have devised means to escape immune surveillance mechanisms, both cytotoxic T lymphocytes (CTL)-mediated and natural killer (NK) cell-mediated, by virtue of several genetic lesions. In approximately 60% of DLBCL clinical samples, the MHC class I complex is not expressed; this is explained in part by (1) biallelic inactivating mutations and/or focal homozygous deletions of the *B2M* gene, which encodes for β2-microglobulin and is required for assembly of the MHC-I complex on the cell surface (29% of cases), and (2) point mutations or genomic loss of the *HLA A, B,* and *C* loci [77]. In the remaining 30–45% of cases, lack of expression or aberrant cytoplasmic localization of the B2M/HLA-I protein complex is observed in the absence of such genetic lesions, suggesting additional mechanisms [78]. Interestingly, the loss of HLA-I expression is infrequently observed in other B-NHL types [77], but it is often associated with FL transformation [38, 79].

Nearly 20% of DLBCL cases carry disruptive point mutations and focal deletions inactivating *CD58*, the ligand for the CD2 receptor expressed on T cells and NK cells [80]. Notably, concurrent loss of HLA-I and CD58 expression is observed in over half of DLBCL samples, suggesting that lymphoma cells co-select these lesions to evade both arms of immune surveillance [78].

Finally, downregulation of MHC class II expression has been reported in 40–50% of samples [5, 81]. This phenotype involves at least in part the genetic inactivation of *CIITA*, the gene encoding for the MHC-II transactivator; *CIITA* was identified as a common target of ASHM in ~23% of DLBCL and can also be implicated in promiscuous chromosomal rearrangements (3% of cases) that were shown to either disrupt the gene or generate dominant-negative fusion proteins [82, 83]. Moreover, CIITA is a functional target of CREBBP, and reduced levels of MHC-II were observed in GC B cells from CREBBP conditional knockout mice, suggesting that CREBBP mutations could also contribute to its downregulated expression [41, 69, 84]. Reduced MHC-II levels were shown to correlate with poor outcome and may thus represent a relevant biomarker [5, 81].

Mutations of FOXO1. The transcription factor *FOXO1* plays central roles during B-cell differentiation and, within the GC, is expressed specifically in the DZ, while its activity is downregulated in the LZ via the phosphatidylinositol 3-kinase (PI3K)/AKT and mTOR cascade. FOXO1 is an essential requirement for sustaining the DZ transcriptional program, in part by cooperating with BCL6. Accordingly, mice engineered to delete FOXO1 specifically in the GC form DZ-less structures [85, 86]. This circuit is disrupted in 8–10% of DLBCL cases that carry somatic mutations of this gene. FOXO1 mutations mainly cluster around a T24 phosphorylation site required for its AKT-mediated nuclear-cytoplasmic translocation and inactivation; other events substitute the initiating methionine of the FOXO1 polypeptide, leading to the synthesis of proteins that utilize a downstream in-frame start codon, and thus also lack the N-terminal nuclear export domain. These events were suggested to prevent the cytoplasmic translocation and inactivation of FOXO1 induced by PI3K signaling [87]. While mutations are preferentially enriched in GCB-DLBCL, aberrant nuclear localization of the FOXO1 protein is observed in both DLBCL phenotypic subgroups (unpublished), implicating a broader involvement for FOXO1 dysregulation in DLBCL pathogenesis. Clearly, additional studies will be needed to dissect the precise mechanism by which FOXO1 mutations contribute to lymphomagenesis, including a systematic examination of their consequences in the context of B cells and the analysis of larger cohorts to confirm the reported preferential enrichment of these mutations in patients with aggressive disease [87, 88].

2.2.4.2 Genetic Lesions Associated with GCB-DLBCL

Chromosomal translocations of BCL2. The *BCL2* proto-oncogene encodes for the founding member of a protein family that governs commitment to programmed cell death at the mitochondrion [89]. *BCL2* is also a direct target of BCL6, which binds to its promoter via the transcriptional co-activator Miz1 and prevents its expression in GC B cells, ensuring the maintenance of a default pro-apoptotic programme [55, 90]. This regulatory axis is disrupted in 30–40% of GCB-DLBCL due to the t(14;18) translocation, which brings the *BCL2* coding exons under the control of potent regulatory elements from the *IG* locus, resulting in its ectopic expression [91]. As a consequence, BCL2 also becomes targeted by multiple AID-mediated somatic mutations, although the significance of these events remains controversial [90, 92]. In line with its ability to confer survival advantage, deregulation of BCL2 has been associated with an inferior outcome [93], particularly when coupled with MYC deregulation (see paragraph on "HGBL-DH").

Chromosomal translocations of MYC. The *MYC* gene encodes for a sequence-specific transcription factor that acts as an amplifier of transcriptional programs associated with numerous biological functions, ranging from proliferation to cell growth, energy metabolism, differentiation, apoptosis [94], and DNA replication independently of its transcriptional activity [95]. In 10–14% of GCB-DLBCLs, the MYC protein is constitutively expressed due to chromosomal translocations that fuse its intact coding exons to the *IG* heavy or light chains loci [96–99]. Besides juxtaposing enhancer elements in close proximity of the MYC locus, a subset of these rearrangements abrogates regulatory sequences bound by BCL6 to negatively modulate its transcription in most GC cells [100]. The presence of MYC-IGH translocations has been linked with worse prognosis in DLBCL [101].

Mutations of the EZH2 methyltransferase. *EZH2* encodes for the enzymatic component of the polycomb repressive complex-2 (PRC2), which is responsible for trimethylating the lysine 27 residue of histone H3 (H3K27me3) at the promoter/enhancer regions of silenced or poised genes [102–104]. In GC B cells, EZH2 facilitates the establishment of bivalent domains [105] in multiple genes that are critical for the termination of the GC reaction (*IRF4, PRDM1*) or for other GC programs (*CDKN1A*) [106, 107]. In line with these essential functions, conditional deletion of *EZH2* in the mouse was sufficient to prevent GC formation and affinity maturation [106, 107].

Somatic heterozygous mutations of the *EZH2* gene have been identified in up to 22% of GCB-DLBCL [108]. The vast majority of these events replace a single evolutionarily conserved residue (Y641) within the protein SET domain, leading to increased levels of H3K27me3 through altered catalytic specificity of EZH2 for its substrates [109–111]. Consistently, expression of the mutant $EZH2^{Y641F}$ allele in the mouse induces GC hyperplasia and, when combined with BCL2 deregulation, accelerates the development of mature B-cell lymphomas [106, 107]. Of note, selective small molecule inhibitors of EZH2 have shown specific activity in preclinical studies particularly in GCB-DLBCL [106, 112, 113], supporting their evaluation in early clinical trials. Indeed, a recent first-in-human phase II trial evaluating a highly selective EZH2 inhibitor showed promising results in patients with FL and, to less extent, relapsed/refractory DLBCL [114].

Mutations of the Gα13 pathway. The positioning and confinement of GC B cells within the B-cell follicle is regulated by the activity of two G-protein-coupled receptors that, among B-cell types, are expressed specifically in the GC: sphingosine-1-phosphate receptor 2 (S1PR2) [115] and the orphan purinergic receptor P2Y, G-protein-coupled 8 (P2RY8) [116]. These receptors recruit two closely related G proteins (Ga12 and Ga13) in response to lipid ligands and stimulate Rho activity via specific guanine nucleotide exchange factors (Rho-GEFs), ultimately suppressing pAKT signaling and cell migration. The importance of the Gα13 inhibitory circuit in the pathogenesis of GCB-DLBCLs is underscored by the presence of recurrent inactivating mutations in several of its components, including *S1PR2, GNA13,* and, more rarely, *ARHGEF1* and *P2RY8* (~20% of cases) (Fig. 2.5) [28, 30, 116]. Consistently, deletion of these genes in the mouse is associated with increased GC B-cell survival and disruption of the GC architecture, followed by dissemination of GC B cells to the lymph and bone marrow; with time, *GNA13, ARHGEF1,* and *S1PR2* [117] knockout mice develop lymphomas exhibiting features of GCB-DLBCL [116]. Disruption of this pathway may thus contribute to malignant transformation by abrogating Gα13-mediated inhibitory signals to both cell migration and AKT signaling.

Mutations of TNFRSF14. TNFRSF14 is a member of the TNF receptor superfamily expressed in both T and B cells, which emanates inflammatory or inhibitory signals depending on its specificity for diverse ligands [118]. In 9–22% of DLBCL, almost exclusively of the GCB type, missense (~50%), nonsense (~40%), and frameshift (2.5%) mutations target the exons encoding for its ectodomain, leading to functional inactivation (Fig. 2.5). Additionally, TNFRSF14 is part of a genomic region that is frequently deleted on chromosome 1p36. A tumor suppressor function for this gene during DLBCL development was recently demonstrated in a BCL2-driven mouse model where silencing of *Tnfrsf14* induced cell autonomous activation of B-cell proliferation and enhanced the development of GC-derived

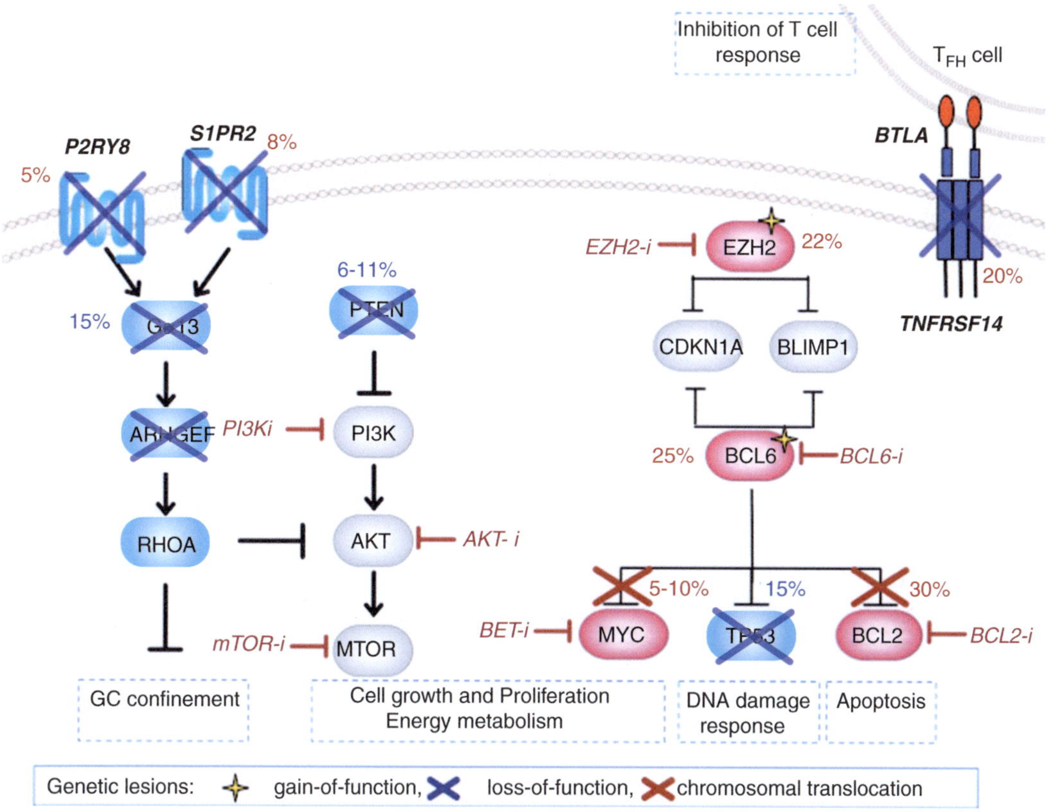

Fig. 2.5 Disrupted signaling pathways in GCB-DLBCL. Genetic lesions preferentially associated with GCB-DLBCL include chromosomal translocations of BCL2 and/or MYC, which cause their ectopic expression in part by bypassing BCL6-mediated transcriptional repression; chromosomal translocations (15% of cases) and point mutations (10% of cases) of BCL6, leading to its deregulated expression; gain-of-function mutations of EZH2 (~20% of cases), which induce epigenetic remodeling in various lymphoma-relevant genes, such as CDKN1A, in part cooperating with BCL6. Additionally, loss of PTEN expression is observed in 55% of cases, as a consequence of genetic deletions (15%) and amplifications of miR17-92 (%), resulting in activation of the PI3K/Akt/mTOR signaling pathway

lymphomas [119]. Loss of *TNFRSF14* contributes to tumorigenesis by inhibiting cell-cell interactions between TNFRSF14 and its ligand BTLA, thus inducing a supportive microenvironmental niche characterized by lymphoid stroma activation and increased recruitment of T follicular-helper cells. Consistent with this model, *TNFRSF14* mutations and BTLA downregulation are largely mutually exclusive in FL, although no studies have investigated this aspect in DLBCL. Of note, administration of soluble HVEM to BTLA-expressing lymphoma cells in vitro was able to restore this circuit and to inhibit cell growth, while local production by modified CAR-T cells in vivo led to the significant reduction of established lymphomas [119].

Other Lesions. While the multitude of genetic alterations associated with DLBCL prevents their comprehensive and detailed description, loss of the tumor suppressor *PTEN*, amplifications of the *REL* gene, and mutations of *SGK1* should be mentioned because of their frequency and/or potential therapeutic implications. Approximately 55% of GCB-DLBCL, as compared to 14% of ABC-DLBCL, lack expression of PTEN [120], due in part to the presence of mutually exclusive 10q chromosomal deletions and amplifications of the oncogenic miR-17-92 micro-RNA cluster (collectively, ~20% of patients) [17]. This pattern was inversely correlated with activation of the PI3K/AKT pathway and sensitivity to pharmacologic PI3K inhibition, uncovering potential therapeutic opportunities

[120]. Also largely restricted to GCB-like DLBCL is the presence of chromosome 2p amplifications encompassing the *REL* gene, which encodes for a subunit of the NF-κB transcription complex. Finally, mutations of *SGK1*, presumably reflecting the aberrant activity of SHM, were found specifically in this phenotypic subgroup. The *SGK1* genes encode for a PI3K-regulated kinase implicated in the control of FOXO transcription factors [121], NF-κB [122], and NOTCH signaling [123], but the functional consequences of these mutations remain unaddressed.

2.2.4.3 Genetic Lesions Associated with ABC-DLBCL

Alterations sustaining constitutive activation of the NF-κB signaling pathway. The genetic hallmark of ABC-DLBCL is the presence of multiple genetic aberrations that lead to the constitutive activation of the NF-κB signaling pathway, downstream of the BCR signaling cascade and the Toll-like receptor (TLR)/IL1R pathway (Fig. 2.6).

Mutations in the BCR signaling pathway. Most ABC-DLBCL cells are characterized by a "chronic active" form of BCR signaling associated with the

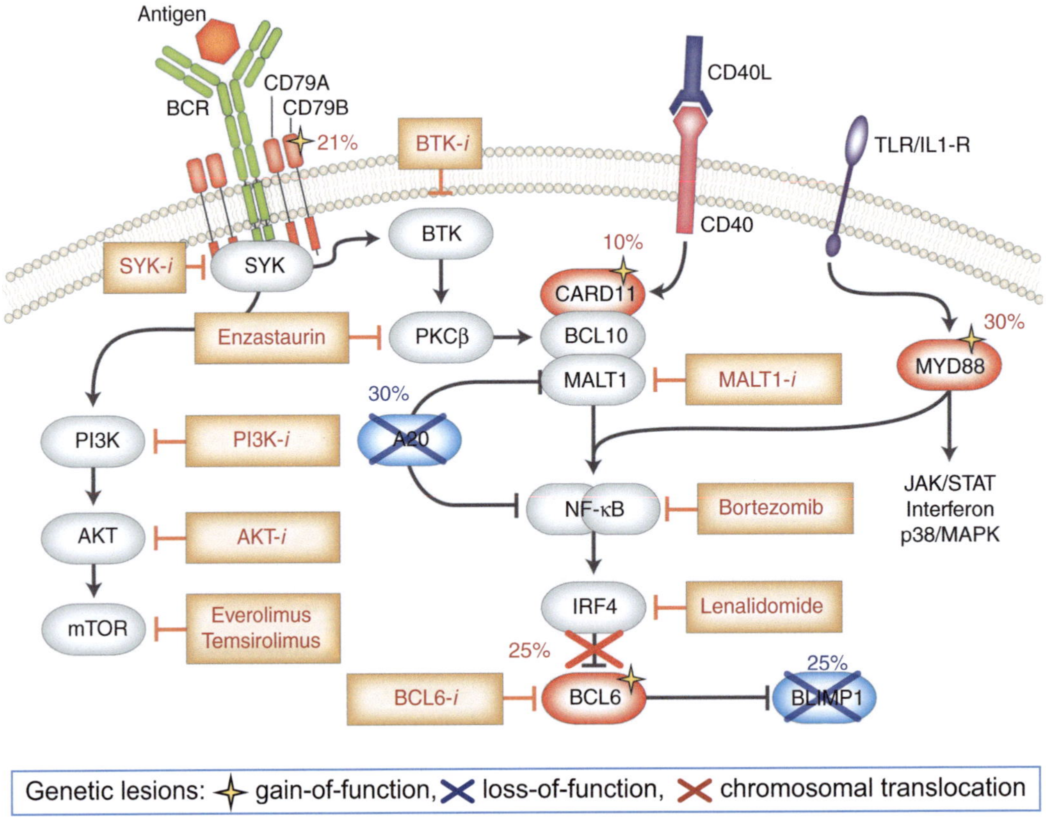

Fig. 2.6 Disrupted signaling pathways in ABC-DLBCL. Multiple genetic alterations cluster around two main biological programs in ABC-DLBCL: constitutive activation of the NF-κB transcription complex and block of plasma cell differentiation. NF-κB activity can be induced by a variety of signals in GC LZ cells, including engagement of the BCR by the antigen, interaction of the CD40 receptor with the CD40L presented by T cells, and TLR activation, which all lead to the upregulated expression of its target genes (e.g., IRF4 and A20). IRF4, in turn, extinguishes the GC program by suppressing BCL6 and thus releasing the expression of the plasma cell master regulator PRDM1/BLIMP1. NF-κB responses are then terminated in part by a negative feedback loop that requires the activity of A20. Subversion of the BCR and NF-κB signaling pathways may fuel malignant transformation by hijacking the anti-apoptotic and pro-proliferative functions of NF-κB while blocking terminal B-cell differentiation through mutually exclusive alterations deregulating BCL6 or inactivation of BLIMP1 (Modified with permission from Pasqualucci and Dalla-Favera, Semin Hematol, 2015) [18]

presence of clustered BCRs on the plasma membrane, similar to those formed in antigen-stimulated B cells. This signaling cascade requires CARD11 and is sustained in part by somatic mutations in the *CD79A/B* genes [124]. In particular, 20% of ABC-DLBCL patients harbor gain-of-function somatic variants in the immunoreceptor tyrosine-based activation motifs (ITAMs) of *CD79B* (or, rarely, *CD79A*) [124]. Most of these events replace the first tyrosine residue (Y196) in the cytoplasmic tail of the two BCR subunits and are thought to maintain BCR signaling chronically active by attenuating the phosphorylation and activation of the Lyn kinase, which is necessary for internalization of the surface BCR and serves as a negative feedback regulator.

In ~9% of ABC-DLBCL, activation of the BCR and NF-κB signaling cascade can be attributed to oncogenic mutations of *CARD11* [125]. The CARD11 protein is a component of the CBM complex that is coordinately recruited to transduce signals emanating from the BCR [126]. Missense mutations typically target the CARD11 coiled-coil domain, facilitating the formation of cytosolic aggregates and the recruitment of downstream effector molecules, ultimately enhancing its ability to transactivate NF-κB target genes [125].

The genetic lesions discussed above maintain, yet do not initiate, chronic active BCR signaling, which instead was recently shown to require engagement by self-antigens [127]. The dependence of ABC-DLBCL from the BCR signaling pathway is underscored by the preferential sensitivity of these tumors to agents that inhibit Bruton's tyrosine kinase (BTK), the molecule linking BCR to NF-κB, even in the absence of mutations targeting CD79A/B [128].

Mutations of the MYD88 gene. MYD88 encodes an adaptor molecule that mediates activation of NF-κB as well as type I interferon responses downstream the TLR signaling pathway [129]. Thirty percent of ABC-DLBCLs carry a hotspot L265P substitution within the protein TIR (Toll/IL1 receptor) domain, which was shown to induce the spontaneous assembly and activation of a protein complex containing the kinases IRAK1 and IRAK4, leading to engagement of the NF-κB signaling pathway [130]. MYD88-mutated DLBCL cases also show autocrine transcriptional activation of the JAK/STAT3 signaling cascade, another distinctive phenotype of ABC-DLBCL required for their survival [130, 131]. The significance of other MYD88 mutations found in both ABC- and GCB-DLBCL remains to be established. Importantly, MYD88-mutant DLBCL are not sensitive to BTK inhibition, but this treatment was exquisitely toxic to tumors carrying concurrent MYD88 and CD79A/B mutations, suggesting functional interaction between these two molecules [128].

Mutations of the TNFAIP3 gene. TNFAIP3 (also called *A20*) encodes a dual function ubiquitin-modification enzyme involved in the termination of NF-κB responses triggered by TLR and BCR stimulation. This protein removes K63-linked regulatory ubiquitins from a number of substrates via its OTU domain and subsequently conjugates K48-linked ubiquitins via its zinc finger domains, targeting these proteins for proteasomal degradation. In line with this, TNFAIP3 knockout mice show abnormally prolonged NF-κB responses associated with an overactive phenotype [132]. Almost one third of ABC-DLBCLs and fewer GCB-DLBCLs harbor biallelic truncating mutations and/or focal deletions that inactivate the function of TNFAIP3, leading to constitutively active NF-κB responses [133, 134]. A tumor suppressor role for this gene in ABC-DLBCL is supported by the observation that enforced expression of wild-type TNFAIP3 in TNFAIP3-null DLBCL cell lines results in cytoplasmic re-localization of the NF-κB complex and suppression of its activity, leading to apoptosis [133, 134].

At lower frequencies, a variety of other genes encoding for NF-κB positive and negative regulators have been found mutated in ABC-DLBCL, overall accounting for more than 50% of cases [133]. It should be considered that, since the BCR emanates signals to multiple downstream effectors besides canonical NF-κB (namely, PI3K, ERK, and NF-AT), the activation of these circuits could also represent vulnerabilities of the tumor cells. This may offer additional therapeutic opportunities based on the design of combinatorial strategies, as supported by the cooperative toxicity observed upon combined inhibition of NF-κB and PI3K [125].

Genetic lesions preventing terminal differentiation. A second pathogenic mechanism in ABC-DLBCL is blockade of post-GC differentiation. Indeed, these tumors derive from a GC B cell that has received signals to commit to plasma cell differentiation but is arrested at the plasma blast developmental stage due to a variety of genetic and epigenetic mechanisms abrogating the function of the plasma cell master regulator *PRDM1/BLIMP1* (Fig. 2.6). In 25% of patients, both copies of the *PRDM1* gene are lost owing to truncating mutations, loss-of-function missense mutations, and/or genomic deletions [135–137]. Another 25% of patients lack BLIMP1 expression as the result of direct transcriptional repression by constitutively active, translocated *BCL6* alleles [135]. Alternative modes of inactivation could explain the absence of BLIMP1 in the remaining large fraction of cases, including epigenetic silencing or high expression of the ETS family factor SPIB. Consistent with this model, conditional ablation of *PRDM1* in mouse GC B cells, either alone or in combination with a constitutively active IκB kinase, leads to the development of DLBCL with ABC-like phenotype [135, 138]. *BCL6* rearrangements and *PRDM1* inactivation are mutually exclusive [34, 35], supporting a complementary role for these lesions in fostering lymphomagenesis.

Other genetic lesions. Additional recurrent alterations include amplifications of the *BCL2* locus, observed in more than one third of patients [5, 17], homozygous deletions or lack of expression of the *CDKN2A/B* tumor suppressor genes (30% of cases) [17], and gains or amplifications of a large region on chromosome 19q (27% of cases), which spans the *SPIB* locus and may contribute to the elevated expression of this protein observed in DLBCL [17].

2.3 High-Grade B-Cell Lymphomas

The fourth edition of the WHO classification of hematolymphoid tumors of 2008 has coined the provisional category of "B-cell lymphoma, unclassifiable, with features intermediate between DLBCL and BL," or so-called grey zone lymphoma [139]. These lymphomas were defined because of their intermediate morphological, immunohistochemical, and genetic features encompassing features of both DLBCL and Burkitt lymphoma. However, this category was poorly reproducible, and, owing to the fact that around 60% of greyzone lymphomas harbor double or triple hits involving *MYC* and *BCL2* and/or *BCL6*, research had mainly focused on the double-/triple-hit subcategory. In the 2017 update of the fourth edition, this provisional category has been replaced by two new categories: high-grade B-cell lymphoma with *MYC* and *BCL2* and/or *BCL6* rearrangements (or HGBL-DH) and high-grade B-cell lymphoma, not otherwise specified (HGBL-NOS), which by definition lacks a double- or triple-hit constellation involving *MYC* but may be *MYC*-rearranged [1]. Most patients with HGBL will present at higher age and with aggressive and/or extensive disease, and bone marrow and extranodal involvements are common, as are elevated lactate dehydrogenase (LDH) levels.

2.3.1 High-Grade B-Cell Lymphoma with *MYC and BCL2 and/or BCL6* Rearrangements (HGBL-DH)

The diagnosis of these tumors as a new WHO category relies exclusively on the presence of rearrangements involving both *MYC* and *BCL2* and/or *BCL6* (previously known as double-hit DLBCL). In contrast, DLBCL featuring high-level amplifications, copy number alterations, or elevated protein expression of MYC will not be included in this category. Therefore, by definition, HGBL-DH encompasses the following morphological cases:

- Tumors with the morphology of DLBCL and a double (DH) or triple hit (TH) (Fig. 2.7a)
- Tumors that, in the former taxonomy, would have been classified as "unclassifiable with features intermediate between DLBCL and BL" harboring dual rearrangements involving *MYC* (Fig. 2.7b)

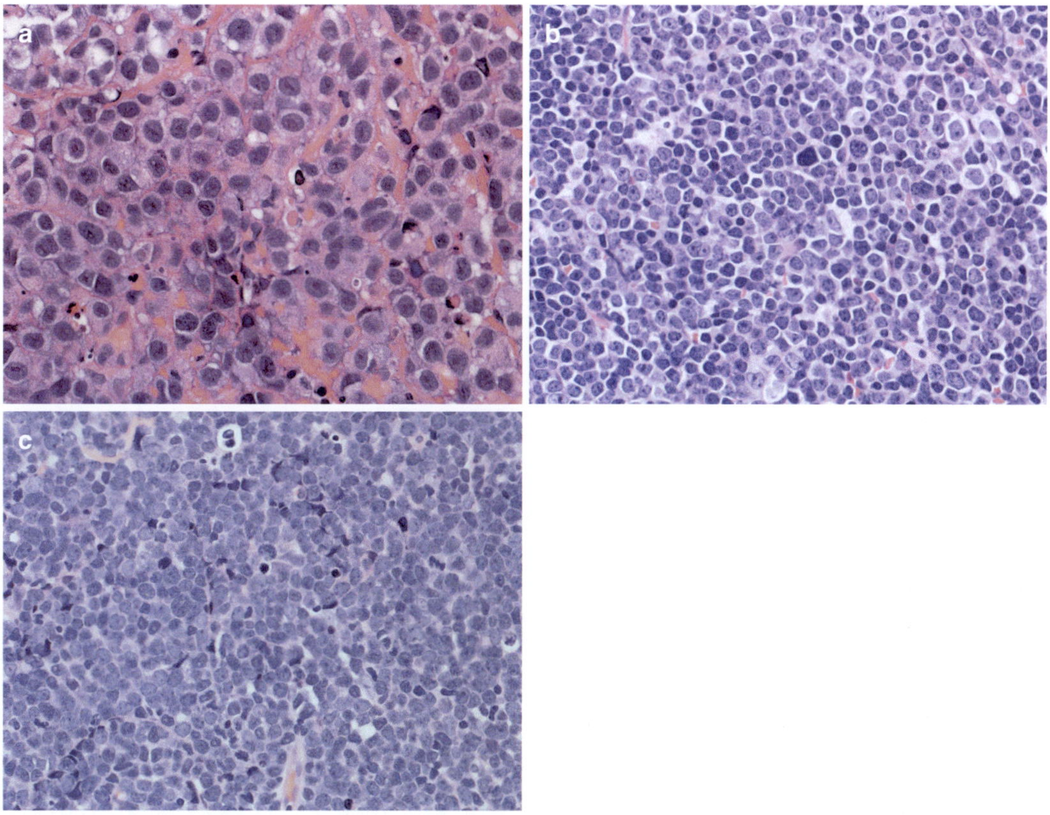

Fig. 2.7 (**a**) High-grade B-cell lymphoma, featuring large tumor cells of varying size and moderately pleomorphic nuclei equivalent to a DLBCL. (**b**) Double-hit DLBCL showing medium-sized cells with narrow cytoplasm and round, only slightly polymorphic nuclei. This tumor would have been classified as "B-cell lymphoma, unclassifiable, with features intermediate between DLBCL and BL" in the 2008 WHO classification. (**c**) High-grade B-cell lymphoma with *MYC/BCL2* translocation, transformed from FL. This tumor features blastoid cells with small to intermediate size and finely dispersed nuclear chromatin

- Cases with blastoid cytomorphology and a double- or triple-hit genetic constitution (Fig. 2.7c)

One important new concept of the updated WHO classification is that DLBCLs with a DH or TH genetic constitution will be reclassified as HGBL-DH. Consequently, all DLBCL would be required to undergo FISH testing in order to identify and classify these cases. The update of the WHO classification, however, does not formally require FISH testing on all DLBCL; therefore, pathologists may preselect cases according to a variety of criteria in order to minimize the efforts inherent to extensive FISH testing.

With the probable exception of cases displaying immunoblastic morphology and cases with a higher number of tumor cells expressing nuclear MYC [140], HGBL—DH/TH are virtually indistinguishable from bona fide DLBCL upon morphology. Cases with blastoid cytomorphology have a lymphoblast-like appearance and, therefore, may require a differential diagnosis with B-cell lymphoblastic leukemia/lymphoma or the blastoid variant of mantle cell lymphoma. More frequently, cases transformed from preexisting or concurrent follicular lymphoma with secondary *MYC* rearrangement will have this appearance. The latter tumors are classified as *transformed follicular lymphomas with dual MYC and BCL2 rearrangements* and blastoid cytomorphology. Finally, tumors previously classified as greyzone lymphomas consist of predominantly medium-sized cells in between the size of Burkitt lymphoma and DLBCL cells, but featuring a more pleomorphic cytology than BL, and will occasionally show a starry-sky pattern [139]. Cases with a *MYC* and *BCL6* double hit are almost exclusively of the GCB type, and, because of their particularly poor clinical outcome, they represent an unmet clinical need within this otherwise favorable prognostic category of DLBCL. Some clinico-pathological differences have been recorded between *MYC-BCL2* and *MYC-BCL6* DH tumors [141, 142].

2.3.2 High-Grade B-Cell Lymphoma Not Otherwise Specified (HGBL-NOS)

This new category mainly includes the former *greyzone or high-grade B-cell lymphomas, unclassifiable, with features intermediate between DLBCL and BL,* which lack a genetic DH or TH constellation. Morphologically, these cases are composed of predominantly medium-sized or blastoid cells with a narrow cytoplasmic rim, round nuclei slightly more pleomorphic than those of Burkitt lymphoma, a finely dispersed nuclear chromatin, and inconspicuous nucleoli, sometimes in combination with a starry-sky pattern (Fig. 2.8). HGBL-NOS often shows a GCB-like GEP, although some cases are of ABC-DLBCL type based on either GEP or immunohistochemical algorithms. By virtue of their definition, these tumors may carry isolated *MYC*, *BCL2*, or *BCL6* rearrangements and may also show dual *BCL2* and *BCL6* rearrangements. It has to be noted that tumors showing the classical morphology of DLBCL and harboring isolated *MYC* rearrangements will continue to be diagnosed as DLBCL and do not fall into the HGBL-NOS category [1].

2.4 Other Lymphomas of Large B Cells and Special Subtypes/Variants

2.4.1 T-Cell/Histiocyte-Rich Large B-Cell Lymphoma

T-cell/histiocyte-rich large B-cell lymphoma (THRLBCL) is defined as a DLBCL variant with few scattered tumor cells and an abundant reactive background consisting of T cells and histiocytes. The median age at presentation is in the sixth to seventh decade of life, but this variant may also be seen in children. There is a male predominance. THRLBCL is a primarily nodal disease and often presents with high-stage and bone

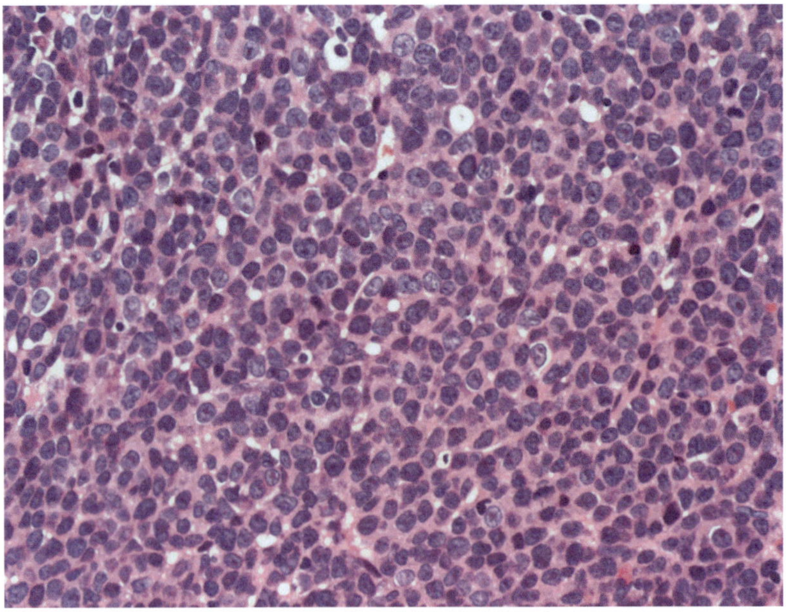

Fig. 2.8 Bone marrow biopsy of a high-grade B-cell lymphoma, NOS, displaying diffuse infiltration by medium-sized blasts. Cytogenetic analysis in this case was positive for a *MYC* translocation, but no alterations of *BCL2* or *BCL6* were seen

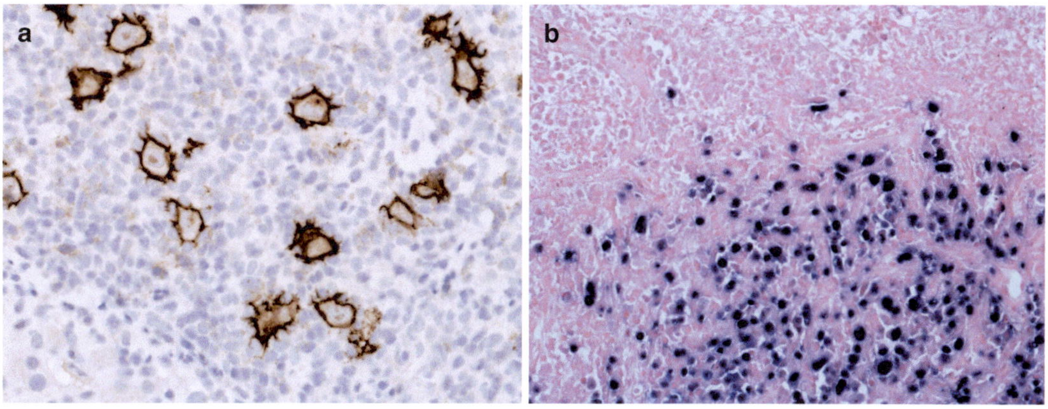

Fig. 2.9 T-cell/histiocyte-rich large B-cell-lymphoma (THRLBCL). In this tumor, rare large B blasts highlighted in a CD20 stain are seen in a background of small and slightly activated reactive T cells and histiocytes (**a**). Of importance, no small B cells are present. (**b**) H&E staining

marrow involvement. On morphology, there is complete effacement of the underlying architecture, with large lymphoid cells scattered in a predominantly reactive background of activated lymphocytes and histiocytes. The tumor cells in THRLBCL make up less than 10% of the whole cell population, without clusters or sheets (Fig. 2.9). Presence of an even focal component of NLPHL excludes de novo THRLBCL (see above). The cytomorphology of the tumor cells is centroblastic, immunoblastic, or LP or HRS cell-like. The tumor cells express pan B-cell markers, are negative for CD30 and CD15, and often co-express BCL6 and EMA. In the background, CD3-positive cells usually express CD8 and TIA1. THRLBCL shows clonally rearranged IG genes, and roughly one quarter of the cases has *BCL2* rearrangements. EBV is negative in the vast majority of cases. In some cases, a biological overlap to progressed variants of nodular lymphocyte predominant Hodgkin lymphoma (NLPHL) is suggested [143]. Malignant lymphomas with features of THRLBCL have been observed in progression of or as secondary lymphomas that develop after NLPHL. Diffuse variants of NLPHL may bear close similarity to THRLBCL, and therefore it is not clear whether predominantly diffuse NLPHL and THRLBCL may be representing a spectrum of the same disease or whether THRLBCL could represent transformation of NLPHL [144, 145]. Cases with T-cell/histiocyte-rich areas in NLPHL are designated as *THRLBCL-like transformation of NLPHL* in the revised fourth edition of the WHO classification.

2.4.2 Intravascular Large B-Cell Lymphoma

Intravascular large B-cell lymphoma (IVLBCL) is a DLBCL subtype in which blastic tumor cells are seen exclusively—or at least predominantly—within the lumina of small-sized blood vessels [146]. The lymphoma is rare, predominantly occurring in older patients with a peak in the seventh decade. IVLBCL can be seen in all organs, but most commonly in the CNS, skin, kidney, lung, and liver. Clinical symptoms are often nonspecific and related to the site of infiltration, such as cerebrovascular dysfunction. Involvement of the bone marrow is rare. A particular variant associated with hemophagocytic syndrome has been described in Asian patients.

Histologically, medium-sized to large lymphoma cells with varying cytological appearance are seen in often dilated lumens of small to intermediate-sized vessels (Fig. 2.10a, b). There may be secondary changes such as thrombosis or endothelial hyperplasia, causing infarction and hemorrhage. The tumor cells express pan B-cell markers and may be positive for CD5, CD10, and/or BCL6. Clonal IGH rearrangements are

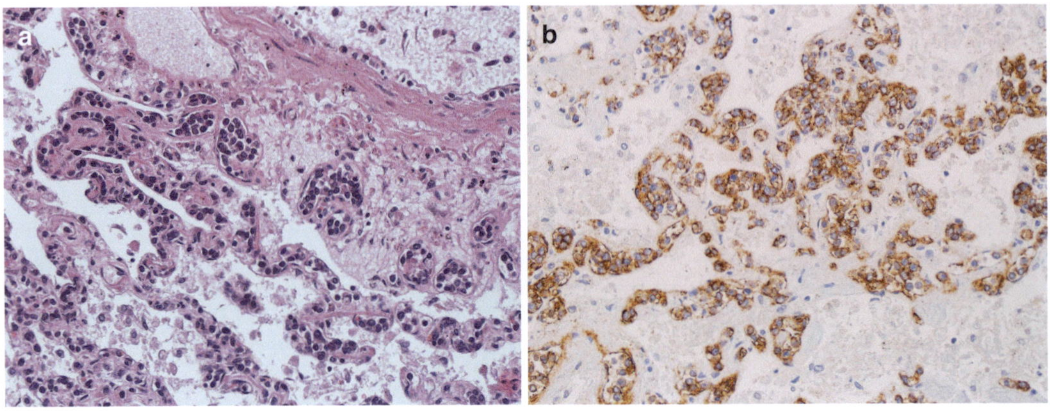

Fig. 2.10 Intravascular large B-cell lymphoma. (**a**) Hematoxylin-eosin (H&E) staining of a lung biopsy showing dense infiltrations of medium- to large-size tumor cells in distended capillary vessels of the alveolar septa. (**b**) CD20 staining of the same sample highlights the intravascular localization of the tumor cells

usually found. The majority of cases show a non-GCB immunophenotype, and no specific cytogenetic alteration has been defined so far [139].

2.4.3 Plasmablastic Lymphoma

Plasmablastic lymphoma (PBL) is defined as a terminally differentiated B-cell neoplasia. Morphologically, it consists of immunoblastic or plasmablastic cells. The negativity of the tumor cells for the CD20 antigen is a hallmark defining feature [139]. PBL frequently occurs in adults with immunodeficiency states (most commonly HIV infection) but may also be seen in the setting of posttransplantation or autoimmune disorders. In addition, these tumors are also diagnosed in patients without any apparent immunodeficiency. PBL frequently arises in extranodal sites, mainly of the head and neck and often in the oral cavity, in which it was primarily described [147]. Other involved locations are the upper respiratory tract, gastrointestinal tract or soft tissues, skin, bone, lung, and lymph nodes. The latter localization is often characteristic in PBL occurring in a post-transplantation setting. Most patients are diagnosed in higher clinical stages (III/IV), but this is less apparent in patients without immunodeficiency. In general, the prognosis is poor.

PBL may demonstrate monomorphic cytological features or plasmacytoid differentiation. The common variant of PBL shows a diffuse proliferation of cohesively growing immunoblasts or plasmablasts, whereas in cases of plasmacytoid differentiation, the cells are rounder with more eccentric nuclei and abundant basophilic cytoplasm. In some cases, a starry-sky pattern may be seen, and there may be extensive necrosis. On immunophenotyping, the tumor cells are negative for CD45, CD20, and PAX5. Expression of CD79A is variable. Plasma cell-associated markers are regularly expressed (CD38, CD138, IRF4/MUM1, and others such as BLIMP1 and XBP1). EMA is frequently positive and CD56 expression may be seen in some cases. The proliferative index is high. BCL2 and BCL6 are usually not expressed [148]. EBV association may be seen in roughly 70% of cases, in most of the tumors with a latency type I pattern. HHV8 is always negative. Genetic analyses frequently show complex karyotypes, and *MYC* translocationsc to the IG genes have been seen in 50% of the cases [149]. These cells express the MYC protein, circumventing the BLIMP1-mediated suppression of its transcription usually encountered in plasma cells.

2.4.4 ALK-Positive Large B-Cell Lymphoma

ALK-positive large B-cell lymphoma is an uncommon subtype of DLBCL that shares with plasmablastic lymphoma its frequent immunoblastic-plasmablastic morphology and protein

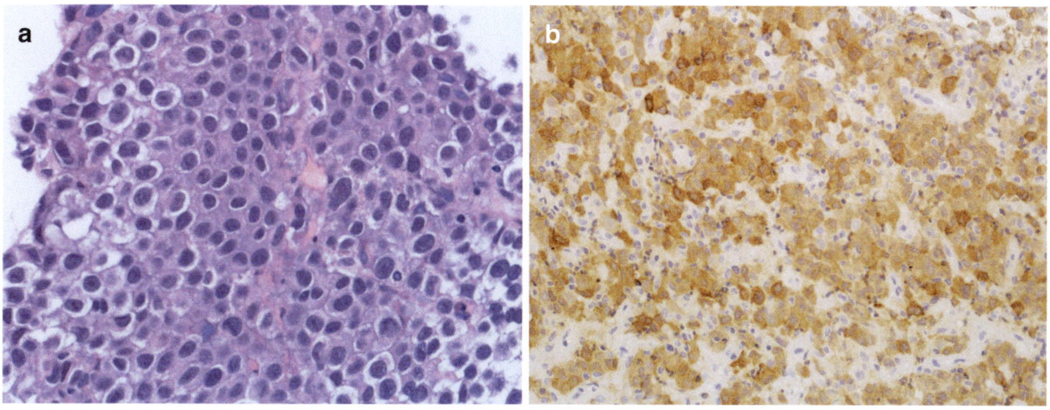

Fig. 2.11 ALK-positive large B-cell lymphoma. (**a**) H&E staining shows large tumor cells reminiscent of immunoblasts with a certain cohesiveness featuring abundant cytoplasm and slightly eccentric nuclei. CD20 negativity of the tumor cells suggested plasmablastic differentiation. (**b**) ALK staining reveals positivity in the cytoplasm of the tumor cells with granular reactivity that is characteristic of an *ALK-CLTC* fusion

expression phenotype. In addition, ALK+ DLBCL strongly expresses the ALK protein. It occurs predominantly in young adults, but there is a broad age range at presentation. Generalized disease is common, and no obvious association with immunodeficiency states has been reported. The majority of patients have high-stage (III/IV) disease, and the tumor is aggressive with short 5-year overall survival.

The tumor cells feature an immunoblastic or plasmablastic appearance with vesicular nuclei and frequently a large central nucleolus (Fig. 2.11a). One characteristic architectural feature is a sinusoidal growth pattern in many cases, creating a differential diagnosis with carcinoma. CD20, CD79A, and PAX5 are usually negative, but the tumor cells express CD45, EMA, IRF4/MUM1, immunoglobulin light chain genes and often IgA. In addition, CD138, BLIMP1, and XBP1 are usually positive. CD30 is negative or only weakly expressed [150]. All cases are EBV- and HHV8-negative. By definition, the ALK kinase is expressed, usually in the cytoplasm with a granular pattern (Fig. 2.11b), and these cases frequently harbor *ALK-CLTC* translocations [150–152]. Tumors with the classical *ALK-NPM* translocation inferring nuclear and cytoplasmic expression of the ALK protein are rare. ALK activation leads to upregulation of the STAT3 pathway, and ALK-positive LBCL express high levels of phospho-STAT3. STAT3, in turn, upregulates MYC and also BLIMP1. Consistently, ALK-positive LBCLs also express the MYC protein, but do not harbor *MYC* translocations [153].

2.4.5 Primary Mediastinal (Thymic) Large B-Cell Lymphoma

Primary mediastinal (thymic) large B-cell lymphoma (PMBCL) is regarded as a distinct subtype of DLBCL with organotypic features. The tumor usually presents in the upper anterior mediastinum of predominantly young adults, with a median age of 35 years and a female to male ratio of 2:1. The tumor can invade into neighboring structures such as the thoracic wall, the pericardium, the pleura, and the lung. Symptoms are related to the often bulky mediastinal mass, such as superior vena cava obstruction, dyspnea, and chest pain [139]. More recently, cases with a gene expression profile of PMBCL have also been described outside the mediastinum [154].

On morphology, the tumor shows a diffuse infiltration of medium-sized to large blastic cells that have a variable cytological appearance (Fig. 2.12) [155]. Centroblastic, immunoblastic, anaplastic, or Hodgkin- and Reed-Sternberg-like cells may occur, and a clear cell morphology is not infrequent [156]. One hallmark feature of

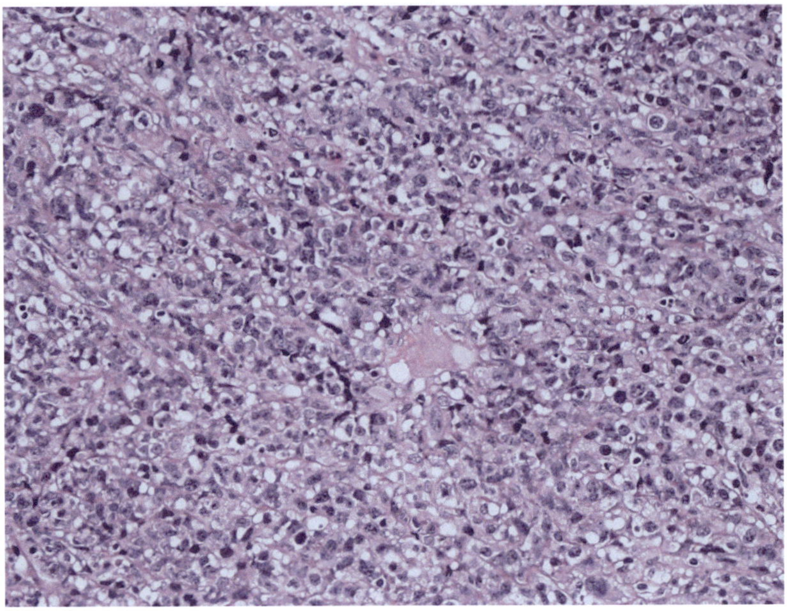

Fig. 2.12 Mediastinal (thymic) large B-cell lymphoma. This biopsy shows large blastic B cells diffusely infiltrating the mediastinal tissue. Note the slight fibrosis in the background

PMBCL is background sclerosis with delicate or coarse collagen fibers encompassing small groups of lymphoma cells in a way "compartmentalizing" the infiltrate. The immunophenotype, although not specific to PMBCL, is characteristic, frequently showing co-expression of CD30 and CD23, with pan B-cell markers and absent expression of MHC class I and II antigens [139]. Another feature characteristic of PMBCL is expression of the MAL protein [157]. PMBCL displays a unique GEP that is closer to that of classical Hodgkin lymphoma and reflects the origin from a thymic, GC-experienced B cell (with particular asteroid morphology) [158, 159].

Molecular Pathogenesis. The core biology of PMBCL is defined by a constellation of somatic mutations, copy number changes, and genomic rearrangements that lead to deregulation of the JAK-STAT and NF-κB signaling pathways, as well as to acquired immune privilege [82, 160–163] (Fig. 2.3).

Constitutive activation of the *JAK-STAT signaling pathway*, a signature identified by gene expression profiling analysis and shared with classical Hodgkin lymphoma (cHL), is the result of both paracrine interleukin receptor-mediated signaling [164] and genetic alterations, including amplification of *JAK2* (>50% of patients) [163, 165], deletions or inactivating mutations of the negative regulators *SOCS1* (45% of cases) [166] and *PTPN1* (22% of cases) [160], and mutations of *STAT6*. Amplification of chromosomal region 9q24 is a genetic hallmark of both PMBCL and cHL and spans multiple genes of possible pathogenic significance, in addition to *JAK2*, namely, *CD274 (PDL1)*, *PDCD1LG2 (PDL2)*, and *JMJD2C*. The latter encodes a demethylase that removes histone H3 lysine 9 trimethylation marks, interfering with the recruitment of HP1α and heterochromatin formation [167]. Interestingly, phosphorylation of JAK2 also contributes to an active chromatin conformation by phosphorylating both histone H3 and HP1α [168]. Thus, activation of JAK-STAT signaling may act synergistically with acquired immune privilege (through PDL1/2) and chromatin remodeling (through JMJD2C) in the pathogenesis of PMBCL [161]. SOCS1 mutations abrogate SOCS box function leading to hyperphosphorylation of JAK2 and STAT5 [166], while mutations of *PTPN1*, encoding a non-receptor member of the protein tyrosine phosphatases superfamily named PTP1B, impair its phosphatase activity causing hyperphosphorylation of STAT molecules.

Consistent with these data, STAT6 phosphorylation has been suggested as a reliable marker for the differential diagnosis of PMBCL from other large cell lymphomas [169]. Finally, recurrent mutations of the transcription factor STAT6 are found in 36% of PMBCL cases, although the exact functional consequences of STAT6 mutations in the DNA binding domain are still a subject of debate.

Another major target of genetic alterations in PMBCL is the *NF-κB signaling pathway* [161], which is maintained constitutively active by a variety of somatic gene mutations and structural genomic changes. These include (1) copy number gains and amplifications of the *REL* gene (>50% of cases), correlated with nuclear localization of the REL protein [170]; (2) inactivating mutations of *TNFAIP3* (36% of cases) [171]; and (3) amplification of the genomic regions encoding for the NF-κB regulators *BCL10* (1p22) and *MALT1* (18q21), observed in a subset of cases [172].

Finally, several genetic lesions impinge on the crosstalk between the tumor cells and the tumor microenvironment [173], leading to *acquired immune privilege* [82]. Among these lesions, the loss of *MHC-II* molecules is a prominent event that, analogous to DLBCL, NOS, has been linked to decreased infiltrating cytotoxic T cells and inferior outcome [5, 81]. Downregulation of surface MHC-II expression in these tumors is explained in part by allelic imbalances of the *HLA-DR* loci on chromosome 6p [174, 175] and by genomic breakpoints and mutations of the MHC class II transactivator gene *CIITA* (38% of samples) [83]. In addition, 20% of PMBCL carry recurrent genomic rearrangements involving the *PDL1/PDL2* genes on the short arm of chromosome 9, which encode for inhibitors of T-cell responses. These rearrangements generate PDL1 and PDL2 gene fusions with various partner genes, leading to elevated protein expression, and may in part explain the unique features of PMBCL, which are characterized by a significant inflammatory infiltrate. The cumulative incidence of genetic alterations that interfere with the interaction between the lymphoma cells and the microenvironment supports a central role for escape from immunosurveillance mechanisms in the pathogenesis of these neoplasms. Importantly, the frequent co-amplification of *JAK2* and *PDL1/2* on chromosome 9p24 suggests that combination therapies with JAK-STAT pathway inhibitors and immune checkpoint inhibitors might have synergistic antitumor activity.

2.4.6 B-Cell Lymphoma, Unclassifiable, with Features Intermediate Between Diffuse Large B-Cell Lymphoma and Classical Hodgkin Lymphoma

B-cell lymphoma, unclassifiable, with features intermediate between DLBCL and CHL (so-called mediastinal greyzone lymphoma, MGZL) still represents a peculiar tumor that shows features of both primary mediastinal large B-cell lymphoma and classical Hodgkin lymphoma. The clinical characteristics of the condition are predominantly determined by the site in which the tumor arises. Usually, there is a large mediastinal mass that can spread to supraclavicular lymph nodes and/or can invade neighboring structures *per continuitatem*, such as the lungs, the surrounding soft tissues, and even bone structures, but that rarely metastasizes to distant sites. Retrospective analyses have shown a poorer clinical outcome of MGZL in comparison with either CHL or PMBCL [176]. There are two more or less distinct morphologies that may be seen. One resembles that of CHL (frequently, of nodular sclerosis type), but, on immunohistochemistry, the B-cell program is greatly preserved as exemplified by strong expression of B-cell-associated antigens including CD20 and CD79a and also reactivity for the B-cell-specific transcription factors OCT-2 and BOB1, while expression of CD15 is usually absent. The other type of MGZL shows the morphology of large B-cell lymphoma with expression of B-cell markers, in which the tumor cells are also uniformly positive for CD30 and often CD15, or are EBV associated [177]. This tumor should be set apart from a composite lymphoma simultaneously showing classical Hodgkin lymphoma and primary large B-cell lymphoma in different areas of the same site or biopsy.

2.4.7 Primary Cutaneous Diffuse Large B-Cell Lymphoma, Leg Type

Primary cutaneous DLBCL, leg type (PCDLBCL, leg type) is a special variant of diffuse large B-cell lymphoma with a characteristic clinical presentation, morphology, and immunophenotype [1]. It usually develops on the lower legs of predominantly female older adults. There is a diffuse infiltration of the skin and subcutaneous tissues by large cells, often centroblasts and immunoblasts, forming large cutaneous nodules [178]. The tumor cells express BCL2, IRF4/MUM1, and FOXP1, while CD10 and BCL6 are negative. A characteristic feature is strong cytoplasmic expression of IgM and MYC protein (without underlying *MYC* rearrangements). Leg-type DLBCL often displays an ABC-type (or non-GCB-type) expression profile. High-level amplifications of the *BCL2* locus have been seen in two thirds of cases along with *CDKN2A* deletion or promoter methylation. Mutation analyses have revealed *MYD88* L265 mutations in 60% of the cases and presence of mutations in genes characteristic of ABC-type DLBCL, such as *CARD11*, *CD79B*, und *TNFAIP3* [179].

2.4.8 Primary Central Nervous System Lymphoma

Primary CNS lymphoma (PCNSL) is a malignant lymphoid neoplasm arising in the brain, spinal cord, or leptomeninges; intraocular lymphoma forms a subset of PCNSL. PCNSL are predominantly diagnosed as large B cell lymphomas [139] and can develop in either immunocompetent or immunosuppressed patients. The affected individuals are in general elderly adults with a slight male predominance while, among immunodeficient patients, HIV-infected individuals, with younger age and clear male predominance at presentation are commonly seen. Histology characteristically reveals a diffuse proliferation of blasts with perivascular growth and—often extensive—necrosis. The tumors are usually composed of immunoblasts or centroblasts. They express pan B-cell antigens, usually BCL2, IRF4/MUM1, and often BCL6 implying a non-GCB immunophenotype [180]. PCNS-DLBCL shares with other lymphomas arising at immune-privileged sites the characteristic downregulation of MHC class II antigens [181]. Virtually all cases of PCNS-DLBCL in immunosuppressed patients are positive for EBERs, and a subset of them also expresses LMP1.

At the molecular level, several lines of investigation support a role for both the NF-κB and JAK/STAT signaling pathways as mediators of pro-survival signals in this tumor type [182]: besides the presence of multiple genetic alterations in NF-κB regulators (see below), interleukin-4 is upregulated at the transcript and protein level within the vascular microenvironment; IL-10 (another first messenger in the JAK/STAT signaling) is increased in the vitreous and cerebrospinal fluid, and increased JAK1 transcripts are detected in the tumor cells [182]. Elevated IL-10 expression alongside activation of JAK/STAT signaling are consistent with aberrant activation of the MYD88 pathway.

Molecular Pathogenesis. The rarity of PCNS-DLBCL and the difficulty in obtaining material for investigational studies has hampered the molecular analysis of this DLBCL subtype. Nonetheless, a number of studies, including recent whole-exome sequencing efforts, have unveiled important genetic features associated with PCNS-DLBCL, including recurrent mutations in genes that are involved in NF-κB pathway activation (e.g., *CARD11*, *CD79/B*, and *MYD88*), cell cycle regulation (*CCND3*), and chromatin structure/histone modifications (*CREBBP*, *KMT2D*, *ARID1A*/B, *SMARCA4*, and *SMARCA5*) [183]. Of these, *MYD88* mutations at the L265 hotspot represent the most common event, accounting for 38–50% of clinical cases [184, 185], followed by *CD79B* (approximately 20% of cases) [186]. PCNS-DLBCL also shows evidence of ASHM in multiple proto-oncogenes with established roles in B-cell development and differentiation, including *PAX5*, *PIM1*, *c-MYC*, and *RhoH/TTF* [187].

Moreover, a critical step in the molecular pathogenesis of PCNSL (and a biomarker of inferior clinical outcome) is inactivation of the *CDKN2A/B* genes, encoding for $p14^{ARF}$ and $p16^{INK4a}$, by either homozygous deletion (40–50% of cases) or hypermethylation (15–30% of cases). BCL6 translocations are detected in 17% of tumors and have been associated with inferior overall survival especially when combined with 6q22 deletions [188]. Other potentially relevant genetic lesions in PCNS-DLBCL comprise recurrent copy number gains of *MALT1* (a potential additional contributor to the aberrant activation of the NF-κB pathway in this disease) [189], chromosome 12 (particularly in the 12q region harboring STAT6, MDM2, and CDK4), and the long arms of chromosomes 1, 7, and 18 [182]; deletions of the short arm of chromosome 6 (which harbors the *HLA* loci) and chromosomes 17 and 18 [188, 190]; and deletions of 6q21-23, detected in 40–60% of cases. The latter encompasses several candidate tumor suppressor genes, among which *PRDM1* [191], *TNFAIP3* (*A20*), and *PTPRK*, a protein tyrosine phosphatase that participates in cell adhesion signaling events [192] may be most relevant. In contrast, mutations in the *TP53* gene are observed in only a small proportion of PCNS-DLBCL specimens.

2.4.9 Epstein-Barr Virus (EBV)-Positive Diffuse Large B-Cell Lymphoma NOS

The update of the fourth edition of the WHO classification has renamed EBV-positive DLBCL because this lymphoma, called *EBV-positive DLBCL of the elderly* in the fourth edition of the classification (2008), can also be seen in younger patients [193]. The name "EBV-positive DLBCL, NOS" was adopted to emphasize the difference from other specific EBV-associated LBCL variants and subtypes. In elderly individuals EBV infection of the tumor cells is explained by an age-related waning of the immune system, whereas its association to DLBCL occurring in the younger age group is not clear [194]. The frequency of EBV-positive DLBCL increases with age and is higher in Japan and Latin America as compared to Europe. Extranodal disease is common, but lymph nodes are affected as well. In younger patients, nodal disease is the most common form of presentation. In both younger and elderly patients, the male gender predominates [195].

Generally, there is a diffuse effacement of the underlying architecture by diffuse infiltrates of blasts, in many cases with extensive necrosis (Fig. 2.13a). A monomorphic subtype characterized by tumor cells resembling centroblasts, immunoblasts, and/or Hodgkin-like cells has been described and set apart from cases where the infiltrate also harbors many reactive bystander cells such as lymphocytes, histiocytes, plasma cells, and eosinophils. Some cases show pleomorphic large cells with several nuclei mimicking Reed-Sternberg cells. The tumor cells usually express pan B-cell markers such as CD20, CD79A, and PAX5. In many cases, co-expression of CD30 and a non-GCB phenotype is common. By definition, in situ hybridization with EBV-encoded small RNAs (EBERs) demonstrates EBV infection in at least 50% of the tumor cells (Fig. 2.13b), although different and lower cutoffs have been used for its definition in the past. LMP1 is usually expressed, and EBNA2 may be positive, consistent with type II latency. As is the case in posttransplantation lymphoproliferative disease (PTLD), the tumor cells are frequently positive for PDL-1 [196], possibly leading to attenuated immune surveillance. In contrast with classical Hodgkin lymphoma, the tumor cells are usually CD15 negative.

EBV-positive DLBCL, NOS, must be differentiated from EBV-associated mucocutaneous ulcer because of the apparently indolent clinical course of the latter.

2.4.10 Primary Effusion Lymphoma

Primary effusion lymphoma (PEL) is a distinct clinico-pathological entity, the hallmark of which is malignant effusion in the pleural or peritoneal

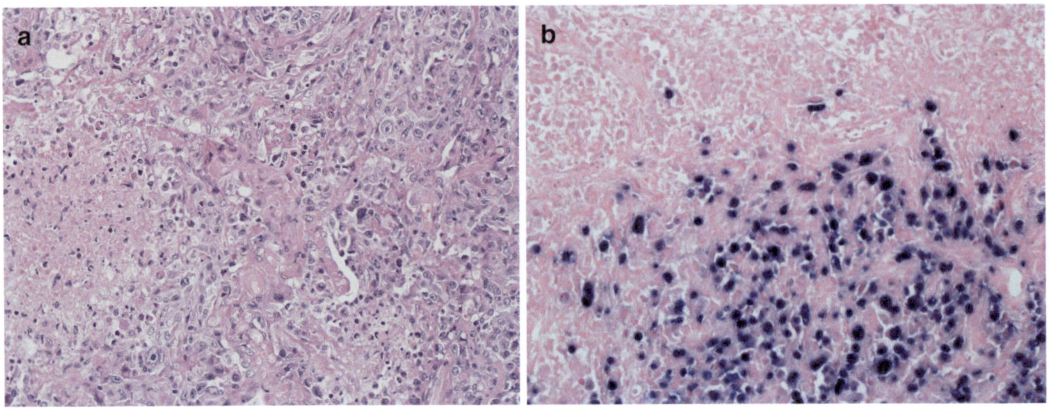

Fig. 2.13 EBV-positive DLBCL, NOS. (**a**) H&E staining of a lung tumor showing blastic tumor cells of varying size and shape, intermingled with some larger Hodgkin-like cells. Note focal necrotic areas. (**b**) EBER in situ hybridization discloses infection in more than 50% of the tumor cell nuclei by the EBV virus

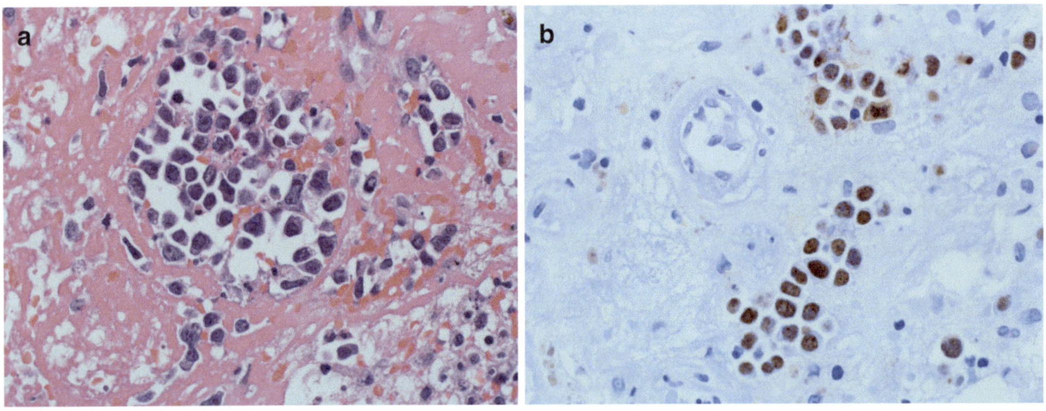

Fig. 2.14 Primary effusion lymphoma (PEL). (**a**) Cytomorphological evaluation of a pleural effusion, disclosing large atypical cells with abundant cytoplasm, irregular nuclei, and prominent nucleoli. (**b**) Nuclear expression of the latency-associated nuclear antigen (LANA) proves infection of the tumor cells by the HHV8/KSHV virus

cavity or in the pericardium (Fig. 2.14a). Infection of the tumor cells by the Kaposi sarcoma herpes/human herpes virus 8 (KSHV/HHV8) (Fig. 2.14b) is characteristic [197, 198]. PEL is a disease of HIV-infected patients and, in this setting, it is also associated with EBV infection. Rare cases of HHV8-positive but EBV-negative cases have been described in immunocompetent patients [199]. PEL associated with HIV infection features malignant effusion without solid tumor infiltrations. Only rarely, there is tumor propagation into the lung, the mediastinum, or regional lymph nodes. On microscopy, centroblastic, immunoblastic, or anaplastic tumor cells are shed into body cavities. The tumor cells are positive for the pan leucocyte antigen (CD45) and activation-associated proteins like HLA-DR and CD30; B-cell specific antigens including immunoglobulins and PAX5 are not expressed. Rarely, aberrant co-expression of T-cell antigens is seen. Characteristically, a nuclear reactivity for the HHV8 latency-associated nuclear antigen (LANA) (Fig. 2.14b) and co-infection with EBV is observed. PEL-like effusion lymphomas without HHV8 may be seen in elderly patients mainly in the peritoneum [200]. Rarely, PEL may manifest as an extrapleural solid tumor without effusion [201]. Immunoglobulin genes are clonally rearranged. Classical cytogenetic analyses have revealed complex karyotypic alterations, but no recurrent aberration has been identified so far.

2.4.11 Diffuse Large B-Cell Lymphoma Associated with Chronic Inflammation

This DLBCL subtype arises in the context of usually long-standing chronic inflammation and involves body cavities or narrow spaces such as the joints. Pyothorax-associated lymphoma (PAL) is the classical form frequently arising in the pleural cavity in the setting of long-standing pyothorax. Most patients are in their fifth to eighth decade, and usually there is a long interval (>20–30 years) between the onset of chronic inflammation and the diagnosis of malignant lymphoma. Most patients present with localized disease [202, 203], and common sites are the pleural cavity, bone, and periarticular soft tissues, with possible invasion of adjacent structures. On histology, the infiltrating blasts are either of centroblastic or immunoblastic type. Immunophenotyping shows the expression of pan B-cell markers and usually a non-GCB expression profile with reactivity for IRF4/MUM1 and negativity for CD10 and BCL6. Occasionally, aberrant expression of T-cell markers may occur [204]. Common genetic features of PAL are *MYC* amplifications, *TP53* mutations, and deletions of *TNFAIP3/A20*. Immunoglobulin genes are clonally rearranged [205, 206].

2.4.12 Lymphomatoid Granulomatosis

Lymphomatoid granulomatosis (LYG) is an angiocentric and angiodestructive lymphoproliferative disorder associated with EBV-positive B-cell blasts in a predominantly reactive background [207]. Most cases of LYG arise in healthy individuals, but the disease can also be seen in immune deficiencies of varying cause, especially iatrogenic immunosuppression. It is usually a disease of adulthood, and most cases occur in the fourth to sixth decade of life, with a male predominance. LYG mainly presents with pulmonary disease and can also manifest in the CNS, skin, liver, and kidneys. In contrast, lymph node, splenic, and bone marrow involvement is uncommon. Presenting clinical symptoms are unspecific. The radiologic hallmark of the disease is bilateral nodular infiltration of the lungs. Histology shows angiocentric and angiodestructive polymorphous infiltrates with lymphocytes, histiocytes, and large atypical lymphoid cells and tissue necrosis [208]. The EBV-associated B cells vary in size and correspond to lymphocytes, blasts, and/or HRS-like cells. Grading of LYG is based on the number of EBV-positive cells. Grade 1 lesions contain a minority of large atypical cells within a rich polymorphous background, and EBER in situ hybridization highlights fewer than five cells per HPF. In grade 3 lesions, the large atypical cells are readily seen and may form smaller or larger aggregates. In case of a uniform infiltration of EBV-positive blasts without the characteristic background of LYG, a diagnosis of EBV-associated DLBCL, NOS, is warranted. On immunophenotyping, the EBV-positive blasts express CD20, PAX5 or CD79a, and CD30 in many cases, but CD15 is negative. LYG frequently shows an EBV latency pattern III with positivity for LMP1, EBNA2, and EBER. Clonal IG rearrangements are usually seen in grades 2 and 3 [209].

2.4.13 HHV8-Positive Diffuse Large B-Cell Lymphoma, NOS

HHV8-positive DLBCL, NOS is a new disease category in the 2016 update of the WHO classification. It forms part of the spectrum of KSHV/HHV8-associated lymphoproliferative disorders and is considered a large B-cell lymphoma that frequently, but not invariably, arises in the background of multicentric Castleman's disease (MCD) [210]. The KSHV/HHV8-positive plasmablasts are usually negative for CD45 and CD20, strongly express the KSHV/HHV8 latency-associated nuclear antigen (LANA), and show monoclonal cytoplasmic IgM/λ staining [211]. They often represent a tumor form of the

KSHV-/HHV8-infected plasmablasts encountered in MCD in HIV-infected individuals.

2.5 Concluding Remarks

During the past decade, our understanding of the pathogenesis of DLBCL, particularly of its most common subtypes DLBCL NOS and PMBCL, has improved substantially, owing in part to the implementation of powerful genomic technologies. We have now identified a number of pathways that are recurrently dysregulated by genetic alterations in this disease and are emerging as central players in tumor development and maintenance. These lesions reveal vulnerabilities in the lymphoma cells, which are often uniquely associated with distinct lymphoma subtypes and could thus be exploited for patient stratification and for the design of more effective, possibly less toxic-targeted therapeutic approaches. Indeed, the information gained from these studies is already being translated into the development and clinical testing (or repositioning) of novel drugs/drug combinations directed against specifically disrupted programs in DLBCL. While these strategies are expected to impact the standard of care for this malignancy, the complexity of the involved pathways and the overall heterogeneity of the disease, which may also involve non-genetic mechanisms, underscores the need of precise patient stratification in order to identify sensitive and resistant cases.

Acknowledgments The authors wish to thank Drs. Annette Staiger and Heike Horn for helpful discussions and editorial help and Dr. Marco Fangazio for help with Figs. 2.5 and 2.6.

References

1. Swerdlow SH, Campo E, Pileri SA, et al. The 2016 revision of the World Health Organization classification of lymphoid neoplasms. Blood. 2016;127:2375–90.
2. Swerdlow SH Campo E, Harris NL, Jaffe ES, Pileri SA, Stein H, Thiele J. WHO classification of haematopoietic and lymphoid tissues. Revised 4th ed. Lyon: IARC; 2017.
3. Swerdlow SH, Campo E, Harris NL, et al. WHO classification of tumors of haematopoietic and lymphoid tissues. In: Bosman FT, Jaffe ES, Lakhani SR, Ohgaki H, editors. World Health Organization of tumor. Lyon: International Agency for Research on Cancer (IARC); 2008.
4. Jaffe ES, Arber DA, Campo E, Harris NL, Quintanilla-Fend L. Hematopathology. Philadelphia: Saunders/Elsevier; 2017.
5. Rosenwald A, Wright G, Chan WC, et al. The use of molecular profiling to predict survival after chemotherapy for diffuse large-B-cell lymphoma. N Engl J Med. 2002;346:1937–47.
6. Engelhard M, Brittinger G, Huhn D, et al. Subclassification of diffuse large B-cell lymphomas according to the Kiel classification: distinction of centroblastic and immunoblastic lymphomas is a significant prognostic risk factor. Blood. 1997;89:2291–7.
7. Lennert K, Feller AC. High grade malignant lymphoma of B-cell type. Histopathology of non-Hodgkin's lymphoma. Berlin: Springer; 1990.
8. Ott G, Ziepert M, Klapper W, et al. Immunoblastic morphology but not the immunohistochemical GCB/nonGCB classifier predicts outcome in diffuse large B-cell lymphoma in the RICOVER-60 trial of the DSHNHL. Blood. 2010;116:4916–25.
9. Horn H, Ziepert M, Becher C, et al. MYC status in concert with BCL2 and BCL6 expression predicts outcome in diffuse large B-cell lymphoma. Blood. 2013;121:2253–63.
10. Johnson NA, Slack GW, Savage KJ, et al. Concurrent expression of MYC and BCL2 in diffuse large B-cell lymphoma treated with rituximab plus cyclophosphamide, doxorubicin, vincristine, and prednisone. J Clin Oncol. 2012;30:3452–9.
11. Perry AM, Alvarado-Bernal Y, Laurini JA, et al. MYC and BCL2 protein expression predicts survival in patients with diffuse large B-cell lymphoma treated with rituximab. Br J Haematol. 2014;165:382–91.
12. Petrella T, Copie-Bergman C, Briere J, et al. BCL2 expression but not MYC and BCL2 coexpression predicts survival in elderly patients with diffuse large B-cell lymphoma independently of cell of origin in the phase 3 LNH03-6B trial. Ann Oncol. 2017;28(5):1042–9.
13. Valera A, Lopez-Guillermo A, Cardesa-Salzmann T, et al. MYC protein expression and genetic alterations have prognostic impact in patients with diffuse large B-cell lymphoma treated with immunochemotherapy. Haematologica. 2013;98:1554–62.
14. Kuppers R, Klein U, Hansmann ML, Rajewsky K. Cellular origin of human B-cell lymphomas. N Engl J Med. 1999;341:1520–9.
15. Alizadeh AA, Eisen MB, Davis RE, et al. Distinct types of diffuse large B-cell lymphoma identified by gene expression profiling. Nature. 2000;403:503–11.
16. Victora GD, Dominguez-Sola D, Holmes AB, Deroubaix S, Dalla-Favera R, Nussenzweig

MC. Identification of human germinal center light and dark zone cells and their relationship to human B-cell lymphomas. Blood. 2012;120:2240–8.

17. Lenz G, Wright GW, Emre NC, et al. Molecular subtypes of diffuse large B-cell lymphoma arise by distinct genetic pathways. Proc Natl Acad Sci U S A. 2008;105:13520–5.
18. Pasqualucci L, Dalla-Favera R. The genetic landscape of diffuse large B-cell lymphoma. Semin Hematol. 2015;52:67–76.
19. Horn H, Staiger AM, Ott G. New targeted therapies for malignant lymphoma based on molecular heterogeneity. Expert Rev Hematol. 2017;10:39–51.
20. Rovira J, Karube K, Valera A, et al. MYD88 L265P mutations, but no other variants, identify a subpopulation of DLBCL patients of activated B-cell origin, extranodal involvement, and poor outcome. Clin Cancer Res. 2016;22:2755–64.
21. Paul U, Richter J, Stuhlmann-Laiesz C, et al. Advanced patient age at diagnosis of diffuse large B-cell lymphoma is associated with molecular characteristics including ABC-subtype and high expression of MYC. Leuk Lymphoma. 2018;59(5):1213–21.
22. Hans CP, Weisenburger DD, Greiner TC, et al. Confirmation of the molecular classification of diffuse large B-cell lymphoma by immunohistochemistry using a tissue microarray. Blood. 2004;103:275–82.
23. Choi WW, Weisenburger DD, Greiner TC, et al. A new immunostain algorithm classifies diffuse large B-cell lymphoma into molecular subtypes with high accuracy. Clin Cancer Res. 2009;15:5494–502.
24. Salles G, Dd J, Xie W, et al. Prognostic significance of immunohistochemical biomarkers in diffuse large B-cell lymphoma: a study from the Lunenburg Lymphoma Biomarker Consortium. Blood. 2011;117:7070–8.
25. Coutinho R, Clear AJ, Owen A, et al. Poor concordance among nine immunohistochemistry classifiers of cell-of-origin for diffuse large B-cell lymphoma: implications for therapeutic strategies. Clin Cancer Res. 2013;19:6686–95.
26. Scott DW, Mottok A, Ennishi D, et al. Prognostic significance of diffuse large B-cell lymphoma cell of origin determined by digital gene expression in formalin-fixed paraffin-embedded tissue biopsies. J Clin Oncol. 2015;33:2848–56.
27. Scott DW, Wright GW, Williams PM, et al. Determining cell-of-origin subtypes of diffuse large B-cell lymphoma using gene expression in formalin-fixed paraffin-embedded tissue. Blood. 2014;123:1214–7.
28. Morin RD, Mendez-Lago M, Mungall AJ, et al. Frequent mutation of histone-modifying genes in non-Hodgkin lymphoma. Nature. 2011;476:298–303.
29. Pasqualucci L, Trifonov V, Fabbri G, et al. Analysis of the coding genome of diffuse large B-cell lymphoma. Nat Genet. 2011;43:830–7.
30. Lohr JG, Stojanov P, Lawrence MS, et al. Discovery and prioritization of somatic mutations in diffuse large B-cell lymphoma (DLBCL) by whole-exome sequencing. Proc Natl Acad Sci U S A. 2012;109:3879–84.
31. Zhang J, Grubor V, Love CL, et al. Genetic heterogeneity of diffuse large B-cell lymphoma. Proc Natl Acad Sci U S A. 2013;110:1398–403.
32. Reddy A, Zhang J, Davis NS, et al. Genetic and functional drivers of diffuse large B cell lymphoma. Cell. 2017;171:481–94 e15.
33. Meng FL, Du Z, Federation A, et al. Convergent transcription at intragenic super-enhancers targets AID-initiated genomic instability. Cell. 2014;159:1538–48.
34. Qian J, Wang Q, Dose M, et al. B cell super-enhancers and regulatory clusters recruit AID tumorigenic activity. Cell. 2014;159:1524–37.
35. Green MR, Gentles AJ, Nair RV, et al. Hierarchy in somatic mutations arising during genomic evolution and progression of follicular lymphoma. Blood. 2013;121:1604–11.
36. Green MR, Kihira S, Liu CL, et al. Mutations in early follicular lymphoma progenitors are associated with suppressed antigen presentation. Proc Natl Acad Sci U S A. 2015;112:E1116–25.
37. Okosun J, Bodor C, Wang J, et al. Integrated genomic analysis identifies recurrent mutations and evolution patterns driving the initiation and progression of follicular lymphoma. Nat Genet. 2014;46:176–81.
38. Pasqualucci L, Khiabanian H, Fangazio M, et al. Genetics of follicular lymphoma transformation. Cell Rep. 2014;6:130–40.
39. Pasqualucci L, Dominguez-Sola D, Chiarenza A, et al. Inactivating mutations of acetyltransferase genes in B-cell lymphoma. Nature. 2011;471:189–95.
40. Goodman RH, Smolik S. CBP/p300 in cell growth, transformation, and development. Genes Dev. 2000;14:1553–77.
41. Zhang J, Vlasevska S, Wells VA, et al. The CREBBP acetyltransferase is a haploinsufficient tumor suppressor in B-cell lymphoma. Cancer Discov. 2017;7:322–37.
42. Bereshchenko OR, Gu W, Dalla-Favera R. Acetylation inactivates the transcriptional repressor BCL6. Nat Genet. 2002;32:606–13.
43. Gu W, Roeder RG. Activation of p53 sequence-specific DNA binding by acetylation of the p53 C-terminal domain. Cell. 1997;90:595–606.
44. Tang Y, Zhao W, Chen Y, Zhao Y, Gu W. Acetylation is indispensable for p53 activation. Cell. 2008;133:612–26.
45. Phan RT, Dalla-Favera R. The BCL6 proto-oncogene suppresses p53 expression in germinal-centre B cells. Nature. 2004;432:635–9.
46. Shilatifard A. The COMPASS family of histone H3K4 methylases: mechanisms of regulation in development and disease pathogenesis. Annu Rev Biochem. 2012;81:65–95.
47. Ortega-Molina A, Boss IW, Canela A, et al. The histone lysine methyltransferase KMT2D sustains a

gene expression program that represses B cell lymphoma development. Nat Med. 2015;21:1199–208.
48. Zhang J, Dominguez-Sola D, Hussein S, et al. Disruption of KMT2D perturbs germinal center B cell development and promotes lymphomagenesis. Nat Med. 2015;21:1190–8.
49. Hatzi K, Melnick A. Breaking bad in the germinal center: how deregulation of BCL6 contributes to lymphomagenesis. Trends Mol Med. 2014;20:343–52.
50. Basso K, Dalla-Favera R. Roles of BCL6 in normal and transformed germinal center B cells. Immunol Rev. 2012;247:172–83.
51. Phan RT, Saito M, Basso K, Niu H, Dalla-Favera R. BCL6 interacts with the transcription factor Miz-1 to suppress the cyclin-dependent kinase inhibitor p21 and cell cycle arrest in germinal center B cells. Nat Immunol. 2005;6:1054–60.
52. Ranuncolo SM, Polo JM, Dierov J, et al. Bcl-6 mediates the germinal center B cell phenotype and lymphomagenesis through transcriptional repression of the DNA-damage sensor ATR. Nat Immunol. 2007;8:705–14.
53. Ranuncolo SM, Polo JM, Melnick A. BCL6 represses CHEK1 and suppresses DNA damage pathways in normal and malignant B-cells. Blood Cells Mol Dis. 2008;41:95–9.
54. Basso K, Saito M, Sumazin P, et al. Integrated biochemical and computational approach identifies BCL6 direct target genes controlling multiple pathways in normal germinal center B cells. Blood. 2010;115:975–84.
55. Ci W, Polo JM, Cerchietti L, et al. The BCL6 transcriptional program features repression of multiple oncogenes in primary B cells and is deregulated in DLBCL. Blood. 2009;113:5536–48.
56. Tunyaplin C, Shaffer AL, Angelin-Duclos CD, Yu X, Staudt LM, Calame KL. Direct repression of prdm1 by Bcl-6 inhibits plasmacytic differentiation. J Immunol. 2004;173:1158–65.
57. Iqbal J, Greiner TC, Patel K, et al. Distinctive patterns of BCL6 molecular alterations and their functional consequences in different subgroups of diffuse large B-cell lymphoma. Leukemia. 2007;21:2332–43.
58. Ye BH, Lista F, Lo Coco F, et al. Alterations of a zinc finger-encoding gene, BCL-6, in diffuse large-cell lymphoma. Science. 1993;262:747–50.
59. Ye BH, Rao PH, Chaganti RS, Dalla-Favera R. Cloning of bcl-6, the locus involved in chromosome translocations affecting band 3q27 in B-cell lymphoma. Cancer Res. 1993;53:2732–5.
60. Baron BW, Nucifora G, McCabe N, Espinosa R 3rd, Le Beau MM, McKeithan TW. Identification of the gene associated with the recurring chromosomal translocations t(3;14)(q27;q32) and t(3;22)(q27;q11) in B-cell lymphomas. Proc Natl Acad Sci U S A. 1993;90:5262–6.
61. Kerckaert JP, Deweindt C, Tilly H, Quief S, Lecocq G, Bastard C. LAZ3, a novel zinc-finger encoding gene, is disrupted by recurring chromosome 3q27 translocations in human lymphomas. Nat Genet. 1993;5:66–70.
62. Butler MP, Iida S, Capello D, et al. Alternative translocation breakpoint cluster region 5′ to BCL-6 in B-cell non-Hodgkin's lymphoma. Cancer Res. 2002;62:4089–94.
63. Ye BH, Chaganti S, Chang CC, et al. Chromosomal translocations cause deregulated BCL6 expression by promoter substitution in B cell lymphoma. EMBO J. 1995;14:6209–17.
64. Pasqualucci L, Migliazza A, Fracchiolla N, et al. BCL-6 mutations in normal germinal center B cells: evidence of somatic hypermutation acting outside Ig loci. Proc Natl Acad Sci U S A. 1998;95:11816–21.
65. Shen HM, Peters A, Baron B, Zhu X, Storb U. Mutation of BCL-6 gene in normal B cells by the process of somatic hypermutation of Ig genes. Science. 1998;280:1750–2.
66. Pasqualucci L, Migliazza A, Basso K, Houldsworth J, Chaganti RS, Dalla-Favera R. Mutations of the BCL6 proto-oncogene disrupt its negative autoregulation in diffuse large B-cell lymphoma. Blood. 2003;101:2914–23.
67. Wang X, Li Z, Naganuma A, Ye BH. Negative autoregulation of BCL-6 is bypassed by genetic alterations in diffuse large B cell lymphomas. Proc Natl Acad Sci U S A. 2002;99:15018–23.
68. Saito M, Gao J, Basso K, et al. A signaling pathway mediating downregulation of BCL6 in germinal center B cells is blocked by BCL6 gene alterations in B cell lymphoma. Cancer Cell. 2007;12:280–92.
69. Jiang Y, Ortega-Molina A, Geng H, et al. CREBBP inactivation promotes the development of HDAC3-dependent lymphomas. Cancer Discov. 2017;7:38–53.
70. Ying CY, Dominguez-Sola D, Fabi M, et al. MEF2B mutations lead to deregulated expression of the oncogene BCL6 in diffuse large B cell lymphoma. Nat Immunol. 2013;14:1084–92.
71. Brescia P, Schneider C, Holmes AB, et al. MEF2B instructs germinal center development and acts as an oncogene in B cell lymphomagenesis. Cancer Cell. 2018;34:453–65.
72. Duan S, Cermak L, Pagan JK, et al. FBXO11 targets BCL6 for degradation and is inactivated in diffuse large B-cell lymphomas. Nature. 2012;481:90–3.
73. Cattoretti G, Pasqualucci L, Ballon G, et al. Deregulated BCL6 expression recapitulates the pathogenesis of human diffuse large B cell lymphomas in mice. Cancer Cell. 2005;7:445–55.
74. Schneider C, Kon N, Amadori L, et al. FBXO11 inactivation leads to abnormal germinal-center formation and lymphoproliferative disease. Blood. 2016;128:660–6.
75. Cerchietti LC, Ghetu AF, Zhu X, et al. A small-molecule inhibitor of BCL6 kills DLBCL cells in vitro and in vivo. Cancer Cell. 2010;17:400–11.
76. Cerchietti LC, Lopes EC, Yang SN, et al. A purine scaffold Hsp90 inhibitor destabilizes BCL-6 and has

specific antitumor activity in BCL-6-dependent B cell lymphomas. Nat Med. 2009;15:1369–76.
77. Fangazio M, Dominguez-Sola D, Tabbo F, et al. Genetic mechanisms of immune escape in diffuse large B cell lymphoma. Blood. 2014;124:1692.
78. Challa-Malladi M, Lieu YK, Califano O, et al. Combined genetic inactivation of beta2-microglobulin and CD58 reveals frequent escape from immune recognition in diffuse large B cell lymphoma. Cancer Cell. 2011;20:728–40.
79. Kridel R, Chan FC, Mottok A, et al. Histological transformation and progression in follicular lymphoma: a clonal evolution study. PLoS Med. 2016;13:e1002197.
80. Moingeon P, Chang HC, Wallner BP, Stebbins C, Frey AZ, Reinherz EL. CD2-mediated adhesion facilitates T lymphocyte antigen recognition function. Nature. 1989;339:312–4.
81. Rimsza LM, Roberts RA, Miller TP, et al. Loss of MHC class II gene and protein expression in diffuse large B-cell lymphoma is related to decreased tumor immunosurveillance and poor patient survival regardless of other prognostic factors: a follow-up study from the Leukemia and Lymphoma Molecular Profiling Project. Blood. 2004;103:4251–8.
82. Mottok A, Woolcock B, Chan FC, et al. Genomic alterations in CIITA are frequent in primary mediastinal large B cell lymphoma and are associated with diminished MHC class II expression. Cell Rep. 2015;13:1418–31.
83. Steidl C, Shah SP, Woolcock BW, et al. MHC class II transactivator CIITA is a recurrent gene fusion partner in lymphoid cancers. Nature. 2011;471:377–81.
84. Hashwah H, Schmid CA, Kasser S, et al. Inactivation of CREBBP expands the germinal center B cell compartment, down-regulates MHCII expression and promotes DLBCL growth. Proc Natl Acad Sci U S A. 2017;114:9701–6.
85. Dominguez-Sola D, Kung J, Wells VA, et al. Role of FOXO1 in germinal center development and lymphomagenesis. Blood. 2014;124:3536.
86. Sander S, Chu VT, Yasuda T, et al. PI3 kinase and FOXO1 transcription factor activity differentially control B cells in the germinal center light and dark zones. Immunity. 2015;43:1075–86.
87. Trinh DL, Scott DW, Morin RD, et al. Analysis of FOXO1 mutations in diffuse large B-cell lymphoma. Blood. 2013;121:3666–74.
88. Morin RD, Assouline S, Alcaide M, et al. Genetic landscapes of relapsed and refractory diffuse large B-cell lymphomas. Clin Cancer Res. 2016;22:2290–300.
89. Hata AN, Engelman JA, Faber AC. The BCL2 family: key mediators of the apoptotic response to targeted anticancer therapeutics. Cancer Discov. 2015;5:475–87.
90. Saito M, Novak U, Piovan E, et al. BCL6 suppression of BCL2 via Miz1 and its disruption in diffuse large B cell lymphoma. Proc Natl Acad Sci U S A. 2009;106:11294–9.
91. Iqbal J, Sanger WG, Horsman DE, et al. BCL2 translocation defines a unique tumor subset within the germinal center B-cell-like diffuse large B-cell lymphoma. Am J Pathol. 2004;165:159–66.
92. Schuetz JM, Johnson NA, Morin RD, et al. BCL2 mutations in diffuse large B-cell lymphoma. Leukemia. 2012;26:1383–90.
93. Barrans SL, Evans PA, O'Connor SJ, et al. The t(14;18) is associated with germinal center-derived diffuse large B-cell lymphoma and is a strong predictor of outcome. Clin Cancer Res. 2003;9:2133–9.
94. Conacci-Sorrell M, McFerrin L, Eisenman RN. An overview of MYC and its interactome. Cold Spring Harb Perspect Med. 2014;4:a014357.
95. Dominguez-Sola D, Ying CY, Grandori C, et al. Non-transcriptional control of DNA replication by c-Myc. Nature. 2007;448:445–51.
96. Dalla-Favera R, Bregni M, Erikson J, Patterson D, Gallo RC, Croce CM. Human c-myc onc gene is located on the region of chromosome 8 that is translocated in Burkitt lymphoma cells. Proc Natl Acad Sci U S A. 1982;79:7824–7.
97. Dalla-Favera R, Martinotti S, Gallo RC, Erikson J, Croce CM. Translocation and rearrangements of the c-myc oncogene locus in human undifferentiated B-cell lymphomas. Science. 1983;219:963–7.
98. Ladanyi M, Offit K, Jhanwar SC, Filippa DA, Chaganti RS. MYC rearrangement and translocations involving band 8q24 in diffuse large cell lymphomas. Blood. 1991;77:1057–63.
99. Karube K, Campo E. MYC alterations in diffuse large B-cell lymphomas. Semin Hematol. 2015;52:97–106.
100. Dominguez-Sola D, Victora GD, Ying CY, et al. The proto-oncogene MYC is required for selection in the germinal center and cyclic reentry. Nat Immunol. 2012;13:1083–91.
101. Copie-Bergman C, Cuillière-Dartigues P, Baia M, et al. *MYC-IG* rearrangements are negative predictors of survival in DLBCL patients treated with immunochemotherapy: a GELA/LYSA study. Blood. 2015;126:2466–74. https://doi.org/10.1182/blood-2015-05-647602.
102. Mahmoudi T, Verrijzer CP. Chromatin silencing and activation by Polycomb and trithorax group proteins. Oncogene. 2001;20:3055–66.
103. Czermin B, Melfi R, McCabe D, Seitz V, Imhof A, Pirrotta V. Drosophila enhancer of Zeste/ESC complexes have a histone H3 methyltransferase activity that marks chromosomal Polycomb sites. Cell. 2002;111:185–96.
104. Cao R, Wang L, Wang H, et al. Role of histone H3 lysine 27 methylation in Polycomb-group silencing. Science. 2002;298:1039–43.
105. Bernstein BE, Mikkelsen TS, Xie X, et al. A bivalent chromatin structure marks key developmental genes in embryonic stem cells. Cell. 2006;125:315–26.
106. Beguelin W, Popovic R, Teater M, et al. EZH2 is required for germinal center formation and somatic

EZH2 mutations promote lymphoid transformation. Cancer Cell. 2013;23:677–92.
107. Caganova M, Carrisi C, Varano G, et al. Germinal center dysregulation by histone methyltransferase EZH2 promotes lymphomagenesis. J Clin Invest. 2013;123:5009–22.
108. Morin RD, Johnson NA, Severson TM, et al. Somatic mutations altering EZH2 (Tyr641) in follicular and diffuse large B-cell lymphomas of germinal-center origin. Nat Genet. 2010;42:181–5.
109. Sneeringer CJ, Scott MP, Kuntz KW, et al. Coordinated activities of wild-type plus mutant EZH2 drive tumor-associated hypertrimethylation of lysine 27 on histone H3 (H3K27) in human B-cell lymphomas. Proc Natl Acad Sci U S A. 2010;107:20980–5.
110. Yap DB, Chu J, Berg T, et al. Somatic mutations at EZH2 Y641 act dominantly through a mechanism of selectively altered PRC2 catalytic activity, to increase H3K27 trimethylation. Blood. 2011;117:2451–9.
111. McCabe MT, Graves AP, Ganji G, et al. Mutation of A677 in histone methyltransferase EZH2 in human B-cell lymphoma promotes hypertrimethylation of histone H3 on lysine 27 (H3K27). Proc Natl Acad Sci U S A. 2012;109:2989–94.
112. Knutson SK, Wigle TJ, Warholic NM, et al. A selective inhibitor of EZH2 blocks H3K27 methylation and kills mutant lymphoma cells. Nat Chem Biol. 2012;8:890–6.
113. McCabe MT, Ott HM, Ganji G, et al. EZH2 inhibition as a therapeutic strategy for lymphoma with EZH2-activating mutations. Nature. 2012;492:108–12.
114. Morschhauser F, Salles GA, McKay P, et al. Interim report from a phase 2 multicenter study of tazemetostat, an EZH2 inhibitor, in patients with relapsed or refractory B-cell non-Hodgkin lymphomas. Hematol Oncol. 2017;35(suppl S2):24–5. https://doi.org/10.1002/hon.2437_3.
115. Green JA, Cyster JG. S1PR2 links germinal center confinement and growth regulation. Immunol Rev. 2012;247:36–51.
116. Muppidi JR, Schmitz R, Green JA, et al. Loss of signalling via Galpha13 in germinal centre B-cell-derived lymphoma. Nature. 2014;516(7530):254–8.
117. Cattoretti G, Mandelbaum J, Lee N, et al. Targeted disruption of the S1P2 sphingosine 1-phosphate receptor gene leads to diffuse large B-cell lymphoma formation. Cancer Res. 2009;69:8686–92.
118. Steinberg MW, Cheung TC, Ware CF. The signaling networks of the herpesvirus entry mediator (TNFRSF14) in immune regulation. Immunol Rev. 2011;244:169–87.
119. Boice M, Salloum D, Mourcin F, et al. Loss of the HVEM tumor suppressor in lymphoma and restoration by modified CAR-T Cells. Cell. 2016;167:405–18 e13.
120. Pfeifer M, Grau M, Lenze D, et al. PTEN loss defines a PI3K/AKT pathway-dependent germinal center subtype of diffuse large B-cell lymphoma. Proc Natl Acad Sci U S A. 2013;110:12420–5.
121. Brunet A, Park J, Tran H, Hu LS, Hemmings BA, Greenberg ME. Protein kinase SGK mediates survival signals by phosphorylating the forkhead transcription factor FKHRL1 (FOXO3a). Mol Cell Biol. 2001;21:952–65.
122. Tai DJ, Su CC, Ma YL, Lee EH. SGK1 phosphorylation of IkappaB Kinase alpha and p300 Up-regulates NF-kappaB activity and increases N-Methyl-D-aspartate receptor NR2A and NR2B expression. J Biol Chem. 2009;284:4073–89.
123. Mo JS, Ann EJ, Yoon JH, et al. Serum- and glucocorticoid-inducible kinase 1 (SGK1) controls Notch1 signaling by downregulation of protein stability through Fbw7 ubiquitin ligase. J Cell Sci. 2011;124:100–12.
124. Davis RE, Ngo VN, Lenz G, et al. Chronic active B-cell-receptor signalling in diffuse large B-cell lymphoma. Nature. 2010;463:88–92.
125. Lenz G, Davis RE, Ngo VN, et al. Oncogenic CARD11 mutations in human diffuse large B cell lymphoma. Science. 2008;319:1676–9.
126. Thome M. CARMA1, BCL-10 and MALT1 in lymphocyte development and activation. Nat Rev Immunol. 2004;4:348–59.
127. Young RM, Wu T, Schmitz R, et al. Survival of human lymphoma cells requires B-cell receptor engagement by self-antigens. Proc Natl Acad Sci U S A. 2015;112:13447–54.
128. Wilson WH, Young RM, Schmitz R, et al. Targeting B cell receptor signaling with ibrutinib in diffuse large B cell lymphoma. Nat Med. 2015;21:922–6.
129. Lin SC, Lo YC, Wu H. Helical assembly in the MyD88-IRAK4-IRAK2 complex in TLR/IL-1R signalling. Nature. 2010;465:885–90.
130. Ngo VN, Young RM, Schmitz R, et al. Oncogenically active MYD88 mutations in human lymphoma. Nature. 2011;470:115–9.
131. Lam LT, Wright G, Davis RE, et al. Cooperative signaling through the signal transducer and activator of transcription 3 and nuclear factor-{kappa}B pathways in subtypes of diffuse large B-cell lymphoma. Blood. 2008;111:3701–13.
132. Boone DL, Turer EE, Lee EG, et al. The ubiquitin-modifying enzyme A20 is required for termination of Toll-like receptor responses. Nat Immunol. 2004;5:1052–60.
133. Compagno M, Lim WK, Grunn A, et al. Mutations of multiple genes cause deregulation of NF-kappaB in diffuse large B-cell lymphoma. Nature. 2009;459:717–21.
134. Kato M, Sanada M, Kato I, et al. Frequent inactivation of A20 in B-cell lymphomas. Nature. 2009;459:712–6.
135. Mandelbaum J, Bhagat G, Tang H, et al. BLIMP1 is a tumor suppressor gene frequently disrupted in activated B cell-like diffuse large B cell lymphoma. Cancer Cell. 2010;18:568–79.
136. Pasqualucci L, Compagno M, Houldsworth J, et al. Inactivation of the PRDM1/BLIMP1 gene in diffuse large B cell lymphoma. J Exp Med. 2006;203:311–7.

137. Tam W, Gomez M, Chadburn A, Lee JW, Chan WC, Knowles DM. Mutational analysis of PRDM1 indicates a tumor-suppressor role in diffuse large B-cell lymphomas. Blood. 2006;107:4090–100.
138. Calado DP, Zhang B, Srinivasan L, et al. Constitutive canonical NF-kappaB activation cooperates with disruption of BLIMP1 in the pathogenesis of activated B cell-like diffuse large cell lymphoma. Cancer Cell. 2010;18:580–9.
139. Swerdlow SH, Campo E, Harris NL, et al. WHO classification of tumours of haematopoetic and lymphoid tissues. Lyon: IARC Press; 2008.
140. Kluk MJ, Ho C, Yu H, et al. MYC immunohistochemistry to identify MYC-driven B-cell lymphomas in clinical practice. Am J Clin Pathol. 2016;145:166–79.
141. Pillai RK, Sathanoori M, van Oss SB, Swerdlow SH. Double-hit B-cell lymphomas with BCL6 and MYC translocations are aggressive, frequently extranodal lymphomas distinct from BCL2 double-hit B-cell lymphomas. Am J Surg Pathol. 2013;37:323–32.
142. Turakhia SK, Hill BT, Dufresne SD, Nakashima MO, Cotta CV. Aggressive B-cell lymphomas with translocations involving BCL6 and MYC have distinct clinical-pathologic characteristics. Am J Clin Pathol. 2014;142:339–46.
143. Delabie J, Vandenberghe E, Kennes C, et al. Histiocyte-rich B-cell lymphoma. A distinct clinicopathologic entity possibly related to lymphocyte predominant Hodgkin's disease, paragranuloma subtype. Am J Surg Pathol. 1992;16:37–48.
144. Boudova L, Torlakovic E, Delabie J, et al. Nodular lymphocyte-predominant Hodgkin lymphoma with nodules resembling T-cell/histiocyte-rich B-cell lymphoma: differential diagnosis between nodular lymphocyte-predominant Hodgkin lymphoma and T-cell/histiocyte-rich B-cell lymphoma. Blood. 2003;102:3753–8.
145. Hartmann S, Doring C, Jakobus C, et al. Nodular lymphocyte predominant Hodgkin lymphoma and T cell/histiocyte rich large B cell lymphoma—endpoints of a spectrum of one disease? PLoS One. 2013;8:e78812.
146. Ponzoni M, Ferreri AJ, Campo E, et al. Definition, diagnosis, and management of intravascular large B-cell lymphoma: proposals and perspectives from an international consensus meeting. J Clin Oncol. 2007;25:3168–73.
147. Delecluse HJ, Anagnostopoulos I, Dallenbach F, et al. Plasmablastic lymphomas of the oral cavity: a new entity associated with the human immunodeficiency virus infection. Blood. 1997;89:1413–20.
148. Montes-Moreno S, Gonzalez-Medina AR, Rodriguez-Pinilla SM, et al. Aggressive large B-cell lymphoma with plasma cell differentiation: immunohistochemical characterization of plasmablastic lymphoma and diffuse large B-cell lymphoma with partial plasmablastic phenotype. Haematologica. 2010;95:1342–9.
149. Valera A, Balague O, Colomo L, et al. IG/MYC rearrangements are the main cytogenetic alteration in plasmablastic lymphomas. Am J Surg Pathol. 2010;34:1686–94.
150. Laurent C, Do C, Gascoyne RD, et al. Anaplastic lymphoma kinase-positive diffuse large B-cell lymphoma: a rare clinicopathologic entity with poor prognosis. J Clin Oncol. 2009;27:4211–6.
151. Gascoyne RD, Lamant L, Martin-Subero JI, et al. ALK-positive diffuse large B-cell lymphoma is associated with Clathrin-ALK rearrangements: report of 6 cases. Blood. 2003;102:2568–73.
152. Pd P, Baens M, van Krieken H, et al. ALK activation by the CLTC-ALK fusion is a recurrent event in large B-cell lymphoma. Blood. 2003;102:2638–41.
153. Valera A, Colomo L, Martinez A, et al. ALK-positive large B-cell lymphomas express a terminal B-cell differentiation program and activated STAT3 but lack MYC rearrangements. Mod Pathol. 2013;26:1329–37.
154. Yuan J, Wright G, Rosenwald A, et al. Identification of primary mediastinal large B-cell lymphoma at nonmediastinal sites by gene expression profiling. Am J Surg Pathol. 2015;39:1322–30.
155. Paulli M, Strater J, Gianelli U, et al. Mediastinal B-cell lymphoma: A study of its histomorphologic spectrum based on 109 cases. Hum Pathol. 1999;30:178–87.
156. Moller P, Lammler B, Eberlein-Gonska M, et al. Primary mediastinal clear cell lymphoma of B-cell type. Virchows Arch A Pathol Anat Histopathol. 1986;409:79–92.
157. Copie-Bergman C, Plonquet A, Alonso MA, et al. MAL expression in lymphoid cells: further evidence for MAL as a distinct molecular marker of primary mediastinal large B-cell lymphomas. Mod Pathol. 2002;15:1172–80.
158. Rosenwald A, Wright G, Leroy K, et al. Molecular diagnosis of primary mediastinal B cell lymphoma identifies a clinically favorable subgroup of diffuse large B cell lymphoma related to Hodgkin lymphoma. J Exp Med. 2003;198:851–62.
159. Savage KJ, Monti S, Kutok JL, et al. The molecular signature of mediastinal large B-cell lymphoma differs from that of other diffuse large B-cell lymphomas and shares features with classical Hodgkin lymphoma. Blood. 2003;102:3871–9.
160. Gunawardana J, Chan FC, Telenius A, et al. Recurrent somatic mutations of PTPN1 in primary mediastinal B cell lymphoma and Hodgkin lymphoma. Nat Genet. 2014;46:329–35.
161. Steidl C, Gascoyne RD. The molecular pathogenesis of primary mediastinal large B-cell lymphoma. Blood. 2011;118:2659–69.
162. Twa DD, Chan FC, Ben-Neriah S, et al. Genomic rearrangements involving programmed death ligands are recurrent in primary mediastinal large B-cell lymphoma. Blood. 2014;123:2062–5.
163. Green MR, Monti S, Rodig SJ, et al. Integrative analysis reveals selective 9p24.1 amplification, increased

PD-1 ligand expression, and further induction via JAK2 in nodular sclerosing Hodgkin lymphoma and primary mediastinal large B-cell lymphoma. Blood. 2010;116:3268–77.
164. Darnell JE Jr, Kerr IM, Stark GR. Jak-STAT pathways and transcriptional activation in response to IFNs and other extracellular signaling proteins. Science. 1994;264:1415–21.
165. Joos S, Otano-Joos MI, Ziegler S, et al. Primary mediastinal (thymic) B-cell lymphoma is characterized by gains of chromosomal material including 9p and amplification of the REL gene. Blood. 1996;87:1571–8.
166. Melzner I, Bucur AJ, Bruderlein S, et al. Biallelic mutation of SOCS-1 impairs JAK2 degradation and sustains phospho-JAK2 action in the MedB-1 mediastinal lymphoma line. Blood. 2005;105:2535–42.
167. Rui L, Emre NC, Kruhlak MJ, et al. Cooperative epigenetic modulation by cancer amplicon genes. Cancer Cell. 2010;18:590–605.
168. Dawson MA, Bannister AJ, Gottgens B, et al. JAK2 phosphorylates histone H3Y41 and excludes HP1alpha from chromatin. Nature. 2009;461:819–22.
169. Guiter C, Dusanter-Fourt I, Copie-Bergman C, et al. Constitutive STAT6 activation in primary mediastinal large B-cell lymphoma. Blood. 2004;104:543–9.
170. Weniger MA, Gesk S, Ehrlich S, et al. Gains of REL in primary mediastinal B-cell lymphoma coincide with nuclear accumulation of REL protein. Genes Chromosomes Cancer. 2007;46:406–15.
171. Schmitz R, Hansmann ML, Bohle V, et al. TNFAIP3 (A20) is a tumor suppressor gene in Hodgkin lymphoma and primary mediastinal B cell lymphoma. J Exp Med. 2009;206:981–9.
172. Wessendorf S, Barth TF, Viardot A, et al. Further delineation of chromosomal consensus regions in primary mediastinal B-cell lymphomas: an analysis of 37 tumor samples using high-resolution genomic profiling (array-CGH). Leukemia. 2007;21:2463–9.
173. Scott DW, Gascoyne RD. The tumour microenvironment in B cell lymphomas. Nat Rev Cancer. 2014;14:517–34.
174. Rigaud G, Moore PS, Taruscio D, et al. Alteration of chromosome arm 6p is characteristic of primary mediastinal B-cell lymphoma, as identified by genome-wide allelotyping. Genes Chromosomes Cancer. 2001;31:191–5.
175. Roberts RA, Wright G, Rosenwald AR, et al. Loss of major histocompatibility class II gene and protein expression in primary mediastinal large B-cell lymphoma is highly coordinated and related to poor patient survival. Blood. 2006;108:311–8.
176. Wilson WH, Pittaluga S, Nicolae A, et al. A prospective study of mediastinal gray-zone lymphoma. Blood. 2014;124:1563–9.
177. Harris NL. Shades of gray between large B-cell lymphomas and Hodgkin lymphomas: differential diagnosis and biological implications. Mod Pathol. 2013;26(Suppl 1):S57–70.
178. Vermeer MH, Geelen FA, van Haselen CW, et al. Primary cutaneous large B-cell lymphomas of the legs. A distinct type of cutaneous B-cell lymphoma with an intermediate prognosis. Dutch Cutaneous Lymphoma Working Group. Arch Dermatol. 1996;132:1304–8.
179. Pham-Ledard A, Prochazkova-Carlotti M, Andrique L, et al. Multiple genetic alterations in primary cutaneous large B-cell lymphoma, leg type support a common lymphomagenesis with activated B-cell-like diffuse large B-cell lymphoma. Mod Pathol. 2014;27:402–11.
180. Camilleri-Broet S, Criniere E, Broet P, et al. A uniform activated B-cell-like immunophenotype might explain the poor prognosis of primary central nervous system lymphomas: analysis of 83 cases. Blood. 2006;107:190–6.
181. Riemersma SA, Jordanova ES, Schop RF, et al. Extensive genetic alterations of the HLA region, including homozygous deletions of HLA class II genes in B-cell lymphomas arising in immune-privileged sites. Blood. 2000;96:3569–77.
182. Rubenstein JL, Treseler P, O'Brien JM. Pathology and genetics of primary central nervous system and intraocular lymphoma. Hematol Oncol Clin North Am. 2005;19:705–17, vii.
183. Vater I, Montesinos-Rongen M, Schlesner M, et al. The mutational pattern of primary lymphoma of the central nervous system determined by whole-exome sequencing. Leukemia. 2015;29:677–85.
184. Montesinos-Rongen M, Godlewska E, Brunn A, Wiestler OD, Siebert R, Deckert M. Activating L265P mutations of the MYD88 gene are common in primary central nervous system lymphoma. Acta Neuropathol. 2011;122:791–2.
185. Gonzalez-Aguilar A, Idbaih A, Boisselier B, et al. Recurrent mutations of MYD88 and TBL1XR1 in primary central nervous system lymphomas. Clin Cancer Res. 2012;18:5203–11.
186. Montesinos-Rongen M, Schafer E, Siebert R, Deckert M. Genes regulating the B cell receptor pathway are recurrently mutated in primary central nervous system lymphoma. Acta Neuropathol. 2012;124:905–6.
187. Montesinos-Rongen M, Van Roost D, Schaller C, Wiestler OD, Deckert M. Primary diffuse large B-cell lymphomas of the central nervous system are targeted by aberrant somatic hypermutation. Blood. 2004;103:1869–75.
188. Cady FM, O'Neill BP, Law ME, et al. Del(6)(q22) and BCL6 rearrangements in primary CNS lymphoma are indicators of an aggressive clinical course. J Clin Oncol. 2008;26:4814–9.
189. Schwindt H, Vater I, Kreuz M, et al. Chromosomal imbalances and partial uniparental disomies in primary central nervous system lymphoma. Leukemia. 2009;23:1875–84.
190. Harada K, Nishizaki T, Kubota H, Harada K, Suzuki M, Sasaki K. Distinct primary central nervous system lymphoma defined by comparative genomic

hybridization and laser scanning cytometry. Cancer Genet Cytogenet. 2001;125:147–50.
191. Courts C, Montesinos-Rongen M, Brunn A, et al. Recurrent inactivation of the PRDM1 gene in primary central nervous system lymphoma. J Neuropathol Exp Neurol. 2008;67:720–7.
192. Nakamura M, Kishi M, Sakaki T, et al. Novel tumor suppressor loci on 6q22-23 in primary central nervous system lymphomas. Cancer Res. 2003;63:737–41.
193. Nicolae A, Pittaluga S, Abdullah S, et al. EBV-positive large B-cell lymphomas in young patients: a nodal lymphoma with evidence for a tolerogenic immune environment. Blood. 2015;126:863–72.
194. Sansoni P, Vescovini R, Fagnoni F, et al. The immune system in extreme longevity. Exp Gerontol. 2008;43:61–5.
195. Oyama T, Yamamoto K, Asano N, et al. Age-related EBV-associated B-cell lymphoproliferative disorders constitute a distinct clinicopathologic group: a study of 96 patients. Clin Cancer Res. 2007;13:5124–32.
196. Chen BJ, Chapuy B, Ouyang J, et al. PD-L1 expression is characteristic of a subset of aggressive B-cell lymphomas and virus-associated malignancies. Clin Cancer Res. 2013;19:3462–73.
197. Cesarman E, Chang Y, Moore PS, Said JW, Knowles DM. Kaposi's sarcoma-associated herpesvirus-like DNA sequences in AIDS-related body-cavity-based lymphomas. N Engl J Med. 1995;332:1186–91.
198. Nador RG, Cesarman E, Chadburn A, et al. Primary effusion lymphoma: a distinct clinicopathologic entity associated with the Kaposi's sarcoma-associated herpes virus. Blood. 1996;88:645–56.
199. Said JW, Tasaka T, Takeuchi S, et al. Primary effusion lymphoma in women: report of two cases of Kaposi's sarcoma herpes virus-associated effusion-based lymphoma in human immunodeficiency virus-negative women. Blood. 1996;88:3124–8.
200. Hermine O, Michel M, Buzyn-Veil A, Gessain A. Body-cavity-based lymphoma in an HIV-seronegative patient without Kaposi's sarcoma-associated herpesvirus-like DNA sequences. N Engl J Med. 1996;334:272–3.
201. Chadburn A, Hyjek E, Mathew S, Cesarman E, Said J, Knowles DM. KSHV-positive solid lymphomas represent an extra-cavitary variant of primary effusion lymphoma. Am J Surg Pathol. 2004;28:1401–16.
202. Nakatsuka S, Yao M, Hoshida Y, Yamamoto S, Iuchi K, Aozasa K. Pyothorax-associated lymphoma: a review of 106 cases. J Clin Oncol. 2002;20:4255–60.
203. Narimatsu H, Ota Y, Kami M, et al. Clinicopathological features of pyothorax-associated lymphoma; a retrospective survey involving 98 patients. Ann Oncol. 2007;18:122–8.
204. Petitjean B, Jardin F, Joly B, et al. Pyothorax-associated lymphoma: a peculiar clinicopathologic entity derived from B cells at late stage of differentiation and with occasional aberrant dual B- and T-cell phenotype. Am J Surg Pathol. 2002;26:724–32.
205. Ando M, Sato Y, Takata K, et al. A20 (TNFAIP3) deletion in Epstein-Barr virus-associated lymphoproliferative disorders/lymphomas. PLoS One. 2013;8:e56741.
206. Yamato H, Ohshima K, Suzumiya J, Kikuchi M. Evidence for local immunosuppression and demonstration of c-myc amplification in pyothorax-associated lymphoma. Histopathology. 2001;39:163–71.
207. Guinee D, Jaffe E, Kingma D, et al. Pulmonary lymphomatoid granulomatosis. Evidence for a proliferation of Epstein-Barr virus infected B-lymphocytes with a prominent T-cell component and vasculitis. Am J Surg Pathol. 1994;18:753–64.
208. Katzenstein AL, Doxtader E, Narendra S. Lymphomatoid granulomatosis: insights gained over 4 decades. Am J Surg Pathol. 2010;34:e35–48.
209. Roschewski M, Wilson WH. Lymphomatoid granulomatosis. Cancer J. 2012;18:469–74.
210. Dupin N, Diss TL, Kellam P, et al. HHV-8 is associated with a plasmablastic variant of Castleman disease that is linked to HHV-8-positive plasmablastic lymphoma. Blood. 2000;95:1406–12.
211. Du MQ, Liu H, Diss TC, et al. Kaposi sarcoma-associated herpesvirus infects monotypic (IgM lambda) but polyclonal naive B cells in Castleman disease and associated lymphoproliferative disorders. Blood. 2001;97:2130–6.

3 Pathology and Molecular Pathogenesis of Burkitt Lymphoma and Lymphoblastic Lymphoma

Hélène A. Poirel, Maria Raffaella Ambrosio, Pier Paolo Piccaluga, and Lorenzo Leoncini

3.1 Burkitt Lymphoma

3.1.1 Introduction

3.1.1.1 Definition

In the updated World Health Organization (WHO) classification of tumors of hematopoietic and lymphoid tissues, Burkitt lymphoma (BL) is defined as a mature highly aggressive B-cell neoplasm that often presents in extranodal sites or as an acute leukemia [1–3]. It is composed of monomorphic medium-sized B-cells with basophilic cytoplasm and numerous mitotic figures and is characterized by MYC protein overexpression (usually due to chromosomal translocation of *MYC* to an immunoglobulin (*IG*) locus) and variable association with Epstein-Barr virus (EBV) infection [3].

H. A. Poirel (✉)
Belgian Cancer Registry and GenHAP, Brussels, Belgium

M. R. Ambrosio · L. Leoncini
Section of Pathology, Department of Medical Biotechnology, University of Siena, Siena, Italy

P. P. Piccaluga
Department of Experimental, Diagnostic, and Specialty Medicine, University of Bologna, Bologna, Italy

3.1.1.2 Cell of Origin

The postulated cell of origin is a mature B-cell during a germinal center (GC) reaction, as indicated by the presence of somatically mutated immunoglobulin genes. More precisely, BL cells seem to derive from the GC dark zone, made up almost exclusively of highly proliferative B-cells that undergo immunoglobulin somatic hypermutation (SHM), as demonstrated by gene expression profiling (GEP) [4–6]. It should be noted however that these previous studies were mainly on sporadic BL, which is usually EBV negative. It has been hypothesized that EBV-associated BL cases derive from a later developmental stage of B-cells than sporadic BL, i.e., post-germinal center/memory B-cells [7]. In fact, in healthy carriers, EBV resides in memory IgM-positive B-cells. Activation of the B-cell receptor (BCR) by malaria infection and/or other pathogens induces the clonal expansion of memory B-cells, which express Epstein-Barr nuclear antigen 1 (EBNA-1) (latency I) and activation-induced cytidine deaminase (AID) when they divide. EBNA-1 expression in this subset of cells allows viral DNA to replicate and may therefore result in the upregulation of hsa-miR-127 and in the shift to the characteristic GC phenotype and reentry into the GC reaction for additional cycles of SHM and division, in an iterative process known as "cyclic reentry." The *MYC-IG* translocations may occur during clonal expansion of

G. Lenz, G. Salles (eds.), *Aggressive Lymphomas*, Hematologic Malignancies,
https://doi.org/10.1007/978-3-030-00362-3_3

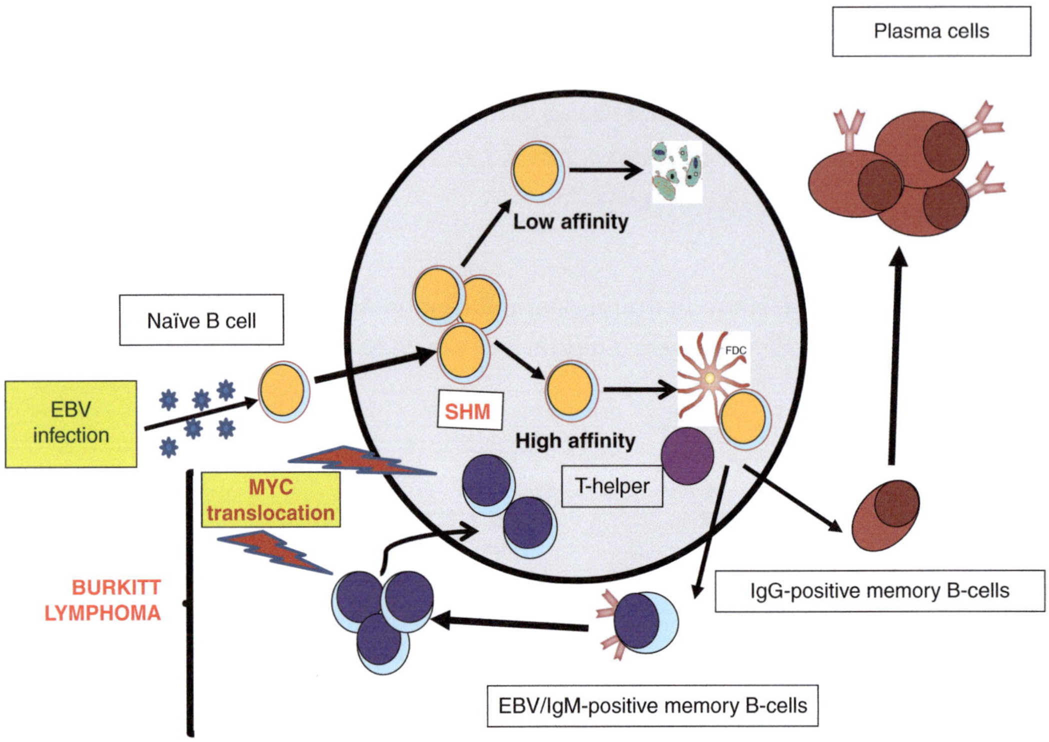

Fig. 3.1 Burkitt lymphoma cell of origin. The postulated cell of origin for sporadic Burkitt lymphoma is a mature B-cell during germinal center reaction, whereas EBV-positive cases seem to derive from a later developmental stage (i.e., post-germinal center/memory B-cells)

activated memory B-cells or when they reenter the GC, being the active form of AID expressed regardless of the B-cell developmental stage [7] (Fig. 3.1).

3.1.1.3 History

BL has often been referred to as "the Rosetta Stone of cancer" because it was the first human cancer for which a viral association was shown and a chromosomal translocation resulting in the activation of an oncogene of clear pathogenic significance was identified. It was also the first tumor to be successfully treated with chemotherapy alone [8]. The first description of BL was probably that of Albert Cook, a missionary doctor in Uganda in 1887: one of Cook's patients in Mulago Hospital (Uganda) was a child with a large jaw tumor, and his illustration of its appearance in his meticulous notes leaves little doubt that this was a case of BL [9]. However, it was Denis Burkitt who provided the first detailed clinical description of the tumor in 1958, which he called "African lymphoma" [10]. He mapped places where children with jaw tumors or large abdominal masses had been seen, plotting the "lymphoma belt" of BL throughout Africa [11]. The high incidence of BL in Equatorial Africa and the peculiar epidemiological features relating the incidence of the tumor to temperature and humidity prompted Anthony Epstein (a young microbiologist) and collaborators to search for a virus in BL specimens, leading to the discovery of the Epstein-Barr virus [12]. In the mid-1960s, several pathologists described lymphomas in Europe and the USA that were indistinguishable at the histological level and, often also clinically, from African BL, and it became clear that this was not a uniquely African disease.

3.1.1.4 Epidemiology

Three epidemiological variants of BL are recognized, differing in their geographical distribution, clinical presentation, molecular genetics, and biological features. This suggests complex biological interactions between the host and the environment.

1. **Endemic BL** (eBL) occurs in Equatorial Africa where it represents the most common childhood malignancy with an incidence peak at 4–7 years and a male to female ratio of 2 to 1. The jaws and other facial bones (orbit) are the site of presentation in about 50% of cases. The central nervous system (CNS) as well as distal ileum, cecum and/or omentum, gonads, kidneys, lung bones, thyroid, salivary glands, and breast may also be involved. eBL is associated with EBV in almost all cases (Fig. 3.2).
2. **Sporadic BL** (sBL) is seen throughout the world, mainly in children and young adults, with a median age in adult patients of 30 years. The male to female ratio is 1.66 to 1. The majority of cases present with abdominal masses (80%) involving the ileocecal region, but bone marrow (20% of cases) and lymph node presentations (more commonly in adults than in children) are also seen. sBL is associated with EBV infection in 30% of cases [13].
3. **Immunodeficiency-associated BL** (iBL) is more common in the setting of human immunodeficiency virus (HIV) infection than in other forms of immunosuppression (posttransplant). In HIV patients, BL appears early in the progression of the disease, when CD4-positive T-cell counts are still high. Nodal and organ localization and bone marrow involvement are frequent. EBV is identified in 25–40% of the patients [13].

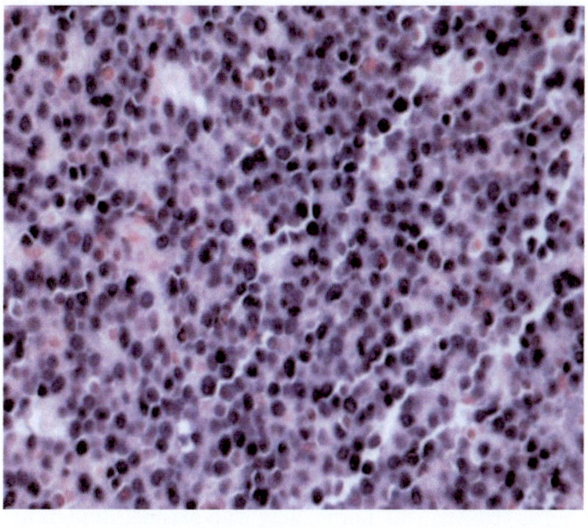

Fig. 3.2 Epstein-Barr virus infection in endemic Burkitt lymphoma. Almost all cases of endemic BL are associated with EBV. EBER-ISH stain; *OM* original magnification, 20×

3.1.2 Pathology, Genetics, and Virology Findings and Their Role in Burkitt Pathogenesis

3.1.2.1 Morphology

Macroscopy

When localized in the head, disruption of teeth, ulcerative and draining lesions of the jaw, and partial obstruction of the airway are observed. Abdominal involvement presents as a huge mass with thickening of the intestinal wall and hemorrhage, often associated with multiple polypoid lesions. Affected lymph nodes are enlarged, with a smooth surface. The cut surface is usually yellow-white to pearl gray and shows a fish-meat-like appearance. Necrotic foci can be seen [3].

Microscopy

Histologically, lymph node architecture is effaced by a characteristically diffuse proliferation, with a distinct starry sky pattern evident at low power magnification. This feature imparts a "moth-eaten" appearance due to the presence of many benign phagocytic histiocytes engulfing the nuclear debris that result from the apoptosis of BL cells. Although the numerous mitoses and high proliferative rate of BL have long been recognized, this tumor also has a significant proportion of cells undergoing apoptosis. The cells are round, medium-sized, with a somewhat uniform appearance, and often seem cohesive. A so-called squaring off of the cytoplasm may be encountered, as the cell border appears to abut one another (Fig. 3.3). The nuclei are uniform and round to oval shaped. The chromatin is clumped, with relatively clear parachromatin and two to five small, centrally located, basophilic nucleoli

(Fig. 3.3a). There is a moderate amount of deeply basophilic cytoplasm that frequently contains lipid vacuoles that are best seen in imprint preparations [3]. The morphologic spectrum of BL is however wider than once thought. Thus, some degree of nuclear irregularity or variations in cell size and shape are accepted for a diagnosis of BL. Atypical morphology may be more common in adult than in pediatric patients and is more often associated with HIV infection (i.e., plasmacytoid appearance) (Fig. 3.3b) and with nodal disease [3].

3.1.2.2 Immunophenotype

The tumor cells typically express moderate to strong membrane IgM with light chain restriction, B-cell antigens (CD19, CD20, CD22, CD79a, PAX5) and germinal center markers (CD10, BCL6). CD38, CD77, and CD43 are also frequently positive [3], whereas BCL2 is usually negative (Fig. 3.4a–c). Almost all BL, including *MYC-IG* translocations negative cases (cf Sect. 1.2.3.2), have strong expression of MYC protein in the majority of cells (Fig. 3.4d). The proliferation rate is very high with nearly 100% of the cells positive for Ki-67 (Fig. 3.4e). The characteristic cytoplasmic lipid vesicles can also be demonstrated by immunohistochemistry on paraffin tissue sections using a monoclonal antibody against adipophilin [14] (Fig. 3.4f). There are very few infiltrating T-cells. T-cell leukemia-1 (TCL-1) is strongly expressed in most pediatric BL. The neoplastic cells are usually negative for CD5, CD23, CD138, and TdT. The immunophenotype may be more variable in sBL in older patients. Aberrant phenotypes such as CD5 expression, lack of CD10, or weak BCL2 expression in a variable number of cells have been described in these cases. However, high BCL2 expression should suggest the presence of an additional *BCL2* breakpoint consistent with a high-grade B-cell lymphoma, with *MYC* and *BCL2* and/or *BCL6* rearrangements (cf Chap. 2). Identifying BL in these cases remains a challenge; however, different scoring systems may be useful. The most feasible are those proposed by Naresh et al. based on morphology, immunohistochemistry, and fluorescent in situ hybridization (FISH) [15, 16].

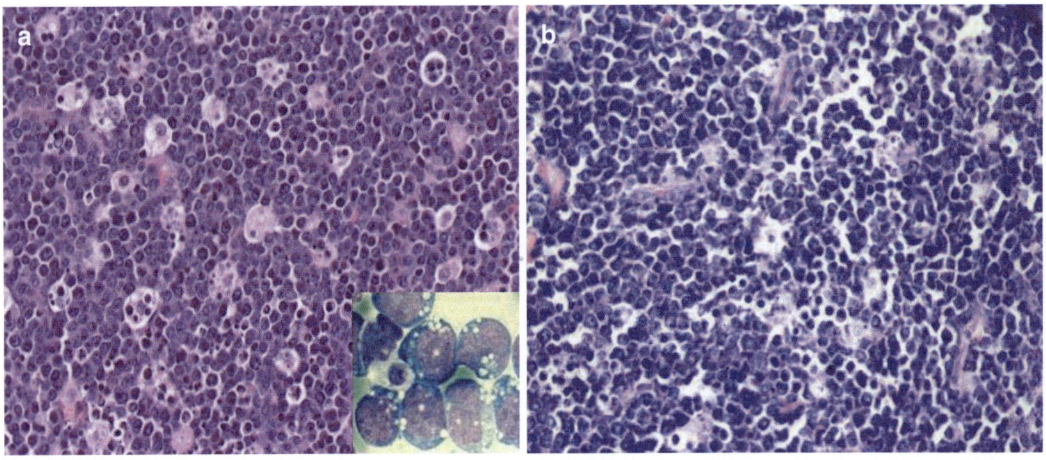

Fig. 3.3 Burkitt lymphoma morphologic and cytologic features. (**a**) A diffuse proliferation of round, medium-sized neoplastic cells with squared-off cytoplasm, uniform nuclei, and clumped chromatin with multiple, centrally located, inconspicuous nucleoli is shown. The typical "starry sky" pattern is evident. The cytoplasm of neoplastic cells contains lipidic vacuoles that are well appreciated on imprint preparations (insert **a**, bottom right). (**b**) Atypical morphology with plasmacytoid differentiation may be present in adult with human immunodeficiency virus (HIV) infection. (**a**, **b**) *HE* Hematoxylin and eosin, OM, 20×

3.1.2.3 Cytogenetics

MYC Rearrangement

At the molecular level, the most consistent factor implicated in the pathogenesis of BL is the translocation of the *MYC* gene (8q24) to one of the *IG* loci, predominantly the heavy chain (*IGH*) locus at the chromosome region 14q32 or the light chain lambda (*IGL*) at 22q11, and, less frequently, the kappa (*IGK*) locus at 2p12 [3]. Most breakpoints originate from aberrant SHM mediated by AID activity. In sporadic and immunodeficiency-associated BL, most breakpoints are close to or within *MYC* gene, whereas in endemic cases most breakpoints are dispersed over several hundred kilobases further upstream of the gene. As a result of translocations, control of normal *MYC* gene expression is lost, leading to constitutive expression of the MYC protein [17].

The product of the *MYC* gene is a global regulator of transcription that affects thousands of genes involved in cell cycle control, cell proliferation, metabolism, regulation of RNA processing, microRNA (miRNA) expression, signal transduction, cell-cell interaction, immune function, and apoptosis. Most importantly, the MYC protein acts as a fail-safe mechanism for the induction of a large number of proapoptotic genes and the transcriptional inhibition of antiapoptotic ones, thereby potentiating cell apoptosis. MYC-driven tumors therefore tend to acquire additional genetic mutations or epigenetic modifications that promote cell survival and shift the balance toward proliferation [18].

Although MYC is well known to be essential for early B-cell development in the bone marrow [19, 20], its role in the germinal center (GC) formation and maintenance and the functional consequence of its deregulated expression in GC have only recently begun to be understood. The GC structure is subdivided into two compartments. After antigenic challenge, B-cells enter the dark zone (DZ) to proliferate and hypermutate their *IG* genes. Mutants with greater affinity for the antigen are positively selected for high affinity in the light zone (LZ) to either differentiate into plasma and memory B-cells. Upon selection, B-cells can reenter the DZ for additional cycles of SHM and division, in an iterative process known as "cyclic reentry" [4, 6].

MYC has a specific bimodal pattern of expression in a small subset of GC B-cells during the GC reaction [4, 5]. The initial expression of MYC required for GC formation is promptly silenced in DZ B-cells as a result of transcriptional repression by BCL6, key transcription regulator for the GC reaction. Through interactions with antigens and T-helper cells, MYC expression is transiently reactivated in a very small subset of LZ B-cells that are primed for DZ reentry to undergo further cycles of proliferation. The role of MYC in cyclic reentry seems to be important in maintaining GC structure through activation of transcriptional programs associated with many of the known functions of MYC. However, MYC must be actively repressed in GC DZ to limit the numbers of cell division before each round of antigen affinity-based selection.

The *MYC-IG* translocation uncouples MYC expression in the GC from the natural process of positive selection in the LZ by bypassing affinity-based selection signals and by alleviating the BCL6-mediated transcriptional repression that normally prevents MYC expression in DZ B-cells. Therefore, by overriding the physiologic control of MYC expression at critical checkpoints in the GC reaction (GC entry and DZ reentry), *MYC-IG* translocations result in an ectopic and constitutive expression of MYC in centroblast cells of the DZ causing a perpetuation of the GC reentry that disturbs normal GC dynamics and significantly increases the risk of lymphomagenesis [4, 5].

11q Aberration

Up to 10% of cases with the clinical, morphologic, and immunophenotypic features of BL lack a demonstrable *MYC* translocation by FISH [3]. Caution is warranted before concluding that these are indeed true *MYC*-negative BL, because the scattering of breakpoints in the *MYC* and *IG* loci, along with small insertions of one locus into the other, can render *MYC* breaks undetectable even if an extensive set of FISH probes is applied (both break-apart and fusion probes for t(8;14)(q24;q32, as well as *IGH*, *IGL*, and *IGK* break-apart probes). However, two pivotal studies by Dave et al. [21] and by Hummel et al. [22], which demonstrated a specific GEP that distinguishes BL from other aggressive mature B-cell lymphomas, revealed that about 10% of cases have the characteristic BL GEP without the typical *MYC* translocation by exhaustive FISH analyses. Although none of the techniques currently used to diagnose genetic changes can unambiguously rule out *MYC* translocations, alternative mechanisms that cause MYC deregulation (such as abnormal expression of miRNAs through direct or indirect mechanisms [18, 23]) may also play a role [17]. In these cases, strict clinical, morphologic, and phenotypic criteria should be used to exclude lymphomas that mimic BL. At least, some of these cases likely represent the new provisional entity "Burkitt-like lymphoma with 11q aberrations" characterized by an interstitial 11q23 gain immediately followed by a telomeric loss at 11q24 [3, 25]. Because this 11q aberration is also detected in *MYC*-rearranged high-grade lymphoma, it cannot be considered as a surrogate for *MYC*-induced lymphomagenesis [25]. Additional studies are needed to better understand such lymphoma with a clinical course similar to classical BL.

Additional Chromosomal Aberrations

Although the karyotype of BL is usually simple, additional chromosomal abnormalities (including gains of 1q, 7q, and 12q and losses of 6q, 13q32–34, and 17p, some of which have been shown to be independently associated with reduced survival [3, 26, 27]) can occur and may influence disease progression.

3.1.2.4 Gene and microRNA Expression Signature

MYC dysregulation through a chromosomal translocation with one of the immunoglobulin gene loci is considered primary in BL while secondary in other *MYC*-rearranged B-cell lymphomas [19]. However, MYC overexpression alone is not sufficient to trigger lymphomagenesis: the proapoptotic properties of MYC in particular have to be counterbalanced. New genomic technologies have uncovered several genomic and epigenetic changes that cooperate with MYC deregulation to generate this highly aggressive lymphoma.

Gene Expression Signature

Studies by Dave et al. [21] and Hummel et al. [22], mainly on sBL samples, have defined a molecular signature of BL that is distinct from that of other lymphomas such as diffuse large B-cell lymphoma (DLBCL). Specifically, the BL signature includes increased expression of *MYC*, *MYC* target genes, and GC B-cell genes with decreased expression of major histocompatibility complex (MHC) class I genes and nuclear factor (NF)-kB target genes. However a gray zone persists in both studies, with unclassifiable cases between BL and DLBCL. Although BL is a relatively homogeneous entity with a molecular profile related to that of GC cells, a study by Piccaluga et al. [28] on eBL, sBL, and iBL identified differences between BL variants: while iBL and eBL appear to be highly related, independent of EBV status, differential expression of genes involved in cell cycle, proliferation, transcription, and nucleic acid metabolism is observed between eBL and sBL. Gene set enrichment revealed an enhancement of the BCR signaling pathway and tumor necrosis factor α (TNFα)/nuclear factor κB (NF-κB), suggesting an active role for chronic antigenic stimulation and infectious agents in eBL pathogenesis and pointing to differences in pathogenetic mechanism between eBL and sBL.

microRNA (miRNA) Signature

BL is characterized by a miRNA expression profile that is distinct from that of DLBCL, which is enriched in MYC- and NF-kB-targeted miRNAs [29]. miRNAs may also act as epigenetic regulators in BL, modulating the pro-survival pathway mediated by PI3K. MYC contributes to activation of PI3K signaling by inducing expression of the mir-17-92 cluster. 13q31 genomic amplification moreover also leads to the upregulation of this cluster [30]. Finally, mir-19a and mir-19b reduce expression of PTEN, which counteracts PI3K activity (Fig. 3.5).

3.1.2.5 Next-Generation Sequencing (NGS) Results

MYC Mutations

In addition to being translocated, MYC is also the most frequently mutated gene in BL (60–70%), [31, 32]. Many of these mutations are likely subject to AID-dependent SHM, due to the high proximity of the *IG* and *MYC* loci in BL. Most *MYC* mutations affect functional domains that either enhance the oncogenic potential of MYC (by different mechanisms, such as increased protein stability and transcriptional function) or impair its ability to induce apoptosis via *BIM* [33] (Fig. 3.4).

Additional Gene Mutations

Recent high-throughput sequencing studies revealed that the genetic landscape of mutations in BL is more complex than might be expected [31, 32, 34, 35]. Aside from *MYC* mutations, about 100 recurrently mutated genes have been identified, including *ID3* (30–75%), *TCF3 (E2A)* (10–25%), and *CCND3*, *TP53*, *CDKN2A*, *ARID1A*, *RHOA*, *PTEN*, *SMARCA4*, *PIK3R1*, *NOTCH1*, *CCNF*, *DDX3*, *GNA13*, *CREBBP*, and *CCT6B*, occurring in 5–40% of BL. The mutational background of BL differs depending on the epidemiological context in which the tumor arises. In sBL (usually EBV negative), the most frequently mutated genes include *MYC*, *ID3*, *TCF3*, *DDX3X*, *CCND3*, and *TP53*. eBL (often EBV positive) has a lower frequency of *TCF3/ID3* mutations (30% versus 70% in sBL) and a higher frequency of mutations in *ARID1A*, *RHOA*, and *CCNF* [36]. Interestingly, in sBL cases, an almost mutual exclusivity has been demonstrated between EBV presence and mutations in *TCF3/ID3*, indicating that TCF3 pathway is more significantly activated in EBV-negative cases [36].

TCF3 Pathway and BCR Signaling

TCF3 is a basic helix-loop-helix (B-HLH) transcription factor that homodimerizes via its HLH domain and uses its basic region to contact DNA within the major groove. TCF3 DNA binding is inhibited by heterodimerization with its negative regulator ID3, an HLH protein that lacks the basic region. TCF3 is rendered constitutively active in BL by somatic inactivating biallelic mutations (mostly in the HLH domain) of ID3 or

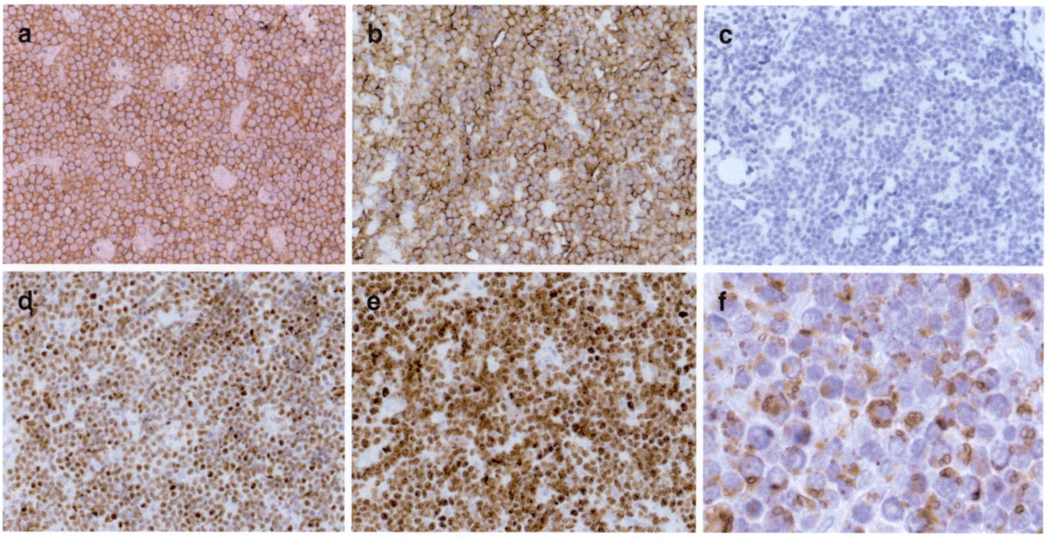

Fig. 3.4 Burkitt lymphoma immunophenotype. The tumor cells typically express CD20 (**a**) and CD10 (**b**), whereas BCL2 is negative (**c**). Almost all cases show a strong expression of MYC protein (**d**) and a very high proliferation rate (**e**). The characteristic cytoplasmic lipid vesicles are shown (**f**). (**a**) CD20 stain; (**b**) CD10 stain; (**c**) BCL2 stain; (**d**) MYC stain; (**e**) Ki-67 stain; (**f**) adipophilin stain. (**a–e**) OM, 20×; (**f**) OM, 63×

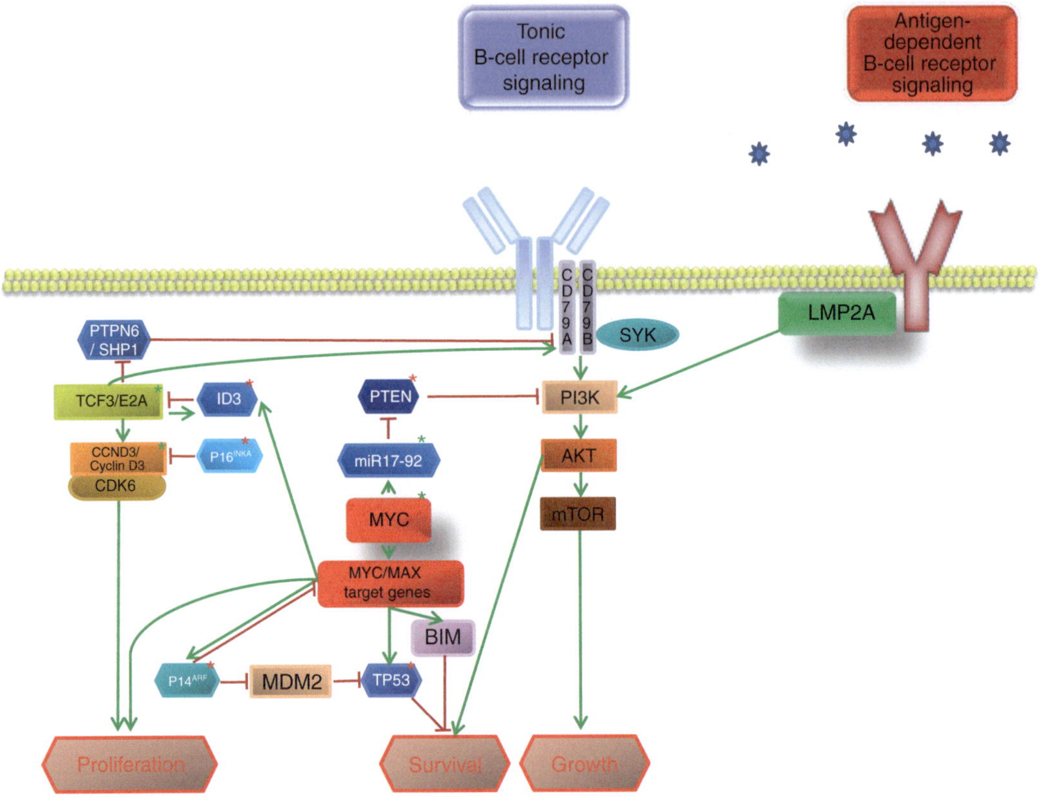

Fig. 3.5 Pathways affected in Burkitt lymphoma. Activating link is mentioned by a green arrow and inactivating link by a red arrow. Gain-of-function mutations are indicated by a green asterisk and loss-of-function mutations by a red asterisk. On the left side of the BCR, activated pathways in EBV-negative BL and on the right side in EBV-positive BL

by somatic activating mutations in the B-HLH domain of TCF3. Both types of mutations result in impaired heterodimerization of ID3 and TCF3 proteins (Fig. 3.5). The resulting deregulated transcriptional activity of TCF3 seems to promote antigen-independent "tonic" BCR signaling by two mechanisms: (1) upregulation of the expression of immunoglobulin chains (heavy and light) on the cell surface and (2) downregulation of *PTPN6*, encoding the SHP1 phosphatase that reduces BCR signaling by dephosphorylating the ITAM motifs of the CD79A and CD79B subunits.

It is noteworthy that the importance of BCR signaling for BL lymphomagenesis was initially suggested by the observation that MYC translocations to the immunoglobulin loci in BL exclusively involve the nonproductively rearranged alleles, indicating that BL cells are selected for BCR expression [37]. The resulting tonic BCR signaling sustains BL cell survival by engaging the phosphoinositide 3-kinase (PI3K) signaling pathway. PI3K signaling represents an essential and pervasive pro-survival mechanism, playing a central role in the development and maintenance of BL. Several additional mechanisms can activate PI3K signaling in BL, including classical inactivating mutations of the inhibitory phosphatase PTEN (7%) and the regulatory subunit PIK3R1, reinforcing the observation of a cooperative role between MYC and PI3K.

The involvement of the PI3K signaling pathway in BL pathogenesis has been elegantly demonstrated in mice engineered to coordinately express MYC and constitutively active PI3K, specifically in B-cells undergoing the GC reaction [38]. The resulting clonal lymphomas phenocopy human BL in terms of their histology, the ongoing SHM of Ig-variable regions, as well as their gene and protein expression signatures. The lymphoma cells also accumulate stabilizing mutations of the phosphorylation motif of cyclin D3, an important regulator of GC B-cell proliferation.

Recent studies have suggested two alternative means of activating BCR signaling, depending on epidemiological context. Whereas sBL is characterized by tonic, intrinsic activation of BCR signaling, eBL, arising in the context of chronic antigen stimulation, is instead characterized by extrinsic, antigen-dependent activation of BCR signaling. The difference in global mutation rate detected in the two BL subtypes is in line with a much lower rate of *TCF3/ID3* mutations in eBL than in sBL cases. We cannot exclude a combination of tonic and extrinsic BCR signaling in the subset of EBV-positive BL with activated TCF3 [39].

TCF3 is also a master regulator of normal GC B-cell differentiation. It upregulates genes expressed in the rapidly dividing centroblasts, the putative cell of origin for BL, while repressing genes expressed in less proliferative centrocytes. Thus TCF3 causes a centroblast-restricted gene expression signature in BL cells, which is exacerbated in cases with *TCF3/ID3* aberrations. The transcriptional program regulated by TCF3 in BL distinguishes normal GC B-cells from blood B-cells, supporting the idea that TCF3 contributes to the BL phenotype by enforcing a GC-derived transcriptional program [32].

CCND3 and Cell Cycle

Part of TCF3's proliferative effect arises from its transactivation CCND3, a D-type cyclin that regulates G1/S cell cycle transition. *CCND3* itself can also be mutated in BL, contributing to its highly proliferative phenotype. Mutations are often located at the threonine residue at position 283 (T283) or the nearby proline (P284) or isoleucine (I290) residues that play a role in cyclin D3 phosphorylation and stability. The *CCND3* mutations serve to uncouple cyclin D3 from the regulatory processes that govern its abundance in normal cells (Fig. 3.4). They occur in 30–40% of sBL and up to 67% of HIV-related BL tumors but are significantly less prevalent in eBL (2.6%). The dearth of *CCND3* mutations in eBL tumors raises the possibility that another cyclin could be induced by EBV, thus removing selective pressure for *CCND3* mutations. The G1/S phase transition is also regulated by the cyclin-dependent kinase inhibitor p16, encoded by the *CDKN2A* gene. BLs harbor deletions or inactivating mutations in *CDKN2A* in 17% of samples, with 8% having both *CCND3* and *CDKN2A* mutations, suggesting that these genetic lesions might cooperatively deregulate the cell cycle in BL. It is noteworthy that the combination of *CCND3* and *ID3* mutations seemed to be associated with a poorer outcome in adult BL. This double hit may be more deleterious because it acts simultaneously on two different pathways that cross-talk to activate the pro-survival PI3 kinase pathway (ID3/TCF3) and to drive cell cycle progression (CCND3/CDK6) [30]. Finally, recurrent R451C mutations in *CCNF*, an atypical cyclin that acts an inhibitor of centrosome reduplication during G2 and protects the cell from genome instability, have recently been identified exclusively in eBL [36].

TP53-Dependent Apoptotic Pathway

To avoid oncogene-induced stress in cells with prolonged MYC expression, autoregulatory mechanisms such as activation of TP53-dependent apoptosis, induction of proapoptotic BIM, and repression of antiapoptotic BCL2 and BCLXL [40] trigger programmed cell death. These proapoptotic effects likely represent a feedback safety mechanism of MYC and must be counterbalanced to allow BL development. Consistent with this, alterations in *TP53* pathway are common in BL, occurring in 55% of sBL and 30% of eBL: either *TP53* mutations or, less frequently, homozygous deletion or inactivating mutations in *p14ARF*, a protein that stabilizes p53. *TP53* and *p14ARF* are usually inactivated in a mutually exclusive manner, in what is considered to be an early event in tumorigenesis [32, 39] (Fig. 3.4).

Other Altered Pathways

Recent studies identified a number of additional genetic mutations targeting other pathways involved in BL lymphomagenesis with overlaps: inactivating mutations targeting the RNA helicase *DDX3X*, the nucleosome remodeling SWI/SNF pathway (*ARID1A* and *SMARCA4* are mutated in a mutually exclusive manner in about 25% of the BL), the focal adhesion pathway (silencing mutations of *GNA13* in nearly 15% of BL but also in some GCB-DLBCL, *ROCK1*, and *RHOA*—exclusively detected in eBL), and recurrent mutations in oncogenes known to be involved in other tumors (*NOTCH1*, *RET*, *BRAF*). Individual BL tumors harbor different combinations of mutations that can give rise to a diversity of molecular phenotypes and that suggest new therapeutic targets [31–34].

3.1.2.6 The Role of Pathogens

EBV

BL was the first human cancer to be associated with the EBV, with the endemic form (eBL) linked to malaria and EBV infection in almost all cases. Epidemiological studies have however shown that malaria and EBV do not fully explain the distribution of eBL in high-risk regions [41]. Both infections are in fact ubiquitous within the lymphoma belt of Africa, suggesting that other etiologic agents may be involved and suggesting BL may be a polymicrobial disease [36, 42]. It is established that EBV latent genes are necessary for the persistence of the viral genome in B-cells (and possibly other cell types) throughout the life of the individual. Latent infection is characterized by maintenance of the genome at constant copy number and expression of a limited number of genes. EBV first infects naïve B-cells and activates a growth program in these cells (also termed latency III), which is characterized by expression of nine latent viral genes. These cells are recognized and targeted by a T-cell-mediated immune response, but a fraction enters the GC, where they express only three latent viral genes (default program or latency II). In proliferating GC B-cells, the process of SHM, which modifies the DNA of the variable region of Ig genes, is activated, and GC B-cells undergo differentiation into memory B-cells or plasma cells. The virus thus gains access to the memory B-cell compartment, its main reservoir during persistence, where no latent viral genes are expressed. This mechanism is thought to allow EBV-infected cells to remain hidden from the immune system, enabling lifelong persistence. Upon receiving certain activation signals (BCR stimulation, hypoxia, TGF-β, DNA damage, chemical agents), the latency of these cells is disrupted, and they divide, expressing EBNA-1 protein (latency I), thereby allowing viral DNA to replicate [43]. The virus reactivates, switching to a lytic phase, with subsequent lysis/death of infected cells and release of virions that infect more cells and enable virus transmission from host to host [44, 45]. The lytic phase can also enhance tumor growth through growth factors and immunosuppressive cytokines. Until recently, BL was considered to be characterized by latency I, classically diagnosed by the detection of EBV-encoded RNAs (EBER) by in situ hybridization (ISH). However, it has now been demonstrated that the latency program elicited by the virus in BL is more complex, with a large number of cases showing a noncanonical latency program with expression of LMP-1/LMP-2A/LMP-2B in a significant proportion of cells along with lytic cycle reactivation [36, 44–46]. LMP-2A participates in the reprogramming of normal B-lymphocytes and enhances *MYC*-driven lymphomagenesis through the activation of PI3K pathway. This suggests that LMP-2A activation of PI3K is an alternative/convergent mechanism to the one driven by *TCF3*/*ID3* mutations [36] (Fig. 3.5).

EBV encodes different products that may be involved in carcinogenesis, including lytic and latent proteins, RNA molecules, and miRNAs. Viral miRNAs regulate both cellular and viral genes, playing important roles in maintaining EBV latency [47]. They provide a potent mechanism for the virus to modulate the cellular environment by regulating host cell growth, survival, apoptosis, and immune evasion. In addition, EBV affects the expression of cellular miRNAs, thereby regulating cellular gene expression, enhancing the pathogenesis of virus- associated diseases [48]. It has been demonstrated that multiple cellular miRNAs are differentially expressed between EBV-positive and EBV-negative BL (hsa-miR-7, hsa-miR-5p, hsa-miR-510, hsa-miR-181d, hsa-miR-609, hsa-miR-574, hsa-miR-197, and has-miR142-5b) and that a subset of viral miRNAs, all belonging to BART-locus, are expressed in EBV-positive BL [44, 45, 49]. Of these, BART6-3p modulates the expression of IL-6 receptor and PTEN in vitro, thus impacting cell proliferation, cell death, and immune escape.

Since EBV is found in other lymphoid and nonlymphoid neoplasms, its direct and specific role in BL pathogenesis remains questionable, and some authors simply considered EBV as a bystander [50]. Early during oncogenesis, viral genes are essential for initiating disease. Progressively, viral genome is lost to escape the immune system, and host mutations accumulate in proto-oncogenic cell. It has been recently demonstrated that EBV may be associated with a larger number of BL cases than previously recognized, including those diagnosed as EBV negative by routine methods [i.e., immunohistochemistry—IHC and EBER-ISH] thanks to a *hit-and-run* mechanism [50]. After eliciting a heritable change in the gene expression pattern of the host cell, the genome of tumor viruses may be completely lost. The cancer cells then accumulate vast numbers of mutations that become the main drivers of oncogenesis, promoting autonomous growth [51]. Thus, it may be inevitable that a cancer, with time, will evolve to be independent from viral gene functions, allowing for viral genome loss. This results in an inverse correlation between the number of viral genes expressed in these tumor cells and their associated cellular mutations [52].

Malaria and Other Pathogens

Malaria is per se a cofactor of BL in conjunction with EBV; in fact, malaria parasites are strong polyclonal stimulators of the B-cell system, thereby increasing the likelihood of chromosomal translocations. Moreover, certain *Plasmodium falciparum* antigens and exposure to a large number of antigens during multiple infections can reactivate EBV from memory B-cells, increasing viral load and consequently the number of EBV-infected B-cells in vivo.

It has been recently found that pathogens other than EBV and malaria are associated with eBL, namely, CMV and KSHV. Their prevalence in areas endemic for EBV, along with their absence in the sporadic cases, suggests that CMV or KSHV could contribute to the chronic antigenic stimulation in the context of which eBL occurs [36]. The presence of these additional cofactors may also induce the EBV lytic cycle through B-cell reactivation, spreading EBV infection out of its natural niche of memory B-cells [44, 45].

A small number of other environmental factors have been proposed to be relevant to the pathogenesis of BL on the basis of apparent space-time clusters and enhanced in vitro transformation of EBV. These include arboviruses and tumor promoters from *Euphorbia tirucalli*, a plant used widely in Africa for a variety of purposes, capable of reactivating the EBV lytic cycle [53].

3.2 Lymphoblastic Lymphoma

3.2.1 Introduction

3.2.1.1 Definition

Lymphoblastic lymphoma (LBL) is a neoplasm of precursor cells (lymphoblasts) of either B- (B-LBL) or T-cell origin (T-LBL), grouped together with acute lymphoblastic leukemia (ALL) of either B- (B-ALL) or T-cell origin (T-ALL) in the last WHO classification. By convention, the word “lymphoma” is used if there is a bulky lesion in the mediastinum or elsewhere, with no or limited infiltration of peripheral blood (PB) and bone marrow (BM). In general, a threshold of 25% BM blasts is used for defining leukemia in the contexte of lymphoma [3, 54]. LBL and ALL show overlapping clinical, pathological, and immunophenotypic features: hence they were considered the same disease (with different clinical presentations) for decades. However, some recent studies showing different molecular profiles suggest different pathogeneses. In the last WHO classification, the precursor lymphoid neoplasms are subdivided into B-lymphoblastic leukemia/lymphoma, not otherwise specified, or B-lymphoblastic leukemia/lymphoma with recurrent genetic abnormalities, and T-lymphoblastic leukemia/lymphoma [55]. Moreover, the natural killer (NK) cell lymphoblastic leukemia/lymphoma as a new provisional entity [3].

3.2.1.2 Cell of Origin

The postulated normal cell of origin is a precursor B- or T-cell in the bone marrow or thymic T-cells at varying stages of differentiation [54, 55].

3.2.1.3 Epidemiology and Etiology

Lymphoblastic lymphoma is a rare disease that accounts for approximately 2% of adult but more than 20% of pediatric non-Hodgkin lymphomas. The overall incidence of LBL is expected to be less than 10% of the total ALL/LBL incidence. In contrast to ALL, T-LBL constitutes the large majority of LBL (~90%). T-LBL occurs more frequently in late childhood, adolescence, and young adulthood, while B-LBL occurs mostly in childhood and to a lesser extent in adulthood. Both B- and T-LBL have male predominance with an overall male/female ratio of 1.4 [54].

T-LBL frequently presents with a mass in the anterior mediastinum, often exhibiting rapid growth and pleural effusion. The most frequent site of involvement in B-LBL are the skin, soft tissue, bone, and lymph nodes, mainly in the head and neck region particularly in children [54].

The causes of LBL as well as ALL are largely unknown. However, several studies suggest an increased risk of ALL associated with several environmental exposures, such as chemicals (pesticides, benzene, oil products, medical drugs) and ionizing radiation. Down syndrome is one congenital conditional known to predispose to the development of ALL, mostly of B-cell lineage. Other germline genetic predispositions to ALL, also of B-cell lineage, have recently been identified by high-throughput sequencing studies. It is noteworthy that the affected genes are frequently also somatically mutated in ALL/LBL: rare, highly penetrant germline variants are reported in *PAX5*, *ETV6*, and *TP53* and common allelic variants in *IKZF1*, *ARID5B*, *CEBPE*, and *CDKN2A* [56]. All these features should be carefully investigated in LBL.

3.2.2 Pathology and Genetics Findings

3.2.2.1 Morphology

The lymphoblasts of LBL are indistinguishable from ALL cells at the cytological analysis of imprints. They range from small cells with scant cytoplasm, condensed nuclear chromatin, and indistinct nucleoli to larger cells with moderate amounts of faintly basophilic cytoplasm, often vacuolated, dispersed chromatin, and multiple prominent nucleoli. The nuclear shape may be round, oval, or convoluted. A few azurophilic cytoplasmic granules may be present. In lymph node sections, LBL is characterized by a diffuse or, less commonly, paracortical pattern. More rarely, particularly in T-LBL, neoplastic cells occur in nodules superficially resembling follicular lymphoma. A single-file pattern of infiltration

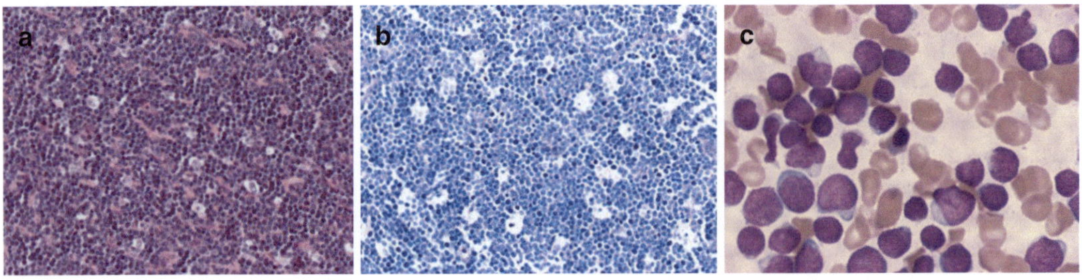

Fig. 3.6 B-Lymphoblastic lymphoma morphologic and cytologic features. (**a**, **b**) Diffuse proliferation of intermediate-sized neoplastic cells with inconspicuous or small nucleoli and scanty, faintly basophilic cytoplasm that typically infiltrate in an Indian file pattern. (**c**) Bone marrow aspirate showing lymphoblasts with variable size and morphology. (**a**) Hematoxylin and eosin; (**b**) Giemsa stain; (**c**) May-Grünewald-Giemsa. (**a**, **b**) OM, 20×; (**c**) OM, 100×

is common (Fig. 3.6). In some circumstances, eosinophils may be present within lymphomatous infiltrate. Mitotic figures are frequent and variable in number. A starry sky pattern or necrotic areas and, in some instances, sclerosis may be seen. There is no correlation between morphology and B or T lineage. Immunophenotyping studies are therefore required to distinguish precursor B-LBL from precursor T-LBL.

Although histological features are usually sufficient to distinguish lymphoblastic from mature B- or T-cell neoplasms, a differential diagnosis with blastoid variant of mantle cell lymphoma, Burkitt lymphoma, or the rare myeloid sarcoma can arise in some cases, particularly in adults, if imprints are unavailable and/or if the biopsy is too small. In these cases, immunophenotyping and molecular genetic studies are critical [57].

Rarely, transformation of low-grade lymphoma such as follicular lymphoma (FL) results in a highly aggressive presentation that is clinically, morphologically, and immunophenotypically reminiscent of B-lymphoblastic leukemia/lymphoma. Transformation may occur during chemotherapy or follow-up of a preexisting FL. Sometimes, patients develop mature high-grade lymphoma, followed by lymphoblastic transformation. In rare cases, FL may be initially diagnosed as a lymphoblastic transformation right from the outset. This rare, highly aggressive variant of FL usually occurs in older patients (median age of around 60 years) than the classical lymphoblastic lymphoma. It is characterized by acquisition of blastic/blastoid morphology, TdT expression, partial or complete loss of immunoglobulin light chain, loss of BCL6, but persistence of PAX5, BCL2, and CD10 expression, and increased proliferation index. The high-grade transformation is usually accompanied by *MYC* gene rearrangement as a critical event in addition to the preexisting *BCL2* deregulation. FL and LBL are usually clonally related. The prognosis is very poor. It is crucial to correctly classify this double-hit lymphoma as high-grade lymphoblastic transformation of FL rather than B-LBL/B-ALL, as the clinical management should be different [58].

3.2.2.2 Immunophenotype

B-LBL

In precursor B-LBL/B-ALL, the B-cell lymphoblasts are virtually always positive for B-cell markers CD19, CD79a, and CD22. They are positive for common acute lymphoblastic leukemia antigen CD10, CD 24, PAX5, and terminal deoxytransferase (TdT) in most cases, while the expression of CD20 and the lineage-independent stem cell antigen CD34 is variable and CD45 may be absent. The following set of antigens defines the stage of differentiation:

- Pro-B stage (CD19+, cytoplasmic CD79a+, cytoplasmic CD22+, and nuclear TdT+)
- "Common" stage (CD10+), which represents the majority of B-LBL [59]
- Pre-B stage (CD20+ and cytoplasmic μ heavy chain+)

Surface immunoglobulin is usually absent, but its presence does not rule out B-LBL, neither does the presence of myeloid antigens CD13 and CD33.

The expression of TdT (characteristics of LBL/ALL) and the lack of surface immunoglobulin (hallmarks of mature B-cell neoplasms) are useful in distinguishing B-LBL from more mature B-cell neoplasms. Negative cyclin D1 and CD5 with concomitant expression of TdT differentiate B-LBL from mantle cell lymphoma. In addition to TdT and MPO, CD19, CD22, CD10, CD79a, and, more recently, LMO2 and SALL4 are useful for the differential diagnosis of T-LBL and myeloid sarcoma [54, 57].

T-LBL

In precursor T-LBL/T-ALL, neoplastic cells are usually TdT positive (Fig. 3.7a) and PAX-5 negative (Fig. 3.7b) with variable expression of CD1a, CD2 to CD5, CD7, and CD8 depending on maturation stage. The only reliable lineage-specific marker is surface CD3 (Fig. 3.7c). CD7 and cytoplasmic CD3 are usually positive. CD4 and CD8 are frequently co-expressed. Besides TdT, the most specific markers are CD99, CD34,

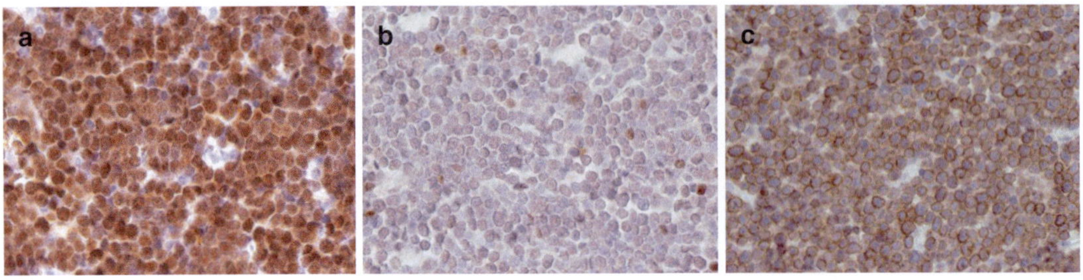

Fig. 3.7 T-Lymphoblastic lymphoma immunophenotype. The tumor cells are typically TdT positive (**a**) and PAX5 negative (**b**); the only reliable lineage-specific marker is CD3 (**c**). (**a**) TdT stain; (**b**) PAX5 stain; (**c**) CD3 stain. (**a**–**c**) OM, 40×

and CD1a. CD10 may be positive. Myeloid-associated antigens CD13 and CD33 are expressed in 19–31% of cases, and their presence does not exclude T-LBL/T-ALL. According to the expression pattern of specific markers, the following categories of T-LBL/T-ALL can be identified:

- Early or pro-T (cCD3+, CD7+, CD2−, CD1a−, CD4−, CD8−, CD34+/−)
- Pre-T (cCD3+, CD7+, CD2+, CD1a−, CD4−, CD8−, CD34+/−)
- Cortical-T (cCD3+, CD7+, CD2+, CD1a+, CD4+, CD8+, CD34−), which represents the majority of T-LBL [59]
- Medullary-T (cCD3+, CD7+, CD2+, CD1a−, CD4+, CD8+, CD34−, and surface CD3+)

T-LBL and T-ALL have almost completely overlapping features, although the lymphomatous counterpart tends to show a more mature immunophenotype than the leukemic one. The differential diagnosis of T-LBL from a peripheral T-cell lymphoma relies on its expression of non-lineage-specific immature markers, such as TdT or CD99 or, in some cases, CD34. Cytoplasmic without surface expression of CD3 is also a relatively specific and useful finding, although it is important to be aware of the fact that this phenotype is best demonstrated by flow cytometry rather than immunohistochemistry. Moreover, CD1a is also a relatively specific feature when positive. Finally, rare cases of LBL express NK-related antigens, such as CD16 and CD57 [54, 57].

3.2.2.3 Genetic Profile

Little is known about the pathogenesis and genetic changes in LBL, due to scant availability of biological material for genetic analysis. The few studies reported in the literature describe certain molecular differences between LBL and ALL.

T-LBL

Four studies have shown that nearly all chromosomal abnormalities reported in T-LBL have previously been reported in T-ALL [60–64]. Cytogenetic abnormalities seem to be frequent in T-LBL patients (50–70%), including pseudodiploidy (25%), deletions (20%), hyperdiploidy, and chromosomal translocations (18% each). The most recurrent cytogenetic abnormalities in T-LBL involve chromosomal loci containing the T-cell receptor (TCR) genes. The 14q11–13 region (containing the TCR-alpha and TCR-delta) as well as the 7q34 (TCR-beta) and 7p14–15 (TCR-gamma) are altered in about 60% of cases [65]. They show chromosomal translocations or cryptic gene rearrangements, usually leading to a transcriptional deregulation of a partner gene due to juxtaposition of the regulatory regions of one of the TCR loci. The most commonly involved genes are the transcription factors *HOX11*(*TLX1*)/10q24 and *HOX11L2*(TLX3)/5q35. Other genes include *TAL1*/1p32, *RBTN1*(*LMO1*)/11p15, *RBTN2*(*LMO2*)/11p13, *LYL1*/19p13, and the cytoplasmic tyrosine kinase *LCK*/1p34.3–35. Importantly, these translocations are not always detected by conventional karyotyping [3, 55].

Other important translocations in T-ALL include *PICALM-MLLT10* -*CALM-AF10*; t(10;11)(p13;q14)-, occurring in 10% of cases, and translocations involving *MLL* (8%), most often with the partner *ENL* at 19p13. Noteworthy, the aberrant expression of *TAL1*, *LYL1*, *HOX11*, *HOX11L2*, *PICALM*, and *MLL* appears to be mutually exclusive, suggesting the existence of nonoverlapping, pathogenically distinct subgroups [3, 57, 66]. *MYC* (8q24.1) translocations can occur in T-ALL but only rarely, with very few unequivocal cases reported in the literature. Similarly, *BCR/ABL1* rearrangements have been occasionally reported in T-LBL [3, 54, 57]. The translocation t(9;17)(q34;q22–23) was described only in T-LBL but not T-ALL [63] and is associated with a dismal prognosis with rapid progressive disease course. Patients with this translocation were reported to present with a mediastinal mass and might have a more aggressive disease course [61, 67]. Although less frequent, the association of T-LBL with myeloproliferative neoplasms should be mentioned. Two different gene rearrangements have been identified in such cases. Cases of T-LBL with myeloid proliferation or hyper-eosinophilia have been reported in patients with t(8;13)(p11;q11) fusing *FGFR1* with *ZMYM2* in the so-called *FGFR1*/8p11 myeloproliferative syndrome. Moreover, two patients with concomitant T-LBL and eosinophilia-associated disorders were shown to bear a FIP1L1-PDGFRA fusion gene. The same gene rearrangement is present in lymphoma and myeloid cells, suggesting a common lymphoid/myeloid stem cell as the target of the original transforming event. The identification of such fusion genes is important since the potential use of tyrosine kinase inhibitors [57].

As classically observed in T-ALL, deletion of the *CDKN2A/CDKN2B* locus at 9p21 seems to be the most frequent genomic imbalance, best detected by molecular karyotyping. Using a single nucleotide polymorphism-based array approach, Schraders et al. [68] detected this deletion in 11 out of 12 cases of pediatric T-LBL. An average of 3–6 genomic imbalances (2–3 losses and 1–3 gains) were identified per case. The two other recurrent genomic imbalances were 13q14 deletion including the *RB1* locus (two cases) and 6q23 gain within the *MYB* locus (two cases).

As in T-ALL, about 60% of T-LBL harbor activating mutations involving the extracellular heterodimerization domain and/or the C-terminal PEST domain of the *NOTCH1* gene, which encodes a transmembrane receptor critical for early T-cell development [69, 70]. In addition, about 18% of cases have mutations in *FBXW7*, a negative regulator of *NOTCH1*, resulting in increased half-life of the NOTCH1 protein [69]. It is noteworthy that *NOTCH1* mutation occurs mutually exclusively from loss of heterozygosity of the long arm of chromosome 6 (LOH 6q) [69]. Whole exome sequencing of a series of five pediatric T-LBL patients identified the recurrently altered genes, *PHF6*, *NOTCH1*, *PAPPA*, *NFIL3*, *MUC4*, *PEDM2*, and *ZNF91*, which can be considered candidates with potential pathogenic relevance for T-LBL [69]. Larger-scale studies are needed to get a genome-wide insight into the genetic basis of T-LBL [71].

B-LBL

Although only a limited number of cytogenetic studies of B-LBL are reported in the literature, the distribution of chromosomal aberrations seems to differ from that of B-ALL. Some of the characteristic cytogenetic changes seen in B-ALL, t(9;22)(q34;q11)/*BCR-ABL* (20–30% in adulthood and 2–4% in childhood) and t(4;11)(q21;q23)/*KMT2A-AFF1* (5–10% in childhood and up to 50% in infants), both of which are associated with an adverse prognosis; t(12;21)(p13;q22)/*ETV6/RUNX1* (~30% in childhood only), associated with a relatively good outcome in children; and t(1;19)(q23;p13)/*TCF3-PBX1* (3–5%), were not detected in B-LBL. Hyperdiploidy does not seem to be as common as in B-ALL, where it is associated with a good clinical outcome, while additional 21 materials—such as trisomy, tetrasomy, or add(21)(q22)—are proportionally more frequent in B-LBL than in B-ALL.

3.2.2.4 Gene Expression Signature

Despite the many similarities between T-ALL and T-LBL, GEP studies have highlighted some subtle differences [72]. While the two malignancies share a large fraction of their transcriptional profile, a subset of genes appears to be differentially expressed between T-LBL and T-ALL. The expression profiles may suggest that thymocytes represent the normal counterpart of T-LBL, while most T-ALL derive from a T-cell progenitor of the bone marrow [64, 65]. This differential signature includes genes involved in cell adhesion, chemotaxis (downregulation of *ARRB2* which reduces chemotaxis), and angiogenesis (upregulation of *EPAS1*, *PTPRB*, and *SLIT2* which promote angiogenesis for local tumoral growth in lymph node), which may play a role in tumor cell localization [73].

No data regarding GEP relative to B-LBL are available yet. It was postulated that differences between B-LBL and B-precursor ALL might be related to overexpression of genes encoding for chemokine receptors CXCR4 and its ligand or other adhesion molecules involved in extramedullary migration and homing [74]. Moreover, GEP revealed the existence of the so-called BCR-ABL1-like B-ALL, a high-risk subtype specially occurring in adolescents and younger adults, which is characterized by kinase-activating alterations. It would be useful to identify such cases in B-ALL as they may benefit from targeted treatments [75].

3.2.2.5 Epigenetics: microRNA (miRNA) Expression Profiling

Nothing is known for LBL; however, distinct miRNA signatures are reported in different ALL subtypes and can be used for the diagnosis, classification, and prognosis of ALL in addition to insights into their pathogenesis [76, 77]. Different examples of miRNA signatures in ALL are listed on Table 3.1. Inappropriate epigenetic regulation of miRNAs may be the initial event that predisposes a precursor ALL cell to transformation. Alternatively, common genetic changes in ALL (such as chromosomal translocations) may be the initial transformation events that lead ALL cells to a more undifferentiated stage, which acquires the epigenetic changes. These effects remain to be assessed in LBL.

Table 3.1 Examples of microRNA signatures in ALL

Effect	microRNA signatures	Reference
Distinction between B- versus T-ALL	miR-16, miR-19b, miR-20a, miR-26a, miR-92, miR-93, miRNA-126, miRNA-128, miR-142-3p, miRNA-146b, miR-148, miR-150, miR-151, miRNA-191, miR-223, miR-342, miR-424, miRNA-425-5p, and miRNA-629	[78] [79]
Favorable clinical outcome	miR-10a, miR-128b, miR-134, miR-214, miR-221, miR-451 miR-484, miR-572, miR-580, miR-624, miR-627, and miR-709	[76] [77]
Unfavorable long-term clinical outcome	miR-9, miR-33, miR-92a, miR-142-3p, miR-146a, miR-181a/c, miR-210, miR-215, miR-369-5p, miR-335, miR-454, miR-496, miR-518d, and miR-599	[76] [77]
Higher relapse and mortality rate, independent of age and ALL type	miR-9–1, miR-9–2, miR-9–3, miR-10b, miR-34b, miR-34c, miR-124a1, miR-124a2, miR-124a3, miR-132, miR-196b, miR-203, and miR-212 (hypermethylation)	[70] [80] [81]
Prediction of prednisone response in pediatric ALL patients	miR-16, miR-18a, miR-193a, miR-218, miR-532, miR-550, miR-625, miR-633, and miR-638	[82]
Regulation of different pathways involved in ALL/LBL pathogenesis	miR-9, miR-10a, miR-34 family, miR-124a, miR-143, miR-152, and miR-196b, mir-200a, miR-203, miR-220b, miR-429, miR-432, miR-503	[77]

References

1. Bennett JM, Catovsky D, Daniel MT, et al. French-American-British (FAB Cooperative Group) Proposals for the classification of the acute leukaemias. Br J Haematol. 1976;33:451–8.
2. Swerdlow SH, Campo E, Harris NL, et al. WHO classification of tumours of haematopoietic and lymphoid tissues. Lyon, France: IARC Press; 2008.

3. Swerdlow SH, Campo E, Harris NL, et al. WHO classification of tumours of haematopoietic and lymphoid tissues. 4th ed. Lyon: IARC Press; 2017.
4. Basso K, Dalla-Favera R. Germinal centres and B cell lymphomagenesis. Nat Rev Immunol. 2015;15(3):172–84. Review.
5. Dominguez-Sola D, Victora GD, Ying CY, Phan RT, Saito M, Nussenzweig MC, Dalla-Favera R. The proto-oncogene MYC is required for selection in the germinal center and cyclic reentry. Nat Immunol. 2012;13(11):1083–91.
6. Victora GD, Dominguez-Sola D, Holmes AB, Deroubaix S, Dalla-Favera R, Nussenzweig MC. Identification of human germinal center light and dark zone cells and their relationship to human B-cell lymphomas. Blood. 2012;120(11):2240–8.
7. Ambrosio MR, Lo Bello G, Amato T, Lazzi S, Piccaluga PP, Leoncini L, Bellan C. The cell of origin of Burkitt lymphoma: germinal centre or not germinal centre? Histopathology. 2016;69(5):885–6.
8. Rowe M, Kelly GL, Bell AI, Rickinson AB. Burkitt's lymphoma: the Rosetta Stone deciphering Epstein-Barr virus biology. Semin Cancer Biol. 2009;19(6):377–88.
9. Magrath I. Epidemiology: clues to the pathogenesis of Burkitt lymphoma. Br J Haematol. 2012;156(6):744–56.
10. Burkitt D. A sarcoma involving the jaws in African children. Br J Surg. 1958;46(197):218–23.
11. Magrath I. Denis Burkitt and the African lymphoma. Ecancermedicalscience. 2009;3:159.
12. Epstein A. Burkitt lymphoma and the discovery of Epstein-Barr virus. Br J Haematol. 2012;156(6):777–9.
13. Van Krieken JHJM. Encyclopedia of pathology. Berlin Heidelberg: Springer-Verlag; 2014.
14. Ambrosio MR, Piccaluga PP, Ponzoni M, Rocca BJ, Malagnino V, Onorati M, De Falco G, Calbi V, Ogwang M, Naresh KN, Pileri SA, Doglioni C, Leoncini L, Lazzi S. The alteration of lipid metabolism in Burkitt lymphoma identifies a novel marker: adipophilin. PLoS One. 2012;7(8):e44315.
15. Disanto MG, Ambrosio MR, Rocca BJ, Ibrahim HA, Leoncini L, Naresh KN. Optimal minimal panels of immunohistochemistry for diagnosis of B-cell lymphoma for application in countries with limited resources and for triaging cases before referral to specialist centers. Am J Clin Pathol. 2016;145(5):687–95.
16. Naresh KN, Ibrahim HA, Lazzi S, Rince P, Onorati M, Ambrosio MR, Bilhou-Nabera C, Amen F, Reid A, Mawanda M, Calbi V, Ogwang M, Rogena E, Byakika B, Sayed S, Moshi E, Mwakigonja A, Raphael M, Magrath I, Leoncini L. Diagnosis of Burkitt lymphoma using an algorithmic approach—applicable in both resource-poor and resource-rich countries. Br J Haematol. 2011;154(6):770–6.
17. Jaffe ES, Arber DA, Campo E, Lee Harris N, Quintanilla-Fend L. Hematopathology. 2nd ed. New York: Elsevier; 2016.
18. De Falco G, Ambrosio MR, Fuligni F, Onnis A, Bellan C, Rocca BJ, Navari M, Etebari M, Mundo L, Gazaneo S, Facchetti F, Pileri SA, Leoncini L, Piccaluga PP. Burkitt lymphoma beyond MYC translocation: N-MYC and DNA methyltransferases dysregulation. BMC Cancer. 2015;15:668.
19. Nguyen L, Papenhausen P, Shao H. The role of c-MYC in B-cell lymphomas: diagnostic and molecular aspects. Genes (Basel). 2017;8(4):E116.
20. Vallespinós M, Fernández D, Rodríguez L, Alvaro-Blanco J, Baena E, Ortiz M, Dukovska D, Martínez D, Rojas A, Campanero MR, Moreno de Alborán I. B Lymphocyte commitment program is driven by the proto-oncogene c-Myc. J Immunol. 2011;186(12):6726–36.
21. Dave SS, Fu K, Wright GW, Lam LT, Kluin P, Boerma EJ, Greiner TC, Weisenburger DD, Rosenwald A, Ott G, Müller-Hermelink HK, Gascoyne RD, Delabie J, Rimsza LM, Braziel RM, Grogan TM, Campo E, Jaffe ES, Dave BJ, Sanger W, Bast M, Vose JM, Armitage JO, Connors JM, Smeland EB, Kvaloy S, Holte H, Fisher RI, Miller TP, Montserrat E, Wilson WH, Bahl M, Zhao H, Yang L, Powell J, Simon R, Chan WC, Staudt LM, Lymphoma/Leukemia Molecular Profiling Project. Molecular diagnosis of Burkitt's lymphoma. N Engl J Med. 2006;354(23):2431–42.
22. Hummel M, Bentink S, Berger H, Klapper W, Wessendorf S, Barth TF, Bernd HW, Cogliatti SB, Dierlamm J, Feller AC, Hansmann ML, Haralambieva E, Harder L, Hasenclever D, Kühn M, Lenze D, Lichter P, Martin-Subero JI, Möller P, Müller-Hermelink HK, Ott G, Parwaresch RM, Pott C, Rosenwald A, Rosolowski M, Schwaenen C, Stürzenhofecker B, Szczepanowski M, Trautmann H, Wacker HH, Spang R, Loeffler M, Trümper L, Stein H, Siebert R, Molecular Mechanisms in Malignant Lymphomas Network Project of the Deutsche Krebshilfe. A biologic definition of Burkitt's lymphoma from transcriptional and genomic profiling. N Engl J Med. 2006;354(23):2419–30.
23. Leucci E, Cocco M, Onnis A, De Falco G, van Cleef P, Bellan C, van Rijk A, Nyagol J, Byakika B, Lazzi S, Tosi P, van Krieken H, Leoncini L. MYC translocation-negative classical Burkitt lymphoma cases: an alternative pathogenetic mechanism involving miRNA deregulation. J Pathol. 2008;216(4):440–50.
24. Salaverria I, Martin-Guerrero I, Wagener R, Kreuz M, Kohler CW, Richter J, Pienkowska-Grela B, Adam P, Burkhardt B, Claviez A, Damm-Welk C, Drexler HG, Hummel M, Jaffe ES, Küppers R, Lefebvre C, Lisfeld J, Löffler M, Macleod RA, Nagel I, Oschlies I, Rosolowski M, Russell RB, Rymkiewicz G, Schindler D, Schlesner M, Scholtysik R, Schwaenen C, Spang R, Szczepanowski M, Trümper L, Vater I, Wessendorf S, Klapper W, Siebert R, Molecular Mechanisms in Malignant Lymphoma Network Project; Berlin-Frankfurt-Münster Non-Hodgkin Lymphoma Group. A recurrent 11q aberration pattern characterizes a subset of MYC-negative high-grade B-cell lymphomas resembling Burkitt lymphoma. Blood. 2014;123(8):1187–98.

25. Havelange V, Ameye G, Théate I, Callet-Bauchu E, Lippert E, Luquet I, Raphaël M, Vikkula M, Poirel HA. The peculiar 11q-gain/loss aberration reported in a subset of MYC-negative high-grade B-cell lymphomas can also occur in a MYC-rearranged lymphoma. Cancer Genet. 2016a;209(3):117–8.
26. Havelange V, Ameye G, Callet-Bauchu E, Dastugue N, Barin C, Penther D, Michaux L, Hagemeijer A, Mugneret F, Poirel HA. Patterns of genomic aberrations suggest that Burkitt lymphomas with complex karyotype remain different from the other aggressive B-cell lymphomas with MYC rearrangement. Genes Chromosomes Cancer. 2013;52(1):81–92.
27. Poirel HA, Cairo MS, Heerema NA, Swansbury J, Aupérin A, Launay E, Sanger WG, Talley P, Perkins SL, Raphael M, McCarthy K, Sposto R, Gerrard M, Bernheim A, Patte C, on behalf of the FAB LMB 96 International Study Committee. Specific cytogenetic abnormalities are associated with a significantly inferior outcome in children and adolescents with mature B-cell non-Hodgkin's lymphoma: results of the FAB/LMB 96 international study. Leukemia. 2009;23(2):323–31.
28. Piccaluga PP, De Falco G, Kustagi M, Gazzola A, Agostinelli C, Tripodo C, Leucci E, Onnis A, Astolfi A, Sapienza MR, Bellan C, Lazzi S, Tumwine L, Mawanda M, Ogwang M, Calbi V, Formica S, Califano A, Pileri SA, Leoncini L. Gene expression analysis uncovers similarity and differences among Burkitt lymphoma subtypes. Blood. 2011;117(13):3596–608.
29. Lenze D, Leoncini L, Hummel M, Volinia S, Liu CG, Amato T, De Falco G, Githanga J, Horn H, Nyagol J, Ott G, Palatini J, Pfreundschuh M, Rogena E, Rosenwald A, Siebert R, Croce CM, Stein H. The different epidemiologic subtypes of Burkitt lymphoma share a homogenous micro RNA profile distinct from diffuse large B-cell lymphoma. Leukemia. 2011;25(12):1869–76.
30. Havelange V, Pepermans X, Ameye G, Théate I, Callet-Bauchu E, Barin C, Penther D, Lippert E, Michaux L, Mugneret F, Dastugue N, Raphaël M, Vikkula M, Poirel HA. Genetic differences between pediatric and adult Burkitt lymphomas. Br J Haematol. 2016b;173(1):137–44.
31. Love C, Sun Z, Jima D, Li G, Zhang J, Miles R, Richards KL, Dunphy CH, Choi WW, Srivastava G, Lugar PL, Rizzieri DA, Lagoo AS, Bernal-Mizrachi L, Mann KP, Flowers CR, Naresh KN, Evens AM, Chadburn A, Gordon LI, Czader MB, Gill JI, Hsi ED, Greenough A, Moffitt AB, McKinney M, Banerjee A, Grubor V, Levy S, Dunson DB, Dave SS. The genetic landscape of mutations in Burkitt lymphoma. Nat Genet. 2012;44(12):1321–5.
32. Schmitz R, Young RM, Ceribelli M, Jhavar S, Xiao W, Zhang M, Wright G, Shaffer AL, Hodson DJ, Buras E, Liu X, Powell J, Yang Y, Xu W, Zhao H, Kohlhammer H, Rosenwald A, Kluin P, Müller-Hermelink HK, Ott G, Gascoyne RD, Connors JM, Rimsza LM, Campo E, Jaffe ES, Delabie J, Smeland EB, Ogwang MD, Reynolds SJ, Fisher RI, Braziel RM, Tubbs RR, Cook JR, Weisenburger DD, Chan WC, Pittaluga S, Wilson W, Waldmann TA, Rowe M, Mbulaiteye SM, Rickinson AB, Staudt LM. Burkitt lymphoma pathogenesis and therapeutic targets from structural and functional genomics. Nature. 2012;490(7418):116–20.
33. Schmitz R, Ceribelli M, Pittaluga S, Wright G, Staudt LM. Oncogenic mechanisms in Burkitt lymphoma. Cold Spring Harb Perspect Med. 2014;4(2):a014282.
34. Richter J, Schlesner M, Hoffmann S, Kreuz M, Leich E, Burkhardt B, Rosolowski M, Ammerpohl O, Wagener R, Bernhart SH, Lenze D, Szczepanowski M, Paulsen M, Lipinski S, Russell RB, Adam-Klages S, Apic G, Claviez A, Hasenclever D, Hovestadt V, Hornig N, Korbel JO, Kube D, Langenberger D, Lawerenz C, Lisfeld J, Meyer K, Picelli S, Pischimarov J, Radlwimmer B, Rausch T, Rohde M, Schilhabel M, Scholtysik R, Spang R, Trautmann H, Zenz T, Borkhardt A, Drexler HG, Möller P, MacLeod RA, Pott C, Schreiber S, Trümper L, Loeffler M, Stadler PF, Lichter P, Eils R, Küppers R, Hummel M, Klapper W, Rosenstiel P, Rosenwald A, Brors B, Siebert R, MMML-Seq Project ICGC. Recurrent mutation of the ID3 gene in Burkitt lymphoma identified by integrated genome, exome and transcriptome sequencing. Nat Genet. 2012;44:1316–20.
35. Greenough A, Dave SS. New clues to the molecular pathogenesis of Burkitt lymphoma revealed through next-generation sequencing. Curr Opin Hematol. 2014;21(4):326–32.
36. Abate F, Ambrosio MR, Mundo L, Laginestra MA, Fuligni F, Rossi M, Zairis S, Gazaneo S, De Falco G, Lazzi S, Bellan C, Rocca BJ, Amato T, Marasco E, Etebari M, Ogwang M, Calbi V, Ndede I, Patel K, Chumba D, Piccaluga PP, Pileri S, Leoncini L, Rabadan R. Distinct viral and mutational spectrum of endemic burkitt lymphoma. PLoS Pathog. 2015;11(10):e1005158.
37. Küppers R. Mechanisms of B-cell lymphoma 7pathogenesis. Nat Rev Cancer. 2005;5(4):251–62. Review.
38. Sander S, Calado DP, Srinivasan L, Köchert K, Zhang B, Rosolowski M, Rodig SJ, Holzmann K, Stilgenbauer S, Siebert R, Bullinger L, Rajewsky K. Synergy between PI3K signaling and MYC in Burkitt lymphomagenesis. Cancer Cell. 2012;22(2):167–79.
39. Amato T, Abate F, Piccaluga P, Iacono M, Fallerini C, Renieri A, De Falco G, Ambrosio MR, Mourmouras V, Ogwang M, Calbi V, Rabadan R, Hummel M, Pileri S, Leoncini L, Bellan C. Clonality analysis of immunoglobulin gene rearrangement by next-generation sequencing in endemic Burkitt lymphoma suggests antigen drive activation of BCR as opposed to sporadic Burkitt lymphoma. Am J Clin Pathol. 2016;145(1):116–27.
40. Cai Q, Medeiros LJ, Xu X, Young KH. *MYC*-driven aggressive B-cell lymphomas: biology, entity, differential diagnosis and clinical management. Oncotarget. 2015;6(36):38591–616.
41. Moormann AM, Snider CJ, Chelimo K. The company malaria keeps: how co-infection with Epstein-Barr

virus leads to endemic Burkitt lymphoma. Curr Opin Infect Dis. 2011;24:435–41.
42. Rochford R, Cannon MJ, Moormann AM. Endemic Burkitt's lymphoma: a polymicrobial disease? Nat Rev Microbiol. 2005;3(2):182–7.
43. Thorley-Lawson DA, Hawkins JB, Tracy SI, Shapiro M. The pathogenesis of Epstein-Barr virus persistent infection. Curr Opin Virol. 2013;3:227–32.
44. Ambrosio MR, Navari M, Di Lisio L, Leon EA, Onnis A, Gazaneo S, Mundo L, Ulivieri C, Gomez G, Lazzi S, Piris MA, Leoncini L, De Falco G. The Epstein Barr-encoded BART-6-3p microRNA affects regulation of cell growth and immuno response in Burkitt lymphoma. Infect Agent Cancer. 2014a;14(9):12.
45. Ambrosio MR, De Falco G, Gozzetti A, Rocca BJ, Amato T, Mourmouras V, Gazaneo S, Mundo L, Candi V, Piccaluga PP, Cusi MG, Leoncini L, Lazzi S. Plasmablastic transformation of a pre-existing plasmacytoma: a possible role for reactivation of Epstein Barr virus infection. Haematologica. 2014b;99(11):e235–7.
46. Arvey A, Ojesina AI, Pedamallu CS, Ballon G, Jung J, et al. The tumor virus landscape of AIDS-related lymphomas. Blood. 2015;125:e14–22.
47. Piccaluga PP, Navari M, De Falco G, Ambrosio MR, Lazzi S, Fuligni F, Bellan C, Rossi M, Sapienza MR, Laginestra MA, Etebari M, Rogena EA, Tumwine L, Tripodo C, Gibellini D, Consiglio J, Croce CM, Pileri SA, Leoncini L. Virus-encoded microRNA contributes to the molecular profile of EBV-positive Burkitt lymphomas. Oncotarget. 2016;7(1):224–40.
48. Navari M, Etebari M, De Falco G, Ambrosio MR, Gibellini D, Leoncini L, Piccaluga PP. The presence of Epstein-Barr virus significantly impacts the transcriptional profile in immunodeficiency-associated Burkitt lymphoma. Front Microbiol. 2015;6:556.
49. Navari M, Fuligni F, Laginestra MA, Etebari M, Ambrosio MR, Sapienza MR, Rossi M, De Falco G, Gibellini D, Tripodo C, Pileri SA, Leoncini L, Piccaluga PP. Molecular signature of Epstein Barr virus-positive Burkitt lymphoma and post-transplant lymphoproliferative disorder suggest different roles for Epstein Barr virus. Front Microbiol. 2014;5:728.
50. Mundo L, Ambrosio MR, Picciolini M, Lo Bello G, Gazaneo S, Del Porro L, Lazzi S, Navari M, Onyango N, Granai M, Bellan C, De Falco G, Gibellini D, Piccaluga PP, Leoncini L. Unveiling another missing piece in EBV-driven lymphomagenesis: EBV-encoded MicroRNAs expression in EBER-negative Burkitt lymphoma cases. Front Microbiol. 2017;8:229.
51. Vereide D, Sugden B. Proof for EBV's sustaining role in Burkitt's lymphomas. Semin Cancer Biol. 2009;19:389–93.
52. Ambrosio MR, Rocca BJ, Ginori A, Mourmouras V, Amato T, Vindigni C, Lazzi S, Leoncini L. A look into the evolution of Epstein-Barr virus-induced lymphoproliferative disorders: a case study. Am J Clin Pathol. 2015;144(5):817–22.
53. Mannucci S, Luzzi A, Carugi A, Gozzetti A, Lazzi S, Malagnino V, Simmonds M, Cusi MG, Leoncini L, van den Bosch CA, De Falco G. Endemic Burkitt lymphoma. Adv Hematol. 2012;2012:149780.
54. Bassan R, Maino E, Cortelazzo S. Lymphoblastic lymphoma: an updated review on biology, diagnosis, and treatment. Eur J Haematol. 2016;96(5):447–60. Review.
55. Paolini S, Gazzola A, Sabattini E, Bacci F, Pileri S, Piccaluga PP. Pathobiology of acute lymphoblastic leukemia. Semin Diagn Pathol. 2011;28(2):124–34.
56. Kratz CP, Stanulla M, Cavé H. Genetic predisposition to acute lymphoblastic leukemia: overview on behalf of the I-BFM ALL Host Genetic Variation Working Group. Eur J Med Genet. 2016;59(3):111–5. Review.
57. Cortelazzo S, Ferreri A, Hoelzer D, Ponzoni M. Lymphoblastic lymphoma. Crit Rev Oncol Hematol. 2017;113:304–17.
58. Geyer JT, Subramaniyam S, Jiang Y, Elemento O, Ferry JA, de Leval L, Nakashima MO, Liu YC, Martin P, Mathew S, Orazi A, Tam W. Lymphoblastic transformation of follicular lymphoma: a clinicopathologic and molecular analysis of 7 patients. Hum Pathol. 2015;46(2):260–71.
59. Oschlies I, Burkhardt B, Chassagne-Clement C, d'Amore ES, Hansson U, Hebeda K, Mc Carthy K, Kodet R, Maldyk J, Müllauer L, Porwit A, Schmatz AI, Tinguely M, Abramov D, Wotherspoon A, Zimmermann M, Reiter A, Klapper W. Diagnosis and immunophenotype of 188 pediatric lymphoblastic lymphomas treated within a randomized prospective trial: experiences and preliminary recommendations from the European childhood lymphoma pathology panel. Am J Surg Pathol. 2011;35(6):836–44. https://doi.org/10.1097/PAS.0b013e318213e90e.
60. Burkhardt B, Bruch J, Zimmermann M, Strauch K, Parwaresch R, Ludwig WD, Harder L, Schlegelberger B, Mueller F, Harbott J, Reiter A. Loss of heterozygosity on chromosome 6q14-q24 is associated with poor outcome in children and adolescents with T-cell lymphoblastic lymphoma. Leukemia. 2006;20:1422–9.
61. Burkhardt B. Paediatric lymphoblastic T-cell leukaemia and lymphoma: one or two diseases? Br J Haematol. 2010;149:653–68.
62. Lones MA, Heerema NA, Le Beau MM, Sposto R, Perkins SL, Kadin ME, Kjeldsberg CR, Meadows A, Siegel S, Buckley J, Abromowitch M, Kersey J, Bergeron S, Cairo MS, Sanger WG. Chromosome abnormalities in advanced stage lymphoblastic lymphoma of children and adolescents: a report from CCG-E08. Cancer Genet Cytogenet. 2007;172:1–11.
63. Sekimizu M, Sunami S, Nakazawa A, Hayashi Y, Okimoto Y, Saito AM, Horibe K, Tsurusawa M, Mori T. Chromosome abnormalities in advanced stage T-cell lymphoblastic lymphoma of children and adolescents: a report from Japanese Paediatric Leukaemia/Lymphoma Study Group (JPLSG) and review of the literature. Br J Haematol. 2011;154(5):612–7.
64. Uyttebroeck A, Vanhentenrijk V, Hagemeijer A, Boeckx N, Renard M, Wlodarska I, Vandenberghe P, Depaepe P, De Wolf-Peeters C. Is there a difference in childhood T-cell acute lymphoblastic leukaemia and

T-cell lymphoblastic lymphoma? Leuk Lymphoma. 2007;48:1745–54.
65. You MJ, Medeiros LJ, Hsi ED. T-lymphoblastic leukemia/lymphoma. Am J Clin Pathol. 2015;144(3):411–22.
66. Baleydier F, Decouvelaere AV, Bergeron J, Gaulard P, Canioni D, Bertrand Y, Lepretre S, Petit B, Dombret H, Beldjord K, Molina T, Asnafi V, Macintyre E. T cell receptor genotyping and HOXA/TLX1 expression define three T lymphoblastic lymphoma subsets which might affect clinical outcome. Clin Cancer Res. 2008;14(3):692–700.
67. Kaneko Y, Frizzera G, Maseki N, Sakurai M, Komada Y, Hiyoshi Y, Nakadate H, Takeda T. A novel translocation, t(9;17)(q34;q23), in aggressive childhood lymphoblastic lymphoma. Leukemia. 1998;2:745–8.
68. Schraders M, Van Reijmersdal SV, Kamping EJ, Van Krieken JH, Van Kessel AG, Groenen PJ, Hoogerbrugge PM, Kuiper RP. High-resolution genomic profiling of pediatric lymphoblastic lymphomas reveals subtle differences with pediatric acute lymphoblastic leukemias in the B-lineage. Cancer Genet Cytogenet. 2009;191:27–33.
69. Bonn BR, Rohde M, Zimmermann M, Krieger D, Oschlies I, Niggli F, et al. Incidence and prognostic relevance of genetic variations in T-cell lymphoblastic lymphoma in childhood and adolescence. Blood. 2013;121:3153–60.
70. Weng AP, Ferrando AA, Lee W, et al. Activating mutations of NOTCH1 in human T cell acute lymphoblastic leukemia. Science. 2004;306(5694):269–71.
71. Bonn BR, Huge A, Rohde M, Oschlies I, Klapper W, Voss R, Makarova O, Rossig C, Jürgens H, Seggewiss J, Burkhardt B. Whole exome sequencing hints at a unique mutational profile of paediatric T-cell lymphoblastic lymphoma. Br J Haematol. 2015;168(2):308–13.
72. Raetz EA, Perkins SL, Bhojwani D, Smock K, Philip M, Carroll WL, et al. Gene expression profiling reveals intrinsic differences between T-cell acute lymphoblastic leukemia and T-cell lymphoblastic lymphoma. Pediatr Blood Cancer. 2006;47:130–40.
73. Basso K, Mussolin L, Lettieri A, Brahmachary M, Lim WK, Califano A, et al. T-cell lymphoblastic lymphoma shows differences and similarities with T-cell acute lymphoblastic leukemia by genomic and gene expression analyses. Genes Chromosomes Cancer. 2011;50:1063–75.
74. Crazzolara R, Kreczy A, Mann G, et al. High expression of the chemokine receptor CXCR4 predicts extramedullary organ infiltration in childhood acute lymphoblastic leukaemia. Br J Haematol. 2001;115(3):545–53.
75. Herold T, Gökbuget N. Philadelphia-like acute lymphoblastic leukemia in adults. Curr Oncol Rep. 2017;19(5):31. https://doi.org/10.1007/s11912-017-0589-2. Review.
76. Agirre X, Martínez-Climent JA, Odero MD, Prósper F. Epigenetic regulation of miRNA genes in acute leukemia. Leukemia. 2012;26(3):395–403.
77. Yeh CH, Moles R, Nicot C. Clinical significance of microRNAs in chronic and acute human leukemia. Mol Cancer. 2016;15(1):37.
78. Fulci V, et al. Characterization of B- and T-lineage acute lymphoblastic leukemia by integrated analysis of MicroRNA and mRNA expression profiles. Genes Chromosomes Cancer. 2009;48(12):1069–82.
79. Luan C, Yang Z, Chen B. The functional role of microRNA in acute lymphoblastic leukemia: relevance for diagnosis, differential diagnosis, prognosis, and therapy. Onco Targets Ther. 2015;8:2903–14.
80. Schotte D, et al. MicroRNA characterize genetic diversity and drug resistance in pediatric acute lymphoblastic leukemia. Haematologica. 2011;96(5):703–11.
81. Nemes K, et al. Expression of certain leukemia/lymphoma related microRNAs and its correlation with prognosis in childhood acute lymphoblastic leukemia. Pathol Oncol Res. 2015;21(3):597–604.
82. Rainer J, et al. Glucocorticoid-regulated microRNAs and mirtrons in acute lymphoblastic leukemia. Leukemia. 2009;23(4):746–52.

4 Pathology and Molecular Pathogenesis of T-Cell Lymphoma

Javeed Iqbal and Laurence de Leval

4.1 Introduction

Peripheral T-cell lymphomas (PTCLs) and natural killer-cell lymphomas (NKCLs) constitute a group of heterogeneous diseases comprising about 10–20% of all non-Hodgkin lymphomas (NHLs). There is substantial geographic variation in the incidence and the subtype prevalence [1, 2], which can be attributed to a combination of genetic and environmental factors. Some PTCL subtypes occur at higher frequency in Asia and Central/South America than in Western countries, especially those induced by the human T-lymphotropic virus 1 (HTLV1) or by the Epstein-Barr virus (EBV) [2]. Conversely, enteropathy-associated T-cell lymphoma (EATL) is predominant in Northern Europe where celiac disease is more prevalent [3] (Fig. 4.1). Despite a plateau observed in the incidence of B-cell lymphoma in the Western world, the incidence of PTCLs has increased in recent years, amounting to 3.8% per annum in the United States [4], sharply augmenting both clinical and research interest. Whether this is due to improved diagnosis, or due to epidemiological changes, is not known. In general, NHL incidence steadily increases with age and is higher in males than females, and similar patterns are also true in PTCL, with the exception of some individual entities that are more common in children or younger adults, such as ALK-positive anaplastic large cell lymphoma (ALK+ALCL) and hepatosplenic T-cell lymphoma (HSTL) [5].

In the World Health Organization (WHO) classification of hematopoietic and lymphoid organs [5, 6], disease entities are defined based on several parameters: morphologic, immunophenotypic, genetic and clinical features, and putative normal cellular counterpart. Application of this principle for the delineation of NK/T-cell neoplasms is more challenging than for the B-cell tumors, reflecting the complexity of the T-cell immunobiology, with numerous functional subsets, and evidence of functional plasticity. Although there is increasing evidence that the cell of origin is a major determinant of PTCL biology [7–10], the cellular derivation of many PTCL entities remains poorly characterized or appears heterogeneous [7]. The cellular composition, cytomorphological features, and immunophenotypic profiles are heterogeneous within disease entities and also significantly overlap across different diseases. The recent application of genome-wide expression profiling (GEP) and

J. Iqbal (✉)
Department of Pathology and Microbiology, University of Nebraska Medical Center, Omaha, NE, USA
e-mail: jiqbal@unmc.edu

L. de Leval (✉)
Institute of Pathology, Lausanne University Hospital (CHUV) and University of Lausanne, Lausanne, Switzerland
e-mail: Laurence.deLeval@chuv.ch

G. Lenz, G. Salles (eds.), *Aggressive Lymphomas*, Hematologic Malignancies,
https://doi.org/10.1007/978-3-030-00362-3_4

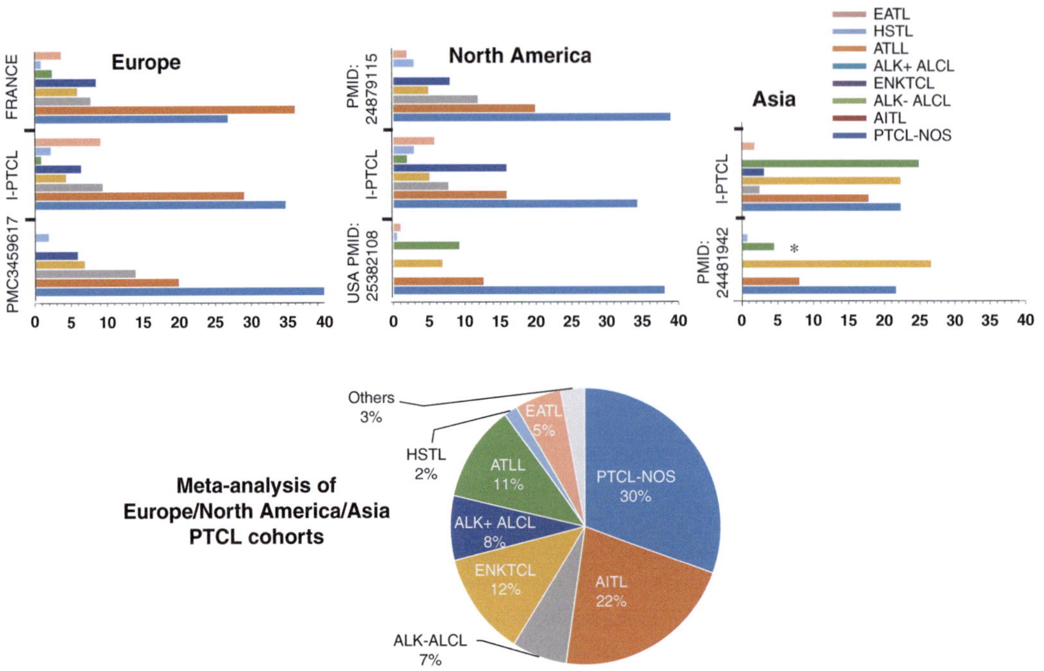

Fig. 4.1 Incidence of PTCL entities. Relative incidence of PTCLs (non-cutaneous) in Europe, North America, and Asia compiled from published data sets with at least 300 cases in (**a**) Europe/France (Laurent et al. J Clin Oncol 2017; Bellei et al. Rev. Bras Hematol Hemoter 2012; Vose et al. JCO, 2008), (**b**) North America/USA (Petrich et al. Br J Haematol 2015; Vose et al. JCO, 2008; Briski et al. Blood Cancer Journal; 2014), (**c**) Asia (Parks et al. Int J Hematol 2014;Vose (Vose et al. JCO, 2008). Meta-analysis of these cohorts revealed that PTCL-NOS is the major PTCL entity in the world, but AITL appears to be more common in France and ENKTL in Asia. *Some of the studies do not include ALK status in ALCL, thus data was not presented

massive parallel/next-generation sequencing (NGS) technologies has markedly accelerated the discovery of new biomarkers, molecular signatures, and cancer-associated mutations. These new data have been included in the revised classification [5] as they refine the diagnostic criteria of some PTCL entities and may be relevant to future clinical management of patients [9, 11]. A striking characteristic of NK/T-cell neoplasms is that the clinical and biological presenting features and disease localization represent relevant diagnostic criteria. In the current classification [5], more than 30 PTCL entities are recognized (Table 4.1) which may present as disseminated (leukemic), predominantly extra-nodal or cutaneous, or predominantly nodal diseases. Some entities are relatively homogeneous and/or well defined, whereas others have poorly defined borders (typically PTCL, not otherwise specified

Table 4.1 2016 WHO classification of mature T- and NK-cell neoplasms

Disseminated/leukemic
T-cell prolymphocytic leukemia
T-cell large granular lymphocytic leukemia
Chronic lymphoproliferative disorder of NK-cells*
Aggressive NK-cell leukemia
Systemic EBV-positive T-cell lymphoma of childhood*
Chronic active EBV infection of T- and NK-cell type, systemic form
Adult T-cell leukemia/lymphoma
Extra-nodal
Extra-nodal NK/T-cell lymphoma, nasal type
Enteropathy-associated T-cell lymphoma
Monomorphic epitheliotropic intestinal T-cell lymphoma
Indolent T-cell lymphoproliferative disorder of the gastrointestinal tract*
Hepatosplenic T-cell lymphoma
Subcutaneous panniculitis-like T-cell lymphoma

Table 4.1 (continued)

Breast implant-associated anaplastic large cell lymphoma*
Cutaneous
Mycosis fungoides
Sezary syndrome
Primary cutaneous CD30+ T-cell lymphoproliferative disorders
Primary cutaneous anaplastic large cell lymphoma
Lymphomatoid papulosis
Primary cutaneous γδ T-cell lymphoma
Primary cutaneous CD8+ aggressive epidermotropic cytotoxic T-cell lymphoma*
Primary cutaneous CD4+ small/medium T-cell lymphoproliferative disorder*
Hydroa vacciniforme-like lymphoproliferative disorder
Severe mosquito bite allergy
Nodal
Peripheral T-cell lymphoma, not otherwise specified
Angioimmunoblastic T-cell lymphoma (AITL)
Follicular T-cell lymphoma
Nodal peripheral T-cell lymphoma with T follicular helper phenotype
Anaplastic large cell lymphoma, ALK-positive
Anaplastic large cell lymphoma, ALK-negative

Adapted from Swerdlow SH et al. WHO Classification of Tumours of Haematopoietic and Lymphoid Tissues, Fourth Edition. Revised [5]

(NOS)) and some are provisional. Among this large number of NK/T-cell lymphoma entities, less than one third of them account for the vast majority of cases, and some entities are extremely rare and/or essentially restricted to certain parts of the world (i.e., the various kinds of childhood EBV-associated lymphoproliferations).

The introduction of targeted immunotherapy (i.e., rituximab) for B-cell lymphomas resulted in remarkable clinical improvement; however, similar improvements in outcomes in PTCL have not been observed over the last three decades (Fig. 4.2) [12–16]. However, depending on the entity and staging, the prognosis can vary widely; thus, accurate diagnosis of PTCL is therefore mandatory. For several reasons, it is highly recommended that the diagnosis should be made by an expert pathologist [17]. PTCLs are not only rare but also heterogeneous, implying limited exposure and experience for most pathologists. The malignant nature of the lymphoproliferation may be difficult to recognize in the infrequent instances where the neoplastic component is rather sparse and obscured by a coexistent reactive infiltrate and architectural distortion is subtle, which may mimic a benign condition. Another confounding element is that PTCLs

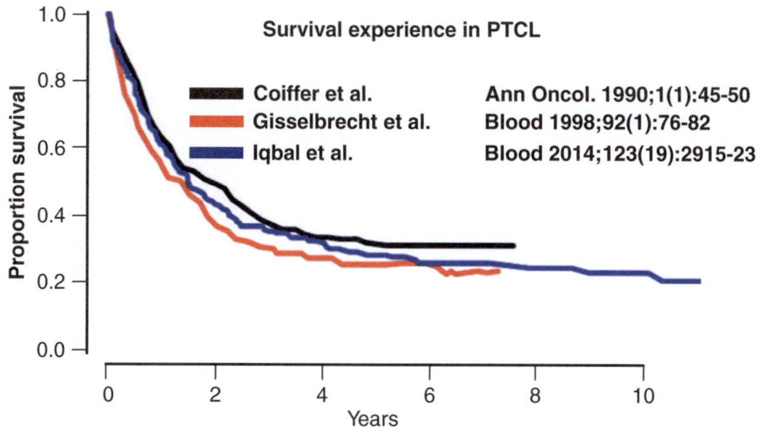

Fig. 4.2 Overall survival of PTCL patients (excluding ALCL) in the last three decades. No significant improvement in overall survival (OS) has been observed since the 1990s. Engauge digitizer software was used to extrapolate data from earlier studies. Survival of PTCL cohorts diagnosed pre-1990 (n = 188), 2000 (n = 228), and 2010 (n = 233) from three earlier studies is shown (Coiffier et al. Ann Oncol. 1990, Gisselbrecht et al. Blood 1998 and Iqbal et al. Blood 2014). Patients were generally treated with anthracycline-containing regimen and are either PTCL-NOS or AITL histological subtypes

may comprise atypical cells resembling Reed-Sternberg cells and/or an expansion of B-cells, misleading toward the diagnosis of Hodgkin or B-cell lymphomas. In France, where a network of expert lymphoma pathologists was created to review lymphoma diagnoses and biopsies from patients with clinically suspected lymphoma, the diagnostic concordance rates (between referral and expert pathologists) for PTCLs were rather low (47–74% for the most frequent entities), except for ALK+ALCL (>80% concordance rate) over a recent time period (2010–2013), highlighting the importance of expert review for diagnoses of PTCL [18]. It is also recommended that the diagnosis of PTCL should rely on an excisional tumor biopsy whenever possible [17] with sufficient tissue for adequate histopathological assessment and additional ancillary techniques, in particular immunohistochemistry and molecular studies that critically contribute to the diagnosis.

After presenting an overview of normal T-cell development and differentiation that is relevant to T-cell lymphoma pathogenesis, we will summarize the pathology, molecular and genetic features of the major NK/T-cell neoplasms.

4.2 Normal T-Cell Differentiation and Relevance to Lymphomagenesis

Many molecular abnormalities in PTCL target genes critical for normal T-cell differentiation and development [19], and thus an overview of normal T-cell development and differentiation is presented here (Fig. 4.3).

T-cell development: T-cells originate from the hematopoietic stem cells (HSC) in the bone marrow [20, 21] and further develop in the thymus, where thymic microenvironment directs differentiation and selection of T-cells [22] for periphery. This tightly regulated phase, also termed β-selection phase, starts with TCR-β chain rearrangement in immature double-negative (DN,

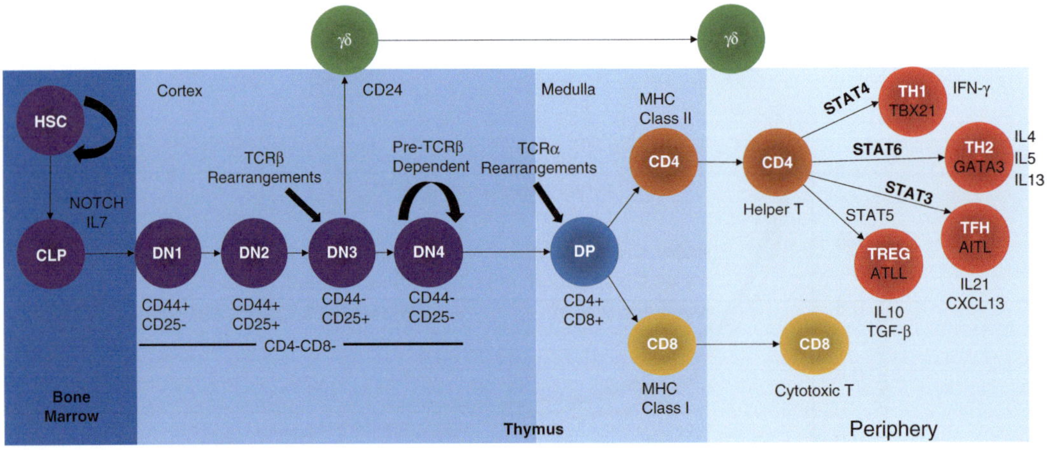

Fig. 4.3 Schematic representation of T-cell development and association with PTCL entities. The hematopoietic stem cells (HSC) in the bone marrow (BM) are the initiating cells for T-cell lymphopoiesis. Common lymphoid progenitor cells (CLP) in BM are directed to T-cell lineage fate via IL7/Notch signaling. Further development of immature precursor T-cells happens in the thymus through a series of tightly regulated steps (double negative (DN (1–4) to double positive (DP)) and differentiate into either single positive CD4+ or CD8+ T-cells. Distinct stages of differentiation (i.e., β selection phase and TCR repertoire phase) can be identified through cell surface receptors (CD44 and CD25) and the rearrangement of TCR genes. T-cells undergo dual selection process, positive selection for compatibility of their TCR with self-MHC molecules and negative selection against autoantigenic peptides, and leave the thymus to form the peripheral T-cell repertoire. Though the vast majority of cells express an αβ TCR, a small subset express an alternative TCR composed of γ and δ chains (γ/δ T-cells) and diverge early place at the DN3a stage in T-cell development and mostly become resident of mucosal sites. Mature CD4+ T-cells can differentiate into different T helper (T_H) subsets (T_{H1}, T_{H2}, T_{FH}, T_{reg}) characterized by expression of transcriptional factors and different cytokine profiles and can represent the normal cell counterpart of different disease entities

$CD4^-/CD8^-$) thymocytes, via productive VDJ rearrangement of TCR-β chain and surface expression of TCRβ, which co-assemble with pre-Tα [23]. The pre-TCR signals are essential for rapid expansion and maturation to the DP ($CD4^+CD8^+$) and rearrangement of the TCR-α chain [24] leading to the mature TCR-αβ receptor expression upon successful rearrangement [25]. The DP thymocytes that recognize self-MHC receive a positive selection signal leading to either CD4 or CD8 T-cells depending on their interaction with either class I or class II MHC, referred to as repertoire selection phase. The TCR repertoire is produced by a series of DNA recombination events that generates 10^{16} to 10^{18} different possible sequences from the VDJ recombination events shaped by the selection by self-antigens. This hyper-variability of the TCR is crucial for recognition of diverse antigens presented by MHC. The TCR includes the α, β, γ, and δ chains, which form α/β or γ/δ heterodimeric receptors that are expressed on the surface of mature T-cells [26]. Both αβ- and γδ-T-cells share similar developmental pathways, but T-cell lineage fate [27] is dependent on the TCR signal strength. This process is regulated by transcription factors (ID3 and Erg), strength of the TCR signaling determined by TCR affinity, with weak TCR signal favoring the αβ lineage T-cells commitment [28]. Other than these signals, Notch and CXCR4 receptors also cooperate with the TCR in determination of lineage fate [28]. Even though γδ T-cells have only a limited repertoire of TCR rearrangements, they have a broad functional armamentarium including cytokines secretion, cytotoxicity, or growth factors [29]. In human, the majority of T-cells express αβ-TCR, whereas 1–5% of the T-cells in the peripheral blood and 20–50% of T-cell in mucosal sites express γδ-TCR [30], and this distribution also reflects in T-NHLs derived from these sites.

T-cell activation: TCR signaling is initiated by the immunological synapses between antigen-presenting cells (APCs) and T-cells with corresponding MHC/peptide interaction with CD4 or CD8 co-receptor. Optimal T-cell activation occurs via T-cell receptor (TCR) in conjunction with CD28 co-receptor engagement. TCR alone cannot effectively signal after it has bound antigen and has to form the TCR complex with the CD3γ, δ, ε, and ζ chains. Once TCRs and CD4 or CD8 molecules bind to MHC/peptide complexes, LCK is activated and subsequently phosphorylates the immunoreceptor tyrosine-based activation motifs (ITAM) in the ζ and ε chains of the CD3 complex. The signaling cascade is extended by phosphorylating LAT, which is a transmembrane adaptor protein associated with GRB2, GADS, and PCLG1 via its four distal tyrosine residues. CD3/TCR activation without co-stimulation induces anergy, in which the T-cell is not able to respond to even high-affinity stimulus. Classically, co-stimulation occurs through CD28, the prototypical costimulatory receptor and founding member of the B7 receptor family. The CD28-mediated activation leads to PI3K, NF-κB, and NFAT activation, augmenting T-cell survival [31]. The negative signals are mediated by competing member CTLA4 which, like CD28, forms heterodimers [32]. CTLA4 shares high-protein homology with CD28 but has some differences that result in affinity and functional changes [32–36]. CTLA4 can prevent CD28 from interacting with src family tyrosine kinases LCK and FYN [37, 38].

The antigen-inexperienced naïve CD4+ T-cells can further differentiate into one of several T-cell subtypes (T_{H1}, T_{H2}, T_{H17}, T_{REG}, and T_{FH}), instructed by distinct environmental cytokines, lineage defining transcription factors, and consequently acquire distinct functions in the adaptive immune system [39]. Though T-cell development and activation are well orchestrated by distinct regulatory genes or pathways, genetic aberrations and/or constitutive activation of these pathways can lead to the development of T-cell neoplasms.

4.3 Angioimmunoblastic T-Cell Lymphoma (AITL) and Other Nodal Lymphomas of Follicular Helper T-Cell Derivation

AITL is the second most common PTCL worldwide (18.5% of the cases in the International T-cell lymphoma project) [2], but most prevalent in North America and Europe where it accounts for up to 35% of non-cutaneous PTCLs, according to a recent epidemiological analysis in France [40–42]. It is defined as a neoplasm of mature T follicular helper (T_{FH}) cells [8] characterized by a systemic disease, a polymorphous infiltrate in lymph nodes with prominent proliferation of vessels and follicular dendritic cells [5, 8]. This disease exhibits variable, often aggressive clinical course, and unfortunately no major improvement in patient care has been achieved over the last three decades (Fig. 4.2).

AITL is usually characterized by generalized peripheral lymphadenopathy, often with extranodal disease and frequent cutaneous involvement. The 2017 WHO classification recognizes two other PTCL entities related to AITL [5], namely, follicular T-cell lymphoma (FTCL) and nodal PTCL with T_{FH} phenotype (T_{FH}-PTCL) [5]. FTCL is a rare T_{FH} neoplasm defined by a predominantly follicular growth pattern [5, 43–45] closely related to AITL as supported by analogies in their cellular derivation and clinical presentation, and documentation that patients with FTCL may relapse with lesions resembling AITL [43, 45]. Nodal PTCL of T_{FH} origin designates a subset of PTCL "unspecified" by morphology showing expression of a T_{FH} phenotype (expression of at least two T_{FH} markers). T_{FH}-PTCL is less frequent than AITL, but not rare, as it is estimated that up to 30% of PTCL unspecified by morphology and formerly considered as PTCL-NOS show a T_{FH} immunophenotype. A common feature of AITL and other nodal T_{FH} lymphomas is the presence of scattered to numerous large B-cell blasts, often infected by EBV [46].

4.3.1 Pathology

The lymph nodes in AITL show complete effacement of architecture, often with perinodal infiltration sparing the peripheral sinus (Fig. 4.4). Less frequently, depleted follicles may be present, or the neoplastic cells infiltrate around hyperplastic GC. The neoplastic cells are typically medium-sized with clear cytoplasm and tend to form small clusters around high endothelial venules admixed with an abundant tumor microenvironment composed of small lymphocytes, histiocytes or epithelioid cells, B-cell immunoblasts, eosinophils, and plasma cells. The relative proportion of the neoplastic and individual reactive components varies widely, and in particular, histiocytes may be prominent and cause confusion with other histiocyte-rich lymphoma entities. The neoplastic cells are mature TCR-αβ $CD4^{+}CD8^{-}$ T-cells that frequently show aberrant loss or reduced expression of CD7, surface CD3 and/or CD4, and may show partial CD30 expression or aberrant co-expression of CD20 [47]. A population of large B-cell blasts, sometimes mimicking Reed-Sternberg cells, usually infected by EBV, is almost invariably present. Irregular proliferation of follicular dendritic cells (FDC) is evidenced in most cases by immunohistochemistry (CD21, CD23, CD35, and CNA42). The neoplastic cells express several markers of T_{FH} cells: CD10, CXCL13, CXCR5, CD154, programmed death-1 (PD-1), inducible costimulatory (ICOS), cytoplasmic SLAM-associated protein (SAP), BCL6, and/or c-MAF [48]. In addition to monoclonal or oligoclonal rearrangement of the TCR genes in the vast majority of cases, a clonal or oligoclonal rearrangement of the immunoglobulin (IG*)* gene(s) is found in up to one third of patients in relationship to increased numbers of B-cell blasts and/or plasma cells.

4.3.2 Molecular Signature

The molecular profile of AITL is dominated by a strong microenvironment imprint, including overexpression of B-cell- and FDC-related genes, chemokines/chemokine receptors, and genes related to extracellular matrix and vascular biology [14, 15, 19, 49] (Fig. 4.5a). The signature contributed by the neoplastic cells, albeit quantitatively minor, is enriched in genes normally expressed by T_{FH} cells. This demonstration of molecular similarities between AITL cells and T_{FH} cells at a genome-wide level definitively established the cellular derivation of AITL from T_{FH} cells [15, 45, 50] (Fig. 4.5b), initially suspected on the basis of expression of single T_{FH} markers in AITL cells, in

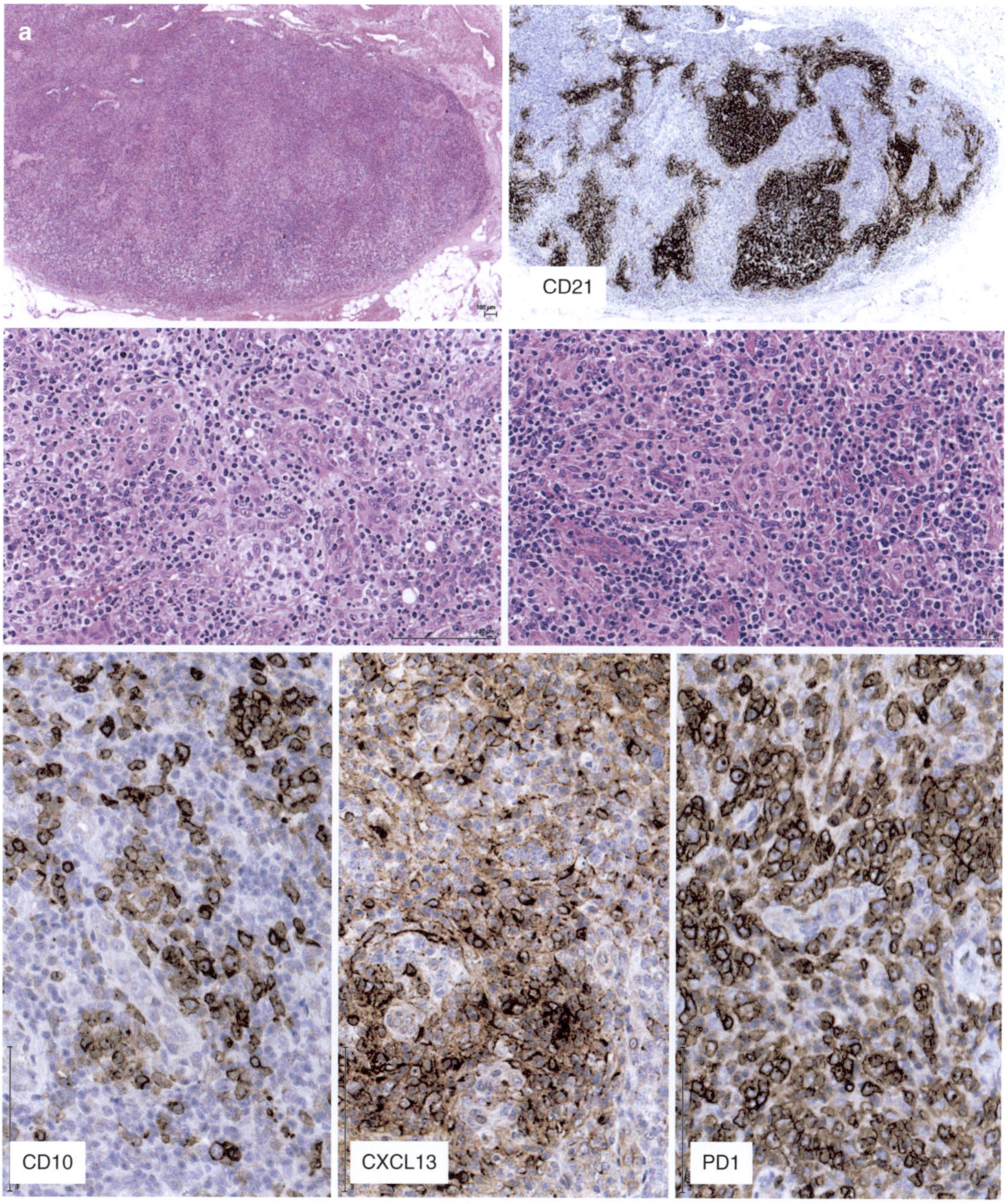

Fig. 4.4 Histopathological features of angioimmunoblastic T-cell lymphoma (AITL) and follicular T-cell lymphoma (F-PTCL). (**a**) AITL. The low-power view of an AITL lymph node shows complete architectural effacement by a diffuse lymphoproliferation (upper left panel), and CD21 highlights a marked expansion of follicular dendritic cells. The case illustrated in the middle left panel shows a lymphoproliferation associated with an increased density of high endothelial veinules and comprising a polymorphous infiltrate among which medium-sized cells with clear cytoplasm that represent the neoplastic component, and a large number of plasma cells. In the case illustrated in the middle right panel, the neoplastic cells are small with minimal atypia and dispersed in a background rich in histiocytes with scattered large blastic cells. Immunohistochemical stains for CD10, CXCL13, and PD1 highlight the neoplastic population. (**b**) F-PTCL. The low-power view of the lymph node shows a vaguely nodular lymphoproliferation (upper left panel), which comprises small dense lymphoid cells interrupted by pale cellular aggregates (upper right panel). Immunohistochemical stains show that the nodules correspond to large follicular structures associated with a CD21+ follicular dendritic cell meshwork and comprising numerous CD20+ B-cells, while CD4 stains the pale aggregates of neoplastic cells

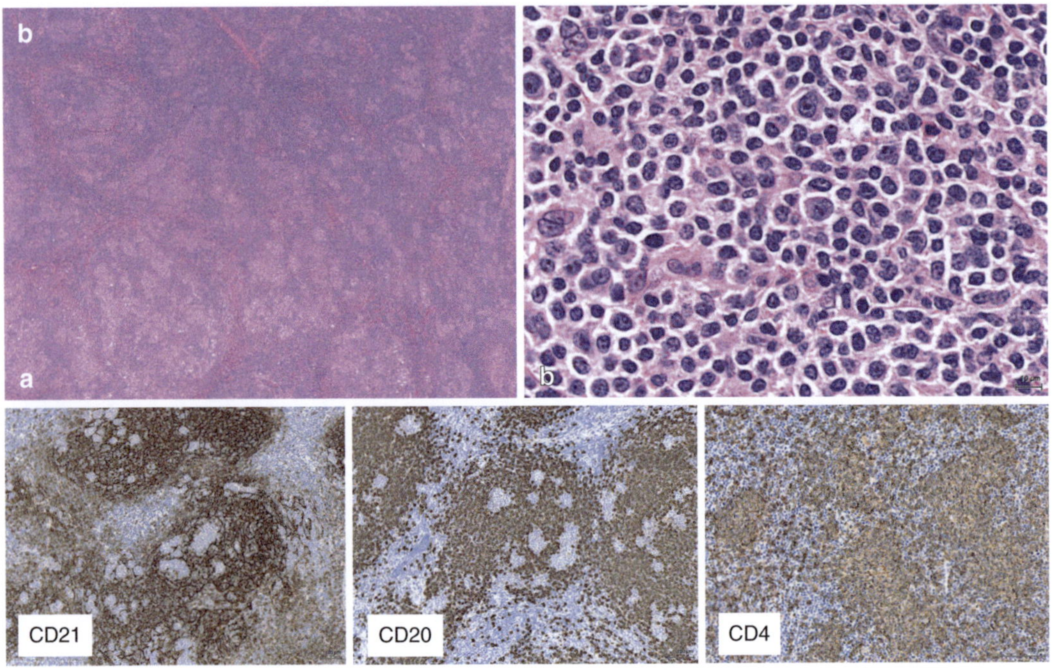

Fig. 4.4 (continued)

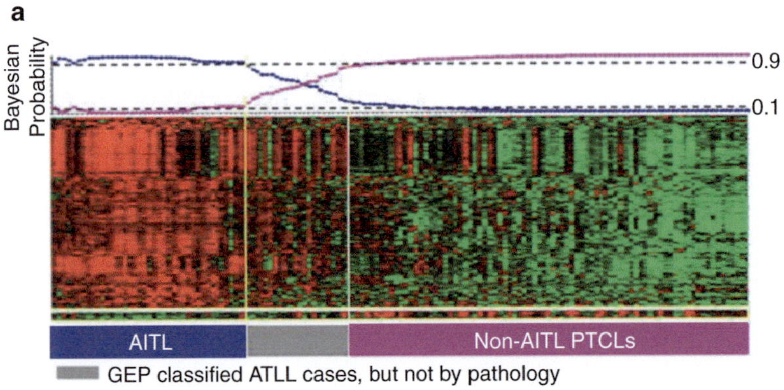

Fig. 4.5 Molecular and genetic features of AITL. (**a**) Gene expression-based molecular predictor identified for AITL. Iqbal et al. used the Bayesian algorithm to distinguish AITL cases from other PTCLs. Genes were selected at significance ($p < 0.001$) and a mean fold difference (>4) between the AITL and other PTCLs. Arbitrary ≥90% threshold probability is used to assign a subgroup, and classification precision was evaluated by the use of leave-one-out cross-validation. Approximately 14% of PTCL-NOS cases showed AITL molecular signature characterized by expression of genes involved in T-cell activation or T_{FH} differentiation and a distinct tumor milieu (adapted from Iqbal et al. Blood 2010). (**b**) T_{FH} genes showed significant association with AITL. A subset of genes that are expressed by T_{FH} cells significantly associate with AITL, but not with PTCL-NOS. Conversely, gene expression signatures of other T-cell subsets (T_{H1}, and T_{H2}) are not enriched in AITL. Standardized expression ranges from low (blue to high (red) (adapted from de Leval et al. Blood 2007). (**c**) Mutational landscape AITL and T_{FH}-like PTCL. Recurrent mutations in epigenetic modifiers and genes related to T-cell receptor signaling were identified by targeted deep sequencing. Case-mutation pairs for which data are not available are indicated by a 0. Mutated genes (rows) are arranged by decreasing order of mutation frequency. Patients (columns) are arranged from left to right based on their mutational status following gene ranking. AITL cases are featured in light gray and T_{FH}-like PTCLs in dark gray (adapted from Vallois et al. Blood 2016)

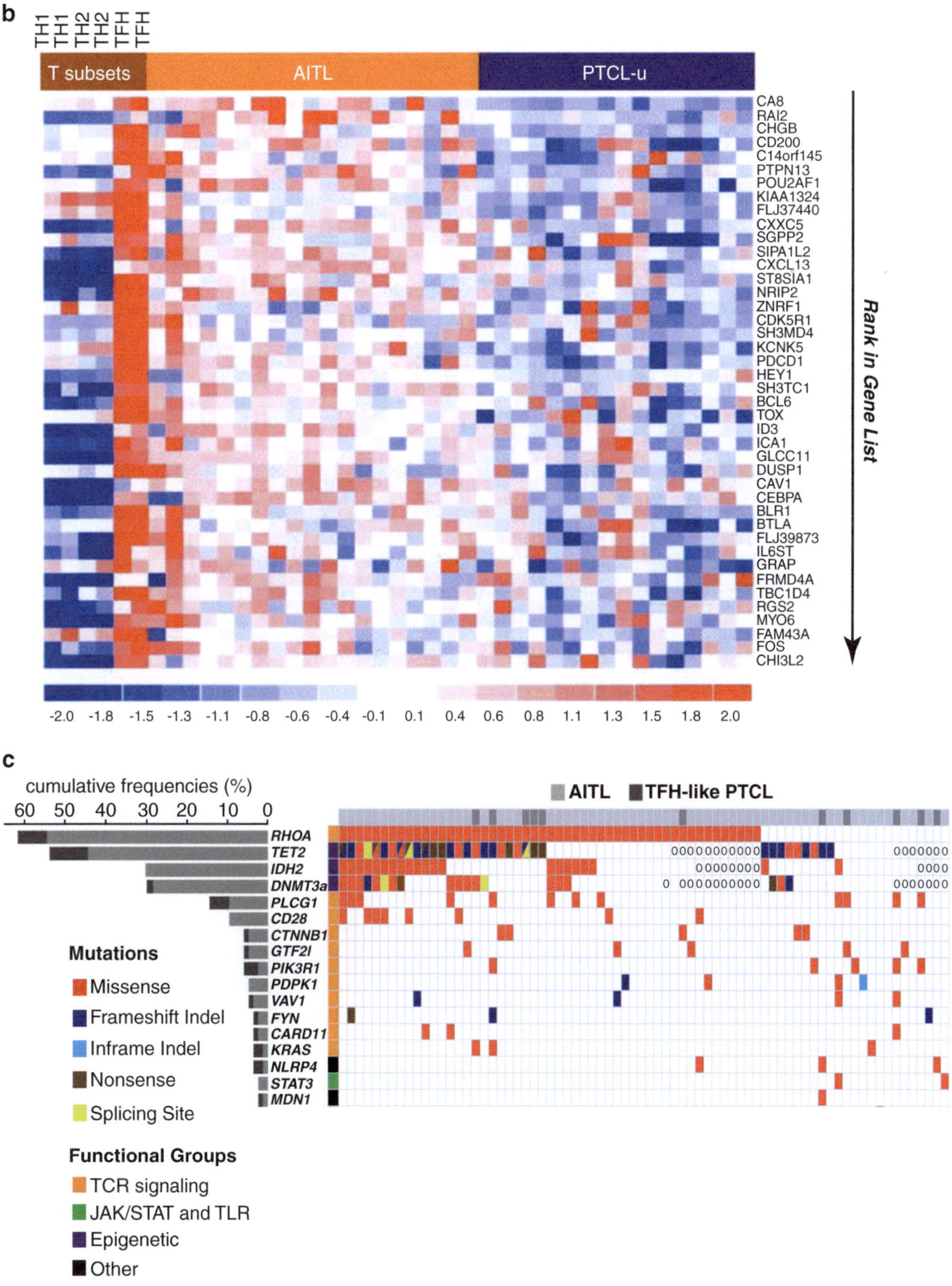

Fig. 4.5 (continued)

particular the CXCL13 chemokine [51]. Analysis of GEP across a variety of PTCL entities indicated that the majority of AITLs clustered together, and robust molecular classifier for AITL was identified, which was dominated by the tumor microenvironment and a complex cytokine profile expressed in the tumor milieu [15]. Further, refinement of these genes signatures [14] reclassified as many as 14–18% of PTCL-NOS cases as AITL. This was further supported by analysis of *IDH2* mutations ($R172^{K/S/T/G/M}$), which are frequent (~33%) in molecularly defined AITL, but not in other PTCL entities [52]. GEP studies identified oncogenic pathways, including the NF-κB pathway, IL-6 signaling, and the TGFβ pathway enriched in AITL compared to other PTCLs [15, 45, 50, 51], but the genetic etiology of these activated pathways is not clear yet. GEP analysis also demonstrated that immunosuppressive tumor microenvironment (TME) predominantly exhibited by tumor-associated dendritic cell gene signatures and macrophage signatures associated with markedly inferior survival in AITL [14], whereas TME exhibiting high B-cell signature was associated with more favorable clinical outcome [14, 15].

Cell of origin: GEP analysis revealed T_{FH} cells as the cellular origin of AITL [15, 45, 50] (Fig. 4.5b). T_{FH} cells are resident T-cells of the germinal center (GC) which are necessary for the formation and maintenance of the GC reaction, a hallmark of adaptive immunity [48]. T_{FH} cells are CD3+ CD4+ cells that express the master transcriptional regulator BCL6; have surface expression of CXCR5, PD-1, and ICOS; and secrete different cytokines and chemokines, in particular CXCL13 and IL-21 [53–55]. IL-21 and/or IL-6 can induce the expression of BCL6 [56]. BCL6 expression is critical for maintaining the T_{FH} transcriptional program [54] via repressing *PRDM1* and the upregulating chemokine receptor *CXCR5*. High-affinity TCR interactions with APCs, especially dendritic cells, are important for T_{FH} cell generation [57]. T_{FH} cells play a major role in supporting and regulating T-cell-dependent B-cell responses in the GC, and their characteristics are retained in AITL neoplastic cells and likely explain the major pathological and biological traits of the disease [48]. AITL features an important reactive cellular background and microenvironment accounted for by the secretion of various soluble factors by T_{FH} cells promoting recruitment, activation, and differentiation of other cells [8, 49]. For example, CXCL13 produced by T_{FH} cells promotes B-cell expansion and plasmacytic differentiation, causing hypergammaglobulinemia and Coombs$^+$ hemolytic anemia commonly found in AITL patients [58]. Other factors incriminated in the pathogenesis of AITL comprise lymphotoxin beta, potentially released by B-cells under CXCL13 stimulation, and several angiogenic mediators.

4.3.3 Molecular Pathogenesis

An increasing number of recurrent genetic aberrations have been identified in AITL and other T_{FH}-derived lymphomas using NGS. Besides *RHOA* which is the most frequently mutated gene, highly recurrent mutations are observed in epigenetic modifier genes and in genes related to the T-cell receptor (TCR) and costimulatory signaling pathways [59–62, 69, 76].

The *RHOA* gene which encodes a small GTPase involved in regulating the actin cytoskeleton, cell adhesion, and distal TCR signaling is most frequently mutated in 60–70% of AITLs and T_{FH}-PTCL [59–62]. No correlation with clinical presentation or outcome was documented. Most *RHOA* mutations are hotspot and generate a *RHOA*^{G17V} dominant-negative variant [59–62]. The substitution of glycine17 with valine prevents the G-box, the domain responsible for stabilizing guanine nucleotide, from binding guanine and performing any of its effector functions. The dominant-negative *RHOA*^{G17V} mutation is particularly perplexing, since a variety of both gain and loss-of-function mutations in *RHOA* are known to occur in other T-cell neoplasms and solid cancers [63]. Nevertheless, the total loss of functional *RHOA* in T-cells by transgenic expression of C3 exotoxin generates a T-acute lymphoblastic leukemia-like disease with thymic enlargement in mice [64]. Experimental works based on mass spectrometry and immunoprecipitation demonstrated that the RHOA^{G17V} protein specifically binds to VAV1, and this interaction enhances the adaptor function of VAV1, ultimately leading to increased TCR signaling [65].

TET2, IDH2, and *DNMT3A*, genes involved in regulating DNA methylation, are mutated in 50–75%, 20–30%, and 20–30% of AITLs, respectively [52, 66–68]. Mono- or biallelic *TET2* and *DNMT3A* mutations are inactivating and distributed along the coding sequences of the genes. Conversely, virtually all *IDH2* mutations are gain-of-function missense at the R172 residue, inducing the production of an oncometabolite (2-hydroxyglutarate) which inhibits various deoxygenases including *TET2* and histone demethylases, resulting in global DNA and histone hypermethylation. Mutations in *TET2* and *DNMT3A* are also found in other PTCL entities, in particular in T_{FH}-PTCLs, but *IDH2* mutations appear to be rather specific for AITL [52, 69]. In AITL, *DNMT3A* and *IDH2* mutations almost always occur in association with *TET2* mutations, which is in contrast with myeloid neoplasms where mutations in these epigenetic modifiers are usually mutually exclusive [59, 60, 67–69]. While *RHOA* and *IDH2* mutations are present in tumor cells only, *TET2* and *DNMT3A* mutations have also been found in hematopoietic progenitors as well as in polyclonal B-cells invariably present in AITL lesions [59, 68, 70–72]. In most cases, *RHOA* mutations are observed in *TET2*-mutated tumors, suggesting cooperation between impaired *RHOA* function supervening on *TET2* loss-of-function contributing to AITL pathogenesis [59]. It was indeed recently demonstrated that loss of *TET2* and *RHOA*^{G17V} expression in mature murine T-cells cooperate to cause abnormal CD4+ T-cell proliferation, aberrant activation of TCR signaling, and an imbalance in differentiation along T_{H17} cells, Tregs, and T_{FH} cells, as a consequence of a synergistic effect inducing deregulation of *FOXO1* gene expression and inactivation of FOXO1 [73].

Mutation-induced activation of the TCR and costimulatory signaling pathways has recently emerged as another oncogenic mechanism in AITL, T_{FH}-PTCL, and PTCL-NOS (Fig. 4.5c). Activating mutations in genes encoding proximal TCR signaling elements (*FYN*), costimulatory receptors (*CD28*), or key intracellular effectors of signal transduction (*PLCG1*) have been discovered in AITL or cutaneous T-cell lymphomas [60, 74–76]. Vallois et al. [62] found that half of the AITL or T_{FH}-PTCL patients carried virtually mutually exclusive mutations in TCR-related genes other than *RHOA*, most frequently in *PLCG1* (14.1%), *CD28* (9.4%, exclusively in AITL), *PI3K* elements (7%), *CTNNB1*(6%), and *GTF2I* (6%). *CARD11* was also mutated in several patients. The vast majority of these variants could be classified as gain-of-function. Although no correlation with clinical features nor a significant impact on survival was observed, the presence of TCR-related mutations correlated with early disease progression [62]. Interestingly, oncogenic TCR activation may result from gene fusions also. For example, the rare t(5;9)(q33;q22) translocation found in about 20% of FTCL and occasionally in AITL [44, 77, 78] produces an ITK-SYK chimeric protein with tyrosine kinase activity which induces a T-cell lymphoproliferative disease in mice [79, 80]. The *CTLA4-CD28* fusion gene recently discovered consists of the extracellular domain of *CTLA4* and the cytoplasmic region of *CD28* and is likely capable of transforming inhibitory signals into stimulatory signals for T-cell activation. It has been reported to occur at very high frequency in AITL and other PTCL as well [81], but this high incidence reported in cases from Asia was not confirmed in other cohorts [82, 83]. Another fusion involving *CD28* (*ICOS-CD28*) and *VAV1* rearrangements which are recurrent in PTCL-NOS (about 10% of the cases) has been shown to drive tumor cell growth [84]. Considering the importance of the TCR pathway to PTCL maintenance from GEP, it follows that mutation of members of this pathway could be relevant to lymphomagenesis and cancer progression.

4.4 Anaplastic Large Cell Lymphomas (ALCL) (Figs. 4.6 and 4.7)

Anaplastic large cell lymphoma, originally termed "Ki-1 lymphoma," was described as a neoplasm composed of clusters of large CD30 (Ki-1)-positive anaplastic cells, often involving lymph nodes in a sinusoidal pattern. Four ALCL

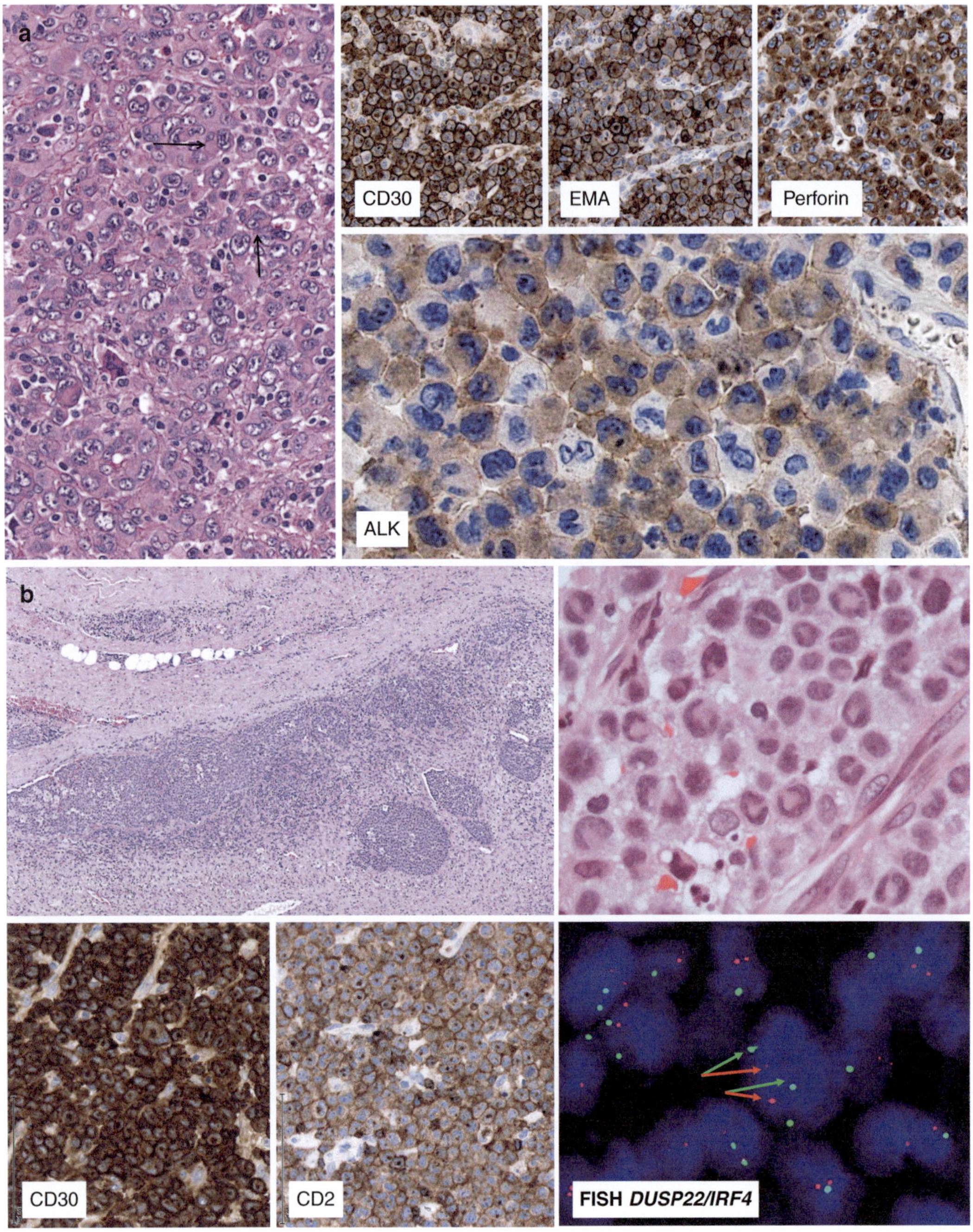

Fig. 4.6 Histopathological features of anaplastic large cell lymphoma (ALCL). (**a**) ALK-positive ALCL. This case presented as an intestinal mass. On a HE stain, this lymphoma comprises diffuse cohesive sheets of large lymphoid cells with abundant cytoplasm and irregular, often horseshoe-shaped nuclei. Several of these show the features of so-called hallmark cells with a prominent paranuclear Golgi region (arrows). The lymphoma cells are strongly positive for CD30, express EMA, and show cytoplasmic positivity for perforin. Immunohistochemistry for ALK produces a cytoplasmic and membrane positivity, which indicates a fusion other than *NPM1-ALK*. (**b**) ALK-negative ALCL with *DUSP22/IRF4* rearrangement. This case manifested as a cutaneous mass with regional lymph node involvement and was considered as a primary cutaneous ALCL. Lymph node involvement was associated to sinusoidal involvement by cohesive sheets of large cells. At high magnification, the tumor comprised many hallmark cells and "doughnut" cells. The lymphoma cells are positive for CD30 and CD2 and are negative for ALK, EMA, and cytotoxic markers (not shown). FISH analysis using break-apart probes spanning the *DUSP22/IRF4* locus shows a biallelic rearrangement

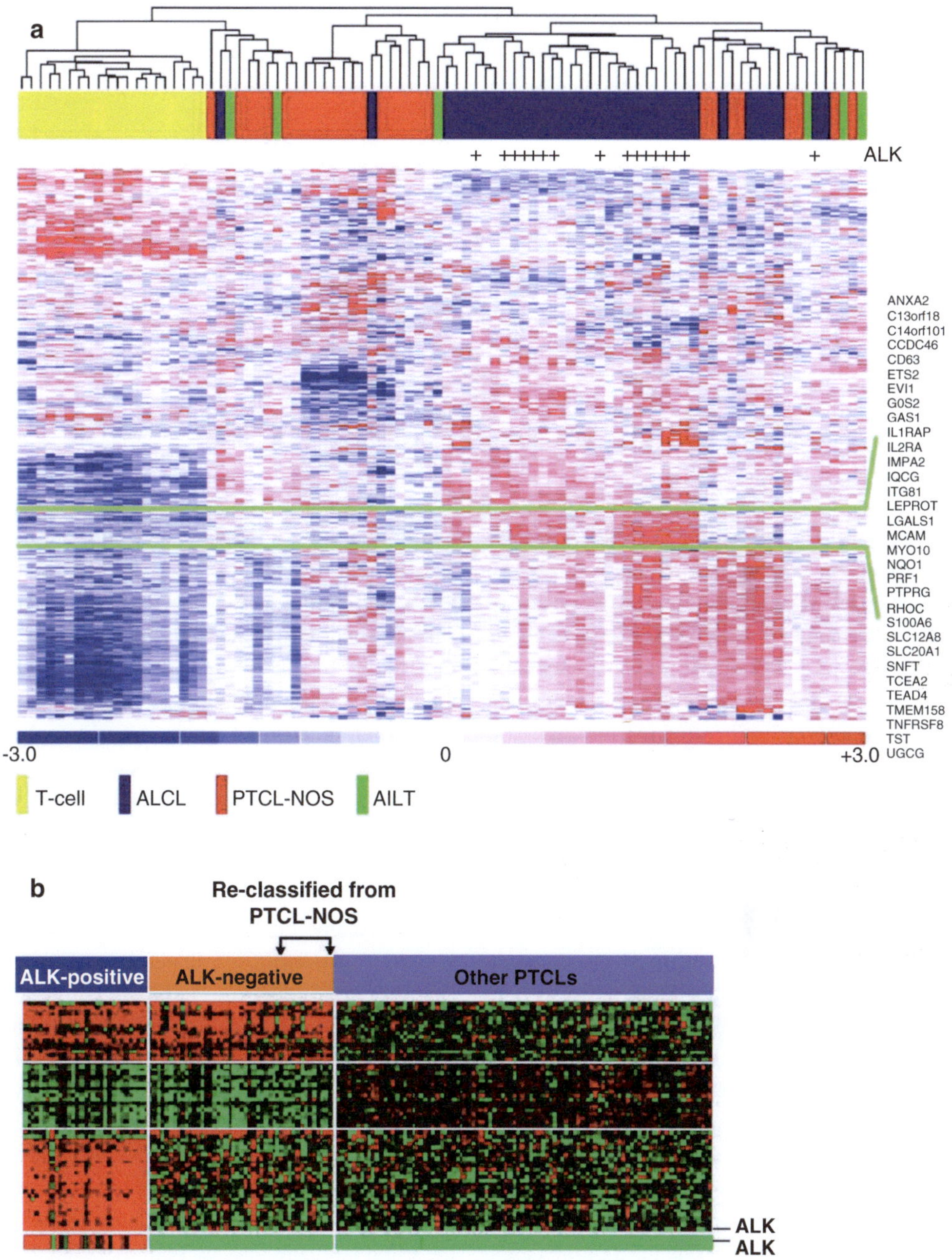

Fig. 4.7 Molecular and genetic features of anaplastic large cell lymphoma (ALCL). (**a**) GEP analysis of ALCL, PTCL entities, and normal T-cells using a predefined 337 gene signature derived from ALCL cell lines altered by ALK and STAT3 KD. This signature showed significant association with ALK+ALCL (adapted from Piva et al., JCO 2010). (**b**) GEP-based molecular predictor for ALK+ALCL and ALK−ALCL and PTCL-NOS cases demonstrating that ALK−ALCL is distinct entity from PTCL-NOS and ALK+ALCL. (re-classified ALCL cases are indicated at the top) (adapted from Iqbal et al. Blood, 2014). (**c**) Overall survival rate in patients with ALCL, stratified by ALK status only (ALK positive, $n = 29$; ALK negative, $n = 67$) and by rearrangements of *ALK DUSP22* and *TP63* triple-negative cases lacking all 3 rearrangements ($N = 40$) (adapted from Feldman et al. Blood. 2011)

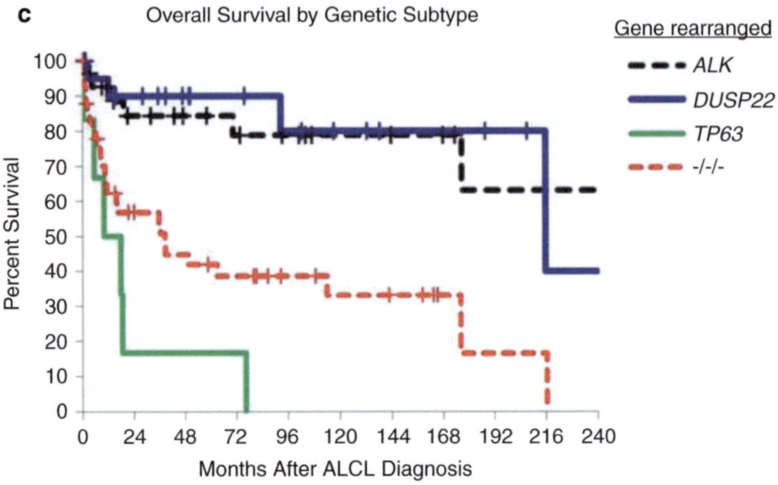

Fig. 4.7 (continued)

entities are currently recognized that differ by their clinical presentation and genetic features, anaplastic lymphoma kinase (ALK)-positive ALCL, ALK-negative ALCL, primary cutaneous ALCL (pcALCL), and breast implant-associated ALCL (BI-ALCL), which is a new provisional entity in the latest classification [5].

4.5 ALK-Positive ALCL

Anaplastic lymphoma kinase (ALK)-positive ALCL represents 7% of PTCL worldwide. It appears to be more common in North America than in Europe and is rather rarely seen in Asia [85]. ALK+ALCL preferentially affects children and young adults, predominantly males, as it represents 10–20% of childhood lymphomas [86]. ALK+ALCL usually presents with lymphadenopathy; mediastinal disease is uncommon, but involvement of other extra-nodal sites (skin, bone, soft tissues) is frequent. However, the bone marrow is involved in less than one third of the cases. Most patients present with stage III or IV disease.

4.5.1 Pathology

ALK+ALCL is a neoplasm of mature T-cells comprising cells that are usually large with abundant cytoplasm and pleomorphic, often horseshoe-shaped nuclei, with a chromosomal translocation involving the *ALK* gene and expression of ALK protein and CD30 (Fig. 4.6a). The neoplastic cells typically involve the sinusoids and infiltrate the lymph node as diffuse sheets. There is frequent fibromyxoid thickening of the capsule, and some cases may show an annular sclerosis, mimicking Hodgkin lymphoma [87]. There is a broad range of cytomorphology, and several variants have been described. All variants contain the so-called hallmark cells which have an eccentric kidney- or horse shoe-shaped nucleus, a prominent Golgi region which appears as a clear, more eosinophilic zone, and abundant, usually basophilic cytoplasm. The classical form (common pattern) (75% of the cases) comprises sheets of large cells, and "hallmark cells" are easily recognized. The small cell variant (comprising small lymphoid cells with irregular nuclei, and fewer larger hallmark cells, which typically tend to cluster around vessels) and the lymphohistiocytic variant (where the neoplastic cells are scattered within a predominant population of reactive histiocytes), each account for <10% of the cases, are often admixed and are both associated with a less favorable outcome [88, 89].

The tumor cells are uniformly strong positive for CD30 on the cell membrane and in the Golgi region and show ALK expression due to rearrangement of the *ALK* gene at 2p23. EMA is positive in the majority of cases, and a subset of cases may express cytokeratins. The tumor cells exhibit an aberrant T-cell immunophenotype with defective expression of the TCR/CD3 complex [90, 91] and pan T-cell antigens, despite a T-cell genotype;

therefore, many cases have an apparent "null" immunophenotype. CD3 is negative in >75% of cases and CD5 and CD7 are often lost. CD2 and CD4 are positive in a significant proportion of cases. CD8 is usually negative, whereas CD43 and CD45 are often positive. Most cases are positive for cytotoxic granule-associated antigens (granzyme, TIA-1, perforin) and exhibit an activated cytotoxic immunophenotype. Although usually negative for CD15, a subset of the cases may be positive for this marker. In the morphologic variants, only the larger cells are highlighted by CD30 and EMA, and in the smaller cells, ALK expression tends to be restricted to the nucleus.

By molecular analysis, ALK+ALCL can usually be shown to be of T-cell origin with a monoclonal rearrangement of the T-cell receptor-β and -γ chains demonstrable by PCR, even in cases with a "null" T-cell phenotype. A recent study [92] presented a model of peripheral ALCL pathogenesis where the malignancy is initiated in early thymocytes, before TCR β-rearrangement, which is bypassed in CD4/NPM-ALK transgenic mice following Notch1 expression. However, TCR is required for thymic egress and development of peripheral murine tumors, yet TCR must be downregulated for T-cell lymphomagenesis. These observations suggest that children affected by ALCL may harbor thymic lymphoma-initiating cells capable of seeding relapse after chemotherapy.

4.5.2 Molecular Signature

In initial GEP analysis, using engineered ALK+ALCL cell lines, the diagnostic signature of systemic ALK+ALCLs was mainly dictated by STAT3 signaling, and a gene subset was able to distinguish primary ALK+ALCL cases from other PTCLs [93] (Fig. 4.7a). Using a more refined GEP analysis in ALK+ALCL, a mRNA classifier with several upregulated transcripts (e.g., *ALK, TNFRSF8 (CD30), MUC1*), T_{H17}-cell-associated molecules (*IL-17A, IL-17F, ROR-γ*), and downregulated transcripts related to TCR components and TCR signaling, was developed that was able to distinguish majority of the cases with >90% probability [15]. An extensive GEP investigation on a well characterized set of ALK+ALCL cases led to identification of gene signature that was able to differentiate ALK+ALCL from ALK−ALCL and showed a concordance with the pathological diagnosis of 100% (31/31) for ALK+ALCL and 94% (30/32) for ALK−ALCL [14]. This signature included some previously defined genes (e.g., *TNFRSF8 [CD30], BATF3, TMOD1*) [94] in ALCL as well as a subset of p53 transcriptional targets. ALK+ALCL cases were enriched for the expression of signatures of HIF1-α target genes, IL10-induced genes, and H-ras/K-ras-induced genes compared with ALK−ALCL, which showed marginal enrichment of PI3K pathway-regulated genes (Fig. 4.7b). The association of T_{H17} cell like gene signature with ALK+ALCL was shown to be regulated by miR-135b [95].

4.5.3 Molecular Pathogenesis and Genetic Features

ALK+ALCLs are characterized by a translocation involving the *ALK* gene on chromosome 2p23, most commonly t(2;5)(p23;q35), which results in a fusion with the nucleophosmin gene (*NPM*) on chromosome 5. The type of translocation determines the subcellular distribution of upregulated ALK; the t(2;5)(p23;q35) translocation produces ALK expression in both the nucleus and the cytoplasm, while less common variant translocations produce a different subcellular distribution (cytoplasmic and/or membranous) of the chimeric protein, which is determined by the translocation partner [96]. There is no prognostic impact according to the type of *ALK* translocation. All translocations juxtapose the cytoplasmic catalytic domain of ALK to a partner protein, forming a chimeric fusion protein inducing ALK phosphorylation and constitutive activation. In vitro, constitutively activated ALK chimeras induce cellular transformation, enhance cell proliferation and survival, and account for the silencing of the T-cell phenotypic markers [97, 98]. GEP analysis demonstrated that C/EBPβ and the anti-apoptotic protein BCL2A1 are absolutely necessary to induce cell transformation and/or to sustain the growth and survival of ALK+ALCL cells [99]. NPM-ALK represents the major oncogenic driver in ALK+ALCL, and accordingly, pharmacologic ALK inhibition has shown efficacy in relapsed/refractory ALK+ALCL patients [100]. The oncogenic properties of ALK are mediated by interaction with downstream molecules that engage intracellular signals, among which the JAK3-STAT3 pathway is of prime importance [101]. The *NPM-ALK* fusion transcript has been detected at low levels in reactive lymph node and normal peripheral blood samples of healthy individuals, suggesting additional cofactors [102] and other genetic alteration required for T-cell transformation. Several studies demonstrated that miR-17 ~ 92 cluster and its paralogues are also highly expressed in ALK+ALCL and may represent important downstream effectors of the ALK oncogenic pathway [103, 104]. No etiologic agent has been linked to ALCL, but there have been case reports of systemic ALK+ALCL presenting with skin lesions occurring after an insect bite [105], suggesting the possible role of inflammatory mediators released upon the bite in eliciting lymphoma development.

4.6 ALK-Negative ALCL

ALK-negative ALCL, introduced as a provisional entity in the 2008 WHO classification, was promoted to a definitive status in the revised edition [5]. This disease is defined as a systemic large cell lymphoma with comparable morphology to classical ALK+ALCL, uniformly strongly positive for CD30 but lacking ALK expression. ALK−ALCL is overall less common than ALK+ALCL; in the international T-cell lymphoma study, it comprised 5.5% of PTCLs worldwide [85]. ALK−ALCL tends to occur in older individuals with less frequent extra-nodal involvement. The distinction from ALK+ALCL is important since the clinical course and prognosis of the patients are worse than for those with ALK+ tumors, but more favorable than those of PTCL-NOS patients [106]. However, recent analyses have highlighted that the prognostic difference between ALK+ and ALK−ALCL might be related to the fact that ALK−ALCL tends to occur in older patients, rather than intrinsically distinct biological properties according to ALK expression [107].

4.6.1 Pathology

By definition the cytomorphologic features overlap with those of the common variant of ALK+ALCL, including the presence of hallmark cells. The diagnostic criteria for ALK−ALCL [108] require (1) the presence of "hallmark cells," (2) a cohesive architecture, and (3) strong CD30 expression in virtually all tumor cells. In most cases, the tumor cells tend to be larger and more pleomorphic than in ALK+ALCL. In addition, the presence of the following criteria is desirable: reduced T-cell surface antigen expression, EMA positivity, and a cytotoxic phenotype and/or a sinusoidal involvement. ALK−ALCL by definition contains no ALK translocation and is negative for ALK protein expression (Fig. 4.6b). Compared to ALK+ALCL, ALK−ALCL has more preserved expression of T-cell antigens, while the expression of cytotoxic markers and of EMA tends to be less frequent. Nuclear expression of PAX5 has been detected in rare cases in association with the presence of extra copies of the gene [109].

4.6.2 Molecular Signature

ALCL, irrespective of ALK status, is molecularly distinct from other PTCLs and expresses a distinct set of transcripts, including CD30 (*TNFRSF8*), *BATF3*, and *TMOD*, and demonstrates low expression of genes associated with TCR signaling [14, 15, 94, 110]. Due to fewer number of cases, it was challenging to generate definitive diagnostic signature for ALK−ALCL, but a refined study used a two-step algorithm to identify ALCL cases from PTCL-NOS first and then within ALCL cases distinguish ALK+ALCL from ALK−ALCL. Using this algorithm, 97% of pathologically defined ALCL cases irrespective of ALK status were identified and reclassified 11% (17 of 150) of PTCL-NOS as ALCL, which upon further review were all ALK−ALCL cases [14]. The signatures distinguishing ALK+ALCL from ALK−ALCL included enrichment of *MYC, IRF4* target, and mTOR genes in ALK−ALCL [94]. Further studies have identified NF-κB and stromal signatures to be predictive of prognosis independent of ALK status in ALCL [111].

4.6.3 Molecular Pathogenesis and Genetic Features

Two types of recurrent translocations were discovered in ALK−ALCL by massive parallel sequencing [112, 113]. The most frequent rearrangements involving the 6p25.3 locus are rather specific to ALK−ALCLs (both systemic and primary cutaneous), and virtually absent in other PTCL entities, and involve either *IRF4* or *DUSP22* (encoding a dual-specificity phosphatase that inhibits TCR signaling) with various partners. The less frequent *TP63* rearrangements encoding fusion proteins homologous to ΔNp63, a dominant-negative p63 isoform that inhibits the p53 pathway, have been detected in systemic ALK−ALCL and PTCL-NOS. The most common rearrangement resulting from inv(3)(q26q28) fuses *TP63* to *TBL1XR1* [112]. Rearrangements of *DUSP22* and *TP63* in ALK−ALCL are mutually exclusive and detected in 19–30% and 7–8% of the cases, respectively [114, 115]. *DUSP22*-rearranged ALCLs have a prognosis similar to ALK+ALCL, while conversely *TP63* rearrangements are associated with a poor outcome (17% 5-year OS), and cases lacking all three genetic markers have an intermediate prognosis [114, 115] (Fig. 4.7c). Interestingly, the genetic heterogeneity seems to imprint phenotypic correlates, as *DUSP22* rearranged cases tend to have very classical morphology with many hallmark cells, usually lack both cytotoxic markers and EMA expression [112] and display higher expression of the chemokine receptor CCR8 [115–117]. A subset of ALK−ALCL is characterized by aberrant expression of *ERBB4*-truncated transcripts carrying intronic 5′ untranslated regions, which appear to have oncogenic properties and can potentially be antagonized pharmacologically [118].

A recent large comprehensive genomic study uncovered diverse mechanisms convergent to induce constitutive oncogenic activation of the JAK/STAT pathway in a substantial proportion of ALK−ALCL [119]. These mechanisms include occasionally co-occurring activating mutations of *STAT3* and *JAK1* in around 40% of the cases and recurrent gene fusions involving a transcription factor (*NFKB2* or *NCOR2*) with tyrosine kinase genes (*ROS1* or *TYK2*) in a small subset of the cases. Therefore, STAT3 activation represents a shared oncogenic mechanism in both ALK+ and ALK−ALCLs. Compared to ALK+ALCL, ALK- tumors have more genomic complexity. Loss at 17p13 (involving *TP53)* or inactivation of *PRDM1* by various mechanisms was found in 42 and 56% of ALK−ALCLs, respectively [120], and these alterations were found to be associated with a more aggressive course [115].

4.7 Primary Cutaneous ALCL

Primary cutaneous (pc)ALCL is a disease entity within the spectrum of primary cutaneous CD30+ lymphoproliferations, along with lymphomatoid papulosis. It is the second most common type of cutaneous T-cell lymphoma (after mycosis fungoides). A history of mycosis fungoides must be excluded, since transformed mycosis fungoides (defined as >25% large cells) is often CD30+ and may mimic pcALCL. pcALCL presents as solitary or less commonly (in 20% of the cases) multiple skin nodule(s) or tumor(s) that may regress and recur and usually carries a good prognosis. Secondary cutaneous involvement by systemic ALK−ALCL has overlapping features, but the distinction is of prime importance given the prognostic implications with systemic ALCL requiring chemotherapy and having a 5-year overall survival (OS) rate of only 49%. Locoregional lymph node involvement may occur and even precede the skin lesions in pcALCL without necessarily indicating an aggressive behavior. Therefore, detailed clinical information is mandatory; involvement of a single peripheral lymph node by ALK−ALCL should always raise the possibility of nodal dissemination of a primary cutaneous lesion before concluding to early-stage systemic disease.

4.7.1 Pathology

In pcALCL, the tumor comprises sheets of large anaplastic, pleomorphic, or immunoblastic T-cells of which the majority express CD30. The neoplastic cells form diffuse infiltrates of cohesive sheets, may display epidermotropism, and can have an inflammatory background. They are usually CD4+, show variable loss of expression of other T-cell antigens, frequently express cytotoxic molecules, and are usually negative for EMA and ALK. At variance with systemic ALCL, pcALCL usually expresses the CLA cutaneous address in antigen.

4.7.2 Genetic and Molecular Features

The genetic features of pcALCL overlap with those of systemic ALK–ALCL, including rearrangements of *DUSP22* in up to 30% of the cases, a feature associated to more pronounced epidermotropism [121, 122], rearrangements of *TYK2* in 13% of the cases [123], occasional *STAT3* mutations [119], and rearrangements of *TP63*. Although pcALCL is classically described as an ALK- form of ALCL, unusual cases of pcALCL expressing ALK and carrying an *ALK* translocation have been reported, which remained confined to the skin and had a very good outcome [124].

4.8 Breast Implant-Associated ALCL

Breast implant-associated ALCL (BI-ALCL) is a very rare form of T-cell lymphoma that arises in association with various kinds of breast implants. The estimated risk is one case for every 500,000–3,000,000 women with breast implants [125]. In the recently revised WHO classification of hematological malignancies, BI-ALCL is introduced as a new provisional disease entity, distinct from the other types of ALCLs already recognized [5]. While the morphological and immunophenotypical features of BI-ALCL are indistinguishable from those of systemic ALK–ALCL, what makes the specificity of this disease is the clinical presentation in association and vicinity with a breast implant. Most cases present as a periprosthetic effusion (seroma or in situ lymphoma), and only a minority of the cases present as a tumor mass infiltrating into the adjacent breast parenchyma, with or without an associated effusion [126–128]. A significant proportion of patients may present with axillary lymphadenopathy which is not proven involved by lymphoma in all instances [126]. Rare cases present with disseminated disease. While most patients have excellent outcome, several studies have highlighted an association between the clinical pattern and disease aggressiveness; for example, most cases presenting as a seroma appear to be cured with surgery alone and infrequently experience recurrences, while the presence of a solid tumor mass is an adverse prognostic factor [126]. A detailed longitudinal analysis of patients who died of BI-ALCL showed locoregional dissemination of the disease to the breast, locoregional lymph nodes, chest, and mediastinum, but no systemic dissemination typical of other lymphomas, hence, suggesting to use a staging system similar in its principles to those applied to solid tumors [126, 129].

4.8.1 Genetic and Molecular Features

Information available on the genetic lesions underlying the development and progression of BI-ALCL and its molecular pathogenesis is limited. *DUSP22* and *TP63* rearrangements were not found in a reported series [127]. Complex karyotypes were observed in cell lines established from three BI-ALCL patients [130]. *STAT3* mutations were found in few cases of BI-ALCL [131].

4.9 Adult T-Cell Lymphoma/Leukemia (Figs. 4.8 and 4.9)

ATLL is a mature T-cell lymphoma that is caused by human T-cell lymphotropic retrovirus type 1 (HTLV-1). The disease distribution parallels that

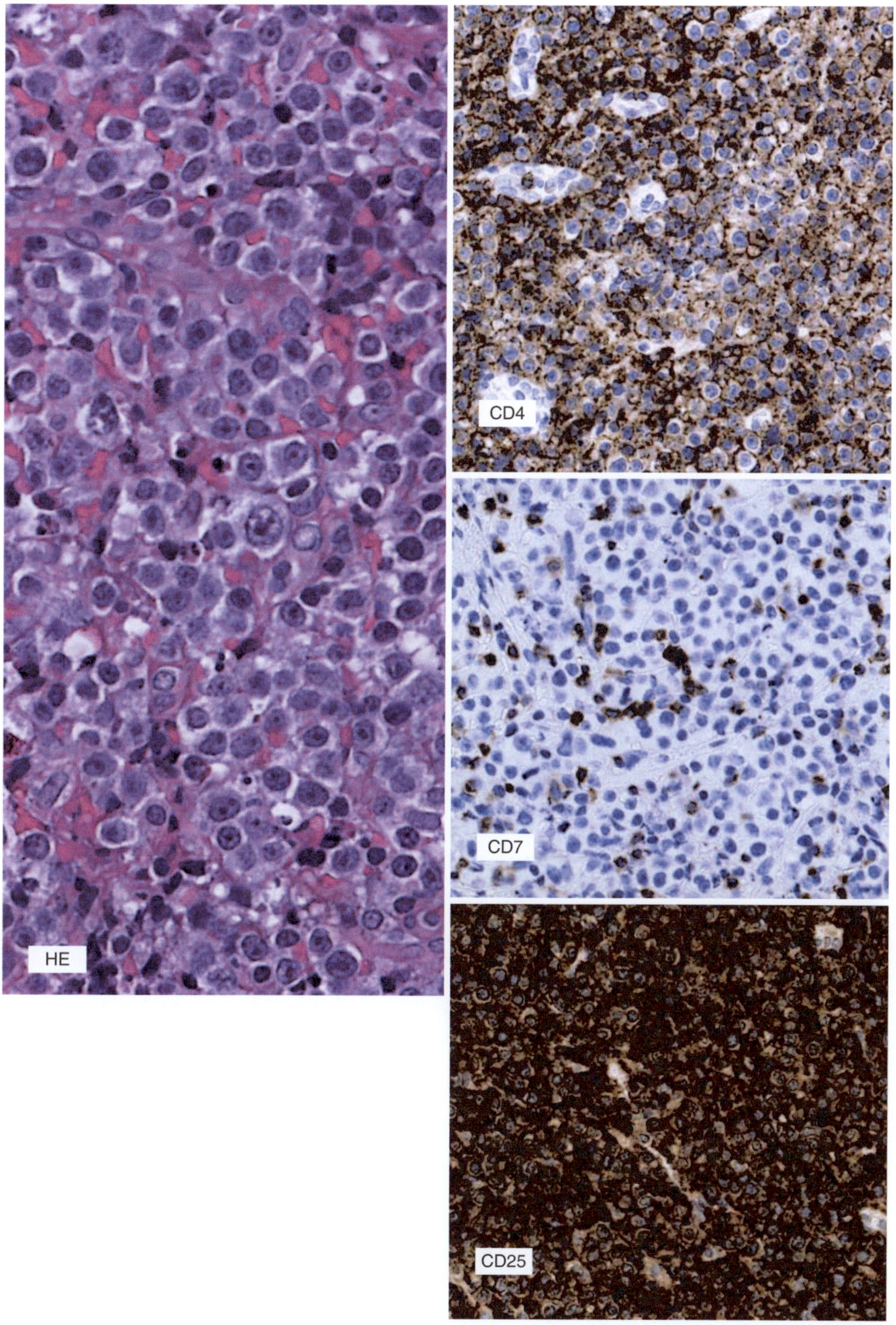

Fig. 4.8 Histopathological features of ATLL. This case with lymphomatous presentation was diagnosed in a middle-aged man with no previous medical history. An abdominal lymph node showed a diffuse involvement by a monotonous population of medium to large lymphoid cells with moderately abundant cytoplasm and slightly irregular nuclei. The lymphoma cells are CD3+ (not shown) CD4+ CD7- CD25+, an immunophenotype characteristic of ATLL. Positivity for HTLV1 was discovered during the clinical work-up

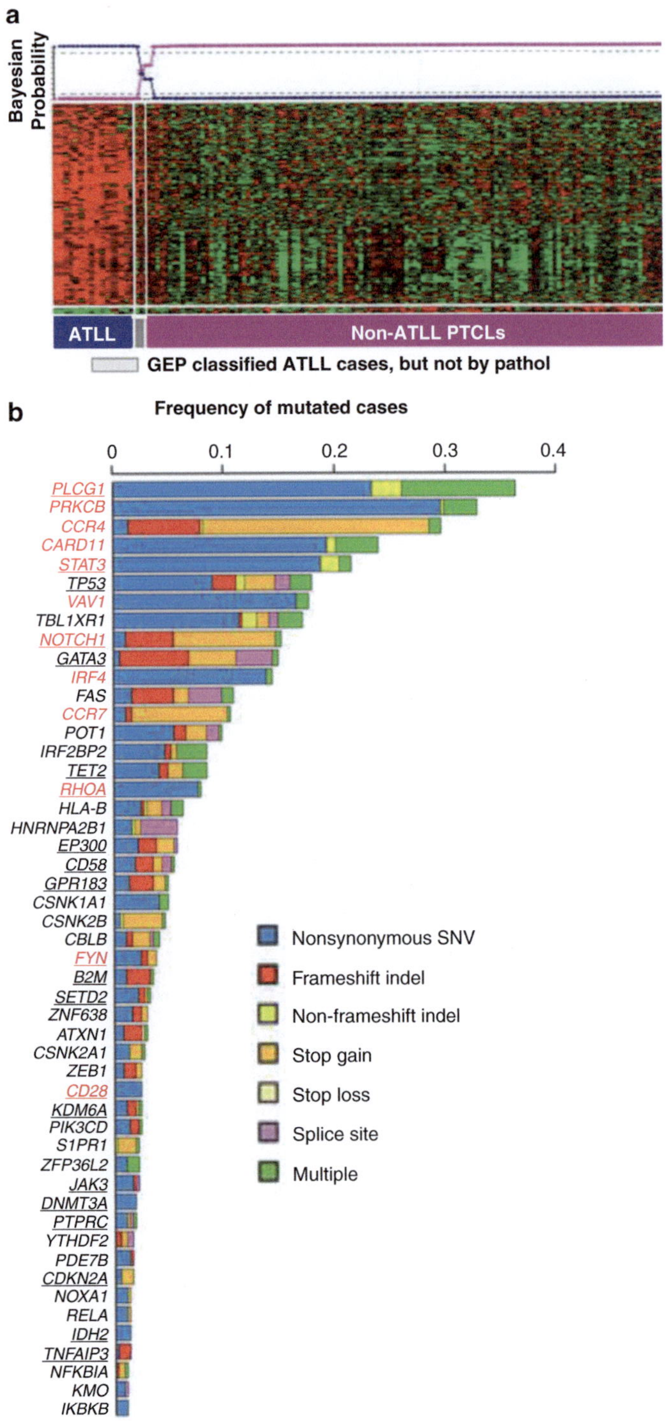

Fig. 4.9 Molecular and genetic features of ATLL. (**a**) Gene expression-based molecular predictor for ATLL versus other PTCLs. The gene signature was derived using Bayesian algorithm and was enriched in genes involved in TCR signaling and HTLV-1-induced genes in T-cells (adapted from Iqbal, et al. Blood, 2010). (**b**) Frequencies and types of somatic mutations identified by targeted capture sequencing in 50 significant genes for 370 ATLL cases ($q < 0.1$). Genes affected by activating mutations are shown in red, and genes previously reported to be altered in other T-cell malignancies are underlined. Significant focal amplifications (red) and deletions (blue) identified by GISTIC 2.0 analysis ($n = 426$). Well-localized regions with 12 or fewer genes <500 kb in size and with residual q value <0.1 are annotated. The number of genes included in each locus is indicated in parentheses. Significantly mutated genes are marked with asterisks. (B-C, adapted from Kataoka, et al. Nat. Genet. 2015)

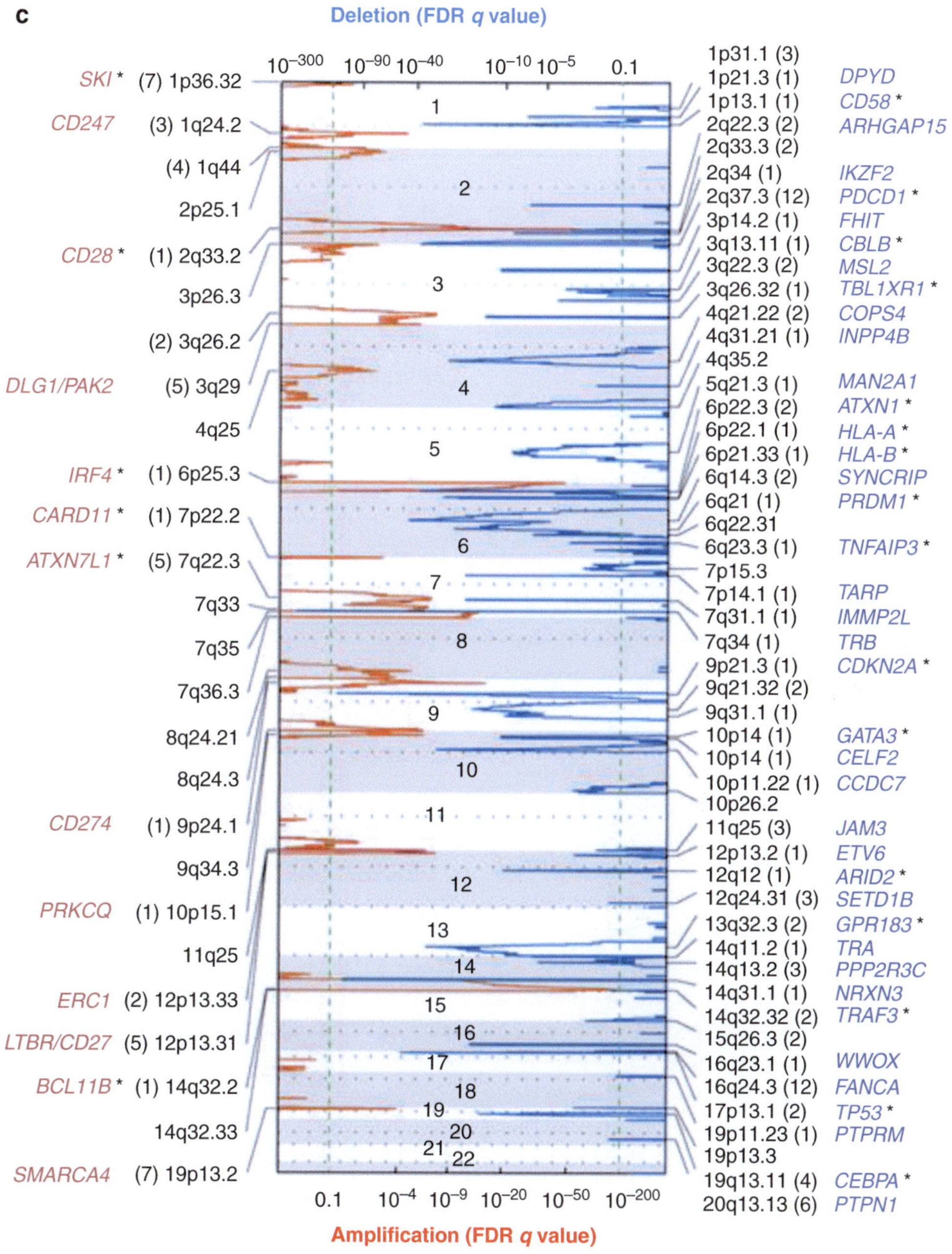

Fig. 4.9 (continued)

of the prevalence of HTLV-1 infection in the population and is endemic in southwest Japan, the Caribbean basin, Central and South America, and Central Africa. The average age at diagnosis is 40–60 years, but comparatively lower in Central and South America than in Japan [132]. The disease encompasses a marked diversity of clinical manifestations: peripheral blood involvement ranging from blood abnormal lymphocytes to lymphocytosis to a frank leukemic picture, widespread lymphadenopathy, hepatomegaly and splenomegaly, hypercalcemia, skin lesions, and involvement of various organs including the gastrointestinal tract and central nervous system. The clinical presentation is classified into four variants (acute and lymphomatous which are highly aggressive and smoldering and chronic which are less aggressive), based on the degree of peripheral blood involvement, type of tissue infiltration, hypercalcemia, and lactate dehydrogenase levels [133]. Most patients present with lymph node and peripheral blood involvement, but no correlation is observed between the abundance of circulating tumor cells and bone marrow involvement.

4.9.1 Pathology

Morphologically, ATLL is characterized by a wide spectrum of morphological appearances including variable patterns of infiltration in the tissues and variable cytological features. In the chronic and smoldering forms, the neoplastic cells tend to be small with minimal atypia, while in the leukemic and lymphomatous presentations, the neoplastic cells are larger and more pleomorphic and may include anaplastic-like or large multinucleated giant cells (Fig. 4.8). Blastoid morphology may be seen in a subset of the cases. In the peripheral blood, the neoplastic cells are typically multilobated and are referred to as "flower cells." In lymph nodes, ATLL infiltrates may be focal or extensive; they may mimic other lymphoma entities and may resemble, for example, AITL by featuring cells with clear cytoplasm and having an associated eosinophilic component; in other cases, they may mimic Hodgkin lymphoma due to the presence of large EBV-positive B-cell blasts likely expanded as a result of the concomitant immune deficiency in ATLL patients. The skin infiltrates are often epidermotropic and may mimic cutaneous T-cell lymphoma.

In most cases, ATLL cells are CD4+ CD8- (but a subset may be CD4- CD8+ or CD4+ CD8+). They express several other T-cell antigens but typically lack CD7 expression. They strongly co-express CD25+, are frequently CCR4+, and may be CD30+ especially in cases with large cell morphology. Expression of Foxp3, a marker for T_{REG} cells, is found in a subset of the cases and often in the neoplastic cells [134, 135]. Thus, it has been suggested that ATLL cells may originate from HTLV-I-infected T_{REG} cells [136]. Recent studies have identified CD45RA (+) T memory stem (TSCM) cells, as the hierarchical apex is capable of reconstituting identical ATLL clones in murine models [137].

4.9.2 Molecular Signature

Many of the molecular features of ATLL are determined by perturbed signaling pathways mediated by HTLV1 infection [138] (Fig. 4.9a). GEP studies have corroborated such findings and demonstrated high expression of *IL2Rα*, *IL2Rβ*, and MHC-II genes in ATLL [139]. Another study using neoplastic lymphoma cells has shown high expression of *TSLC1/CADM1, CAV1*, and *PTGDS* compared to normal T-cells [140]. Leukemic ATLL cells have increased expression of unique genes including *TNFSF11, RGS13, MAFb, CSPG2, C/EBP-α*, and *TCF4*, and gene associated with cell cycle (*CDC2, cyclin B*), hypercalcemia (*RANKL, PTHLH*), tyrosine kinase signaling (*SYK, LYN*), and anti-apoptosis (*BIRC5*) [141]. We identified a unique mRNA signature for ATLL, which is distinct from other PTCL entities and included many of the transcripts induced by TAX viral oncoprotein [15] or involved in TCR signaling. At least 3% of PTCL-NOS cases exhibited similar signature, which were seropositive for HTLV1, but had no integrated HTLV-1 proviral genome in the tumor cells. GSEA revealed enrichment of TCR signaling genes, RARγ target signature but not T_{REG}-related gene signatures [15].

4.9.3 Molecular Pathogenesis and Genetic Features

Without a doubt, HTLV1 is involved in ATLL lymphomagenesis, but most neoplastic cells do not express oncogenic viral protein TAX and only express antisense gene product HBZ [142]. However both HTLV1 Tax and HBZ act as major drivers of T-cell transformation and induce chronic proliferation, apoptotic resistance, multiple organ invasion, and drug resistance [143]. TAX oncoprotein has been shown to activate multiple signaling pathways in infected T-cells, which acquire further genetic and epigenetic changes for neoplasm transformation [138]. Despite these observations, the low rate of ATLL incidence in HTLV1-infected population suggests that HTLV1 itself is not sufficient, but other genetic events are the likely driving force fueling the clonal progression of tumor cells. A comprehensive genetic study has shown deletions of the *NRXN3* locus (14q31.1 fragile site) in 60% of cases [63] and a number of driver abnormalities enriched in components of the TCR pathway, the most common being in *PLCG1* (36%) and *PRKCB* (33%) which are the two most common mutated genes overall (Fig. 4.9b). *CARD11* was also frequently mutated (24%) or amplified (12%), and 8% of the cases had focal small internal deletions within the protein's auto-inhibitory domain. Other changes include hotspot mutations in *VAV1* (18%), some of which are known to be activating by altering auto-inhibitory domains, and in *FYN* (4%), many in the C-terminal auto-inhibitory region. Signaling from CD28 is expected to be frequently enhanced by several mechanisms, including focal gains (71%), which are often high-level amplifications (23%), mutations in hotspots that could increase activity; and tandem duplications leading to expression of CD28 sequences from the *CTLA4* or *ICOS* promoter and occasionally substituting the extracellular domain with that of *ICOS* or *CTLA4*. Since CTLA4 binds CD80 and CD86 more strongly than CD28, this results in stronger signaling from the retained CD28 intracellular domain. Since CTLA4 binds CD80 and CD86 more strongly than CD28, this results in stronger signaling from the retained CD28 intracellular domain. Mutations in *CCR4* (29%) and *CCR7* (11%) almost always result in truncation of the intracellular C-terminal tail, which prevents internalization upon stimulation with ligand and thereby enhances chemotaxis [144]. *CCR4* is expressed at a high level in ATLL [144–146] and likely contributes to the frequent skin involvement in this disease. Mogamulizumab, a monoclonal antibody to CCR4, has been approved in Japan for the treatment of ATLL and has shown efficacy [147, 148] in PTCL-NOS and CTCL [149]. In contrast to these gain-of-function mutations in *CCR4* and *CCR7*, apparent loss-of-function mutations are frequent (28%) in *GPR183* (*EBI2*), which responds to 7α, 25-dihydroxycholesterol and may promote retention in the lymph node by positioning the cells adjacent to follicles [150].

4.10 Cutaneous T-Cell Lymphomas

CTCL encompasses several disease entities characterized by neoplastic T-cell proliferations that are by definition largely confined to the skin at the time of diagnosis [151] (Table 4.1). Altogether, CTCL largely outnumber primary cutaneous lymphomas of B-cell derivation. Within CTCL, the most common subtypes are mycosis fungoides (MF) and Sezary syndrome (SS) accounting for about 75% of the cases, followed by primary cutaneous CD30+ lymphoproliferative disorders, while other entities are distinctively rare [152].

Mycosis fungoides is the most common type of CTCL; it is characterized by epidermotropic infiltrates of small- to medium-sized lymphocytes with cerebriform nuclei. The disease affects mainly adults and elderly patients with a male predominance but can also be observed in children. The disease has an indolent clinical course with slow progression over years from cutaneous patches to more infiltrated plaques and tumors at a later stage. Early-stage lesions are often distributed in sun-protected areas. Histologically, patch lesions show a lichenoid infiltrate of lymphocytes and histiocytes in the dermis, with a component of atypical lymphocytes with cerebriform nuclei and pericellular haloes infiltrating the epidermis in the basal layer. More infiltrated lesions comprise a more diffuse infiltrate with intraepidermal collections of atypical cells (Pautrier microabcesses). At the stage of tumors, ulceration may be seen, and epidermotropic features may not be apparent any more. Histological transformation defined as >25% large lymphoid cells may occur at the tumor stage. Uncommon histological variants (folliculotropic MF, pagetoid reticulosis, and granulomatous slack skin) are associated with distinct clinical presentations. In MF the neoplastic cells are usually CD2+ CD3+ CD4+ CD5+ CD8-, often lack CD7 and express TCRalphabeta. CD30 expression is not uncommon, especially in large cell transformation. The cell of origin is resident memory T-cells homing to the skin [153].

Sezary syndrome (SS) is a rare and aggressive disease defined by a triad consisting of erythroderma, generalized lymphadenopathy, and the presence of clonal T-cells with cerebriform nuclei (Sezary cells) in the skin, lymph nodes, and peripheral blood. SS and MF are closely related diseases—and MF patients may uncommonly develop and erythrodermic stage without fulfilling the criteria for SS—but they are considered distinct diseases based on different biology and different cell of origin, SS being derived from central memory T-cells [153]. The neoplastic cells in SS are usually CD3+ CD4+ CD8- typically lacking CD7 or CD26 expression. The cutaneous lymphocyte antigen (CLA) is expressed in most cases of SS, as it is in MF. In the skin and lymph nodes, the neoplastic cell infiltrate is usually monotonous, with effacement of the architecture in lymph nodes. In the skin, the features may overlap with those seen in MF, but epidermotropism may be absent. Bone marrow involvement can be present, usually patchy and interstitial.

4.10.1 Molecular Signature

Numerous GEP studies have compared various CTCL subtypes to those of normal T-cells, normal skin, and inflammatory skin conditions and often resulted in discrepancies in GEP signatures, which can be attributed to cell population selection or small sample number in these studies (reviewed by Dulmage et.al [154]). Most GEP studies were performed on common clinical variants (i.e., MF or SS), commonly overexpressed genes in these variants but not in normal T-cells, including *TWIST1*, *PLS3* (plastin 3), and two NK-cell markers, *NCR1* (NKp46) and *KIR3DL2* [155]. Several gene expression changes are seen in both MF and SS (*TWIST1, CD52, PTPRCAP, JUNB, TOX)*, and still others show differential expression between MF and SS (*EPHA4, STAT4*) [156]. GSEA showed the upregulated genes to be enriched in cell cycle control, *MYC* transcriptional activation, immune system regulation, and chemokine signaling [156]. Several genes with critical roles in TCR, cytokine, and chemokine signaling are strongly upregulated (≥5×). These include *CD3G*, *RAC2*, *PRKCQ*, and *HRAS* (TCR signaling) and chemokine receptors *CCR4* and *CCR8*, *IL6R*, and *IL2RG*. *IL2RG* encodes the IL-2 receptor common gamma chain, which is a subunit of six cytokine receptors including receptors for IL-15 and IL-21, which are important autocrine factors in CTCL. Upregulated transcripts for transcription factors include *TOX* (~19-fold increase), which has been suggested as a specific biomarker for MF and SS. There is evidence for a pathogenic role for *TOX* in CTCL by downregulating the cell cycle inhibitory proteins CDKN1B and –C [157], and RUNX3 [158] which may act as a tumor suppressor gene in CTCL [159].

4.10.2 Molecular Pathogenesis and Genetic Features

The specialized homing of neoplastic cells in the skin may reveal the role of tumor microenvironment in disease progression. However, tumor intrinsic features are essential to maintain the survival advantage, and distinctive pathognomonic chromosomal alterations have been observed in CTCL [160–163], with loss of 17p in ~40% of cases, including smaller deletions at 17p13.1 encompassing *TP53* in >50% SS cases. In addition, deletions at 9p21.3 that include *CDKN2A* occur in ~50% of cases and are often homozygous. Loss of *CDKN2A* and *TP53* is expected to confer resistance to apoptosis and cellular senescence and enhances proliferation and genomic instability. Other aberrations inducing the loss of cell cycle regulators include deletion at 13q14.2 (*RB1*) and 12p13.1 (*CDKN1B*). Another apoptosis regulator that is commonly deleted or mutated is *FAS* (10q23.3, which also includes *PTEN*). Loss of *FAS* is expected to interfere with activation-induced cell death (AICD), an important homeostatic mechanism in T-cells. Genes involved in chromatin remodeling are frequently affected. A focused deletion on 1p36.1 includes *ARID1A*, which also shows a mutation in ~10% of cases. Together, ~40–60% of cases have either deletion or mutation of *ARID1A*. *ARID5B* is also frequently (~40%) included in deletions within 10q and *ARID3A* in deletions of distal 19p [162].

Other SWItch/sucrose mon-fermentable (SWI/SNF) components are also frequently affected by deletions. In particular, *SMARCC1* at 3p21.31 was included in deletions of <4 Mb in 21% of tumors. Deletions or mutations affecting *ARID1A*, *ARID5B*, or *SMARCC1* occurred in 61% of cases. Other genes mutated in CTCL also have roles in enhancer function. For example, mutations in *MLL2*, *MLL3*, and *MLL4* (*KDM2D*, *-C*, and *-B*) occur in SS although the frequencies vary considerably among reports [161, 162]. Alterations affecting DNA methylation are also common in CTCL. Focal deletions at 2p23.3, sometimes homozygous, likely target de novo DNA methyltransferase *DNMT3A* in ~20–35% in CTCL [160, 161]; deleterious mutations also occur. Mutations and deletions also occur in *TET* family genes, essentially affecting *TET1*, whereas *TET2* mutations are uncommon [161].

4.11 Hepatosplenic T-Cell Lymphoma (HSTL) (Fig. 4.10)

HSTL is a very rare and aggressive entity originally described as "hepatosplenic γδ T-cell lymphoma" because most cases derive from γδ T-cells. Since there are rare cases with an αβ

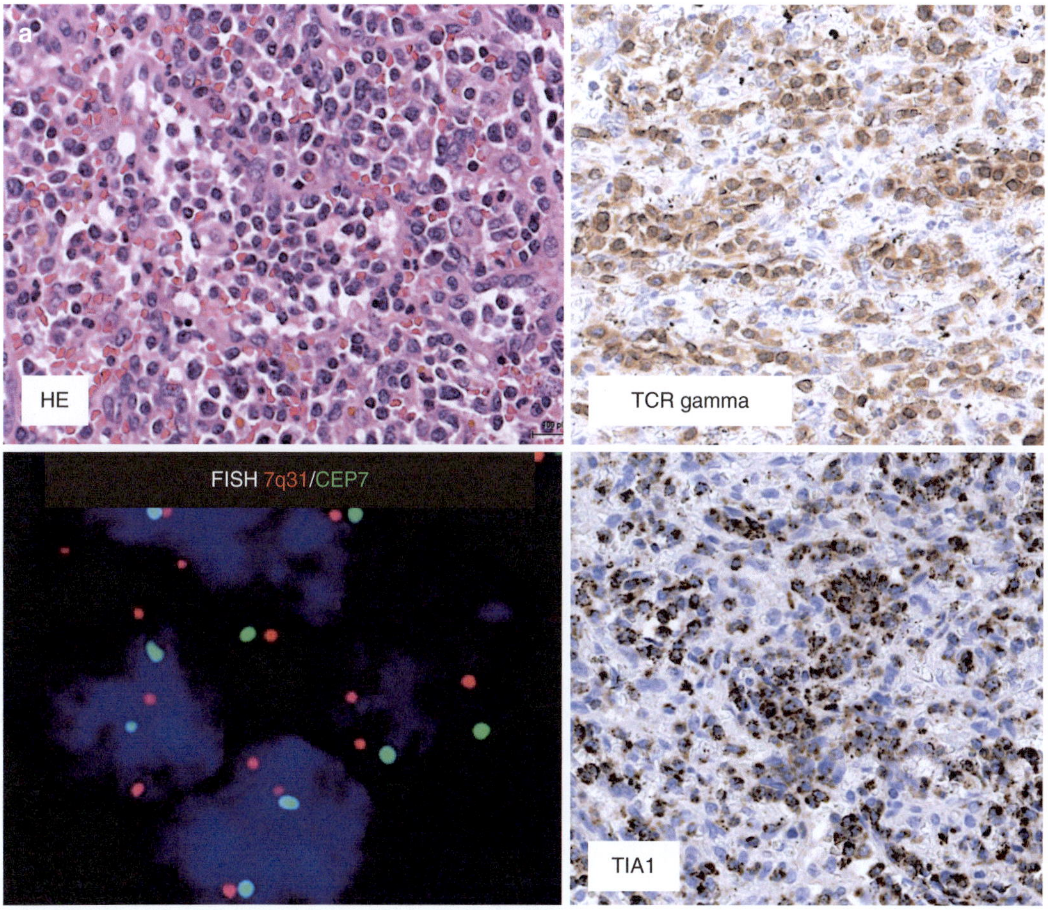

Fig. 4.10 Hepatosplenic T-cell lymphoma (HSTL). (**a**) Histopathology of a splenectomy specimen showing intra-sinusoidal involvement by medium-sized lymphoid cells in the splenic white pulp. The lymphoma cells are positive for TCR gamma expression, and this immunostain emphasizes the intravascular distribution of the neoplastic cells, which are also positive for TIA1. Iso7q demonstrated here by FISH is a major genetic abnormality in HSTL. (**b**) Recurrent mutation is chromatin modifiers in HSTL. Bars colored by most damaging mutation in each gene-sample pair (adapted from McKinney et al. Cancer Discovery 2017)

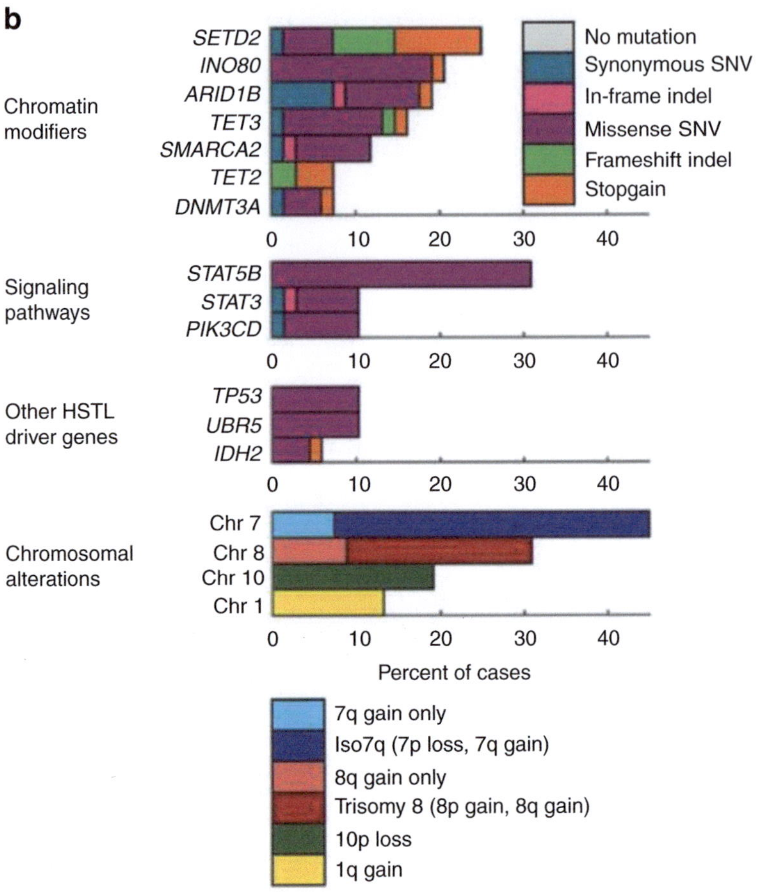

Fig. 4.10 (continued)

phenotype and similar clinicopathologic and molecular features, the entity was simply renamed (hepatosplenic T-cell lymphoma) [164]. HSTL predominantly affects young male adults; in about 20% of the cases, it occurs in the setting of chronic immune suppression or prolonged antigenic stimulation, particularly in solid organ transplant recipients, and about 10% of the patients have a history of inflammatory bowel disease that may have required treatment by azathioprine and/or anti-TNF-alpha conjugates [165–167]. The disease typically presents with hepatosplenomegaly, thrombocytopenia, and systemic symptoms without lymphadenopathy or peripheral blood involvement.

4.11.1 Pathology

HSTL comprises a monotonous infiltrate of atypical medium-sized lymphoid cells (Fig. 4.10a). A subset of cases may show more pleomorphic or blastoid morphology. Splenomegaly results from the enlargement of the red pulp while the white pulp is rather atrophic [168]. The lymphoma cells expand the red pulp cords and distend the sinusoids. A sinusoidal pattern of infiltrate is also seen in the liver and bone marrow. HSTL is thought to derive from functionally immature cytotoxic γδ T-cells of the splenic pool with vδ1 gene usage. The usual immunophenotype is CD3+ CD5− CD56+ CD4−/CD8− TCRγδ+ with a nonactivated cytotoxic profile (Fig. 4.10a) [168].

4.11.2 Molecular Pathogenesis and Genetic Features

Isochromosome 7 is observed in majority of the cases (Fig. 4.10a), both in cases with a γδ or αβ phenotype [169, 170] resulting in (1) deletion of the short arm of chromosome 7 which may lead to the loss of tumor suppressor genes located on 7p, as well as loss of *TRB@* gene at 7p15 and (2) duplication of the long arm most likely causing overexpression of oncogenes located on 7q, as well as the *TRG@* gene at 7q35 [171]. Isochromosome 7q is usually thought to be the primary abnormality of this disease with a tendency to multiply the i(7)(q10) during disease progression; it may be accompanied by trisomy 8 and loss of a sex chromosome, which seem also to be associated with progression of the disease [169, 172]. Isochromosome 7q is not specific for HSTL, as it is indeed one of the most common isochromosomes in malignant disorders (acute myeloid and lymphoblastic leukemias, myelodysplastic syndromes, and Wilms tumor) and in the spectrum of NK/T-cell malignancies and ALK–ALCLs [173].

Whole-exome sequencing analysis of a large series of HSTL (Fig. 4.10b) showed frequent mutations in chromatin-modifying genes (*SETD2*, *INO80*, and *ARID1B*) in 62% of cases and also in *STAT5B* (31%), *STAT3* (9%), and *PIK3CD* (9%) [174]. *SETD2* encodes a major chromatin modifier and catalyzes trimethylation of Lys-36 of histone H3 (H3K36me3) [173, 174]; thus, epigenetic imbalance widely governs the molecular pathways in HSTL.

4.11.3 Molecular Signature

Irrespective of TCR cell lineage, these lymphomas have unique gene signatures and in general form a distinct hierarchical cluster [164] but exhibit close association with ENKTCL [16]. The differentially expressed transcripts reflect the characteristic distribution of the neoplastic cells in the liver and spleen with high expression of metabolic and B-cell-related genes, mainly from stromal components. Overall, there were differences in expression of cytotoxicity genes compared with NKCL and/or other non-hepatosplenic cytotoxic PTCLs [175]. Other GEP studies have identified a unique gene signature that can distinguish hepatosplenic γδ-TCL from other αβ-TCL and γδ-TCL [175]. Travert et al. also performed GEP analysis on a subset of HSTL and showed overexpression of genes encoding NK-cell-associated molecules and oncogenes (*FOS* and *VAV3*). The study also showed low expression of AIM1 due to promoter hypermethylation and decitabine treatment that induced a significant increase in AIM1 transcript [164].

4.12 Intestinal T-Cell Lymphomas

Primary intestinal T-cell lymphomas formerly designated as enteropathy-associated T-cell lymphomas (EATL) type I and type II are derived from intraepithelial T lymphocytes and overall account for 5–8% of PTCLs and 10–25% of all primary intestinal lymphomas [3, 6, 176, 177]. These diseases tend to occur in adults older than 50 years, with a slight male preponderance. Symptoms may include anorexia, weight loss, diarrhea, abdominal pain, malaise, and fever, but many cases present with acute symptoms due to intestinal perforation, obstruction, or bleeding. The tumor usually develops in the small intestine, most often in the jejunum, ileum, or duodenum, or as multifocal intestinal lesions. Primary intestinal T-cell lymphomas have a poor prognosis, with <20% 5-year survival [6, 178]. Besides these primary intestinal diseases, the intestines may be involved by virtually any T-cell lymphoma entity at presentation or during disease course, especially EBV-associated ENKTL. Moreover a peculiar form of indolent clonal intestinal T-cell lymphoproliferative disorder was recently recognized.

4.12.1 Pathology (Fig. 4.11)

The two subtypes of EATL previously considered as variants of the same disease have been

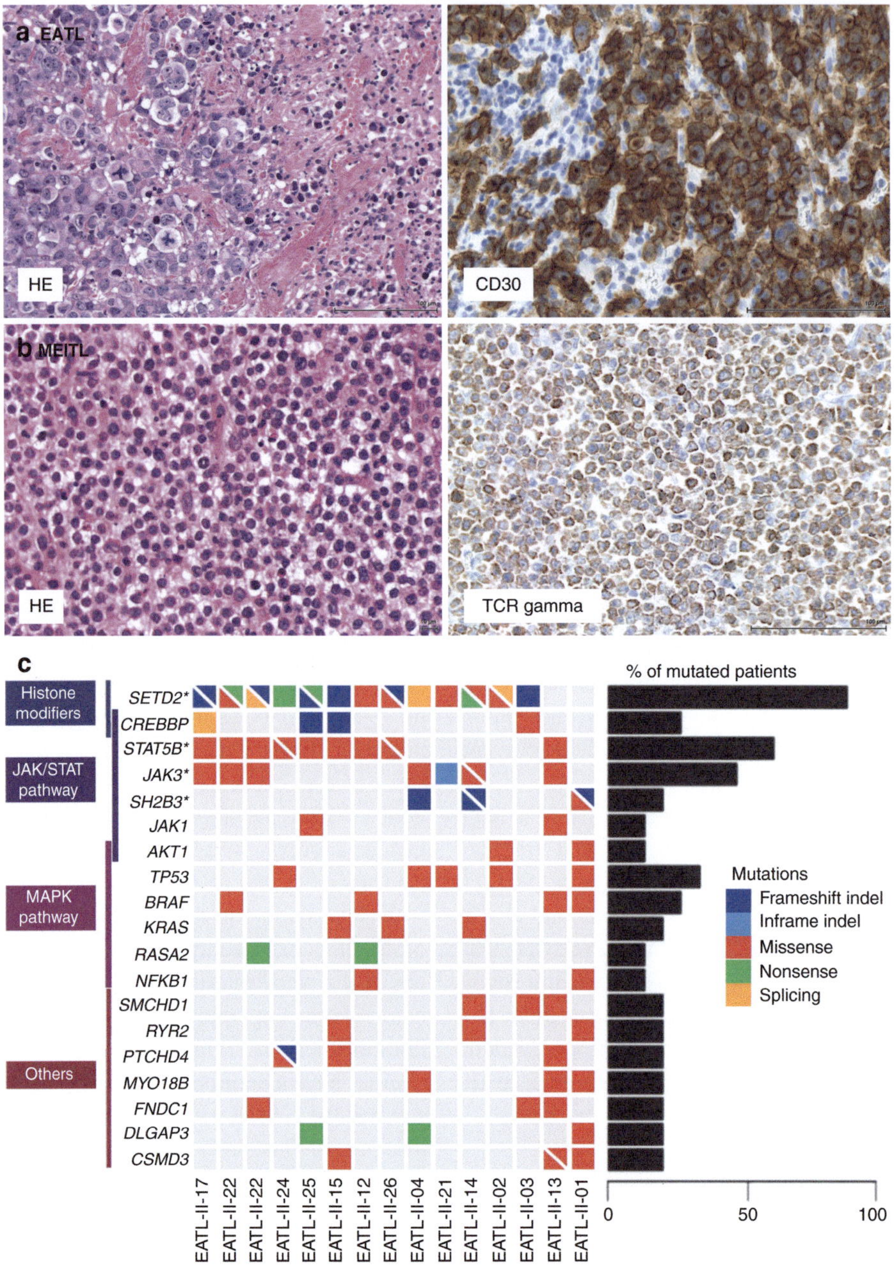

Fig. 4.11 Histopathological and genetic features of primary intestinal T-cell lymphomas. (**a**) Enteropathy-associated T-cell lymphoma (EATL) in a patient with history of celiac disease; the tumor is presented as an ulcerated mass and is composed of large pleomorphic and somewhat anaplastic cells, which are strongly positive for CD30. (**b**) Monomorphic epitheliotropic intestinal T-cell lymphoma (MEITL) composed of monotonous medium-sized cells, expressing the gamma chain of the TCR. (**c**) Most frequent mutation and pathways perturbed in MEITL. Epigenetic modification and JAK-STAT pathway are more frequently altered pathways in this rare entity (adapted from Roberti et al., Nat Commun. 2016). (**d**) An extended cohort of EATL (type I $n = 41$) and MEITL (EATL type II $n = 23$) showed a higher frequency of *SETD2* alterations in MEITL and similar mutation profile in other genes in these entities: type I frequency (purple; left); type II frequency (orange; right) (adapted from Moffitt et al., JEM 2017). (**e**) The Circos diagram summarizes the somatically acquired genetic variants in MEITL genomes detected by WES. From outermost to innermost tracks: (1) ideogram representing chromosomes oriented clockwise, with centromeres indicated in red; (2, 3) plot of somatic copy number alterations and relative frequency, gains (red) and losses (blue); (4) neutral LOH distribution; (5) distribution of somatic mutations and different mutation types across the genome colored by type of alteration (adapted from Roberti et al., Nat Commun. 2016)

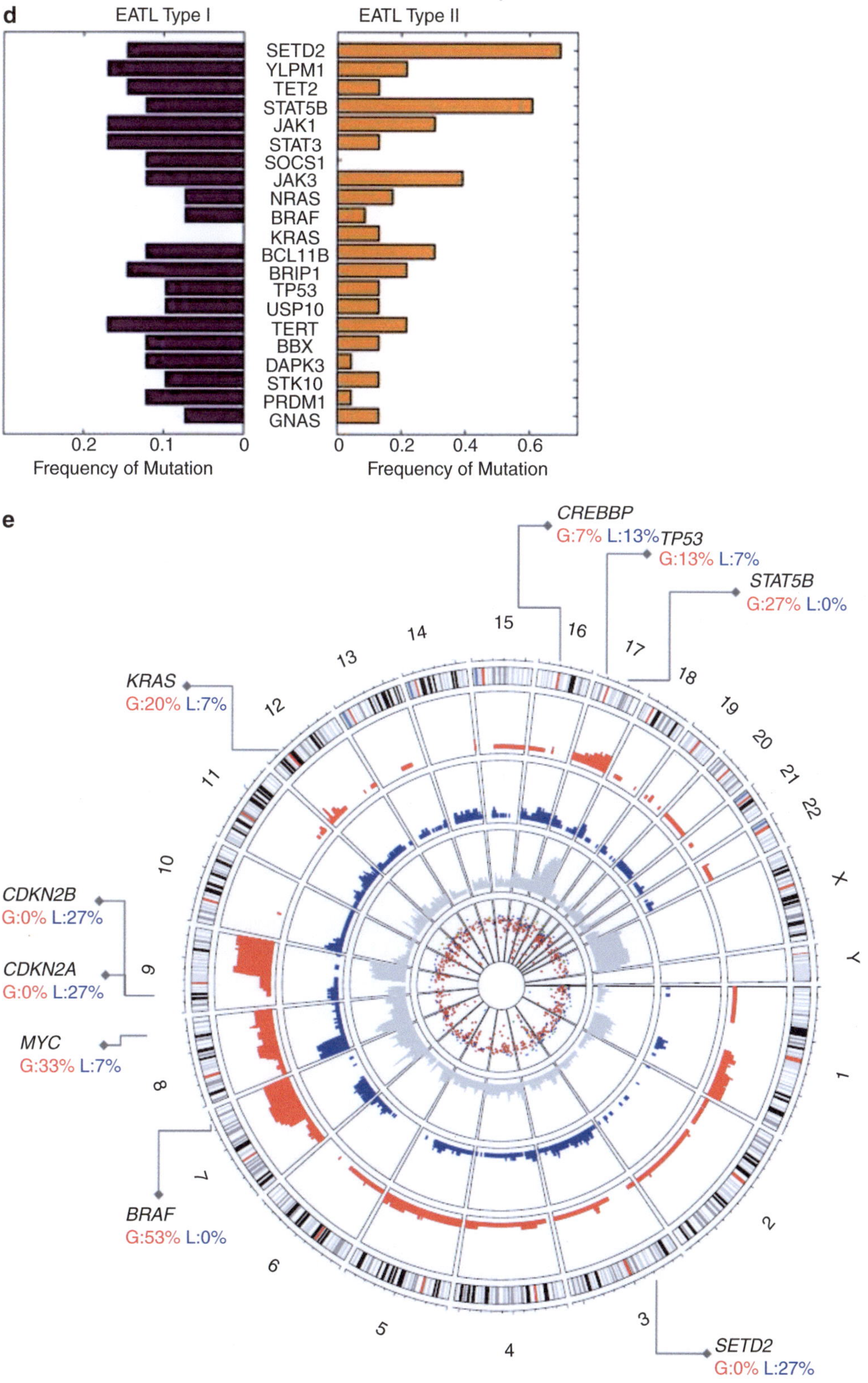

Fig. 4.11 (continued)

Table 4.2 Characteristics of primary intestinal T-cell lymphomas

	Enteropathy-associated T-cell lymphoma (EATL)	Monomorphic epitheliotropic intestinal T-cell lymphoma (MEITL)
Epidemiology	Northern Europe, association with celiac disease (CD) HLA-DQ2/−DQ8: >90%	Celiac disease uncommon HLA-DQ2/−DQ8: nl frequency
Morphology	Pleomorphic, medium to large size, some cases anaplastic Inflammation, necrosis common	Monomorphic, small to medium size, epitheliotropic No inflammation, no necrosis
Distant mucosa	Enteropathy	Increased IEL, no atrophy
Immuno-phenotype	CD3+, CD5−, CD8−/+, CD56- frequently CD30+ Cytotoxic activated MATK+ <40% of tumor cells	CD3+, CD5−, CD8+/−, CD56+/− CD30- Cytotoxic activated MATK+ >80% tumor cells Co-expression of B-cell antigens (20%)
TCR expression	Usually αβTCR	γδTCR (Vδ1) > αβTCR
Genomic imbalances	+1q32.2-q41, +5q34-q35.2 +9q −16q21.1	+8q24 (*MYC*) +9q −16q21.1
Epigenetics	*SETD2* mut. rare	*SETD2* inactivation (>90%)
JAK/STAT pathway	*JAK1* mut (20–50%) *JAK3* mut (10%) *STAT3* mut (20%) *STAT5B* mut (rare)	*JAK1* mut (10–20%) *JAK3* mut (35–50%) *STAT3* mut (10%) *STAT5B* mut (50–65%)
MAPK pathway	*KRAS NRAS BRAF* mut (20%)	*BRAF KRAS NRAS* mut (50%)
GRP signaling		*GNAI2* mut (24%)

reclassified as two distinct disease entities (WHO 2017) due to differences in epidemiological, clinical, histological, and genetic features (Table 4.2) [6], i.e., former type I EATL is now simply designated as EATL, and former type II EATL was renamed monomorphic epitheliotropic intestinal T-cell lymphoma (MEITL).

EATL is most common overall, comprising about 80–90% of cases, and is more prevalent in Western populations, especially in Northern Europe where celiac disease is more prevalent. EATL occurs as a complication of gluten-sensitive enteropathy, but less than half of the patients have a known history of celiac disease. In patients with symptomatic celiac disease, the development of EATL may be preceded by refractory celiac disease (RCD) (RCD I, comprising increased polyclonal IEL with normal immunophenotype, or RCD II, characterized by monoclonal IEL with an aberrant immunophenotype) or chronic ulcerative jejunitis (multifocal ulcerated microlymphomas). In around half of the patients, EATL represents the first manifestation of enteropathy. It is composed of pleomorphic, medium to large, occasionally anaplastic lymphoid cells. Extensive necrosis and a high mitotic rate are common (Fig. 4.11a). A polymorphic inflammatory infiltrate rich in histiocytes and eosinophils is frequently present, sometimes obscuring the lymphoma cells, and indeed the disease was initially reported as "malignant histiocytosis of the small intestine" [179]. The neoplastic cells are usually CD3+, CD5-, CD4-, CD8-, and CD56- and diffusely express cytotoxic markers with an activated profile (expression of TIA1 and granzyme B and/or perforin) [180]. Most cases are CD30+ (Fig. 4.11a), and interestingly complete remission was reported recently in a patient with CD30+ EATL, after brentuximab vedotin administration [47, 180, 181]. The neoplastic cells are EBV-negative and usually express TCRαβ+ and the intraepithelial homing integrin CD103 [178].

MEITL is overall very rare [3]. It comprises <20% of primary intestinal T-cell lymphomas, is rare in Western populations, and represents the more prevalent intestinal T-cell lymphoma type in Asian-Pacific studies [5, 182]. Although this remains controversial, most studies suggest the lack of association with celiac disease in the majority of type II EATL cases [3, 178, 183]. Typically, it comprises a monomorphic proliferation of medium-sized cells, without necrosis and inflammation [184]. At the periphery of the central tumor zone, the neoplastic cells spread to the adjacent mucosa by featuring marked epitheliotropism [185, 186]. The neoplastic cells are usually CD3+, CD5-, CD7+, CD4-/CD8+, CD30-, and CD56+, with an activated cytotoxic immunophenotype. EBV is negative. Aberrant expression of CD20 and/or other B-cell markers may be seen in up to 25% of the cases. The megakaryocyte-associated tyrosine kinase (MATK) was reported as a specific marker of MEITL [186, 187]. MEITL appears heterogeneous in terms of TCR expression, and the majority of the cases are of γδ origin (Fig. 4.11b) [185]. Increased IEL in distant mucosa can be frequently identified upon careful examination and have an immunophenotype that is either concordant or variably discordant with that of the invasive tumor [185, 186, 188, 189].

4.12.2 Molecular Pathogenesis and Genetic Features (Table 4.2)

Comparative genomic hybridization (CGH)-based studies have shown that EATL and MEITL share common recurrent chromosomal imbalances, and also distinctive genetic alterations [190–192]. Both are cytogenetically characterized by chromosome 9q gains and almost mutually exclusive losses of 16q12.1. Gain of chromosome 7 and losses of 8p22–23.2, 16q21.1, 11q14.1- q14.2, and 9p21.2-p21.3 are also frequent in both diseases. Conversely, MEITL is characterized by significantly more frequent gains of the *MYC* oncogene locus and less frequent gains of chromosomes 1q and 5q as compared with EATL, suggesting two distinct genetic pathways. Additionally the loss of 3p21.31 has been reported as recurrent in MEITL, but not in EATL.

A few studies have examined the mutational landscape of these lymphomas, by targeted or by whole-exome sequencing. While some studies have examined both EATL and MEITL [193, 194], a few were primarily focused on MEITL [195–197], and overall MEITL appears to be better characterized than EATL (Fig. 4.11c–e). Whole-exome sequencing analysis of a series of MEITL led to the discovery of highly recurrent alterations of the tumor suppressor *SETD2* gene encoding a nonredundant H3K36-specific trimethyltransferase, in the majority of the cases (14/15) (93%) [196]. *SETD2* alterations were often biallelic, mainly by loss-of-function mutations and/or loss of the corresponding locus (3p21.31). The latter finding was generated from CNV analysis of the exome sequences and confirmed by a FISH assay that we designed to specifically interrogate the *SETD2* locus. *SETD2* alterations are found in both γδ and αβ-expressing tumors and consistently correlated with defective SETD2 expression and H3K36 trimethylation evaluated by immunohistochemistry. In a subsequent study, Moffitt et al. confirmed that *SETD2* was the most frequently silenced gene in MEITL and identified *SETD2* alterations in a small percentage of EATL as well [194] (Fig. 4.11d). These authors also modeled the effects of *SETD2* loss in vivo by developing a T-cell-specific knockout mouse, and these mice manifested an expansion of γδ T-cells, indicating novel roles for *SETD2* in T-cell development and lymphomagenesis. Interestingly, *SETD2* is also most frequently mutated gene (about one third of the cases) in HSTL [174], an entity having in common with MEITL to be highly aggressive and often derived from γδ T-cells. In another study, *GNAI2* was identified as a frequently mutated gene in MEITL(24% of the cases) [195]. Collectively, sequencing studies of EATL and MEITL have pointed at recurrent mutation-induced activation of the JAK/STAT pathway in these tumors. Recurrent mutations of *STAT5B* in MEITL were first reported by Kucuk C et al. and found to occur exclusively in cases of γδ origin [198]. The study by Nairismagi et al. and Roberti et al. further substantiated almost constant mutation-induced alterations in the JAK-STAT pathway in MEITL, mainly affecting *STAT5B* (60–65%), *JAK3* (35–46%), and *SH2B*3 (20%) [195, 196]. In a targeted NGS analysis of 34 intestinal T-cell lymphomas (comprising EATLs, MEITLs, and other T-cell lymphomas), Nicolae et al. reported JAK/STAT pathway mutations in 67.6% of cases (with *STAT5B* and *JAK3* most frequently mutated in 26.5% and 27.3% of cases) in all intestinal PTCL subtypes with a higher prevalence in MEITL, regardless of αβ and γδ origin, and RAS pathway gene alterations in 24.2% of cases [193]. A high percentage of cases showed co-occurring mutations in both the JAK/STAT and RAS pathway. Moffitt AB et al. also found evidence of overlapping genetic alterations in EATL and MEITL, with frequent mutations in MAPK signaling pathway (*TP53*, *BRAF*, and *KRAS*) indicating shared mechanisms underlying their pathogenesis [194].

4.13 Indolent Intestinal T-Cell Lymphoproliferations

"Indolent T-cell lymphoproliferative disorder of the gastrointestinal tract" was coined to designate clonal T-cell proliferations, with indolent clinical course after long-term monitoring [199]. The small number of such cases reported in the literature [199–202] occurred more commonly in males at a median age of 48.5 years (range, 15–77 years). Patients presented with chronic diarrhea, weight loss, abdominal pain, and/or rectal bleeding. Endoscopic findings include mucosal erythema, erosions or small ulcerations, and in some instances small polyps without mass lesions. Patients usually had multiple lesions along the gastrointestinal tract, most commonly in the small intestines and colon. Rare cases have evidence of distant disease, with liver or bone marrow infiltrates, proven with biopsy and/or detection of monoclonal *TCR* rearrangement.

Mucosal biopsies reveal a dense infiltrate of small, monotonous lymphoid cells expanding the lamina propria and displacing the epithelial structures without signs of destruction. Villous atrophy is commonly present [199, 200, 202]. The infiltrate is composed of CD3+ T-cells, either CD4+ (more commonly) or CD8+, or in rare instances CD4-/CD8-. CD8-positive cases have a cytotoxic profile [199, 203], and some cases show loss of expression CD5 and/or CD7. CD56, CD103, and EBV are not detected. The variations observed in the immunophenotype do not appear to translate into any relevant clinical correlation. Ki67 proliferation index is in the range of 5–10%. *STAT3* mutations or evidence of STAT3 activation has not been found [199]. Some CD4+ cases occurred in patients with associated autoimmune disease [202].

The differential diagnosis includes inflammatory conditions, such as ulcerative colitis, but more challenging is to not misdiagnose an indolent T-cell lymphoproliferation as lymphoma, and indeed among the cases reported in the literature, several patients have received chemotherapy for presumed T-cell lymphoma; the diagnosis was then revisited after the lesions persisted without significant progression or resolution under treatment. The condition is clinically indolent, and most patients are alive with persistent disease after several years of follow-up. Complete remissions have been reported in two cases [199], and death from disease progression has been reported at 132 and 176 months after diagnosis in two patients [200, 201].

4.14 Extra-nodal NK/T-Cell Lymphoma (ENKTCL)

ENKTCL is not exceptional in Western countries, but predominantly affects middle-aged men in Asia, Mexico, and South America [204]. It presents as tumors or destructive lesions in the nasal cavity, maxillary sinuses, or palate and, despite a localized presentation in most patients, tends to relapse locally or at other extra-nodal sites, such as the skin, and has an overall 40–50% 5-year survival rate. "Extranasal NK/T-cell lymphomas" otherwise similar to the nasal NKTCL may present in other localizations, especially in the skin, gastrointestinal tract, or testis, and tend to have a more adverse clinical outcome [204]. Aggressive NK-cell leukemia, also EBV-associated and derived from NK-cells, is regarded as the systemic form of NKTCL [205].

4.14.1 Pathology (Fig. 4.12)

ENKTCL ranges from monomorphic small-/medium-sized to large cell lymphomas and is characterized by frequent features of angioinvasion and angiocentrism, and common necrosis,

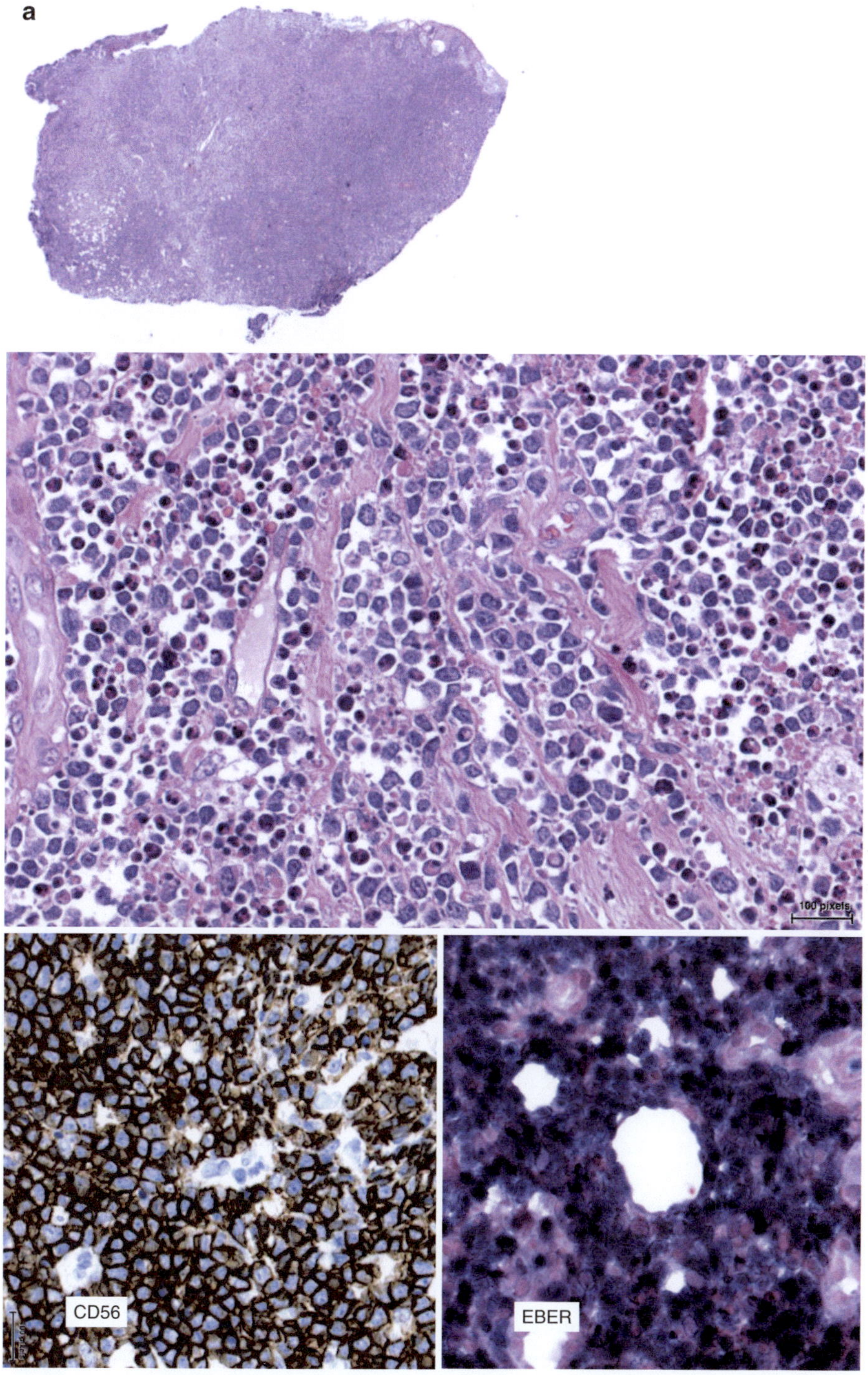

Fig. 4.12 Extra-nodal NK/T-cell lymphoma (ENKTCL). (**a**) Histopathological features of a case presenting as an ulcerated mass of the gingiva; low-power view of the biopsy shows massive infiltration of the subepithelial soft tissues and surface ulceration. At higher magnification, the lymphoma comprises a proliferation of medium to large slightly pleomorphic cells, with abundant apoptotic debris and foci of necrosis. The lymphoid cells are strongly positive for CD56 and most nuclei stain for Epstein-Barr virus-encoded RNAs (EBERs) as shown by in situ hybridization. (**b**) Gene mutations identified in ENKTCL. The mutations are classified into the categories indicated at left: *I* RNA helicase, *II* tumor suppressors, *III* JAK-STAT pathway, *IV* epigenetic modifiers, *V* others, *VI* RNA helicase family (adapted from Jian E. al. Nat Genet. 2015)

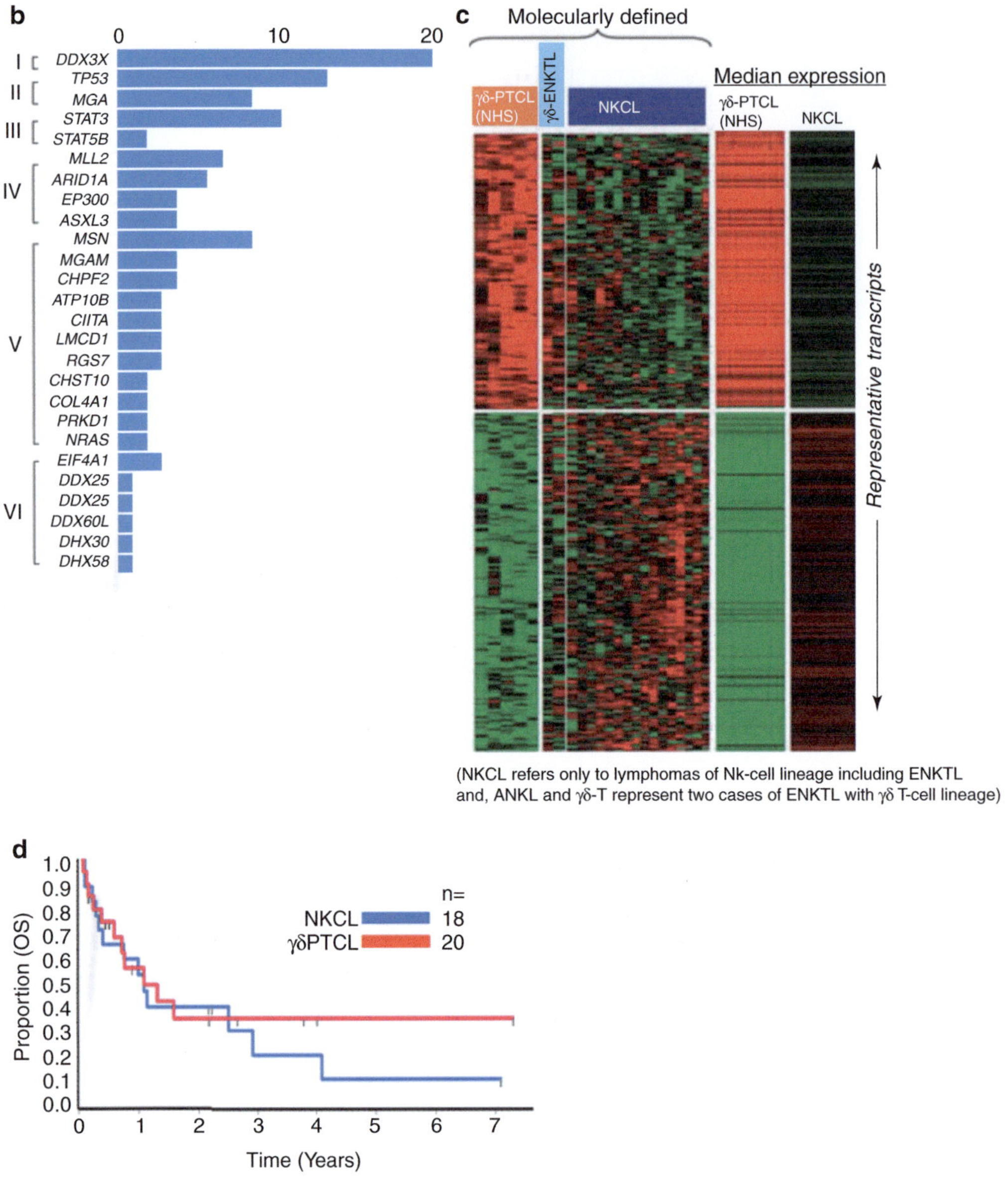

Fig. 4.12 (continued)

accounting for frequent diagnostic difficulties on small biopsies. In cases where the neoplastic cells are admixed with an inflammatory component and/or in small biopsies, the lesions may be mistaken for a reactive process. Pseudoepitheliomatous hyperplasia of the overlying epithelium in mucosal localizations is another source of diagnostic difficulties. The neoplastic cells usually express cytoplasmic CD3 (CD3ε+); are CD2+, CD5-, CD7+, CD16+/− and CD56+; and have an activated cytotoxic profile. A subset of cases are negative for CD56 which is not specific for ENKTCL, as most cases are derived from NK-cells; however, up to 38% of the cases derived from clonal T-cells with a γδ or more rarely αβ TCR configuration. By definition, all cases are associated with EBV, which is best demonstrated by in situ hybridization [6]. EBV infection in ENKTCL is characterized by a type II latency program with expression of EBERs,

LMP1, and EBNA2 [206]. Recently, several studies have documented consistent PD-L1 expression by ENKTCL neoplastic cells in the vast majority of the cases [207], and recent reports indicate that antagonization of PD1-PD-L1 interactions might represent a therapeutic option for ENKTCL patients refractory to standard lines of therapy [208].

4.14.2 Molecular Signature

The molecular signature of ENKTCL, irrespective of the cellular derivation, is distinct from that of other PTCLs and is characterized by high expression of transcripts associated with NK-cell-associated receptors (e.g., killer cell immunoglobulin- or lectin-like receptor (KIR or KLR), cytotoxic markers (e.g., GZMB, GZMH), and distinct chemokine signatures, TCRδ mRNA, but not CD16 (FCGR3A)). It was also noted that non-hepatosplenic γδ-TCL showed a very similar gene expression profile to NKTCL [15], suggesting that these two diseases are highly similar and may use the same oncogenic mechanisms during neoplastic transformation. A subsequent mRNA signature was able to delineate NK and γδ-T-cell lineage in these tumors. Compared to normal NK-cells, ENKTCL is characterized by activation of PDGFRA, JAK/STAT, MYC, AKT, and NF-KB pathways [206, 209–211], and NK-cell lines have been shown to be sensitive to STAT3 and NOTCH inhibition.

4.14.3 Molecular Pathogenesis and Genetic Features

EBV is clonally present in an episomal form in the tumor cells and exerts oncogenic effects through the production of cytokines such as IL-9 and IL-10 and the upregulation of IP10/MIP2 chemokines that may contribute to vascular damage and secondary necrosis [212], while TNF-α production may explain the common hematophagocytic syndrome. ENKTCL usually bears complex recurrent genomic aberrations [206]. Partial deletion of chromosome 6 (6q21–25) is a recurrent aberration in ENKTCL. Several candidate tumor suppressor genes, such as *PRDM1*, *ATG5*, *AIM1*, and *HACE1*, are mapping to that region, and their inactivation by deletion and/or methylation might be involved in lymphomagenesis [206, 211]. ENKTL is characterized by constitutive activation of the JAK/STAT pathway [210], and activating *JAK3* mutations are detected in up to one third of the cases [213, 214], but a report showed that *JAK3* mutations are not frequent in NKTCLs, at least in Japan [215]. This marked difference in mutation frequency requires additional investigation. In a recent whole-exome sequencing analysis [216], the most frequent mutations involved *DDX3X,* an RNA helicase that has been found to be recurrently methylated as well [198], but understanding the precise role of *DDX3X* in the pathogenesis of ENKTCL needs further exploration. This study also confirms the frequent *TP53 and STAT3* mutations and demonstrated mutations affecting epigenetic modifiers. Similar to the γδ T-cell-derived tumors, JAK-STAT pathway plays a pathogenetic role in ENKTL [217] (Fig. 4.12b).

4.15 PTCL Not Otherwise Specified (PTCL-NOS)

PTCL-NOS is a heterogeneous entity of both nodal and extra-nodal mature T-cell neoplasms that do not correspond to any of the more specific entities. The disease generally occurs in adults and has an aggressive clinical course [218]. Importantly, neoplasms with a T_{FH} immunophenotype are now excluded from the PTCL-NOS category. In many publications, PTCL-NOS is reported as the most common PTCL entity; however, with the current more stringent criteria including the exclusion of T_{FH} neoplasms, PTCL-NOS appears to be outnumbered by AITL and related T_{FH} tumors [18].

4.15.1 Pathology (Fig. 4.13a–c)

In PTCL-NOS, lymph nodes usually are diffusely involved. While a small subset of the cases show monomorphic cytology, most cases are typically pleomorphic. Most cases consist predominantly

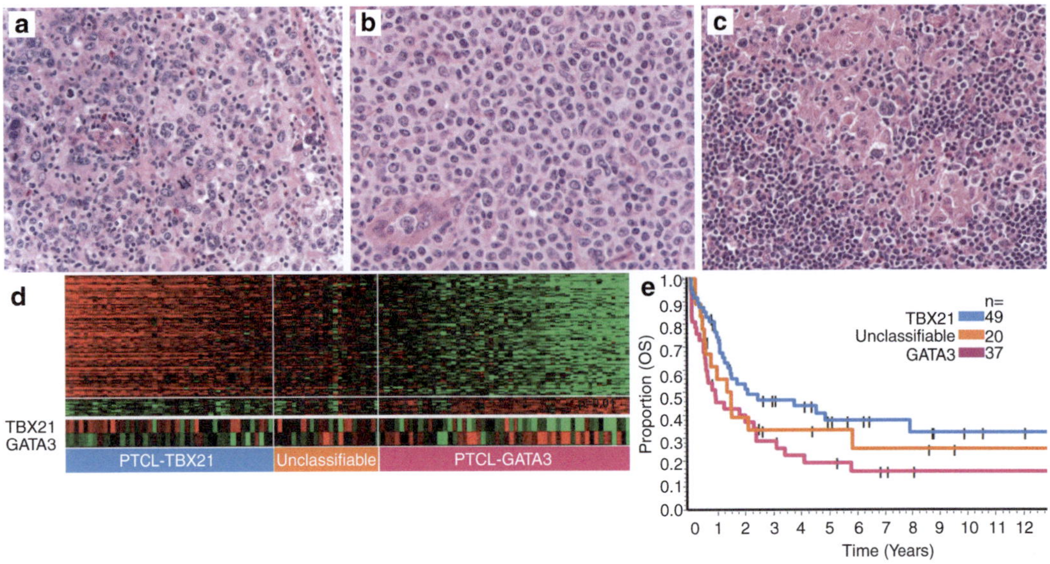

Fig. 4.13 Pathological heterogeneity of peripheral T-cell lymphoma (**a–c**). Three different cases are shown, (**a**) characterized by markedly pleomorphic morphology and eosinophilia, (**b**) composed of monotonous medium-sized cells with few reactive cells, and (**c**) containing numerous histiocytes (lymphoepithelioid lymphoma). Molecular subgroups within PTCL-NOS with prognostic difference (**d–e**): GEP identified two major molecular subgroups within PTCL-NOS. Bayesian predictor for the PTCL-GATA3 and PTCL-TBX21 subgroups was derived using PTCL-NOS cases; LOOCV was used for classification precision. Overall survival (OS) analysis of molecularly defined GATA3 and TBX21 subgroups showed significant difference in clinical outcome ($P = 0.01$) (adapted from Iqbal et al. Blood 2014)

of medium-sized or large cells with irregular nuclei containing prominent nucleoli and many mitoses. High endothelial venules are usually increased. Many cases comprise an admixture of small lymphocytes, eosinophils, histiocytes, B-cells, and plasma cells. Many cases are CD4+ CD8-, a subset are CD4-CD8+, and more rarely tumors are either double(−) or -positive for CD4 and CD8. Most cases derive from T cells expressing an αβ-TCR, a minority are of γδ origin, or TCR-silent. The lymphoma cells usually express several T-cell-associated antigens, but one or several of these (most commonly CD5 or CD7, more rarely CD3 or CD2) may show reduced or absent expression. Expression of CD20 or other B-cell markers (CD19, CD79a, PAX5) has been documented in rare cases of PTCL-NOS, but co-expression of several of them seems exceptional [219–221]. CD30 is often detected in a variable proportion of tumor cells [47]. Up to 50% of PTCL-NOS are EBV-positive usually in a small subset of cells, likely bystander B-cells, and this feature has been associated with a poor survival [222]. A subset of PTCL-NOS (15–40% of cases), most commonly CD8+, feature a cytotoxic immunophenotype. The rare lymphoepithelioid variant, comprising a proliferation of small cytotoxic CD8+ neoplastic T-cells in association with an abundant epithelioid cell background, may have a better prognosis [223, 224]. All cases of CD4+ non-cytotoxic "unspecified" PTCLs should be investigated for the expression of T_{FH} markers, since PTCL of T_{FH} cell origin are now classified in the group of AITL and related neoplasms.

4.15.2 Molecular Signature

Several GEP studies of PTCL-NOS identified distinct clusters, but their biological significance was not clear and largely reflected characteristics of the tumor microenvironment [45, 50, 225], and either association with activated CD4^{+}

or $CD8^+$ T-cell gene expression signatures [50]. Molecular prognosticators showed association of NF-κB activation with a favorable clinical outcome, whereas high proliferation gene signature was associated with poor clinical outcome [226, 227]. Though no consensus in biological significance was observed in these studies, which may be due to either platform differences or differences in the patient populations profiled, nevertheless, multiple molecular subgroups within nodal PTCL-NOS [228] were anticipated. Using a large cohort of PTCL-NOS cases and rigorous pathology review and GEP analysis, we identified two novel molecular subgroups within PTCL-NOS showing distinct signaling pathways and different prognosis [14]. They are characterized by high expression of either TBX21 (T_{H1} master regulator) or GATA3 (T_{H2} master regulator) and corresponding target genes at both mRNA and protein levels. The "PTCL-GATA3" subgroup was associated with poor clinical outcome and the lack of a prominent microenvironment signature (Fig. 4.13d–e). It was associated with high *MYC* and proliferation signatures, whereas the NF-κB pathway was enriched in the TBX21 subgroup, which may likely explain the favorable outcome associated with the NF-κB pathway reported in the previous study [227]. Our study also suggested that the TBX21 subgroup (49% of PTCL-NOS) may contain a subset with high cytotoxic signature, which is associated with a poorer clinical outcome than compared to the rest of the TBX21 subgroup. This adverse outcome of the GATA3 subgroup is further supported by an independent study using immunohistochemistry for GATA3 expression [229]. The T_{H1} polarization is induced by exposure to IFNγ and IL-12, leading to STAT1 and *STAT4* activation and induction of *TBX21* expression. *TBX21* upregulates the production of IFNγ leading to a positive feedback loop through both autocrine and paracrine mechanisms. T_{H2} polarization, however, is induced by exposure to IL-4, leading to STAT6 activation and upregulation of *GATA3*. Though there is great plasticity between the different T-cell helper subsets, T_{H1} and T_{H2} identities are relatively stable because they have built-in positive feedback loops to maintain the current polarization and inhibit all other helper lineages.

4.15.3 Genetic Features

As anticipated, the genetic features of PTCL are heterogeneous with significant overlap with other PTCL subtypes. There are fewer genomic studies in PTCL-NOS, and even the results generated from conventional cytogenetic, karyotyping, or array-based hybridization platforms are difficult to interpret. Nevertheless structural alterations are found in the majority of PTCL-NOS, more commonly in tumors with large cell morphology, cytological grade, and chromosomal gains of 7q and 8q identified in majority of PTCL-NOS (reviewed by de Leval et al.) [230]. Two genes on chromosome 7 (*CDK6* at 7q22 and *CARMA1* at 7p22), have been shown to be effected by chromosomal genes and may have pathogenic role in PTCL-NOS [231, 232].

Chromosomal breaks involving the *TCR* gene loci (mostly the *A/B TCR* locus at 14q11.2) have been reported in rare cases of PTCL-NOS, but the translocation partner(s) has been identified in only occasional cases [173, 231, 233, 234]. The t(14;19)(q11;q13) translocation involves the poliovirus receptor-related 2 gene (*PVRL2*) and induces overexpression of both *PVRL2* and *BCL3* mRNAs [235, 236]. The multiple myeloma oncogene-1/interferon regulatory factor-4 (*IRF4*) was recently identified as the gene partner in chromosomal translocations involving the *TCRA* gene in the t(6;14)(p25;q11.2) translocation in three cases of clinically aggressive cytotoxic PTCL-NOS, involving the bone marrow and skin or presenting with massive splenomegaly (Fig. 4.12) [237, 238]. *TP63* rearrangements encoding fusion proteins homologous to ΔNP63, (a dominant-negative p63 isoform that inhibits the p53 pathway reported in a subset of ALK-ALCLs) are detected in less than 10% of PTCL-NOS as well, and are associated with an aggressive clinical course and bad outcome [113]. A high-resolution genomic analysis of the two molecular subgroups of PTCL-NOS (TBX21 and GATA3) revealed significant differences in the profile of copy number aberrations (CNAs), with higher genomic complexity in the PTCL-GATA3 subgroup, suggesting different oncogenic pathways for tumorigenesis [239].

Scanty data are available so far regarding the mutational landscape of PTCL-NOS. Some mutations that are frequent in AITL (see above) are also detected in PTCL-NOS but at lower frequencies. A study using a limited capture panel of known mutated genes [240] reported frequent mutations in epigenetic regulators including *MLL2*, *KDM6A*, *MLL*, *TET2,* and *DNMT3A*. Cases showing alterations in histone methyltransferase genes (*MLL*, *MLL2*, or *KDM6A*) were associated with poor clinical outcome (P = 0.0198). Recent studies have identified *VAV1* fusion transcripts that have the common theme of deleting the terminal SH2 domain, thus eliminating an autoregulatory domain and possibly causing constitutive VAV1 activation [61, 241]. A small deletion affecting intron 25 extending to exon 26 of *VAV1* is detected in number of PTCL cases resulting in the abnormal splicing of exon 25, again leading to a protein that is constitutively active. Thus, VAV1 activation could be a significant pathogenetic mechanism in this group of lymphomas. In future studies, it is anticipated that the integration of GEP data with mutational profiles would support defining genetic subgroups with recurrent lesions and well-defined expression profiles.

4.16 Conclusion

With the advent of high-throughput genomic analysis, molecular description has aided in PTCL diagnosis and provided a deeper understanding of their intrinsic biology. Therapeutic interventions especially targeting epigenome have shown early promise reference, but accurate diagnosis of PTCL is a prerequisite for selecting the most appropriate treatment regimen for patients in future clinical trials [242]. PTCL is rare and heterogenous, and more collaborative international efforts are required to identify molecular features that can decipher molecular subgroups of PTCLs for better understanding.

Acknowledgments The authors would like to acknowledge Tayla Heavican in preparation of this manuscript. We would also like to thank many esteemed investigators in T-cell lymphoma biology, whose work was cited in this paper.

References

1. Rudiger T, Weisenburger DD, Anderson JR, et al. Peripheral T-cell lymphoma (excluding anaplastic large-cell lymphoma): results from the Non-Hodgkin's Lymphoma Classification Project. Ann Oncol. 2002;13(1):140–9.
2. Vose J, Armitage J, Weisenburger D, International TCLP. International peripheral T-cell and natural killer/T-cell lymphoma study: pathology findings and clinical outcomes. J Clin Oncol Off J Am Soc Clin Oncol. 2008;26(25):4124–30.
3. Delabie J, Holte H, Vose JM, et al. Enteropathy-associated T-cell lymphoma: clinical and histological findings from the international peripheral T-cell lymphoma project. Blood. 2011;118(1):148–55.
4. Wang SS, Vose JM. Epidemiology and prognosis of T-cell lymphoma. New York: Springer Science; 2013.
5. Swerdlow SH, Campo E, Harris NL, et al. WHO classification of tumours of haematopoietic and lymphoid tissues, vol. 2. 4th ed. Revised; 2017.
6. Swerdlow SH, Campo E, Harris NL, et al. WHO classification of tumours of haematopoietic and lymphoid tissues. 4th ed; 2008.
7. de Leval L, Gaulard P. Cellular origin of T-cell lymphomas. Blood. 2014;123(19):2909–10.
8. de Leval L, Gisselbrecht C, Gaulard P. Advances in the understanding and management of angioimmunoblastic T-cell lymphoma. Br J Haematol. 2010;148(5):673–89.
9. Gaulard P, de Leval L. Pathology of peripheral T-cell lymphomas: where do we stand? Semin Hematol. 2014;51(1):5–16.
10. Swerdlow SH, Campo E, Pileri SA, et al. The 2016 revision of the World Health Organization classification of lymphoid neoplasms. Blood. 2016;127(20):2375–90.
11. Pileri SA, Piccaluga PP. New molecular insights into peripheral T cell lymphomas. J Clin Invest. 2012;122(10):3448–55.
12. Croziera JA, Shera T, Yangb D, et al. Persistent disparities among patients with T-cell Non-Hodgkin Lymphomas and B-cell Diffuse Large Cell Lymphomas over 40 years: a SEER database review. Clin Lymphoma Myeloma Leuk. 2015;15(10):578–85.

13. Xu B, Liu P. No survival improvement for patients with angioimmunoblastic T-cell lymphoma over the past two decades: a population-based study of 1207 cases. PLoS One. 2014;9(3):e92585.
14. Iqbal J, Wright G, Wang C, et al. Gene expression signatures delineate biological and prognostic subgroups in peripheral T-cell lymphoma. Blood. 2014;123(19):2915–23.
15. Iqbal J, Weisenburger DD, Greiner TC, et al. Molecular signatures to improve diagnosis in peripheral T-cell lymphoma and prognostication in angioimmunoblastic T-cell lymphoma. Blood. 2010;115(5):1026–36.
16. Iqbal J, Weisenburger DD, Chowdhury A, et al. Natural killer cell lymphoma shares strikingly similar molecular features with a group of non-hepatosplenic gammadelta T-cell lymphoma and is highly sensitive to a novel aurora kinase A inhibitor in vitro. Leukemia. 2011;25(2):348–58.
17. d'Amore F, Gaulard P, Trumper L, et al. Peripheral T-cell lymphomas: ESMO Clinical Practice Guidelines for diagnosis, treatment and follow-up. Ann Oncol. 2015;26(Suppl 5):v108–15.
18. Laurent C, Baron M, Amara N, et al. Impact of expert pathologic review of lymphoma diagnosis: study of patients from the French lymphopath network. J Clin Oncol. 2017;35(18):2008–17.
19. Iqbal J, Wilcox R, Naushad H, et al. Genomic signatures in T-cell lymphoma: how can these improve precision in diagnosis and inform prognosis? Blood Rev. 2016;30(2):89–100.
20. Schmitt TM, Zuniga-Pflucker JC. Induction of T cell development from hematopoietic progenitor cells by delta-like-1 in vitro. Immunity. 2002;17(6):749–56.
21. Wu L. T lineage progenitors: the earliest steps en route to T lymphocytes. Curr Opin Immunol. 2006;18(2):121–6.
22. Ladi E, Yin X, Chtanova T, Robey EA. Thymic microenvironments for T cell differentiation and selection. Nat Immunol. 2006;7(4):338–43.
23. Groettrup M, Ungewiss K, Azogui O, et al. A novel disulfide-linked heterodimer on pre-T cells consists of the T cell receptor beta chain and a 33 kd glycoprotein. Cell. 1993;75(2):283–94.
24. Abbey JL, O'Neill HC. Expression of T-cell receptor genes during early T-cell development. Immunol Cell Biol. 2008;86(2):166–74.
25. Starr TK, Jameson SC, Hogquist KA. Positive and negative selection of T cells. Annu Rev Immunol. 2003;21:139–76.
26. Turner SJ, Doherty PC, McCluskey J, Rossjohn J. Structural determinants of T-cell receptor bias in immunity. Nat Rev Immunol. 2006;6(12): 883–94.
27. Hayes SM, Shores EW, Love PE. An architectural perspective on signaling by the pre-, alphabeta and gammadelta T cell receptors. Immunol Rev. 2003;191:28–37.
28. Kreslavsky T, Gleimer M, Garbe AI, von Boehmer H. alphabeta versus gammadelta fate choice: counting the T-cell lineages at the branch point. Immunol Rev. 2010;238(1):169–81.
29. Vantourout P, Hayday A. Six-of-the-best: unique contributions of gammadelta T cells to immunology. Nat Rev Immunol. 2013;13(2):88–100.
30. Silva-Santos B, Serre K, Norell H. gammadelta T cells in cancer. Nat Rev Immunol. 2015;15(11):683–91.
31. Smith-Garvin JE, Koretzky GA, Jordan MS. T cell activation. Annu Rev Immunol. 2009;27:591–619.
32. Collins AV, Brodie DW, Gilbert RJ, et al. The interaction properties of costimulatory molecules revisited. Immunity. 2002;17(2):201–10.
33. van der Merwe PA, Bodian DL, Daenke S, Linsley P, Davis SJ. CD80 (B7-1) binds both CD28 and CTLA-4 with a low affinity and very fast kinetics. J Exp Med. 1997;185(3):393–403.
34. Linsley PS, Brady W, Grosmaire L, Aruffo A, Damle NK, Ledbetter JA. Binding of the B cell activation antigen B7 to CD28 costimulates T cell proliferation and interleukin 2 mRNA accumulation. J Exp Med. 1991;173(3):721–30.
35. Linsley PS, Brady W, Urnes M, Grosmaire LS, Damle NK, Ledbetter JA. CTLA-4 is a second receptor for the B cell activation antigen B7. J Exp Med. 1991;174(3):561–9.
36. Linsley PS, Greene JL, Brady W, Bajorath J, Ledbetter JA, Peach R. Human B7-1 (CD80) and B7-2 (CD86) bind with similar avidities but distinct kinetics to CD28 and CTLA-4 receptors. Immunity. 1994;1(9):793–801.
37. Hu H, Rudd CE, Schneider H. Src kinases Fyn and Lck facilitate the accumulation of phosphorylated CTLA-4 and its association with PI-3 kinase in intracellular compartments of T-cells. Biochem Biophys Res Commun. 2001;288(3):573–8.
38. Berg M, Zavazava N. Regulation of CD28 expression on CD8+ T cells by CTLA-4. J Leukoc Biol. 2008;83(4):853–63.
39. O'Shea JJ, Paul WE. Mechanisms underlying lineage commitment and plasticity of helper CD4+ T cells. Science. 2010;327(5969):1098–102.
40. de Leval L, Parrens M, Le Bras F, et al. Angioimmunoblastic T-cell lymphoma is the most common T-cell lymphoma in two distinct French information data sets. Haematologica. 2015;100(9):e361–4.
41. Ellin F, Landstrom J, Jerkeman M, Relander T. Real-world data on prognostic factors and treatment in peripheral T-cell lymphomas: a study from the Swedish Lymphoma Registry. Blood. 2014;124(10):1570–7.
42. Petrich AM, Helenowski IB, Bryan LJ, Rozell SA, Galamaga R, Nabhan C. Factors predicting survival in peripheral T-cell lymphoma in the USA: a population-based analysis of 8802 patients in the modern era. Br J Haematol. 2015;168(5):708–18.
43. de Leval L, Savilo E, Longtine J, Ferry JA, Harris NL. Peripheral T-cell lymphoma with follicular involvement and a CD4+/bcl-6+ phenotype. Am J Surg Pathol. 2001;25(3):395–400.

44. Huang Y, Moreau A, Dupuis J, et al. Peripheral T-cell lymphomas with a follicular growth pattern are derived from follicular helper T cells (TFH) and may show overlapping features with angioimmunoblastic T-cell lymphomas. Am J Surg Pathol. 2009;33(5):682–90.
45. de Leval L, Rickman DS, Thielen C, et al. The gene expression profile of nodal peripheral T-cell lymphoma demonstrates a molecular link between angioimmunoblastic T-cell lymphoma (AITL) and follicular helper T (TFH) cells. Blood. 2007;109(11):4952–63.
46. Nicolae A, Pittaluga S, Venkataraman G, et al. Peripheral T-cell lymphomas of follicular T-helper cell derivation with Hodgkin/Reed-Sternberg cells of B-cell lineage: both EBV-positive and EBV-negative variants exist. Am J Surg Pathol. 2013;37(6): 816–26.
47. Bossard C, Dobay MP, Parrens M, et al. Immunohistochemistry as a valuable tool to assess CD30 expression in peripheral T-cell lymphomas: high correlation with mRNA levels. Blood. 2014;124(19):2983–6.
48. Gaulard P, de Leval L. Follicular helper T cells: implications in neoplastic hematopathology. Semin Diagn Pathol. 2011;28(3):202–13.
49. Gaulard P, de Leval L. The microenvironment in T-cell lymphomas: emerging themes. Semin Cancer Biol. 2014;24:49–60.
50. Piccaluga PP, Agostinelli C, Califano A, et al. Gene expression analysis of angioimmunoblastic lymphoma indicates derivation from T follicular helper cells and vascular endothelial growth factor deregulation. Cancer Res. 2007;67(22):10703–10.
51. Grogg KL, Attygalle AD, Macon WR, Remstein ED, Kurtin PJ, Dogan A. Angioimmunoblastic T-cell lymphoma: a neoplasm of germinal-center T-helper cells? Blood. 2005;106(4):1501–2.
52. Cairns RA, Iqbal J, Lemonnier F, et al. IDH2 mutations are frequent in angioimmunoblastic T-cell lymphoma. Blood. 2012;119(8):1901–3.
53. Johnston RJ, Poholek AC, DiToro D, et al. Bcl6 and Blimp-1 are reciprocal and antagonistic regulators of T follicular helper cell differentiation. Science. 2009;325(5943):1006–10.
54. Nurieva RI, Chung Y, Martinez GJ, et al. Bcl6 mediates the development of T follicular helper cells. Science. 2009;325(5943):1001–5.
55. Yu D, Rao S, Tsai LM, et al. The transcriptional repressor Bcl-6 directs T follicular helper cell lineage commitment. Immunity. 2009;31(3):457–68.
56. Nurieva RI, Chung Y, Hwang D, et al. Generation of T follicular helper cells is mediated by interleukin-21 but independent of T helper 1, 2, or 17 cell lineages. Immunity. 2008;29(1):138–49.
57. Fazilleau N, McHeyzer-Williams LJ, Rosen H, McHeyzer-Williams MG. The function of follicular helper T cells is regulated by the strength of T cell antigen receptor binding. Nat Immunol. 2009;10(4):375–84.
58. Yu H, Shahsafaei A, Dorfman DM. Germinal-center T-helper-cell markers PD-1 and CXCL13 are both expressed by neoplastic cells in angioimmunoblastic T-cell lymphoma. Am J Clin Pathol. 2009;131(1):33–41.
59. Sakata-Yanagimoto M, Enami T, Yoshida K, et al. Somatic RHOA mutation in angioimmunoblastic T cell lymphoma. Nat Genet. 2014;46(2):171–5.
60. Palomero T, Couronne L, Khiabanian H, et al. Recurrent mutations in epigenetic regulators, RHOA and FYN kinase in peripheral T cell lymphomas. Nat Genet. 2014;46(2):166–70.
61. Yoo HY, Sung MK, Lee SH, et al. A recurrent inactivating mutation in RHOA GTPase in angioimmunoblastic T cell lymphoma. Nat Genet. 2014;46(4):371–5.
62. Vallois D, Dobay MP, Morin RD, et al. Activating mutations in genes related to TCR signaling in angioimmunoblastic and other follicular helper T-cell-derived lymphomas. Blood. 2016;128(11):1490–502.
63. Kataoka K, Nagata Y, Kitanaka A, et al. Integrated molecular analysis of adult T cell leukemia/lymphoma. Nat Genet. 2015;47(11):1304–15.
64. Cleverley SC, Costello PS, Henning SW, Cantrell DA. Loss of Rho function in the thymus is accompanied by the development of thymic lymphoma. Oncogene. 2000;19(1):13–20.
65. Fujisawa M, Sakata-Yanagimoto M, Nishizawa S, et al. Activation of RHOA-VAV1 signaling in angioimmunoblastic T-cell lymphoma. Leukemia. 2018;32(3):694–702.
66. Lemonnier F, Couronne L, Parrens M, et al. Recurrent TET2 mutations in peripheral T-cell lymphomas correlate with TFH-like features and adverse clinical parameters. Blood. 2012;120(7):1466–9.
67. Couronne L, Bastard C, Bernard OA. TET2 and DNMT3A mutations in human T-cell lymphoma. N Engl J Med. 2012;366(1):95–6.
68. Odejide O, Weigert O, Lane AA, et al. A targeted mutational landscape of angioimmunoblastic T-cell lymphoma. Blood. 2014;123(9):1293–6.
69. Wang C, McKeithan TW, Gong Q, et al. IDH2R172 mutations define a unique subgroup of patients with angioimmunoblastic T-cell lymphoma. Blood. 2015;126(15):1741–52.
70. Quivoron C, Couronne L, Della Valle V, et al. TET2 inactivation results in pleiotropic hematopoietic abnormalities in mouse and is a recurrent event during human lymphomagenesis. Cancer Cell. 2011;20(1):25–38.
71. Schwartz FH, Cai Q, Fellmann E, et al. TET2 mutations in B cells of patients affected by angioimmunoblastic T-cell lymphoma. J Pathol. 2017;242(2):129–33.
72. Nguyen TB, Sakata-Yanagimoto M, Asabe Y, et al. Identification of cell-type-specific mutations in nodal T-cell lymphomas. Blood Cancer J. 2017;7(1):e516.

73. Zang S, Li J, Yang H, et al. Mutations in 5-methylcytosine oxidase TET2 and RhoA cooperatively disrupt T cell homeostasis. J Clin Invest. 2017;127(8):2998–3012.
74. Manso R, Sanchez-Beato M, Monsalvo S, et al. The RHOA G17V gene mutation occurs frequently in peripheral T-cell lymphoma and is associated with a characteristic molecular signature. Blood. 2014;123(18):2893–4.
75. Lee SH, Kim JS, Kim J, et al. A highly recurrent novel missense mutation in CD28 among angioimmunoblastic T-cell lymphoma patients. Haematologica. 2015;100(12):e505–7.
76. Rohr J, Guo S, Huo J, et al. Recurrent activating mutations of CD28 in peripheral T-cell lymphomas. Leukemia. 2016;30(5):1062–70.
77. Streubel B, Vinatzer U, Willheim M, Raderer M, Chott A. Novel t(5;9)(q33;q22) fuses ITK to SYK in unspecified peripheral T-cell lymphoma. Leukemia. 2006;20(2):313–8.
78. Attygalle AD, Feldman AL, Dogan A. ITK/SYK translocation in angioimmunoblastic T-cell lymphoma. Am J Surg Pathol. 2013;37(9):1456–7.
79. Pechloff K, Holch J, Ferch U, et al. The fusion kinase ITK-SYK mimics a T cell receptor signal and drives oncogenesis in conditional mouse models of peripheral T cell lymphoma. J Exp Med. 2010;207(5):1031–44.
80. Dierks C, Adrian F, Fisch P, et al. The ITK-SYK fusion oncogene induces a T-cell lymphoproliferative disease in mice mimicking human disease. Cancer Res. 2010;70(15):6193–204.
81. Yoo HY, Kim P, Kim WS, et al. Frequent CTLA4-CD28 gene fusion in diverse types of T-cell lymphoma. Haematologica. 2016;101(6):757–63.
82. Gong Q, Wang C, Rohr J, Feldman AL, Chan WC, McKeithan TW. Comment on: frequent CTLA4-CD28 gene fusion in diverse types of T-cell lymphoma, by Yoo et al. Haematologica. 2016;101(6):e269–70.
83. D Vallois AD, Lemonnier F, Fataccioli V, Ortonne N, Allen G, Tournilhac O, Delarue R, Rousselet-Chapeau M, Fabiani B, Llamas-Gutierrez F, Ko YH, Kataoka K, Gaulard P, de Leval L. Tanslocations involving CD28 are rare in peripheral T-cell lymphomas. Hematol Oncol. 2017;35(S2):164–5.
84. Boddicker RL, Razidlo GL, Dasari S, et al. Integrated mate-pair and RNA sequencing identifies novel, targetable gene fusions in peripheral T-cell lymphoma. Blood. 2016;128(9):1234–45.
85. Vose J, Armitage J, Weisenburger D, International T-Cell Lymphoma Project. International peripheral T-cell and natural killer/t-cell lymphoma study: pathology findings and clinical outcomes. J Clin Oncol. 2008;26(25):4124–30.
86. Stein H, Foss HD, Durkop H, et al. CD30(+) anaplastic large cell lymphoma: a review of its histopathologic, genetic, and clinical features. Blood. 2000;96(12):3681–95.
87. Vassallo J, Lamant L, Brugieres L, et al. ALK-positive anaplastic large cell lymphoma mimicking nodular sclerosis Hodgkin's lymphoma: report of 10 cases. Am J Surg Pathol. 2006;30(2):223–9.
88. Lamant L, de Reynies A, Duplantier MM, et al. Gene-expression profiling of systemic anaplastic large-cell lymphoma reveals differences based on ALK status and two distinct morphologic ALK+ subtypes. Blood. 2007;109(5):2156–64.
89. Lamant L, McCarthy K, d'Amore E, et al. Prognostic impact of morphologic and phenotypic features of childhood ALK-positive anaplastic large-cell lymphoma: results of the ALCL99 study. J Clin Oncol. 2011;29(35):4669–76.
90. Bonzheim I, Geissinger E, Roth S, et al. Anaplastic large cell lymphomas lack the expression of T-cell receptor molecules or molecules of proximal T-cell receptor signaling. Blood. 2004;104(10):3358–60.
91. Geissinger E, Sadler P, Roth S, et al. Disturbed expression of the T-cell receptor/CD3 complex and associated signaling molecules in CD30+ T-cell lymphoproliferations. Haematologica. 2010;95(10):1697–704.
92. Malcolm TI, Villarese P, Fairbairn CJ, et al. Anaplastic large cell lymphoma arises in thymocytes and requires transient TCR expression for thymic egress. Nat Commun. 2016;7:10087.
93. Piva R, Agnelli L, Pellegrino E, et al. Gene expression profiling uncovers molecular classifiers for the recognition of anaplastic large-cell lymphoma within peripheral T-cell neoplasms. J Clin Oncol. 2010;28(9):1583–90.
94. Agnelli L, Mereu E, Pellegrino E, et al. Identification of a 3-gene model as a powerful diagnostic tool for the recognition of ALK-negative anaplastic large-cell lymphoma. Blood. 2012;120(6):1274–81.
95. Matsuyama H, Suzuki HI, Nishimori H, et al. miR-135b mediates NPM-ALK-driven oncogenicity and renders IL-17-producing immunophenotype to anaplastic large cell lymphoma. Blood. 2011;118(26):6881–92.
96. de Leval L, Gaulard P. Tricky and terrible T-cell tumors: these are thrilling times for testing: molecular pathology of peripheral T-cell lymphomas. Hematology Am Soc Hematol Educ Program. 2011;2011:336–43.
97. Amin HM, Lai R. Pathobiology of ALK+ anaplastic large-cell lymphoma. Blood. 2007;110(7):2259–67.
98. Ambrogio C, Martinengo C, Voena C, et al. NPM-ALK oncogenic tyrosine kinase controls T-cell identity by transcriptional regulation and epigenetic silencing in lymphoma cells. Cancer Res. 2009;69(22):8611–9.
99. Piva R, Pellegrino E, Mattioli M, et al. Functional validation of the anaplastic lymphoma kinase signature identifies CEBPB and BCL2A1 as critical target genes. J Clin Invest. 2006;116(12):3171–82.

100. Richly H, Kim TM, Schuler M, et al. Ceritinib in patients with advanced anaplastic lymphoma kinase-rearranged anaplastic large-cell lymphoma. Blood. 2015;126(10):1257–8.
101. Chiarle R, Voena C, Ambrogio C, Piva R, Inghirami G. The anaplastic lymphoma kinase in the pathogenesis of cancer. Nat Rev Cancer. 2008;8(1):11–23.
102. Maes B, Vanhentenrijk V, Wlodarska I, et al. The NPM-ALK and the ATIC-ALK fusion genes can be detected in non-neoplastic cells. Am J Pathol. 2001;158(6):2185–93.
103. Liu C, Iqbal J, Teruya-Feldstein J, et al. MicroRNA expression profiling identifies molecular signatures associated with anaplastic large cell lymphoma. Blood. 2013;122(12):2083–92.
104. Spaccarotella E, Pellegrino E, Ferracin M, et al. STAT3-mediated activation of microRNA cluster 17~92 promotes proliferation and survival of ALK-positive anaplastic large cell lymphoma. Haematologica. 2014;99(1):116–24.
105. Lamant L, Pileri S, Sabattini E, Brugieres L, Jaffe ES, Delsol G. Cutaneous presentation of ALK-positive anaplastic large cell lymphoma following insect bites: evidence for an association in five cases. Haematologica. 2010;95(3):449–55.
106. Savage KJ, Harris NL, Vose JM, et al. ALK- anaplastic large-cell lymphoma is clinically and immunophenotypically different from both ALK+ALCL and peripheral T-cell lymphoma, not otherwise specified: report from the International Peripheral T-Cell Lymphoma Project. Blood. 2008;111(12):5496–504.
107. Sibon D, Fournier M, Briere J, et al. Long-term outcome of adults with systemic anaplastic large-cell lymphoma treated within the Groupe d'Etude des Lymphomes de l'Adulte trials. J Clin Oncol. 2012;30(32):3939–46.
108. Attygalle AD, Cabecadas J, Gaulard P, et al. Peripheral T-cell and NK-cell lymphomas and their mimics; taking a step forward—report on the lymphoma workshop of the XVIth meeting of the European Association for Haematopathology and the Society for Hematopathology. Histopathology. 2014;64(2):171–99.
109. Feldman AL, Law ME, Inwards DJ, Dogan A, McClure RF, Macon WR. PAX5-positive T-cell anaplastic large cell lymphomas associated with extra copies of the PAX5 gene locus. Mod Path. 2010;23(4):593–602.
110. Bisig B, de Reynies A, Bonnet C, et al. CD30-positive peripheral T-cell lymphomas share molecular and phenotypic features. Haematologica. 2013;98(8):1250–8.
111. Abate F, Todaro M, van der Krogt JA, et al. A novel patient-derived tumorgraft model with TRAF1-ALK anaplastic large-cell lymphoma translocation. Leukemia. 2015;29(6):1390–401.
112. Feldman AL, Dogan A, Smith DI, et al. Discovery of recurrent t(6;7)(p25.3;q32.3) translocations in ALK-negative anaplastic large cell lymphomas by massively parallel genomic sequencing. Blood. 2011;117(3):915–9.
113. Vasmatzis G, Johnson SH, Knudson RA, et al. Genome-wide analysis reveals recurrent structural abnormalities of TP63 and other p53-related genes in peripheral T-cell lymphomas. Blood. 2012;120(11):2280–9.
114. Pedersen MB, Hamilton-Dutoit SJ, Bendix K, et al. DUSP22 and TP63 rearrangements predict outcome of ALK-negative anaplastic large cell lymphoma: a Danish cohort study. Blood. 2017;130(4):554–7.
115. Parrilla Castellar ER, Jaffe ES, Said JW, et al. ALK-negative anaplastic large cell lymphoma is a genetically heterogeneous disease with widely disparate clinical outcomes. Blood. 2014;124(9):1473–80.
116. King RL, Dao LN, McPhail ED, et al. Morphologic features of ALK-negative anaplastic large cell lymphomas with DUSP22 rearrangements. Am J Surg Pathol. 2016;40(1):36–43.
117. Xing X, Flotte TJ, Law ME, et al. Expression of the chemokine receptor gene, CCR8, is associated with DUSP22 rearrangements in anaplastic large cell lymphoma. Appl Immunohistochem Mol Morphol. 2015;23(8):580–9.
118. Scarfo I, Pellegrino E, Mereu E, et al. Identification of a new subclass of ALK-negative ALCL expressing aberrant levels of ERBB4 transcripts. Blood. 2016;127(2):221–32.
119. Crescenzo R, Abate F, Lasorsa E, et al. Convergent mutations and kinase fusions lead to oncogenic STAT3 activation in anaplastic large cell lymphoma. Cancer Cell. 2015;27(4):516–32.
120. Boi M, Rinaldi A, Kwee I, et al. PRDM1/BLIMP1 is commonly inactivated in anaplastic large T-cell lymphoma. Blood. 2013;122(15):2683–93.
121. Wada DA, Law ME, Hsi ED, et al. Specificity of IRF4 translocations for primary cutaneous anaplastic large cell lymphoma: a multicenter study of 204 skin biopsies. Mod Path. 2011;24(4):596–605.
122. Onaindia A, Montes-Moreno S, Rodriguez-Pinilla SM, et al. Primary cutaneous anaplastic large cell lymphomas with 6p25.3 rearrangement exhibit particular histological features. Histopathology. 2015;66(6):846–55.
123. Velusamy T, Kiel MJ, Sahasrabuddhe AA, et al. A novel recurrent NPM1-TYK2 gene fusion in cutaneous CD30-positive lymphoproliferative disorders. Blood. 2014;124(25):3768–71.
124. Oschlies I, Lisfeld J, Lamant L, et al. ALK-positive anaplastic large cell lymphoma limited to the skin: clinical, histopathological and molecular analysis of 6 pediatric cases. A report from the ALCL99 study. Haematologica. 2013;98(1):50–6.
125. Brody GS, Deapen D, Taylor CR, et al. Anaplastic large cell lymphoma occurring in women with breast implants: analysis of 173 cases. Plast Reconstr Surg. 2015;135(3):695–705.
126. Clemens MW, Medeiros LJ, Butler CE, et al. Complete surgical excision is essential for the

management of patients with breast implant-associated anaplastic large-cell lymphoma. J Clin Oncol. 2016;34(2):160–8.
127. Laurent C, Delas A, Gaulard P, et al. Breast implant-associated anaplastic large cell lymphoma: two distinct clinicopathological variants with different outcomes. Ann Oncol. 2016;27(2):306–14.
128. Miranda RN, Aladily TN, Prince HM, et al. Breast implant-associated anaplastic large-cell lymphoma: long-term follow-up of 60 patients. J Clin Oncol. 2014;32(2):114–20.
129. Clemens MW, Horwitz SM. NCCN consensus guidelines for the diagnosis and management of breast implant-associated anaplastic large cell lymphoma. Aesthet Surg J. 2017;37(3):285–9.
130. Lechner MG, Megiel C, Church CH, et al. Survival signals and targets for therapy in breast implant-associated ALK—anaplastic large cell lymphoma. Clin Cancer Res. 2012;18(17):4549–59.
131. Di Napoli A, Jain P, Duranti E, et al. Targeted next generation sequencing of breast implant-associated anaplastic large cell lymphoma reveals mutations in JAK/STAT signalling pathway genes, TP53 and DNMT3A. Br J Haematol. 2018;180(5):741–4.
132. Oliveira PD, Kachimarek AC, Bittencourt AL. Early onset of HTLV-1 Associated Myelopathy/Tropical Spastic Paraparesis (HAM/TSP) and Adult T-Cell Leukemia/Lymphoma (ATL): systematic search and review. J Trop Pediatr. 2018;64(2):151–61.
133. Shimoyama M. Diagnostic criteria and classification of clinical subtypes of adult T-cell leukaemia-lymphoma. A report from the Lymphoma Study Group (1984-87). Br J Haematol. 1991;79(3): 428–37.
134. Karube K, Ohshima K, Tsuchiya T, et al. Expression of FoxP3, a key molecule in CD4CD25 regulatory T cells, in adult T-cell leukaemia/lymphoma cells. Br J Haematol. 2004;126(1):81–4.
135. Roncador G, Garcia JF, Garcia JF, et al. FOXP3, a selective marker for a subset of adult T-cell leukaemia/lymphoma. Leukemia. 2005;19(12):2247–53.
136. Kohno T, Yamada Y, Akamatsu N, et al. Possible origin of adult T-cell leukemia/lymphoma cells from human T lymphotropic virus type-1-infected regulatory T cells. Cancer Sci. 2005;96(8):527–33.
137. Nagai Y, Kawahara M, Hishizawa M, et al. T memory stem cells are the hierarchical apex of adult T-cell leukemia. Blood. 2015;125(23):3527–35.
138. Jeang KT, Giam CZ, Majone F, Aboud M. Life, death, and tax: role of HTLV-I oncoprotein in genetic instability and cellular transformation. J Biol Chem. 2004;279(31):31991–4.
139. Alizadeh AA, Bohen SP, Lossos C, et al. Expression profiles of adult T-cell leukemia-lymphoma and associations with clinical responses to zidovudine and interferon alpha. Leuk Lymphoma. 2010;51(7):1200–16.
140. Sasaki H, Nishikata I, Shiraga T, et al. Overexpression of a cell adhesion molecule, TSLC1, as a possible molecular marker for acute-type adult T-cell leukemia. Blood. 2005;105(3):1204–13.
141. Pise-Masison CA, Radonovich M, Dohoney K, et al. Gene expression profiling of ATL patients: compilation of disease related genes and evidence for TCF-4 involvement in BIRC5 gene expression and cell viability. Blood. 2009;113(17):4016–26.
142. Gaudray G, Gachon F, Basbous J, Biard-Piechaczyk M, Devaux C, Mesnard JM. The complementary strand of the human T-cell leukemia virus type 1 RNA genome encodes a bZIP transcription factor that down-regulates viral transcription. J Virol. 2002;76(24):12813–22.
143. Yamagishi M, Watanabe T. Molecular hallmarks of adult T cell leukemia. Front Microbiol. 2012;3:334.
144. Nakagawa M, Schmitz R, Xiao W, et al. Gain-of-function CCR4 mutations in adult T cell leukemia/lymphoma. J Exp Med. 2014;211(13):2497–505.
145. Yoshie O, Fujisawa R, Nakayama T, et al. Frequent expression of CCR4 in adult T-cell leukemia and human T-cell leukemia virus type 1-transformed T cells. Blood. 2002;99(5):1505–11.
146. Harasawa H, Yamada Y, Hieshima K, et al. Survey of chemokine receptor expression reveals frequent co-expression of skin-homing CCR4 and CCR10 in adult T-cell leukemia/lymphoma. Leuk Lymphoma. 2006;47(10):2163–73.
147. Ishida T, Joh T, Uike N, et al. Defucosylated anti-CCR4 monoclonal antibody (KW-0761) for relapsed adult T-cell leukemia-lymphoma: a multicenter phase II study. J Clin Oncol. 2012;30(8):837–42.
148. Iyama S, Sato T, Ohnishi H, et al. A multicenter retrospective study of mogamulizumab efficacy in adult T-cell leukemia/lymphoma. Clin Lymphoma Myeloma Leuk. 2017;17(1):23–30 e22.
149. Briski R, Feldman AL, Bailey NG, et al. The role of front-line anthracycline-containing chemotherapy regimens in peripheral T-cell lymphomas. Blood Cancer J. 2014;4:e214.
150. Li J, Lu E, Yi T, Cyster JG. EBI2 augments Tfh cell fate by promoting interaction with IL-2-quenching dendritic cells. Nature. 2016;533(7601):110–4.
151. Willemze R, Jaffe ES, Burg G, et al. WHO-EORTC classification for cutaneous lymphomas. Blood. 2005;105(10):3768–85.
152. Bradford PT, Devesa SS, Anderson WF, Toro JR. Cutaneous lymphoma incidence patterns in the United States: a population-based study of 3884 cases. Blood. 2009;113(21):5064–73.
153. Campbell JJ, Clark RA, Watanabe R, Kupper TS. Sezary syndrome and mycosis fungoides arise from distinct T-cell subsets: a biologic rationale for their distinct clinical behaviors. Blood. 2010;116(5):767–71.
154. Dulmage BO, Geskin LJ. Lessons learned from gene expression profiling of cutaneous T-cell lymphoma. Br J Dermatol. 2013;169(6):1188–97.
155. Michel L, Jean-Louis F, Begue E, Bensussan A, Bagot M. Use of PLS3, Twist, CD158k/KIR3DL2, and

NKp46 gene expression combination for reliable Sezary syndrome diagnosis. Blood. 2013;121(8):1477–8.
156. Lee CS, Ungewickell A, Bhaduri A, et al. Transcriptome sequencing in Sezary syndrome identifies Sezary cell and mycosis fungoides-associated lncRNAs and novel transcripts. Blood. 2012;120(16):3288–97.
157. Huang Y, Su MW, Jiang X, Zhou Y. Evidence of an oncogenic role of aberrant TOX activation in cutaneous T-cell lymphoma. Blood. 2015;125(9): 1435–43.
158. Dulmage BO, Akilov O, Vu JR, Falo LD, Geskin LJ. Dysregulation of the TOX-RUNX3 pathway in cutaneous T-cell lymphoma. Oncotarget. 2015.
159. Haider A, Steininger A, Ullmann R, et al. Inactivation of RUNX3/p46 promotes cutaneous T-cell lymphoma. J Invest Dermatol. 2016;136(11):2287–96.
160. Choi J, Goh G, Walradt T, et al. Genomic landscape of cutaneous T cell lymphoma. Nat Genet. 2015;47(9):1011–9.
161. da Silva Almeida AC, Abate F, Khiabanian H, et al. The mutational landscape of cutaneous T cell lymphoma and Sezary syndrome. Nat Genet. 2015;47(12):1465–70.
162. Kiel MJ, Sahasrabuddhe AA, Rolland DC, et al. Genomic analyses reveal recurrent mutations in epigenetic modifiers and the JAK-STAT pathway in Sezary syndrome. Nat Commun. 2015;6:8470.
163. Ichiyama K, Chen T, Wang X, et al. The methylcytosine dioxygenase Tet2 promotes DNA demethylation and activation of cytokine gene expression in T cells. Immunity. 2015;42(4):613–26.
164. Travert M, Huang Y, de Leval L, et al. Molecular features of hepatosplenic T-cell lymphoma unravels potential novel therapeutic targets. Blood. 2012;119(24):5795–806.
165. Belhadj K, Reyes F, Farcet JP, et al. Hepatosplenic gammadelta T-cell lymphoma is a rare clinicopathologic entity with poor outcome: report on a series of 21 patients. Blood. 2003;102(13):4261–9.
166. Yabe M, Medeiros LJ, Tang G, et al. Prognostic factors of hepatosplenic T-cell lymphoma: clinicopathologic study of 28 cases. Am J Surg Pathol. 2016;40(5):676–88.
167. Thai A, Prindiville T. Hepatosplenic T-cell lymphoma and inflammatory bowel disease. J Crohns Colitis. 2010;4(5):511–22.
168. Farcet JP, Gaulard P, Marolleau JP, et al. Hepatosplenic T-cell lymphoma: sinusal/sinusoidal localization of malignant cells expressing the T-cell receptor gamma delta. Blood. 1990;75(11):2213–9.
169. Alonsozana EL, Stamberg J, Kumar D, et al. Isochromosome 7q: the primary cytogenetic abnormality in hepatosplenic gammadelta T cell lymphoma. Leukemia. 1997;11(8):1367–72.
170. Macon WR, Levy NB, Kurtin PJ, et al. Hepatosplenic alphabeta T-cell lymphomas: a report of 14 cases and comparison with hepatosplenic gammadelta T-cell lymphomas. Am J Surg Pathol. 2001;25(3):285–96.
171. Wlodarska I, Martin-Garcia N, Achten R, et al. Fluorescence in situ hybridization study of chromosome 7 aberrations in hepatosplenic T-cell lymphoma: isochromosome 7q as a common abnormality accumulating in forms with features of cytologic progression. Genes Chromosomes Cancer. 2002;33(3):243–51.
172. Jonveaux P, Daniel MT, Martel V, Maarek O, Berger R. Isochromosome 7q and trisomy 8 are consistent primary, non-random chromosomal abnormalities associated with hepatosplenic T gamma/delta lymphoma. Leukemia. 1996;10(9):1453–5.
173. Feldman AL, Law M, Grogg KL, et al. Incidence of TCR and TCL1 gene translocations and isochromosome 7q in peripheral T-cell lymphomas using fluorescence in situ hybridization. Am J Clin Pathol. 2008;130(2):178–85.
174. McKinney M, Moffitt AB, Gaulard P, et al. The genetic basis of hepatosplenic T-cell lymphoma. Cancer Discov. 2017;7(4):369–79.
175. Miyazaki K, Yamaguchi M, Imai H, et al. Gene expression profiling of peripheral T-cell lymphoma including gammadelta T-cell lymphoma. Blood. 2009;113(5):1071–4.
176. Lee MY, Tsou MH, Tan TD, Lu MC. Clinicopathological analysis of T-cell lymphoma in Taiwan according to WHO classification: high incidence of enteropathy-type intestinal T-cell lymphoma. Eur J Haematol. 2005;75(3):221–6.
177. Verbeek WH, Van De Water JM, Al-Toma A, Oudejans JJ, Mulder CJ, Coupe VM. Incidence of enteropathy—associated T-cell lymphoma: a nation-wide study of a population-based registry in The Netherlands. Scand J Gastroenterol. 2008;43(11):1322–8.
178. Malamut G, Chandesris O, Verkarre V, et al. Enteropathy associated T cell lymphoma in celiac disease: a large retrospective study. Dig Liver Dis. 2013;45(5):377–84.
179. Isaacson P, Wright DH. Intestinal lymphoma associated with malabsorption. Lancet. 1978;1(8055):67–70.
180. Sabattini E, Pizzi M, Tabanelli V, et al. CD30 expression in peripheral T-cell lymphomas. Haematologica. 2013;98(8):e81–2.
181. Khalaf WF, Caldwell ME, Reddy N. Brentuximab in the treatment of CD30-positive enteropathy-associated T-cell lymphoma. J Natl Compr Cancer Netw. 2013;11(2):137–40; quiz 140.
182. van de Water JM, Cillessen SA, Visser OJ, Verbeek WH, Meijer CJ, Mulder CJ. Enteropathy associated T-cell lymphoma and its precursor lesions. Best Pract Res Clin Gastroenterol. 2010;24(1):43–56.
183. Malamut G, Afchain P, Verkarre V, et al. Presentation and long-term follow-up of refractory celiac disease: comparison of type I with type II. Gastroenterology. 2009;136(1):81–90.
184. Chott A, Haedicke W, Mosberger I, et al. Most CD56+ intestinal lymphomas are CD8+CD5-T-cell

lymphomas of monomorphic small to medium size histology. Am J Pathol. 1998;153(5):1483–90.
185. Chan JK, Chan AC, Cheuk W, et al. Type II enteropathy-associated T-cell lymphoma: a distinct aggressive lymphoma with frequent gammadelta T-cell receptor expression. Am J Surg Pathol. 2011;35(10):1557–69.
186. Tan SY, Chuang SS, Tang T, et al. Type II EATL (epitheliotropic intestinal T-cell lymphoma): a neoplasm of intra-epithelial T-cells with predominant CD8alphaalpha phenotype. Leukemia. 2013;27(8):1688–96.
187. Tan SY, Ooi AS, Ang MK, et al. Nuclear expression of MATK is a novel marker of type II enteropathy-associated T-cell lymphoma. Leukemia. 2011;25(3):555–7.
188. Akiyama T, Okino T, Konishi H, et al. CD8+, CD56+ (natural killer-like) T-cell lymphoma involving the small intestine with no evidence of enteropathy: clinicopathology and molecular study of five Japanese patients. Pathol Int. 2008;58(10):626–34.
189. Takeshita M, Nakamura S, Kikuma K, et al. Pathological and immunohistological findings and genetic aberrations of intestinal enteropathy-associated T cell lymphoma in Japan. Histopathology. 2011;58(3):395–407.
190. Deleeuw RJ, Zettl A, Klinker E, et al. Whole-genome analysis and HLA genotyping of enteropathy-type T-cell lymphoma reveals 2 distinct lymphoma subtypes. Gastroenterology. 2007;132(5):1902–11.
191. Tomita S, Kikuti YY, Carreras J, et al. Genomic and immunohistochemical profiles of enteropathy-associated T-cell lymphoma in Japan. Mod Pathol. 2015;28(10):1286–96.
192. Ko YH, Karnan S, Kim KM, et al. Enteropathy-associated T-cell lymphoma—a clinicopathologic and array comparative genomic hybridization study. Hum Pathol. 2010;41(9):1231–7.
193. Nicolae A, Xi L, Pham TH, et al. Mutations in the JAK/STAT and RAS signaling pathways are common in intestinal T-cell lymphomas. Leukemia. 2016;30(11):2245–7.
194. Moffitt AB, Ondrejka SL, McKinney M, et al. Enteropathy-associated T cell lymphoma subtypes are characterized by loss of function of SETD2. J Exp Med. 2017;214(5):1371–86.
195. Nairismagi ML, Tan J, Lim JQ, et al. JAK-STAT and G-protein-coupled receptor signaling pathways are frequently altered in epitheliotropic intestinal T-cell lymphoma. Leukemia. 2016;30(6):1311–9.
196. Roberti A, Dobay MP, Bisig B, et al. Type II enteropathy-associated T-cell lymphoma features a unique genomic profile with highly recurrent SETD2 alterations. Nat Commun. 2016;7:12602.
197. Kucuk C, Jiang B, Hu X, et al. Activating mutations of STAT5B and STAT3 in lymphomas derived from gammadelta-T or NK cells. Nat Commun. 2015;6:6025.
198. Kucuk C, Hu X, Jiang B, et al. Global promoter methylation analysis reveals novel candidate tumor suppressor genes in natural killer cell lymphoma. Clin Cancer Res. 2015;21(7):1699–711.
199. Perry AM, Warnke RA, Hu Q, et al. Indolent T-cell lymphoproliferative disease of the gastrointestinal tract. Blood. 2013;122(22):3599–606.
200. Carbonnel F, d'Almagne H, Lavergne A, et al. The clinicopathological features of extensive small intestinal CD4 T cell infiltration. Gut. 1999;45(5):662–7.
201. Margolskee E, Jobanputra V, Lewis SK, Alobeid B, Green PH, Bhagat G. Indolent small intestinal CD4+ T-cell lymphoma is a distinct entity with unique biologic and clinical features. PLoS One. 2013;8(7):e68343.
202. Malamut G, Meresse B, Kaltenbach S, et al. Small intestinal CD4+ T-cell lymphoma is a heterogenous entity with common pathology features. Clin Gastroenterol Hepatol. 2014;12(4):599–608 e591.
203. Leventaki V, Manning JT Jr, Luthra R, et al. Indolent peripheral T-cell lymphoma involving the gastrointestinal tract. Hum Pathol. 2014;45(2):421–6.
204. Au WY, Weisenburger DD, Intragumtornchai T, et al. Clinical differences between nasal and extranasal natural killer/T-cell lymphoma: a study of 136 cases from the International Peripheral T-Cell Lymphoma Project. Blood. 2009;113(17):3931–7.
205. Kwong YL. The diagnosis and management of extranodal NK/T-cell lymphoma, nasal-type and aggressive NK-cell leukemia. J Clin Exp Hematop. 2011;51(1):21–8.
206. Huang Y, de Leval L, Gaulard P. Molecular underpinning of extranodal NK/T-cell lymphoma. Best practice & research. Clin Haematol. 2013;26(1):57–74.
207. Kim WY, Jung HY, Nam SJ, et al. Expression of programmed cell death ligand 1 (PD-L1) in advanced stage EBV-associated extranodal NK/T cell lymphoma is associated with better prognosis. Virchows Arch. 2016;469(5):581–90.
208. Lai J, Xu P, Jiang X, Zhou S, Liu A. Successful treatment with anti-programmed-death-1 antibody in a relapsed natural killer/T-cell lymphoma patient with multi-line resistance: a case report. BMC Cancer. 2017;17(1):507.
209. Coppo P, Gouilleux-Gruart V, Huang Y, et al. STAT3 transcription factor is constitutively activated and is oncogenic in nasal-type NK/T-cell lymphoma. Leukemia. 2009;23(9):1667–78.
210. Huang Y, de Reynies A, de Leval L, et al. Gene expression profiling identifies emerging oncogenic pathways operating in extranodal NK/T-cell lymphoma, nasal type. Blood. 2010;115(6):1226–37.
211. Iqbal J, Kucuk C, Deleeuw RJ, et al. Genomic analyses reveal global functional alterations that promote tumor growth and novel tumor suppressor genes in natural killer-cell malignancies. Leukemia. 2009;23(6):1139–51.

212. Teruya-Feldstein J, Jaffe ES, Burd PR, et al. The role of Mig, the monokine induced by interferon-gamma, and IP-10, the interferon-gamma-inducible protein-10, in tissue necrosis and vascular damage associated with Epstein-Barr virus-positive lymphoproliferative disease. Blood. 1997;90(10):4099–105.
213. Koo GC, Tan SY, Tang T, et al. Janus kinase 3-activating mutations identified in natural killer/T-cell lymphoma. Cancer Discov. 2012;2(7):591–7.
214. Bouchekioua A, Scourzic L, de Wever O, et al. JAK3 deregulation by activating mutations confers invasive growth advantage in extranodal nasal-type natural killer cell lymphoma. Leukemia. 2014;28(2):338–48.
215. Kimura H, Karube K, Ito Y, et al. Rare occurrence of JAK3 mutations in NK cell neoplasms in Japan. Leuk Lymphoma. 2014;55(4):962–3.
216. Jiang L, Gu ZH, Yan ZX, et al. Exome sequencing identifies somatic mutations of DDX3X in natural killer/T-cell lymphoma. Nat Genet. 2015;47(9):1061–6. Epub ahead of print.
217. Dybkaer K, Iqbal J, Zhou G, et al. Genome wide transcriptional analysis of resting and IL2 activated human natural killer cells: gene expression signatures indicative of novel molecular signaling pathways. BMC Genomics. 2007;8:230.
218. Schmitz N, de Leval L. How I manage peripheral T-cell lymphoma, not otherwise specified and angioimmunoblastic T-cell lymphoma: current practice and a glimpse into the future. Br J Haematol. 2017;176(6):851–66.
219. Matnani RG, Stewart RL, Pulliam J, Jennings CD, Kesler M. Peripheral T-cell lymphoma with aberrant expression of CD19, CD20, and CD79a: case report and literature review. Case Rep Hematol. 2013;2013:183134.
220. Yao X, Teruya-Feldstein J, Raffeld M, Sorbara L, Jaffe ES. Peripheral T-cell lymphoma with aberrant expression of CD79a and CD20: a diagnostic pitfall. Mod Pathol. 2001;14(2):105–10.
221. Rahemtullah A, Longtine JA, Harris NL, et al. CD20+ T-cell lymphoma: clinicopathologic analysis of 9 cases and a review of the literature. Am J Surg Pathol. 2008;32(11):1593–607.
222. Dupuis J, Emile JF, Mounier N, et al. Prognostic significance of Epstein-Barr virus in nodal peripheral T-cell lymphoma, unspecified: a Groupe d'Etude des Lymphomes de l'Adulte (GELA) study. Blood. 2006;108(13):4163–9.
223. Yamashita Y, Nakamura S, Kagami Y, et al. Lennert's lymphoma: a variant of cytotoxic T-cell lymphoma? Am J Surg Pathol. 2000;24(12):1627–33.
224. Geissinger E, Odenwald T, Lee SS, et al. Nodal peripheral T-cell lymphomas and, in particular, their lymphoepithelioid (Lennert's) variant are often derived from CD8(+) cytotoxic T-cells. Virchows Arch. 2004;445(4):334–43.
225. Martinez-Delgado B. Peripheral T-cell lymphoma gene expression profiles. Hematol Oncol. 2006;24(3):113–9.
226. Cuadros M, Dave SS, Jaffe ES, et al. Identification of a proliferation signature related to survival in nodal peripheral T-cell lymphomas. J Clin Oncol. 2007;25(22):3321–9.
227. Martinez-Delgado B, Cuadros M, Honrado E, et al. Differential expression of NF-kappaB pathway genes among peripheral T-cell lymphomas. Leukemia. 2005;19(12):2254–63.
228. Ballester B, Ramuz O, Gisselbrecht C, et al. Gene expression profiling identifies molecular subgroups among nodal peripheral T-cell lymphomas. Oncogene. 2006;25(10):1560–70.
229. Wang T, et al. GATA-3 expression identifies a high-risk subset of PTCL, NOS with distinct molecular and clinical features. Blood. 2014;123(19):3007–15.
230. de Leval L, Bisig B, Thielen C, Boniver J, Gaulard P. Molecular classification of T-cell lymphomas. Crit Rev Oncol Hematol. 2009;72(2):125–43.
231. Nagel S, Leich E, Quentmeier H, et al. Amplification at 7q22 targets cyclin-dependent kinase 6 in T-cell lymphoma. Leukemia. 2008;22(2):387–92.
232. Fujiwara SI, Yamashita Y, Nakamura N, et al. High-resolution analysis of chromosome copy number alterations in angioimmunoblastic T-cell lymphoma and peripheral T-cell lymphoma, unspecified, with single nucleotide polymorphism-typing microarrays. Leukemia. 2008;22(10):1891–8.
233. Nelson M, Horsman DE, Weisenburger DD, et al. Cytogenetic abnormalities and clinical correlations in peripheral T-cell lymphoma. Br J Haematol. 2008;141(4):461–9.
234. Gesk S, Martin-Subero JI, Harder L, et al. Molecular cytogenetic detection of chromosomal breakpoints in T-cell receptor gene loci. Leukemia. 2003;17(4):738–45.
235. Almire C, Bertrand P, Ruminy P, et al. PVRL2 is translocated to the TRA@ locus in t(14;19)(q11;q13)-positive peripheral T-cell lymphomas. Genes Chromosomes Cancer. 2007;46(11):1011–8.
236. Martin-Subero JI, Wlodarska I, Bastard C, et al. Chromosomal rearrangements involving the BCL3 locus are recurrent in classical Hodgkin and peripheral T-cell lymphoma. Blood. 2006;108(1):401–2; author reply 402-403.
237. Feldman AL, Law M, Remstein ED, et al. Recurrent translocations involving the IRF4 oncogene locus in peripheral T-cell lymphomas. Leukemia. 2009;23(3):574–80.
238. Somja J, Bisig B, Bonnet C, Herens C, Siebert R, de Leval L. Peripheral T-cell lymphoma with t(6;14)(p25;q11.2) translocation presenting with massive splenomegaly. Virchows Arch. 2014;464(6):735–41.
239. Heavican TB, Yu J, Bouska A, Greiner TC, Lachel CM, Wang C, Dave BJ, Amador CC, Fu K, Vose JM, Weisenburger DD, Gascoyne RD, Hartmann S, Pedersen MB, Wilcox R, Teh BT, Lim ST, Ong

CK, Seto M, Berger F, Rosenwald A, Ott G, Campo E, Rimsza LM, Jaffe ES, Braziel RM, d'Amore FA, Inghirami G, Bertoni F, Staudt L, McKeithan TW, Pileri SA, Chan WC, Iqbal J. Molecular subgroups of peripheral T-cell lymphoma evolve by distinct genetic pathways. 58th ASH Annual Meeting and Exposition, San Diego, CA; 2106.

240. Schatz JH, Horwitz SM, Teruya-Feldstein J, et al. Targeted mutational profiling of peripheral T-cell lymphoma not otherwise specified highlights new mechanisms in a heterogeneous pathogenesis. Leukemia. 2015;29(1):237–41.

241. Abate F, da Silva-Almeida AC, Zairis S, et al. Activating mutations and translocations in the guanine exchange factor VAV1 in peripheral T-cell lymphomas. Proc Natl Acad Sci U S A. 2017;114(4):764–9.

242. Coiffier B, Federico M, Caballero D, et al. Therapeutic options in relapsed or refractory peripheral T-cell lymphoma. Cancer Treat Rev. 2014;40(9):1080–8.

Part II

Standard of Care of Aggressive Lymphomas

5 Standard of Care in First-Line Therapy of DLBCL

Greg Nowakowski, Fabian Frontzek, and Norbert Schmitz

5.1 Introduction

Diffuse large B-cell lymphoma (DLBCL) is the most common lymphoma entity accounting for about 40% of the global lymphoma burden [1]. Approximately 60% of patients are cured with frontline chemoimmunotherapy, with most relapses occurring within the first 2 years from diagnosis. While some of the patients with relapsed disease can be salvaged with aggressive chemotherapy and transplant approaches, the majority of patients who relapse after modern frontline therapy will succumb to the disease [2, 3]. Not surprisingly, a great effort has been undertaken to improve outcomes of frontline treatment and increase cure rates in newly diagnosed DLBCL. DLBCL is unique with respect to the number and the quality of studies providing level 1 evidence which treatment should be considered. In addition to unmet clinical needs, two factors resulted in successful development of randomized studies in DLBCL: it is a common lymphoma enabling fast accrual to prospective studies and it runs an aggressive clinical course allowing for relatively quick readout of study endpoints. However, it is now recognized that DLBCL is a molecularly diverse disease, with several distinct molecular subtypes showing different outcomes and responsiveness to therapy [4]. These molecular subtypes described in Chap. 2 will drive future developments of novel therapies in DLBCL. Nonetheless, the large diversity of the clinical presentation of DLBCL including increasing patient age, comorbidities, and performance status will remain important variables affecting therapy selection and outcomes.

5.2 Current Standard Therapy

The current chemotherapy backbone, the anthracycline-based CHOP (cyclophosphamide, doxorubicin, vincristine, prednisolone) regimen first described in 1976 [5] demonstrated its curative potential in a number of early studies. In the 1980s and 1990s of the last century, major efforts of clinical investigators focused on intensification of chemotherapy in order to increase cure rates. Disappointingly, intensification of cytotoxic therapy failed to improve treatment outcome in a pivotal randomized study [6]. Consequently, it became apparent that novel approaches rather than escalation of classical cytotoxic therapy were needed. Such a novel approach and major breakthrough were the

G. Nowakowski
Mayo Clinic, Rochester, MN, USA
e-mail: Nowakowski.Grzegorz@mayo.edu

F. Frontzek · N. Schmitz (✉)
Department of Medicine A, Hematology, Oncology, Hemostaseology and Pneumonology, University Hospital of Muenster, Muenster, Germany
e-mail: Fabian.Frontzek@ukmuenster.de; Norbert.Schmitz@ukmuenster.de; n.schmitz@asklepios.com

G. Lenz, G. Salles (eds.), *Aggressive Lymphomas*, Hematologic Malignancies,
https://doi.org/10.1007/978-3-030-00362-3_5

development of chemoimmunotherapy. The addition of rituximab, a monoclonal anti-CD20 antibody, to CHOP chemotherapy in the early 2000s represented the first major advance in DLBCL management since decades. A number of large, randomized pivotal trials demonstrated consistent benefit of adding rituximab to CHOP or CHOP-like chemotherapy with respect to progression-free and overall survival. Importantly, improvement in progression-free survival translated to a consistent overall survival benefit of approximately 15% in both younger and older populations [7–11]. Long-term outcome reports and population-based studies showed results concordant with the randomized studies, hence initiating the "rituximab era" in therapy of DLBCL. R-CHOP or R-CHOP-like chemotherapy became the standard treatment approach in DLBCL. Currently, the vast majority of novel combinations for up-front treatment of DLBCL incorporate new molecules into a backbone of chemoimmunotherapy rather than using these molecules alone or in more experimental combinations.

5.3 Prognostic Factors in Patients Treated with R-CHOP or R-CHOP-Like

While the development of rituximab-containing chemoimmunotherapy improved overall outcome, significant variation in survival persisted and resulted in the renewed interest in identification of clinical and molecular factors behind. The International Prognostic Index (IPI, comprised of age, LDH, stage, more than one extranodal site, and performance status) retains its prognostic significance in R-CHOP-treated patients [12] and is a useful tool in cross-trial evaluation of outcomes. Variations of the IPI, developed in the rituximab era, such as the revised IPI (R-IPI) and the National Comprehensive Cancer Network-IPI (NCCN-IPI) have been proposed and validated [13, 14]. The R-IPI reassessed clinical prognostic variables in a population-based cohort of DLBCL patients treated almost uniformly with rituximab. While the original components of the IPI remain prognostically significant, three groups, rather than the original five, emerged [13]. Importantly, patients with low R-IPI of 0 achieved long-term disease control and survival of over 90%. The NCCN-IPI, based on an analysis of 1650 adults with DLBCL and validated using a Canadian cohort of over 1100 patients, identified age, lactate dehydrogenase (LDH), sites of involvement, Ann Arbor stage, and ECOG performance status as the key prognostic variables [14]. When compared to the original IPI, the NCCN-IPI was better able to distinguish high-risk and low-risk subgroups. A direct comparison of IPI, R-IPI, and NCCN-IPI in a large and independent cohort of patients with DLBCL has not been reported. While the newer prognostic indices may have advantages, an important point in favor of staying with the original IPI is that comparison across different trials over time is possible without adjustments.

In addition to clinical risk factors, molecular differences in DLBCL have been used to define new prognostic subgroups. DLBCL is a heterogeneous disease consisting of several morphological, immunophenotypic, and molecular subtypes [1] with unique biology and differences in clinical outcome [15, 16]. These biological entities are discussed in more detail in Chap. 2. In terms of clinical outcomes, the relevant subgroups include:

- *The "germinal center (GC)," "activated B cell" (ABC or non-GC), and "unclassifiable" subtype of DLBCL originally identified by gene expression profiling (GEP).* The clinical significance of determining the cell of origin (COO) was evident in both CHOP- and R-CHOP-treated patient cohorts where information on molecular subtypes had been collected retrospectively: ABC-DLBCL had a substantially inferior outcome [17]. Data from prospective studies using NanoString technology [18] or the Hans classifier [19, 20] failed to confirm the prognostic impact of COO subtyping. It should also be pointed out that COO classification is not fully applicable to uncommon DLBCL variants like histiocyte-/T-cell-rich DLBCL or primary mediastinal DLBCL, since these tumors show different molecular signatures and were generally excluded from studies on the role of COO in DLBCL.

- *MYC, BCL2, and BCL6 deregulation. MYC* is rearranged in 6–16% of DLBCL cases and said to confer an adverse prognosis [21, 22]. It is widely accepted that the concurrent rearrangement of MYC and *BCL2* or *BCL6* genes (resulting in so-called double-hit or triple-hit lymphomas) substantially contributes to poor outcome. The new WHO classification defines lymphomas with concomitant *MYC* and *BCL2* (and/or *BCL6*) rearrangements as a new biologic entity termed "high-grade B-cell lymphoma with rearrangements of MYC and BCL2 and/or BCL6 " [23], comprising approximately 5% of DLBCL; HGBL with rearrangements of MYC and/or BCL2/BCL6 are associated with poor outcomes when treated with R-CHOP [24] and most other treatment regimens.
- *MYC and BCL2 protein expression.* Up to one-third of DLBCL patients have protein overexpression of both MYC and BCL2 ("dual protein"-expressing lymphomas, DEL) also reported to result in inferior outcomes [24–27].
- A number of other genetic and epigenetic lesions have been described and also may contribute to poor outcome in DLBCL [16, 28, 29].

The initial studies in DLBCL patients harboring dual *MYC* and *BCL2/BCL6* rearrangements demonstrated that double-hit or triple-hit lymphomas (DHL and THL) are rarely cured with R-CHOP. While subsequent reports showed better outcomes in prospectively identified patients, results with R-CHOP remain poor. A single-center review of 129 patients reported a 2-year disease-free survival of 33% following R-CHOP. More intensive regimens were variably effective, and consolidative ASCT (performed only in patients achieving complete remission) was not significantly beneficial [30]. Another retrospective analysis from various American centers similarly reported that R-CHOP was inferior to all intensive regimens with a hazard ratio of 0.53 and less than 20% long-term survival; again, ASCT consolidation was not beneficial [31]. Preliminary results of a phase II NCI study of DA-EPOCH-R in *MYC*-associated lymphomas are promising, with a PFS of 87% but, however, with very short follow-up [32]. To date, there are no prospective trials powered to study the effects of alternative, mostly more aggressive, therapies in DHL. Therefore, recommendations to use intensive, Burkitt lymphoma-like therapy especially in younger patients with good performance status document clinicians' despair rather than evidence-based medicine.

5.4 Improving on R-CHOP

Attempts to improve R-CHOP have taken several avenues , including the addition of other cytotoxic drugs (CHOEP, DA-EPOCH), testing alternative polychemotherapy with moderate increases of anthracycline and cyclophosphamide (R-ACVBP), adding new agents onto an R-CHOP backbone (XR-CHOP, where X is a new agent), testing dose-dense delivery of R-CHOP (R-CHOP-14) with growth factor support, or integrating alternative anti-CD20 antibodies. Only one trial to date has demonstrated a survival advantage. In patients with IPI 1, the R-ACVBP regimen had a 3-year OS of 92% versus 84% ($p = 0.007$) for R-CHOP, but widespread use is likely to be limited by the increased toxicity of ACVBP in older patients and limited global availability of vindesine. Etoposide added to CHOP either as a fixed dose of 100 mg/sqm i.v. (CHOEP) [33] or in a dose-escalating fashion guided by the leukocyte nadir of the previous treatment course as stipulated in the DA-EPOCH-R regimen had impressive activity in phase II settings, but has not randomly been tested against R-CHOP (R-CHOEP) or failed to improve outcomes in the US intergroup study (CALGB 50303) comparing DA-EPOCH-R to R-CHOP in unselected patients [34]. The DA-EPOCH-R was more toxic with more vincristine-associated neuropathy and neutropenic complications but no better than R-CHOP in terms of disease control and survival. The analysis of molecular and high IPI subtypes is ongoing but unlikely to show significant positive results considering the number of patients with high-risk features and the overall negative results.

Based on experimental findings and retrospective observations that lenalidomide and ibrutinib appear to have selective activity in relapsed ABC-DLBCL as compared to GC-DLBCL, prospective randomized trials designed to assess the activity of both molecules in treatment-naive DLBCL, enriched for ABC-DLBCL, when added to R-CHOP-21 have been performed. Results are not yet available. Lenalidomide has an overall response rate of 53% in relapsed/refractory ABC-DLBCL versus 9% in GC-DLBCL ($p = 0.006$), with COO designation via an IHC algorithm [35]. Addition of lenalidomide to R-CHOP in two phase II trials showed improved PFS compared to historical controls specifically for the ABC-DLBCL subtype [36, 37]. These results prompted a US intergroup randomized phase II trial, powered to have sufficient ABC-DLBCL patients on both arms, and a phase III trial sponsored by industry, both of which compare R-CHOP to R-CHOP plus lenalidomide (NCT01856192, NCT02285062).

Ibrutinib is a BTK inhibitor showing inhibition of DLBCL in vitro [38] and clinically as a single agent [39] also preferentially in ABC subtype. A small phase I/II study showed impressive results when ibrutinib was combined with R-CHOP [40]. Based on these findings, a worldwide study randomizing patients (with ABC-DLBCL defined by the Hans classifier) to R-CHOP or R-CHOP combined with ibrutinib has been completed, but no results are currently available (NCT01855750). A smaller phase II study testing the feasibility and toxicity of R-CHOEP plus ibrutinib is accruing patients (NCT03399513). Another large phase III trial compared the combination of the proteasome inhibitor bortezomib and R-CHOP with R-CHOP and showed no benefit to this approach in all DLBCL subtypes [20]. Despite encouraging preclinical data, there was also no evidence of benefit to the addition of bortezomib in ABC-DLBCL as defined by GEP [41].

Ofatumumab [42] and obinutuzumab [43] are alternative anti-CD20 antibodies with experimental characteristics different from rituximab. Unfortunately, in DLBCL, neither antibody showed superiority to rituximab when studied prospectively in phase III studies. While ofatumumab was tested against rituximab in the relapsed setting only [42], a large phase III study was performed comparing R-CHOP with O(binutuzumab)-CHOP in newly diagnosed patients with DLBCL [44]. No significant difference in any clinically relevant endpoint (EFS, OS) was observed between R-CHOP- and O-CHOP-treated patients. The German High-Grade Lymphoma Study Group (DSHNHL) performed a number of phase II studies investigating the role of different dosing and scheduling of rituximab in combination with CHOP [45–48]. Overall, only one of these studies showed a significantly better EFS and OS when compared to retrospective data from the RICOVER-60 trial [46]. The improvement demonstrated by administering rituximab on days −4, 0, 10, 29, 57, 99, 155, and 239 instead of day 1 of each chemotherapy cycle, however, was largely restricted to men aged 60–80 years with poor prognosis. No benefit was shown when 12 instead of 6 rituximab infusions were administered to young, high-risk patients [48] or when patients of all risk groups aged 18–80 years received an extra infusion of rituximab on day 8 of the first cycles of R-CHOP [49].

5.4.1 Radiotherapy as Part of First-Line Therapy in DLBCL

In contrast to most other study groups, all study protocols of the German High-Grade Lymphoma Study Group for first-line treatment of patients with aggressive B-cell lymphoma stipulated local radiotherapy (RT) for patients with bulky or extranodal disease who had achieved CR, CRu, or PR after chemotherapy. Of note, these studies did not use PET or PET/CT to define remission status. In patients mostly with advanced disease (stages III–IV, 60% of patients) or IPI 1–4 (IPI 2–4, 77%), a retrospective comparison of patients aged 60–80 years receiving or not receiving RT to bulky and extralymphatic disease suggested a survival benefit for patients with bulky disease treated with chemo- and radiotherapy [50]. Data from randomized studies addressing the role of RT in advanced stage DLBCL are not available. Likewise, the role of PET to spare RT in patients with early PET-negative remission has not been investigated in a randomized study so far. RT in patients with limited disease is discussed elsewhere in this article.

5.4.2 High-Dose Chemotherapy/Autologous Stem Cell Transplantation for Consolidation

Four prospective randomized studies addressed the question if high-dose therapy followed by autologous stem cell transplantation (HDT/AST) improves outcome of young, high-risk patients with aggressive B-cell lymphoma in the era of rituximab. Three of these studies did not find a survival benefit of HDT/SCT when compared to R-CHOP [51], R-(Mega)CHOP-14 [52], or R-CHOEP-14 [33]. The American study (Southwest Oncology Group trial 9704) compared eight courses of R-CHOP to six courses of R-CHOP followed by HDT/SCT [53]. No difference in OS was found between treatment arms. The authors, however, conclude that HDT/AST is beneficial for patients with high-risk disease because PFS and OS differed significantly from R-CHOP-treated patients. This interpretation has been questioned by the Fondazione Italiana Linfomi (FIL) and the DSHNHL because of statistical concerns [54]. Taken together, in the rituximab era, HDT/AST does not improve survival of younger patients with aaIPI 2 and 3. Accordingly, consolidation of CR and PR patients with HDT/AST has largely been abandoned.

5.4.3 Maintenance Therapy in DLBCL

An alternative approach to trying to improve on R-CHOP has been the introduction of maintenance therapy post R-CHOP particularly in high-risk patients. The PRELUDE trial, which randomized high-intermediate and high-risk DLBCL patients 2:1 to either oral enzastaurin or placebo, focused on patients with IPI 3–5 in complete response following R-CHOP induction [55]. There was no difference in disease-free survival; overall outcomes were better than expected in both groups with 70% long-term DFS and OS despite IPI 3–5 at baseline. The similarly designed PILLAR study showed no advantage to 1 year of everolimus maintenance vs. placebo [56]. In contrast, the use of lenalidomide maintenance (25 mg/day for 3 weeks followed by 1 week rest over 2 years) was associated with a PFS but no survival advantage [57]. Rituximab maintenance [58] also did not result in improvement of outcome. Interestingly, if only male patients were considered, they did significantly better with than without maintenance supporting earlier observations that particularly older male patients show faster clearance of rituximab than females [59]. In summary, as of 2018, CHOP or CHOP-like chemotherapy in combination with standard-dose rituximab without maintenance remains a standard therapy for DLBCL regardless of the molecular subtype.

5.5 Risk of CNS Relapse and Prophylaxis

Patients with CNS relapse have an extremely poor prognosis; in most cases, their life expectancy does not exceed a couple of months [60]. On the other hand, progression or relapse in the CNS is relatively rare in patients with DLBCL; a strategy administering prophylaxis of CNS disease to every patient with DLBCL therefore would be inadequate. Accordingly, clinical risk models have been developed in order to describe subgroups of DLBCL patients with high risk of CNS disease. Such patients were considered for prophylaxis usually consisting of intrathecal (IT) methotrexate (MTX) or combinations of MTX with cytosine arabinoside and prednisolone. Because risk models for patients treated with CHOP or R-CHOP differed substantially [60–62], we set out to develop the CNS International Prognostic Index (CNS-IPI) which was developed in patients treated on studies of the DSHNHL and validated in an independent cohort of patients from British Columbia [63]. The CNS-IPI comprises all individual IPI factors (age, LDH, ECOG performance status, stage, and extranodal involvement) and involvement of the kidneys and/or adrenal glands. The 2-year rates for development of CNS relapse are estimated at 0.6% for patients in the low-risk group, 3.4% for the intermediate-risk group, and 10.2% for the high-risk group. Meanwhile the CNS-IPI has been validated not only by the patient cohort from BC but also by other groups from Australia and Denmark [64]. Furthermore, an algorithm on how to use the CNS-IPI in order to diagnose and to initiate prophylaxis against CNS relapse has been developed [65]. Patients with high risk of CNS relapse should undergo imaging of the brain (preferentially by gadolinium-enhanced MR) and a lumbar puncture. If signs of CNS disease are found, patients should be switched to a state-of-the-art CNS protocol. Patients testing negative for CNS disease but with bone marrow, testicular, or kidney involvement should receive prophylaxis preferentially using systemic MTX before and after R-CHOP. Because some studies observed an increase of CNS disease in patients with double-/triple-hit lymphoma, also these patients may receive systemic MTX [66]. In contrast to most chemotherapeutic agents, small molecules such as lenalidomide and ibrutinib cross the blood-brain barrier and have been used to treat primary CNS lymphoma [67, 68]. It remains to be seen if patients treated on the randomized studies comparing R-CHOP with R-CHOP plus lenalidomide or ibrutinib, respectively, show reduced incidences of CNS involvement as compared to the patients treated with R-CHOP only. Patients with simultaneous lymph node and/or organ involvement as well as CNS disease have a particularly poor prognosis. Combining R-CHOP with systemic MTX, high-dose Ara-C, and other CNS-penetrating agents seems feasible, but success rates are moderate. Best results are reported from studies involving high-dose therapy with cytotoxic drugs crossing the blood-brain barrier and autologous stem cell transplantation [66, 67].

5.6 Therapy of Limited-Stage Disease

There is an ongoing debate whether patients with limited-stage DLBCL should receive full immunochemotherapy (six courses of R-CHOP identical to patients with more advanced disease) or show better results and/or less toxicity after administration of only three courses of R-CHOP followed by local radiotherapy. Problems in this group of patients begin with the definition of limited-stage disease. While S8736, the SWOG study setting the standard of care in the pre-rituximab era [69], enrolled patients with stage I and II disease including patients with bulky stage I (>10 cm in diameter) as well as patients with systemic symptoms, most recent studies excluded such patients. Furthermore, the definition of bulky disease varies from study to study with tumors from 5 to 10 cm in greatest diameter defined to represent bulky disease. In the rituximab era, a later phase II study by SWOG reported excellent PFS and OS after three courses of R-CHOP and local radiotherapy. However, the authors themselves state that both the previous (SWOG S8736) and the new study are characterized by a pattern of continuing late relapses dampening the enthusiasm for implementation of abbreviated (immuno)chemotherapy in limited-stage DLBCL [70]. A recently published French study [71] reported on 334 patients with stage I/II non-bulky DLBCL (bulk defined by tumor >7 cm in diameter) based on PET scan who received 4 courses of R-CHOP-14 followed by PET/CT. If the PET/CT after four cycles of R-CHOP showed a metabolic CR, patients were randomized to RT or observation. Five-year EFS and OS (96% vs. 92%) were not significantly different. The authors conclude that R-CHOP alone is not inferior to R-CHOP followed by RT in patients with non-bulky limited-stage DLBCL. The DSHNHL performed two studies in limited-stage DLBCL. The FLYER study randomized patients with IPI 0 and without bulky disease to four or six courses of CHOP in combination with six rituximab infusions. Results are not yet available, but warnings pointing to possible inferiority of four courses of R-CHOP did not appear. The UNFOLDER study randomized patients with IPI 0 and bulky disease and patients with IPI 1 to 6 x R-CHOP-21 or R-CHOP-14 with or without RT. The treatment arm without RT was closed prematurely, but the final analysis of the study is pending. Taken together, the evidence available today would recommend to administer 4–6 cycles of R-CHOP to patients with IPI 0 and IPI 1 with or without bulky disease. Probably, most patients can be spared RT, especially if PET negativity is documented after four cycles of R-CHOP.

5.7 Therapy of DLBCL in the Elderly

Clinical experience and results from prospective randomized trials demonstrate that six or eight cycles of standard R-CHOP can be difficult to administer without severe, sometimes life-threatening, side effects in patients beyond 65 years [72]. Several analyses show that especially patients beyond 75 years of age tolerate R-CHOP less well than younger patients with increased toxicities (infection, polyneuropathy, cardiac failure) leading to dose reductions, omission of cytotoxic agents, and administration of less cycles than planned and finally resulting in decreased survival. In order to avoid such problems, a number of strategies have been evaluated. Since anthracyclines significantly contribute to the morbidity and mortality of R-CHOP, reducing the dose of doxorubicin [73], substituting etoposide for doxorubicin [74], and combining bendamustine with rituximab are among the most popular strategies to avoid severe toxicities in the elderly. The French study by Peyrade et al. administered standard-dose rituximab, 400 mg/sqm of cyclophosphamide, 25 mg/sqm of doxorubicin, and 1 mg/sqm of vincristine, all on day 1, and 40 mg/sqm on days 1–5 to 150 patients with DLBCL over the age of 80 years. Two-year OS was 59%, and 2-year PFS was 47% [73]. A study from BCCA substituted etoposide for doxorubicin in patients with contraindications for doxorubicin [74]. Five-year OS after R-CEOP was 49% as compared to 64% in patients treated with R-CHOP. Bendamustine has been widely used in indolent lymphoma; studies in relapsed and refractory DLBCL suggest acceptable efficacy with moderate toxicity [75]. A phase II study combining rituximab with bendamustine as first-line therapy in patients beyond the age of 80 years or patients unfit to receive R-CHOP has been completed; results are not yet available. Probably, the optimal approach in order to judge the tolerability of standard therapy in old and frail patients would be applying a standardized geriatric/comorbidity score to each patient deemed unfit to receive R-CHOP. Furthermore, administration of pre-phase therapy (1 mg of vincristine and 5 days of prednisolone) and vigorous supportive care including the regular use of G-CSF especially in older patients and antibiotic and antiviral prophylaxis will help to avoid inferior results due to dose reductions, prolongation of the therapeutic interval, omission of effective drugs, or premature end of therapy. Of course, some patients will remain who cannot tolerate standard R-CHOP. In such patients, palliative care may at least partly alleviate pain and other symptoms caused by lymphomatous infiltrates for weeks or months.

5.8 Summary

In 2018, the standard of care for patients newly diagnosed with DLBCL consists of six courses of R-CHOP. In patients with IPI 0, four courses of R-CHOP may be enough. There is no definitive scientific evidence that other or higher doses of chemotherapy necessitating transplantation, the addition of radiotherapy, new molecules or antibodies, or consolidation with any therapeutic agent will improve outcome. ACVBP may improve outcome in DLBCL patients with IPI 1; the favorable results reported with DA-EPOCH-R and R-CHOEP-14 cause some investigators to continue using these regimens in high-risk patients. Large prospective, randomized trials investigating the addition of targeted therapies to R-CHOP have been completed; results, however, are not yet available. A plethora of new drugs has been developed and is under investigation in relapsed disease and to a lesser extent also as part of first-line therapy.

Results of prospective studies randomizing patients to R-CHOP vs. R-CHOP plus new agent are eagerly awaited especially for those patients where clinical and molecular risk factors herald poor prognosis with R-CHOP alone.

References

1. Swerdlow SH, Campo E, Harris NL, Jaffe ES. WHO classification of tumours of haematopoietic and lymphoid tissues. Revised 4th ed. Lyon: IARC Publications; 2017.
2. Glass B, Hasenkamp J, Wulf G, Dreger P, Pfreundschuh M, Gramatzki M, et al. Rituximab after lymphoma-directed conditioning and allogeneic stem-cell transplantation for relapsed and refractory aggressive non-Hodgkin lymphoma (DSHNHL R3): an open-label, randomised, phase 2 trial. Lancet Oncol. 2014;15(7):757–66.
3. Glass B, Dohm AJ, Truemper LH, Pfreundschuh M, Bleckmann A, Wulf GG, et al. Refractory or relapsed aggressive B-cell lymphoma failing (R)-CHOP: an analysis of patients treated on the RICOVER-60 trial. Ann Oncol. 2017;28(12):3058–64.
4. Swerdlow SH, Campo E, Pileri SA, Harris NL, Stein H, Siebert R, et al. The 2016 revision of the World Health Organization classification of lymphoid neoplasms. Blood. 2016;127(20):2375–90.
5. McKelvey EM, Gottlieb JA, Wilson HE, Haut A, Talley RW, Stephens R, et al. Hydroxyldaunomycin (Adriamycin) combination chemotherapy in malignant lymphoma. Cancer. 1976;38(4):1484–93.
6. Fisher RI, Gaynor ER, Dahlberg S, Oken MM, Grogan TM, Mize EM, et al. Comparison of a standard regimen (CHOP) with three intensive chemotherapy regimens for advanced non-Hodgkin's lymphoma. N Engl J Med. 1993;328(14):1002–6.
7. Sehn LH, Donaldson J, Chhanabhai M, Fitzgerald C, MacPherson N, O'Reilly SE, et al. Introduction of combined CHOP-rituximab therapy dramatically improved outcome of diffuse large B-cell lymphoma (DLBC) in British Columbia (BC). Blood. 2003;102(11):88a.
8. Coiffier B, Lepage E, Briere J, Herbrecht R, Tilly H, Bouabdallah R, et al. CHOP chemotherapy plus rituximab compared with CHOP alone in elderly patients with diffuse large-B-cell lymphoma. N Engl J Med. 2002;346(4):235–42.
9. Pfreundschuh M, Trumper L, Osterborg A, Pettengell R, Trneny M, Imrie K, et al. CHOP-like chemotherapy plus rituximab versus CHOP-like chemotherapy alone in young patients with good-prognosis diffuse large-B-cell lymphoma: a randomised controlled trial by the MabThera International Trial (MInT) Group. Lancet Oncol. 2006;7(5):379–91.
10. Pfreundschuh M, Kloess M, Zeynalava E, Lengfelder E, Franke A, Reiser M, et al. Six vs. eight cycles of bi-weekly CHOP-14 with or without rituximab for elderly patients with diffuse large B-cell lymphoma (DLBCL): results of the completed RICOVER-60 trial of the German high-grade non-Hodgkin lymphoma study group (DSHNHL). Blood. 2006;108:205 abstract.
11. Habermann TM, Weller EA, Morrison VA, Gascoyne RD, Cassileth PA, Cohn JB, et al. Rituximab-CHOP versus CHOP alone or with maintenance rituximab in older patients with diffuse large B-cell lymphoma. J Clin Oncol. 2006;24(19):3121–7.
12. Ziepert M, Hasenclever D, Kuhnt E, Glass B, Schmitz N, Pfreundschuh M, et al. Standard International prognostic index remains a valid predictor of outcome for patients with aggressive CD20+ B-cell lymphoma in the rituximab era. J Clin Oncol. 2010;28(14):2373–80.
13. Sehn LH, Berry B, Chhanabhai M, Fitzgerald C, Gill K, Hoskins P, et al. The revised International Prognostic Index (R-IPI) is a better predictor of outcome than the standard IPI for patients with diffuse large B-cell lymphoma treated with R-CHOP. Blood. 2007;109(5):1857–61.
14. Zhou Z, Sehn LH, Rademaker AW, Gordon LI, Lacasce AS, Crosby-Thompson A, et al. An enhanced International Prognostic Index (NCCN-IPI) for patients with diffuse large B-cell lymphoma treated in the rituximab era. Blood. 2014;123(6):837–42.
15. Sehn LH, Gascoyne RD. Diffuse large B-cell lymphoma: optimizing outcome in the context of clinical and biologic heterogeneity. Blood. 2015;125(1):22–32.
16. Pasqualucci L, Dalla-Favera R. The genetic landscape of diffuse large B-cell lymphoma. Semin Hematol. 2015;52(2):67–76.
17. Lenz G, Staudt LM. Aggressive lymphomas. N Engl J Med. 2010;362(15):1417–29.
18. Staiger AM, Ziepert M, Horn H, Scott DW, Barth TFE, Bernd HW, et al. Clinical impact of the cell-of-origin classification and the MYC/BCL2 dual expresser status in diffuse large B-cell lymphoma treated within prospective clinical trials of the German high-grade non-Hodgkin's lymphoma study group. J Clin Oncol. 2017;35(22):2515–26.
19. Cunningham D, Hawkes EA, Jack A, Qian W, Smith P, Mouncey P, et al. Rituximab plus cyclophosphamide, doxorubicin, vincristine, and prednisolone in patients with newly diagnosed diffuse large B-cell non-Hodgkin lymphoma: a phase 3 comparison of dose intensification with 14-day versus 21-day cycles. Lancet. 2013;381(9880):1817–26.
20. Davies AJ, Caddy J, Maishman T, Barrans S, Mamot C, Care M, et al. A prospective randomised trial of targeted therapy for diffuse large B-cell lymphoma (DLBCL) based upon real-time gene expression profiling: the Remodl-B Study of the UK NCRI and SAKK Lymphoma Groups (ISRCTN51837425). Blood. 2015;126(23):812.
21. Dave SS, Fu K, Wright GW, Lam LT, Kluin P, Boerma EJ, et al. Molecular diagnosis of Burkitt's lymphoma. N Engl J Med. 2006;354(23):2431–42.

22. Barrans S, Crouch S, Smith A, Turner K, Owen R, Patmore R, et al. Rearrangement of MYC is associated with poor prognosis in patients with diffuse large B-cell lymphoma treated in the era of rituximab. J Clin Oncol. 2010;28(20):3360–5.
23. Swerdlow S, Campo E, Harris N, Jaffe ES, Pileri A, Stein H, et al. WHO classification of tumours of haematopoietic and lymphoid tissues. 4th ed. Lyon: IARC; 2008.
24. Hu S, Xu-Monette ZY, Tzankov A, Green T, Wu L, Balasubramanyam A, et al. MYC/BCL2 protein coexpression contributes to the inferior survival of activated B-cell subtype of diffuse large B-cell lymphoma and demonstrates high-risk gene expression signatures: a report from The International DLBCL Rituximab-CHOP Consortium Program. Blood. 2013;121(20):4021–31; quiz 250
25. Perry AM, Alvarado-Bernal Y, Laurini JA, Smith LM, Slack GW, Tan KL, et al. MYC and BCL2 protein expression predicts survival in patients with diffuse large B-cell lymphoma treated with rituximab. Br J Haematol. 2014;165(3):382–91.
26. Johnson NA, Slack GW, Savage KJ, Connors JM, Ben-Neriah S, Rogic S, et al. Concurrent expression of MYC and BCL2 in diffuse large B-cell lymphoma treated with rituximab plus cyclophosphamide, doxorubicin, vincristine, and prednisone. J Clin Oncol. 2012;30(28):3452–9.
27. Green TM, Young KH, Visco C, Xu-Monette ZY, Orazi A, Go RS, et al. Immunohistochemical double-hit score is a strong predictor of outcome in patients with diffuse large B-cell lymphoma treated with rituximab plus cyclophosphamide, doxorubicin, vincristine, and prednisone. J Clin Oncol. 2012;30(28):3460–7.
28. Young RM, Shaffer AL 3rd, Phelan JD, Staudt LM. B-cell receptor signaling in diffuse large B-cell lymphoma. Semin Hematol. 2015;52(2):77–85.
29. Jiang Y, Melnick A. The epigenetic basis of diffuse large B-cell lymphoma. Semin Hematol. 2015;52(2):86–96.
30. Puvvada SD, Stiff PJ, Leblanc M, Cook JR, Couban S, Leonard JP, et al. Outcomes of MYC-associated lymphomas after R-CHOP with and without consolidative autologous stem cell transplant: subset analysis of randomized trial intergroup SWOG S9704. Br J Haematol. 2016;174(5):686–91.
31. Petrich AM, Gandhi M, Jovanovic B, Castillo JJ, Rajguru S, Yang DT, et al. Impact of induction regimen and stem cell transplantation on outcomes in double-hit lymphoma: a multicenter retrospective analysis. Blood. 2014;124(15):2354–61.
32. Dunleavy K, Fanale M, LaCasce A, Noy A, Caimi P, Parekh S, et al. Preliminary report of a multicenter prospective phase II study of DA-EPOCH-R in MYC-rearranged aggressive B-cell lymphoma. Blood. 2014;124:abstract 395.
33. Schmitz N, Nickelsen M, Ziepert M, Haenel M, Borchmann P, Schmidt C, et al. Conventional chemotherapy (CHOEP-14) with rituximab or high-dose chemotherapy (MegaCHOEP) with rituximab for young, high-risk patients with aggressive B-cell lymphoma: an open-label, randomised, phase 3 trial (DSHNHL 2002-1). Lancet Oncol. 2012;13(12):1250–9.
34. Wilson WH, Sin-Ho J, Pitcher BN, Hsi ED, Friedberg J, Cheson B, et al. Phase III randomized study of R-CHOP versus DA-EPOCH-R and molecular analysis of untreated diffuse large B-cell lymphoma: CALGB/Alliance 50303. Blood. 2016;128(22):469.
35. Hernandez-Ilizaliturri FJ, Deeb G, Zinzani PL, Pileri SA, Malik F, Macon WR, et al. Higher response to lenalidomide in relapsed/refractory diffuse large B-cell lymphoma in nongerminal center B-cell-like than in germinal center B-cell-like phenotype. Cancer. 2011;117(22):5058–66.
36. Nowakowski GS, LaPlant B, Macon WR, Reeder CB, Foran JM, Nelson GD, et al. Lenalidomide combined with R-CHOP overcomes negative prognostic impact of non-germinal center B-cell phenotype in newly diagnosed diffuse large B-cell lymphoma: a phase II study. J Clin Oncol. 2015;33(3):251–7.
37. Vitolo U, Chiappella A, Franceschetti S, Carella AM, Baldi I, Inghirami G, et al. Lenalidomide plus R-CHOP21 in elderly patients with untreated diffuse large B-cell lymphoma: results of the REAL07 open-label, multicentre, phase 2 trial. Lancet Oncol. 2014;15(7):730–7.
38. Yang Y, Shaffer AL 3rd, Emre NC, Ceribelli M, Zhang M, Wright G, et al. Exploiting synthetic lethality for the therapy of ABC diffuse large B cell lymphoma. Cancer Cell. 2012;21(6):723–37.
39. Wilson WH, Young RM, Schmitz R, Yang Y, Pittaluga S, Wright G, et al. Targeting B cell receptor signaling with ibrutinib in diffuse large B cell lymphoma. Nat Med. 2015;21(8):922–6.
40. Younes A, Thieblemont C, Morschhauser F, Flinn I, Friedberg JW, Amorim S, et al. Combination of ibrutinib with rituximab, cyclophosphamide, doxorubicin, vincristine, and prednisone (R-CHOP) for treatment-naive patients with CD20-positive B-cell non-Hodgkin lymphoma: a non-randomised, phase 1b study. Lancet Oncol. 2014;15(9):1019–26.
41. Leonard JP, Kolibaba KS, Reeves JA, Tulpule A, Flinn IW, Kolevska T, et al. Randomized phase II study of R-CHOP with or without bortezomib in previously untreated patients with non-germinal center B-cell-like diffuse large B-cell lymphoma. J Clin Oncol. 2017;35(31):3538–46.
42. van Imhoff GW, McMillan A, Matasar MJ, Radford J, Ardeshna KM, Kuliczkowski K, et al. Ofatumumab versus rituximab salvage chemoimmunotherapy in relapsed or refractory diffuse large B-cell lymphoma: The ORCHARRD Study. J Clin Oncol. 2017;35(5):544–51.
43. Mossner E, Brunker P, Moser S, Puntener U, Schmidt C, Herter S, et al. Increasing the efficacy of CD20 antibody therapy through the engineering of a new type II anti-CD20 antibody with enhanced direct and immune effector cell-mediated B-cell cytotoxicity. Blood. 2010;115(22):4393–402.
44. Vitolo U, Trneny M, Belada D, Burke JM, Carella AM, Chua N, et al. Obinutuzumab or rituximab plus cyclophosphamide, doxorubicin, vincristine, and

prednisone in previously untreated diffuse large B-cell lymphoma. J Clin Oncol. 2017;35(31):3529–37.
45. Murawski N, Pfreundschuh M, Zeynalova S, Poeschel V, Hanel M, Held G, et al. Optimization of rituximab for the treatment of DLBCL (I): dose-dense rituximab in the DENSE-R-CHOP-14 trial of the DSHNHL. Ann Oncol. 2014;25(9):1800–6.
46. Pfreundschuh M, Poeschel V, Zeynalova S, Hanel M, Held G, Schmitz N, et al. Optimization of rituximab for the treatment of diffuse large B-cell lymphoma (II): extended rituximab exposure time in the SMARTE-R-CHOP-14 trial of the German high-grade non-Hodgkin lymphoma study group. J Clin Oncol. 2014;32(36):4127–33.
47. Pfreundschuh M, Murawski N, Zeynalova S, Ziepert M, Loeffler M, Hanel M, et al. Optimization of rituximab for the treatment of DLBCL: increasing the dose for elderly male patients. Br J Haematol. 2017;179(3):410–20.
48. Schmitz N, Nickelsen M, Ziepert M, Haenel M, Viardot A, Dreyling MH, et al. Optimization of rituximab for treatment of DLBCL in young, high-risk patients-results of the dense-R-CHOEP trial of the German high-grade lymphoma study group. Blood. 2015;126(23):474.
49. Lugtenburg PJ, Brown PDN, van der Holt B, D'Amore F, Koene HR, Berenschot HW, et al. Randomized phase III study on the effect of early intensification of rituximab in combination with 2-weekly CHOP chemotherapy followed by rituximab or no maintenance in patients with diffuse large B-cell lymphoma: results from a HOVON-Nordic Lymphoma Group study. J Clin Oncol. 2016;34(15):7504.
50. Held G, Murawski N, Ziepert M, Fleckenstein J, Poschel V, Zwick C, et al. Role of radiotherapy to bulky disease in elderly patients with aggressive B-cell lymphoma. J Clin Oncol. 2014;32(11):1112–8.
51. Le Gouill S, Milpied NJ, Lamy T, Delwail V, Gressin R, Guyotat D, et al. First-line rituximab (R) high-dose therapy (R-HDT) versus R-CHOP14 for young adults with diffuse large B-cell lymphoma: preliminary results of the GOELAMS 075 prospective multicenter randomized trial. J Clin Oncol. 2011;29(15):8003.
52. Chiappella A, Martelli M, Angelucci E, Brusamolino E, Evangelista A, Carella AM, et al. Rituximab-dose-dense chemotherapy with or without high-dose chemotherapy plus autologous stem-cell transplantation in high-risk diffuse large B-cell lymphoma (DLCL04): final results of a multicentre, open-label, randomised, controlled, phase 3 study. Lancet Oncol. 2017;18(8):1076–88.
53. Stiff PJ, Unger JM, Cook JR, Constine LS, Couban S, Stewart DA, et al. Autologous transplantation as consolidation for aggressive non-Hodgkin's lymphoma. N Engl J Med. 2013;369(18):1681–90.
54. Schmitz N, Ziepert M, Vitolo U, German High-Grade Non-Hodgkin's Lymphoma Study Group, Fondazione Italiana Linfomi. The role of myeloablation for lymphoma. N Engl J Med. 2014;370(6):574–5.
55. Crump M, Leppa S, Fayad L, Lee JJ, Di Rocco A, Ogura M, et al. Randomized, double-blind, phase III trial of enzastaurin versus placebo in patients achieving remission after first-line therapy for high-risk diffuse large B-cell lymphoma. J Clin Oncol. 2016;34(21):2484–92.
56. Witzig TE, Tobinai K, Rigacci L, Ikeda T, Vanazzi A, Hino M, et al. Adjuvant everolimus in high-risk diffuse large B-cell lymphoma: final results from the PILLAR-2 randomized phase III trial. Ann Oncol. 2018;29(3):707–14.
57. Thieblemont C, Tilly H, Gomes da Silva M, Casasnovas RO, Fruchart C, Morschhauser F, et al. Lenalidomide maintenance compared with placebo in responding elderly patients with diffuse large B-cell lymphoma treated with first-line rituximab plus cyclophosphamide, doxorubicin, vincristine, and prednisone. J Clin Oncol. 2017;35(22):2473–81.
58. Jaeger U, Trneny M, Melzer H, Praxmarer M, Nawarawong W, Ben Yehuda D, et al. Rituximab maintenance for patients with aggressive B-cell lymphoma in first remission: results of the randomized NHL13 trial. Haematologica. 2015;100(7):955–63.
59. Muller C, Murawski N, Wiesen MH, Held G, Poeschel V, Zeynalova S, et al. The role of sex and weight on rituximab clearance and serum elimination half-life in elderly patients with DLBCL. Blood. 2012;119(14):3276–84.
60. Boehme V, Schmitz N, Zeynalova S, Loeffler M, Pfreundschuh M. CNS events in elderly patients with aggressive lymphoma treated with modern chemotherapy (CHOP-14) with or without rituximab: an analysis of patients treated in the RICOVER-60 trial of the German High-Grade Non-Hodgkin Lymphoma Study Group (DSHNHL). Blood. 2009;113(17):3896–902.
61. Hollender A, Kvaloy S, Nome O, Skovlund E, Lote K, Holte H. Central nervous system involvement following diagnosis of non-Hodgkin's lymphoma: a risk model. Ann Oncol. 2002;13(7):1099–107.
62. Villa D, Connors JM, Shenkier TN, Gascoyne RD, Sehn LH, Savage KJ. Incidence and risk factors for central nervous system relapse in patients with diffuse large B-cell lymphoma: the impact of the addition of rituximab to CHOP chemotherapy. Ann Oncol. 2010;21(5):1046–52.
63. Schmitz N, Zeynalova S, Nickelsen M, Kansara R, Villa D, Sehn LH, et al. CNS International Prognostic Index: a risk model for CNS relapse in patients with diffuse large B-cell lymphoma treated with R-CHOP. J Clin Oncol. 2016;34(26):3150–6.
64. El-Galaly TC, Villa D, Michaelsen TY, Hutchings M, Mikhaeel NG, Savage KJ, et al. The number of extranodal sites assessed by PET/CT scan is a powerful predictor of CNS relapse for patients with diffuse large B-cell lymphoma: an international multicenter study of 1532 patients treated with chemoimmunotherapy. Eur J Cancer. 2017;75:195–203.
65. Schmitz N, Nickelsen M, Savage KJ. Central nervous system prophylaxis for aggressive B-cell lymphoma who, what, and when? Hematol Oncol Clin N. 2016;30(6):1277–91.

66. Savage KJ, Slack GW, Mottok A, Sehn LH, Villa D, Kansara R, et al. Impact of dual expression of MYC and BCL2 by immunohistochemistry on the risk of CNS relapse in DLBCL. Blood. 2016;127(18):2182–8.
67. Lionakis MS, Dunleavy K, Roschewski M, Widemann BC, Butman JA, Schmitz R, et al. Inhibition of B cell receptor signaling by ibrutinib in primary CNS lymphoma. Cancer Cell. 2017;31(6):833–43 e5.
68. Houillier C, Choquet S, Touitou V, Martin-Duverneuil N, Navarro S, Mokhtari K, et al. Lenalidomide monotherapy as salvage treatment for recurrent primary CNS lymphoma. Neurology. 2015;84(3):325–6.
69. Miller TP, Dahlberg S, Cassady JR, Adelstein DJ, Spier CM, Grogan TM, et al. Chemotherapy alone compared with chemotherapy plus radiotherapy for localized intermediate- and high-grade non-Hodgkin's lymphoma. N Engl J Med. 1998;339(1):21–6.
70. Persky DO, Unger JM, Spier CM, Stea B, LeBlanc M, McCarty MJ, et al. Phase II study of rituximab plus three cycles of CHOP and involved-field radiotherapy for patients with limited-stage aggressive B-cell lymphoma: Southwest Oncology Group study 0014. J Clin Oncol. 2008;26(14):2258–63.
71. Lamy T, Damaj G, Soubeyran P, Gyan E, Cartron G, Bouabdallah K, et al. R-CHOP 14 with or without radiotherapy in nonbulky limited-stage diffuse large B-cell lymphoma. Blood. 2018;131(2):174–81.
72. Zettl F, Ziepert M, Altmann B, Zeynalova S, Loeffler M, Schmitz N, et al. Age-dependent analysis of toxicity, mortality, and implementation of an anti-infective prophylaxis in 1171 elderly patients (pts) with aggressive B-cell lymphoma (aNHL): data from consecutive phase II and III trials of the DSHNHL. J Clin Oncol. 2016;34(15):7539.
73. Peyrade F, Jardin F, Thieblemont C, Thyss A, Emile JF, Castaigne S, et al. Attenuated immunochemotherapy regimen (R-miniCHOP) in elderly patients older than 80 years with diffuse large B-cell lymphoma: a multicentre, single-arm, phase 2 trial. Lancet Oncol. 2011;12(5):460–8.
74. Moccia AA, Schaff K, Hoskins P, Klasa R, Savage KJ, Shenkier T, et al. R-CHOP with etoposide substituted for doxorubicin (R-CEOP): excellent outcome in diffuse large B cell lymphoma for patients with a contraindication to anthracyclines. Blood. 2009;114(22):170.
75. Vacirca JL, Acs PI, Tabbara IA, Rosen PJ, Lee P, Lynam E. Bendamustine combined with rituximab for patients with relapsed or refractory diffuse large B cell lymphoma. Ann Hematol. 2014;93(3):403–9.

6 Standard of Care Relapsed DLBCL

Kayane Mheidly, Roch Houot, Michael Scordo, and Craig Moskowitz

6.1 Introduction

At least 50% of patients with diffuse large B-cell lymphoma (DLBCL) experience long-term disease-free survival [1, 2]. Although the addition of anti-CD20 monoclonal antibody rituximab (R) to conventional chemotherapy has dramatically improved event-free survival (EFS) and overall survival (OS) in DLBCL [3], a significant proportion of patients are refractory or relapse following first-line treatment.

Patients with DLBCL are considered primary refractory if they have no response or if they experience on or within 3 months of completion of primary therapy [4]. The incidence of primary refractory DLBCL is between 5 and 10%. Patients with DLBCL are considered to have relapsed disease if lymphoma recurs beyond 3 months after achieving an initial objective response. Most relapses occur during the first 2–3 years following treatment, with less than 4% of relapses occurring after 5 years [5].

Relapses are rarely identified solely based on routine imaging. Most of the relapses are associated with B symptoms (i.e., fever, night sweats, and/or weight loss) and other symptoms such as cytopenias, lymphadenopathy, splenomegaly, hepatomegaly, and/or extranodal tumors [6]. Whenever possible, a biopsy should be performed to confirm the relapse before proceeding to salvage therapy, particularly for late relapses, or when intensive consolidation is planned.

The outcome of relapsed DLBCL depends on several factors. The secondary age-adjusted International Prognostic Index at the initiation of second-line therapy (sAAIPI) comprises three of the IPI risk factors: LDH, Ann Arbor stage, and Karnofsky performance status. The sAAIPI predicts outcome for patients with relapsed or primary refractory DLBCL and is a powerful prognostic instrument to predict response to salvage chemotherapy [7]. Time to relapse (within the first 12 months following first-line treatment) is also an independent prognostic factor for progression-free survival (PFS) and OS [3, 4, 8, 9].

K. Mheidly
Department of Clinical Hematology, Rennes University Hospital, University of Rennes, CHU de Rennes Pontchaillou, Rennes, France

R. Houot (✉)
Department of Clinical Hematology, Rennes University Hospital, Inserm 1236, University of Rennes, CHU de Rennes Pontchaillou, Rennes, France
e-mail: roch.houot@chu-rennes.fr

M. Scordo
Adult Bone Marrow Transplant Service, Department of Medicine, Memorial Sloan Kettering Cancer Center, New York, NY, USA
e-mail: scordom@mskcc.org

C. Moskowitz
Memorial Sloan Kettering Cancer Center, Weill Medical College of Cornell University, New York, NY, USA
e-mail: moskowic@mskcc.org

G. Lenz, G. Salles (eds.), *Aggressive Lymphomas*, Hematologic Malignancies,
https://doi.org/10.1007/978-3-030-00362-3_6

Patients with chemorefractory DLBCL, defined as progressive or stable disease after therapy or relapse less than 12 months from ASCT, have poor outcome with a median OS of 6.6 months [10].

6.2 Second-Line Treatment

6.2.1 Induction/Salvage Therapy

Two randomized trials evaluated the efficacy of different salvage regimens in patients with relapsed DLBCL and eligible to ASCT (Table 6.1).

The CORAL study, a phase III, multicenter, randomized trial, compared R-ICE (rituximab, ifosfamide, carboplatin, and etoposide) versus R-DHAP (rituximab, dexamethasone, high-dose cytarabine, and cisplatin), followed by ASCT in 396 patients between ages 18 and 65 years, with relapsed DLBCL. Similar response rates were observed after three cycles of R-ICE (63%) or R-DHAP (64%). Three-year PFS and OS were not significantly different between the two treatment arms [3]. However, when analyzing the outcome of these patients according to the cell of origin (COO), there was a significantly higher CR rate (49% vs. 31%, respectively, $P = 0.035$) and PFS (52% vs. 32% at 3 years, respectively, $P = 0.0108$) in the germinal center B (GCB)-like DLBCL subset for patients treated with R-DHAP compared to R-ICE [11].

The NCIC-CTG LY.12 study [12] randomized 619 patients with relapsed/refractory aggressive lymphoma (89% of patients had DLBCL) to receive either a treatment with gemcitabine, dexamethasone, and cisplatin (GDP) or DHAP as salvage therapy. Patients with DLBCL also received rituximab (71% DLBCL) followed by high-dose chemotherapy and ASCT for responding patients. In this study, treatment with GDP was non-inferior but was associated with fewer adverse events, better preservation of patient-reported quality of life, and less frequent hospitalization (Table 6.1).

Other treatments with gemcitabine-containing regimens have low toxicities and similar efficacy (Table 6.1). In a prospective phase II study, 49 patients not eligible to ASCT received R-GemOx (rituximab, gemcitabine, and oxaliplatin). The overall response rate (ORR) was 61% with a complete remission (CR)/unconfirmed CR rate of 44%. The 5-year PFS rate was 13%, while the 5-year OS rate was 14% [13].

The combination of bendamustine and rituximab was also tested in patients with relapsed DLBCL (Table 6.1). Fifty-nine patients were treated prospectively with rituximab and bendamustine. The ORR was 62.7% with a CR rate of 37.3%. The median PFS was 6.7 months (95% CI, 3.6–13 months) [14].

Since no salvage chemotherapy regimens have demonstrated superior efficacy over the

Table 6.1 Salvage chemotherapy regimen tested in R/R DLBCL patients

Regimen	References	Phase	Patients (*n*)	RR	CR	OS	PFS
GDP vs. DHAP	[12]		619	45.1% vs. 44.1% $P = 0.005$	13.5% vs. 14.3%	39% (4-year OS) vs. 39% $P = 0.78$	26% (4-year EFS) vs. 28% $P = 0.95$
R-ICE vs. R-DHAP	[3]		396	63% vs. 64%	36% vs. 40%	47% (3-year OS) vs. 51% $P = 0.48$	31% (3-year PFS) vs. 42% $P = 0.44$
GDP	[15]		51	53%	23%	9 months (median OS)	3 months (median PFS)
R-GemOx	[13]		49	61%	44%	14% (5-year OS)	13% (5-year PFS)
R-bendamustine	[14]		59	63%	37%		6.7 months (median PFS)

GDP gemcitabine, dexamethasone, cisplatin, *DHAP* dexamethasone, high-dose cytarabine, cisplatin, *ICE* ifosfamide, carboplatin, etoposide, *R-GemOx* rituximab, gemcitabine, oxaliplatin, *CR* complete response, *ORR* overall response rate, *PFS* progression-free survival, *OS* overall survival

others, the choice of the chemotherapy regimen is largely based on their toxicity profile and individual institutional practice, the practice of each center.

The role of rituximab in combination with salvage chemotherapy may be questioned for patients who have relapsed after a rituximab-containing regimen. In a retrospective cohort of 414 patients (78% DLBCL) initially treated with R-CHOP, the incorporation of rituximab to salvage chemotherapy (R-positive cohort) increased ORR (45.6% for R-positive cohort vs. 25% for R-negative cohort, $P = 0.0003$) and the rate of CR (15.7% vs. 4.2%, $P =$). The percentage of patients undergoing hematopoietic stem cell transplantation was also significantly higher in the R-positive cohort (51.9% vs. 31.3%, $P = 0.0004$). In patients who responded to rituximab in the first-line treatment, there was an overall survival benefit to re-treatment with rituximab in the second line [16].

6.2.2 Consolidation

6.2.2.1 Autologous Stem Cell Transplantation

The pivotal PARMA study randomized patients to salvage chemotherapy alone versus high-dose therapy and autologous stem cell transplantation (HDT-ASCT) and demonstrated superior OS and EFS in patients who underwent up-front HDT-ASCT [17]. This trial established HDT-ASCT as the standard of care in transplant-eligible patients <60 years old with relapsed, chemosensitive aggressive NHL treated with curative intent. The PARMA trial did not enroll patients >60 years old, and there are no published studies comparing HDT-ASCT and salvage therapy in this specific population. Several retrospective cohort studies examined this issue in patients ≥60 years old and demonstrated acceptable results, suggesting that age alone should not be considered an absolute contraindication to HDT-ASCT [18, 19]. However, it must be noted that PFS, OS, and non-relapse mortality (NRM) outcomes appear inferior to those seen in patients <60 years old in these studies.

Patients whose disease fails to achieve at least a partial remission following standard platinum-containing salvage chemotherapy have poor overall outcomes after HDT-ASCT [20]. Demonstrating chemosensitivity to salvage therapy prior to HDT-ASCT remains the most important prognostic factor impacting outcomes after ASCT [7, 21]. In the modern era, assessing chemosensitivity to salvage therapy is routinely done with fluorodeoxyglucose positron emission tomography (FDG-PET). Multiple groups have shown that patients with a negative FDG-PET prior to HDT-ASCT have more favorable outcomes when compared to patients with a positive FDG-PET [22–24]. These results have remained consistent even when assessing FDG-PET response using the contemporary Deauville scale [25].

6.2.2.2 Peripheral Blood Versus (vs.) Bone Marrow Stem Cells

Growth factor-mobilized peripheral blood stem cells (PBSC) have become the standard and preferred stem cell source for ASCT due to more rapid engraftment, improved quality of life and costs, and a reduced need for supportive care measures when compared to bone marrow harvested stem cells [26–28]. Over the years, there has been considerable debate regarding the impacts of lymphoma cell contamination in mobilized PBSC products; however, in vivo malignant cell purging is not routinely practiced [29].

6.2.2.3 Choice of ASCT Conditioning Regimen

Historically, the choice of conditioning regimen for HDT-ASCT in patients with relapsed, chemosensitive DLBCL was guided by institutional practice, as there have been no direct comparative studies. For years, centers more often relied on total-body irradiation (TBI)-based regimens, though chemotherapy-only myeloablative conditioning (MAC) regimens such as carmustine, etoposide, cytarabine, and melphalan (BEAM) and cyclophosphamide, carmustine, and etoposide (CBV) are now more commonly utilized [30]. Early phase studies incorporating radioimmunotherapy (RIT) agents, such as I^{131} tositumomab, into the BEAM platform showed promising results; however, the pivotal phase III trial completed by the BMT Clinical Trial Network (BMT CTN) showed no advantage when compared to rituximab and BEAM [31, 32]. In a large, retrospective registry analysis using data from the Center for International Blood and Marrow Transplantation (CIBMTR), ASCT patients receiving regimens containing higher doses of carmustine incurred more serious toxicities and had poorer overall survival, whereas BEAM conditioning appeared to result in the most favorable outcomes [33]. In early phase studies, investigators reported encouraging results with novel combinations such as the replacement of carmustine with bendamustine in BEAM regimen, known as BeEAM; however, in the absence of prospective, randomized studies, rituximab and BEAM remain the most commonly utilized conditioning regimens for patients with DLBCL [34].

Patients with relapsed, chemosensitive primary or secondary central nervous system lymphoma (CNSL), which is most often of DLBCL histology, have decidedly benefited from HDT-ASCT. Specifically, transplant-eligible patients conditioned with the highly CNS penetrant agents, thiotepa, busulfan, and cyclophosphamide (TBC), had durable long-term remission and often cure in multiple retrospective studies [35–38]. Relapsed DLBCL involving the CNS may therefore represent a very unique population that should be strongly considered for TBC-conditioned ASCT.

6.2.2.4 The Role of Radiotherapy

The role of radiotherapy (RT) has been largely undefined for patients with relapsed DLBCL proceeding to HDT-ASCT. Given that the majority of treatment failures after ASCT occur at previously involved bulky sites, RT remains a potentially important consolidation strategy in high-risk patients, though the timing, schedule, and dose of RT in the peri-ASCT period are unclear [39]. Most centers utilize consolidative RT after ASCT to allow for recovery from the effects of HDT and to mitigate unnecessary toxicities [40]. However, this approach may result in the inability to deliver the intended RT treatment plan given the variable toxicity experienced by patients recently completing HDT. Some centers have successfully integrated RT as part of a combined-modality conditioning regimen prior to ASCT, ensuring that patients receive planned RT prior to ASCT. A study of 164 patients with relapsed/refractory DLBCL receiving salvage involved-field radiation therapy (IFRT) given twice daily for a total dose of 30 Gy to sites of disease >5 cm or to sites of residual disease of >2 cm demonstrated favorable 5-year PFS and OS of 53% and 58%, respectively. Additionally, there was enhanced disease control in sites of bulky or residual disease, few relapses within the RT fields, and an acceptable toxicity profile [40]. In a subsequent study, it was shown that while FDG-PET-positive patients after salvage therapy had poor overall survival after ASCT, disease-specific survival and OS were improved in a subset of these patients if they received combined-modality conditioning pre-ASCT [41].

6.2.2.5 Allogeneic Hematopoietic Cell Transplantation

The use of allogeneic hematopoietic cell transplantation (allo-HCT) has the potential added advantage of the graft-versus-lymphoma effect [42, 43]. It is most often considered in patients who relapse after HDT-ASCT or high-risk patients with a specific contraindication to ASCT, such as persistent bone marrow involvement. Even in patients previously treated with rituximab, the addition of rituximab to salvage therapy for relapse after HDT-ASCT was shown to improve CR and OS rates [44].

More contemporary, non-randomized studies have compared first HDT-ASCT with MAC allogeneic hematopoietic cell transplantation (allo-HCT) for patients with relapsed DLBCL. One group compared patients undergoing ASCT with those undergoing T-cell-depleted MAC allo-HCT and showed a markedly higher risk of non-relapse mortality (NRM) and similar overall survival among all patients [45]. In a multicenter, retrospective CIBMTR analysis published in 2010, patients undergoing allo-HCT had similar risk of disease progression though had significantly higher non-relapse mortality (NRM) and overall mortality, particularly within the first year after

HCT, when compared to patients that underwent ASCT. Long-term PFS and OS were more favorable in the ASCT group overall mostly due to early treatment-related deaths [46]. While neither study demonstrated differences in relapse or progression, patients treated with allo-HCT generally had poorer-risk disease [47].

Given the unfavorable NRM with myeloablative conditioning (MAC), the use of reduced intensity conditioning (RIC) and non-myeloablative (NMA) conditioning regimens has been studied extensively in DLBCL, particularly for older patients and those that relapsed after ASCT. Despite high relapse rates in early studies, patients with chemosensitive disease prior to allo-HCT had PFS rates of up to 54% at 3 years [47]. In the largest study comparing MAC and RIC/NMA completed on behalf of the CIBMTR, relapse or progression rates were lower for patients receiving MAC than RIC and NMA (26% vs. 38% vs. 40%, $P = 0.031$); however, NRM was significantly higher in MAC than RIC and NMA (56% vs. 47% vs. 36%, $P = 0.007$) leading to similar OS in both cohorts. Additionally, multivariate analysis showed that Karnofsky performance status <90 and chemoresistance to salvage therapy were associated with poorer survival, while patients transplanted in later years had improved survival [48].

The incidence of graft-versus-host disease (GVHD), particularly chronic GVHD, has also been challenging after allo-HCT for relapsed DLBCL. In an effort to reduce high incidence of GVHD, many centers began incorporating alemtuzumab into their RIC regimens [49, 50]. This method resulted in reduced risk of both acute and chronic GVHD, though at the expense of an increased risk of progression or relapse in prospective series [51].

These data highlight an ongoing debate in the field regarding the use of MAC vs. RIC/NMA, as well as optimal conditioning regimen in patients undergoing allo-HCT who relapsed after ASCT. This is reflected in the most recent evidence-based review provided by the American Society of Blood and Marrow Transplantation, which could not provide a consensus recommendation regarding the use of MAC vs. RIC/NMA due to insufficient high-quality data [52]. Similarly, the optimal conditioning and GVHD preventive regimens for patients undergoing allo-HCT are unknown. These decisions ultimately involve a detailed assessment of patient and disease-related risk factors.

6.2.3 Maintenance

6.2.3.1 Rituximab Maintenance

In the CORAL study, 242 patients underwent a second randomization after ASCT between rituximab maintenance (every 2 months for 1 year) and surveillance [53]. The 4-year EFS after ASCT was not significantly different between the two groups (52% vs. 53%, respectively). Therefore, rituximab maintenance in R/R DLBCL is not recommended. Similarly, in a second randomization after ASCT in a large, prospective study, Haioun and colleagues showed no significant difference in survival for those patients who received rituximab maintenance versus observation [54].

6.2.3.2 Lenalidomide Maintenance

In an open-label, multicenter phase II trial, 46 patients with chemosensitive relapses of DLBCL who were not eligible for ASCT or who had relapsed after ASCT received maintenance with lenalidomide [55]. Lenalidomide maintenance started within 2 months from the end of salvage chemotherapy and lasted until lymphoma progression or unacceptable toxicity. One-year PFS was of 70% (95% CI 57–83) and 3-year OS was 71%. However, there is insufficient data to recommend lenalidomide maintenance in R/R DLBCL.

6.3 Second Relapse and Beyond

6.3.1 Chemotherapy

In DLBCL patients who have failed a first salvage therapy, third-line treatments are not well established. A follow-up study from the CORAL trial evaluated the outcome and prognostic factors of 203 patients who failed second-line chemotherapy [56]. In the intent-to-treat analysis, overall response rate to third-line chemotherapy was 39%, with 27% CR or uCR, and 12% PR. Among the 203 patients, 64 (31.5%) were eventually transplanted. Interestingly, patients who shifted from DHAP-type to ICE-type or vice versa could achieve a favorable response (with ~43% OR and ~25% CR), demonstrating that a significant percentage of patients can still be rescued by standard chemotherapy.

6.3.2 New Drugs

A phase II/III, multicenter, randomized study was initiated to compare the efficacy and safety of lenalidomide as single agent versus investigator's choice (IC) (gemcitabine, rituximab, etoposide, or oxaliplatin monotherapy) in relapsed/refractory DLBCL. Twenty-five patients were included in each subgroup (GCB or non-GCB) who received either lenalidomide or IC. A significant benefit in PFS and OS was observed for lenalidomide vs. IC in non-GCB (ABC) patients ($P < 0.05$).

In a phase I/II clinical trial that involved 80 subjects with relapsed or refractory DLBCL, ibrutinib induced an objective response of 37% (14/38) in the ABC subset versus 5% (1/20) in the GCB subset ($P = 0.0106$) [57].

Chimeric antigen receptor T-cell (CAR-T) therapy may also have efficacy in this population of patients. In the ZUMA-1 trial, 101 refractory DLBCL patients were treated with CD19-CAR-T (Ref: Neelapu, ICML-14, 2017). This therapy achieved a CR rate of 57%, which was sevenfold higher than historical controls (8% in the SCHOLAR-1 study, ref). The 6-month OS was 80% compared to the 55% in SCHOLAR-1 study. In July 2017, the US Food and Drug Administration (US FDA) recommended approval of CAR-T therapy (CTL019, Novartis) for the treatment of relapsed or refractory pediatric and young adult patients with B-cell acute lymphoblastic leukemia. This will likely soon be followed by applications for approval of CTL019 therapy for the treatment of relapsed or refractory DLBCL.

There are many new agents being studied in this setting including inhibitors of BTK, BCL-2, histone deacetylase, BET, PD1, and PDLI; these drugs are commonly combined. For example, a recent study with nivolumab and ibrutinib showed promising activity in Richter's transformation. Antibody-drug conjugates (ADCs) that bind to CD30, CD19, or CD79 have reasonable single-agent activity, and a large phase II study adding an CD19 ADC to R-ICE chemotherapy is ongoing. Lastly, novel bi-specific monoclonal antibodies such as bi-specific T-cell engagers (BiTES) and dual-affinity retargeting antibodies (DARTs) have shown reasonable single-agent response rates, and clinical research studies continue to accrue (Fig. 6.1).

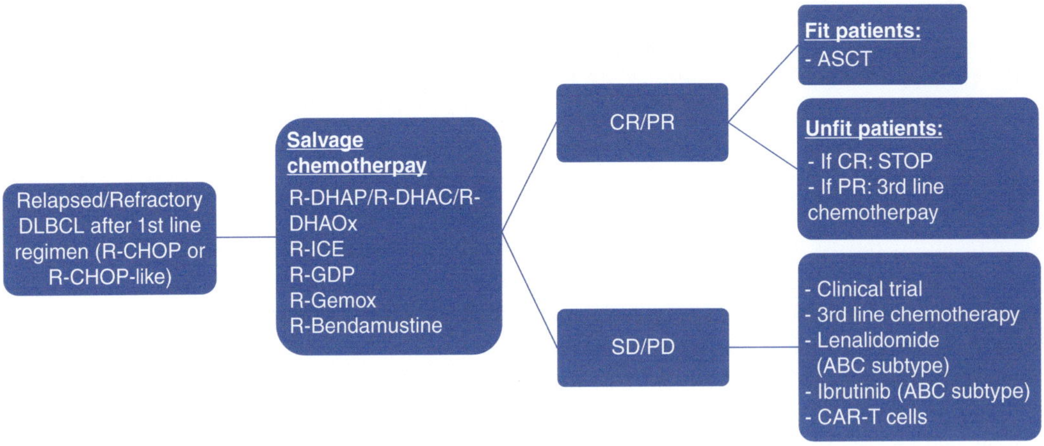

Fig. 6.1 Standard of care relapsed/refractory DLBCL

6.4 Conclusion

In the post-rituximab era, significant improvements in all outcomes were seen for patients undergoing up-front induction therapy for DLBCL. For those with relapsed DLBCL in the post-rituximab era, marked improvements in long-term survival have been more elusive. It is clear that chemosensitivity to salvage therapy as measured by FDG-PET remains the single most important prognostic factor in achieving cure and that consolidative HDT-ASCT remains the standard of care for many patients. While RIC increased access to allo-HCT for many older patients, there are many challenges that remain, including reducing NRM and GVHD. Areas of active and ongoing research include the incorporation of novel agents such as monoclonal antibodies, antibody-drug conjugates, and small molecule inhibitors [e.g., Bruton's tyrosine kinase inhibitors, PI3 kinase inhibitors, etc.] into both salvage platforms, conditioning regimens for ASCT and in post-ASCT maintenance. Moreover, it remains to be seen how these and other promising approaches such as cellular therapies, including bi-specific T-cell engagers (BITEs) and CAR-T, will impact the scope of practice [58–62].

References

1. Feugier P, Van Hoof A, Sebban C, et al. Long-term results of the R-CHOP study in the treatment of elderly patients with diffuse large B-cell lymphoma: a study by the Groupe d'Etude des Lymphomes de l'Adulte. J Clin Oncol. 2005;23(18):4117–26. https://doi.org/10.1200/JCO.2005.09.131.
2. Pfreundschuh M, Trümper L, Osterborg A, et al. CHOP-like chemotherapy plus rituximab versus CHOP-like chemotherapy alone in young patients with good-prognosis diffuse large-B-cell lymphoma: a randomised controlled trial by the MabThera International Trial (MInT) Group. Lancet Oncol. 2006;7(5):379–91. https://doi.org/10.1016/S1470-2045(06)70664-7.
3. Gisselbrecht C, Glass B, Mounier N, et al. Salvage regimens with autologous transplantation for relapsed large B-cell lymphoma in the rituximab era. J Clin Oncol. 2010;28(27):4184–90. https://doi.org/10.1200/JCO.2010.28.1618.
4. Telio D, Fernandes K, Ma C, et al. Salvage chemotherapy and autologous stem cell transplant in primary refractory diffuse large B-cell lymphoma: outcomes and prognostic factors. Leuk Lymphoma. 2012;53(5):836–41. https://doi.org/10.3109/10428194.2011.643404.
5. Larouche J-F, Berger F, Chassagne-Clément C, et al. Lymphoma recurrence 5 years or later following diffuse large B-cell lymphoma: clinical characteristics and outcome. J Clin Oncol. 2010;28(12):2094–100. https://doi.org/10.1200/JCO.2009.24.5860.
6. Cohen JB, Behera M, Thompson CA, Flowers CR. Evaluating surveillance imaging for diffuse large B-cell lymphoma and Hodgkin lymphoma. Blood. 2017;129(5):561–4. https://doi.org/10.1182/blood-2016-08-685073.
7. Hamlin PA, Zelenetz AD, Kewalramani T, et al. Age-adjusted international prognostic index predicts autologous stem cell transplantation outcome for patients with relapsed or primary refractory diffuse large B-cell lymphoma. Blood. 2003;102(6):1989–96. https://doi.org/10.1182/blood-2002-12-3837.
8. Guglielmi C, Gomez F, Philip T, et al. Time to relapse has prognostic value in patients with aggressive lymphoma enrolled onto the Parma trial. J Clin Oncol. 1998;16(10):3264–9. https://doi.org/10.1200/JCO.1998.16.10.3264.
9. Hitz F, Connors JM, Gascoyne RD, et al. Outcome of patients with primary refractory diffuse large B cell lymphoma after R-CHOP treatment. Ann Hematol. 2015;94(11):1839–43. https://doi.org/10.1007/s00277-015-2467-z.
10. Crump M, Neelapu S, Farooq U, et al. Outcomes in refractory aggressive diffuse large B cell lymphoma (DLBCL): results from the International SCHOLAR-1 Study. Clin Lymphoma Myeloma Leuk. 2016;16:S101. https://doi.org/10.1016/j.clml.2016.07.147.
11. Thieblemont C, Briere J, Mounier N, et al. The germinal center/activated B-cell subclassification has a prognostic impact for response to salvage therapy in relapsed/refractory diffuse large B-cell lymphoma: a bio-CORAL study. J Clin Oncol. 2011;29(31):4079–87. https://doi.org/10.1200/JCO.2011.35.4423.
12. Crump M, Kuruvilla J, Couban S, et al. Randomized comparison of gemcitabine, dexamethasone, and cisplatin versus dexamethasone, cytarabine, and cisplatin chemotherapy before autologous stem-cell transplantation for relapsed and refractory aggressive lymphomas: NCIC-CTG LY.12. J Clin Oncol. 2014;32(31):3490–6. https://doi.org/10.1200/JCO.2013.53.9593.
13. Mounier N, El Gnaoui T, Tilly H, et al. Rituximab plus gemcitabine and oxaliplatin in patients with refractory/relapsed diffuse large B-cell lymphoma who are not candidates for high-dose therapy. A phase II Lymphoma Study Association trial. Haematologica. 2013;98(11):1726–31. https://doi.org/10.3324/haematol.2013.090597.
14. Ohmachi K, Niitsu N, Uchida T, et al. Multicenter phase II study of bendamustine plus rituximab in patients with relapsed or refractory diffuse large

B-cell lymphoma. J Clin Oncol. 2013;31(17):2103–9. https://doi.org/10.1200/JCO.2012.46.5203.
15. Crump M, Baetz T, Couban S, et al. Gemcitabine, dexamethasone, and cisplatin in patients with recurrent or refractory aggressive histology B-cell non-Hodgkin lymphoma: a phase II study by the National Cancer Institute of Canada Clinical Trials Group (NCIC-CTG). Cancer. 2004;101(8):1835–42. https://doi.org/10.1002/cncr.20587.
16. Baetz T, Chen BE, Couban S, et al. Addition of rituximab to salvage chemotherapy in aggressive CD20+ lymphoma prior to autologous stem cell transplant (ASCT): a cohort comparison from the NCIC CTG study LY.12. Blood. 2014;124(21):1712.
17. Philip T, Guglielmi C, Hagenbeek A, et al. Autologous bone marrow transplantation as compared with salvage chemotherapy in relapses of chemotherapy-sensitive non-Hodgkin's lymphoma. N Engl J Med. 1995;333(23):1540–5. https://doi.org/10.1056/NEJM199512073332305.
18. Buadi FK, Micallef IN, Ansell SM, et al. Autologous hematopoietic stem cell transplantation for older patients with relapsed non-Hodgkin's lymphoma. Bone Marrow Transplant. 2006;37(11):1017–22. https://doi.org/10.1038/sj.bmt.1705371.
19. Jantunen E, Itälä M, Lehtinen T, et al. Early treatment-related mortality in adult autologous stem cell transplant recipients: a nationwide survey of 1482 transplanted patients. Eur J Haematol. 2006;76(3):245–50. https://doi.org/10.1111/j.1600-0609.2005.00605.x.
20. Sehn LH, Gascoyne RD. Diffuse large B-cell lymphoma: optimizing outcome in the context of clinical and biologic heterogeneity. Blood. 2015;125(1):22–32. https://doi.org/10.1182/blood-2014-05-577189.
21. Cortelazzo S, Rambaldi A, Rossi A, et al. Intensification of salvage treatment with high-dose sequential chemotherapy improves the outcome of patients with refractory or relapsed aggressive non-Hodgkin's lymphoma. Br J Haematol. 2001;114(2):333–41. http://www.ncbi.nlm.nih.gov/pubmed/11529852. Accessed 28 Jun 2017.
22. Filmont J-E, Gisselbrecht C, Cuenca X, et al. The impact of pre- and post-transplantation positron emission tomography using 18-fluorodeoxyglucose on poor-prognosis lymphoma patients undergoing autologous stem cell transplantation. Cancer. 2007;110(6):1361–9. https://doi.org/10.1002/cncr.22911.
23. Dickinson M, Hoyt R, Roberts AW, et al. Improved survival for relapsed diffuse large B cell lymphoma is predicted by a negative pre-transplant FDG-PET scan following salvage chemotherapy: research paper. Br J Haematol. 2010;150(1):39–45. https://doi.org/10.1111/j.1365-2141.2010.08162.x.
24. Roland V, Bodet-Milin C, Moreau A, et al. Impact of high-dose chemotherapy followed by auto-SCT for positive interim [18F] FDG-PET diffuse large B-cell lymphoma patients. Bone Marrow Transplant. 2011;46(3):393–9. https://doi.org/10.1038/bmt.2010.130.
25. Sauter CS, Matasar MJ, Meikle J, et al. Prognostic value of FDG-PET prior to autologous stem cell transplantation for relapsed and refractory diffuse large B-cell lymphoma. Blood. 2015;125(16):2579–81. https://doi.org/10.1182/blood-2014-10-606939.
26. Ottinger HD, Beelen DW, Scheulen B, Schaefer UW, Grosse-Wilde H. Improved immune reconstitution after allotransplantation of peripheral blood stem cells instead of bone marrow. Blood. 1996;88(7):2775–9. http://www.ncbi.nlm.nih.gov/pubmed/8839875.
27. Vellenga E, van Agthoven M, Croockewit AJ, et al. Autologous peripheral blood stem cell transplantation in patients with relapsed lymphoma results in accelerated haematopoietic reconstitution, improved quality of life and cost reduction compared with bone marrow transplantation: the Hovon 22 study. Br J Haematol. 2001;114(2):319–26. http://www.ncbi.nlm.nih.gov/pubmed/11529850. Accessed 28 Jun 2017.
28. Vose JM, Sharp G, Chan WC, et al. Autologous transplantation for aggressive non-Hodgkin's lymphoma: results of a randomized trial evaluating graft source and minimal residual disease. J Clin Oncol. 2002;20(9):2344–52. https://doi.org/10.1200/JCO.2002.09.138.
29. Jacobsen E, Freedman A. B-cell purging in autologous stem-cell transplantation for non-Hodgkin lymphoma. Lancet Oncol. 2004;5(12):711–7. https://doi.org/10.1016/S1470-2045(04)01646-8.
30. Friedberg JW. Relapsed/refractory diffuse large B-cell lymphoma. Hematology Am Soc Hematol Educ Program. 2011;2011(1):498–505. https://doi.org/10.1182/asheducation-2011.1.498.
31. Vose JM, Bierman PJ, Enke C, et al. Phase I trial of iodine-131 tositumomab with high-dose chemotherapy and autologous stem-cell transplantation for relapsed non-Hodgkin's lymphoma. J Clin Oncol. 2005;23(3):461–7. https://doi.org/10.1200/JCO.2005.05.117.
32. Vose JM, Carter S, Burns LJ, et al. Phase III randomized study of rituximab/carmustine, etoposide, cytarabine, and melphalan (BEAM) compared with iodine-131 tositumomab/BEAM with autologous hematopoietic cell transplantation for relapsed diffuse large B-cell lymphoma: results from the BMT CTN 0401 trial. J Clin Oncol. 2013;31(13):1662–8. https://doi.org/10.1200/JCO.2012.45.9453.
33. Chen Y-B, AA L, Logan BR, et al. Impact of conditioning regimen on outcomes for patients with lymphoma undergoing high-dose therapy with autologous hematopoietic cell transplantation. Biol Blood Marrow Transplant. 2015;21(6):1046–53. https://doi.org/10.1016/j.bbmt.2015.02.005.
34. Visani G, Malerba L, Stefani PM, et al. BeEAM (bendamustine, etoposide, cytarabine, melphalan) before autologous stem cell transplantation is safe and effective for resistant/relapsed lymphoma patients. Blood. 2011;118(12):3419–25. https://doi.org/10.1182/blood-2011-04-351924.
35. Cote GM, Hochberg EP, Muzikansky A, et al. Autologous stem cell transplantation with thiotepa,

busulfan, and cyclophosphamide (TBC) conditioning in patients with CNS involvement by non-Hodgkin lymphoma. Biol Blood Marrow Transplant. 2012;18(1):76–83. https://doi.org/10.1016/j.bbmt.2011.07.006.

36. Chen Y-B, Batchelor T, Li S, et al. Phase 2 trial of high-dose rituximab with high-dose cytarabine mobilization therapy and high-dose thiotepa, busulfan, and cyclophosphamide autologous stem cell transplantation in patients with central nervous system involvement by non-Hodgkin lymphoma. Cancer. 2015;121(2):226–33. https://doi.org/10.1002/cncr.29023.
37. Welch MR, Sauter CS, Matasar MJ, et al. Autologous stem cell transplant in recurrent or refractory primary or secondary central nervous system lymphoma using thiotepa, busulfan and cyclophosphamide. Leuk Lymphoma. 2015;56(2):361–7. https://doi.org/10.3109/10428194.2014.916800.
38. Scordo M, Bhatt V, Hsu M, et al. A comprehensive assessment of toxicities in patients with central nervous system lymphoma undergoing autologous stem cell transplantation using thiotepa, busulfan, and cyclophosphamide conditioning. Biol Blood Marrow Transplant. 2017;23(1):38–43. https://doi.org/10.1016/j.bbmt.2016.09.024.
39. Dhakal S, Bates JE, Casulo C, et al. Patterns and timing of failure for diffuse large B-cell lymphoma after initial therapy in a cohort who underwent autologous bone marrow transplantation for relapse. Int J Radiat Oncol Biol Phys. 2016;96(2):372–8. https://doi.org/10.1016/j.ijrobp.2016.05.021.
40. Hoppe BS, Moskowitz CH, Filippa DA, et al. Involved-field radiotherapy before high-dose therapy and autologous stem-cell rescue in diffuse large-cell lymphoma: long-term disease control and toxicity. J Clin Oncol. 2008;26(11):1858–64. https://doi.org/10.1200/JCO.2007.15.4773.
41. Hoppe BS, Moskowitz CH, Zhang Z, et al. The role of FDG-PET imaging and involved field radiotherapy in relapsed or refractory diffuse large B-cell lymphoma. Bone Marrow Transplant. 2009;43(12):941–8. https://doi.org/10.1038/bmt.2008.408.
42. Mandigers CMPW, Verdonck LF, Meijerink JPP, Dekker AW, Schattenberg AVMB, Raemaekers JMM. Graft-versus-lymphoma effect of donor lymphocyte infusion in indolent lymphomas relapsed after allogeneic stem cell transplantation. Bone Marrow Transplant. 2003;32(12):1159–63. https://doi.org/10.1038/sj.bmt.1704290.
43. Bishop MR, Dean RM, Steinberg SM, et al. Clinical evidence of a graft-versus-lymphoma effect against relapsed diffuse large B-cell lymphoma after allogeneic hematopoietic stem-cell transplantation. Ann Oncol. 2008;19(11):1935–40. https://doi.org/10.1093/annonc/mdn404.
44. Calvo-Villas JM, Martín A, Conde E, et al. Effect of addition of rituximab to salvage chemotherapy on outcome of patients with diffuse large B-cell lymphoma relapsing after an autologous stem-cell transplantation. Ann Oncol. 2010;21(9):1891–7. https://doi.org/10.1093/annonc/mdq035.
45. Aksentijevich I, Jones RJ, Ambinder RF, Garrett-Mayer E, Flinn IW. Clinical outcome following autologous and allogeneic blood and marrow transplantation for relapsed diffuse large-cell non-Hodgkin's lymphoma. Biol Blood Marrow Transplant. 2006;12(9):965–72. https://doi.org/10.1016/j.bbmt.2006.05.018.
46. Lazarus HM, Zhang M-J, Carreras J, et al. A comparison of HLA-identical sibling allogeneic versus autologous transplantation for diffuse large B cell lymphoma: a report from the CIBMTR. Biol Blood Marrow Transplant. 2010;16(1):35–45. https://doi.org/10.1016/j.bbmt.2009.08.011.
47. Papageorgiou SG, Cwynarski K, Kottaridis PD. The role of allogeneic haematopoietic progenitor cell transplantation in patients with diffuse large B-cell non-Hodgkin lymphomas (DLBCL). Bone Marrow Transplant. 2013;48(10):1271–8. https://doi.org/10.1038/bmt.2012.266.
48. Bacher U, Klyuchnikov E, Le-Rademacher J, et al. Conditioning regimens for allotransplants for diffuse large B-cell lymphoma: myeloablative or reduced intensity? Blood. 2012;120(20):4256–62. https://doi.org/10.1182/blood-2012-06-436725.
49. Faulkner RD, Craddock C, Byrne JL, et al. BEAM-alemtuzumab reduced-intensity allogeneic stem cell transplantation for lymphoproliferative diseases: GVHD, toxicity, and survival in 65 patients. Blood. 2004;103(2):428–34. https://doi.org/10.1182/blood-2003-05-1406.
50. Morris E, Thomson K, Craddock C, et al. Outcomes after alemtuzumab-containing reduced-intensity allogeneic transplantation regimen for relapsed and refractory non-Hodgkin lymphoma. Blood. 2004;104(13):3865–71. https://doi.org/10.1182/blood-2004-03-1105.
51. Sauter CS, Chou JF, Papadopoulos EB, et al. A prospective study of an alemtuzumab containing reduced-intensity allogeneic stem cell transplant program in patients with poor-risk and advanced lymphoid malignancies. Leuk Lymphoma. 2014;55(12):2739–47. https://doi.org/10.3109/10428194.2014.894185.
52. Oliansky DM, Czuczman M, Fisher RI, et al. The role of cytotoxic therapy with hematopoietic stem cell transplantation in the treatment of diffuse large B cell lymphoma: update of the 2001 evidence-based review. Biol Blood Marrow Transplant. 2011;17(1):18–9. https://doi.org/10.1016/j.bbmt.2010.07.008.
53. Gisselbrecht C, Schmitz N, Mounier N, et al. Rituximab maintenance therapy after autologous stem-cell transplantation in patients with relapsed CD20(+) diffuse large B-cell lymphoma: final analysis of the collaborative trial in relapsed aggressive lymphoma. J Clin Oncol. 2012;30(36):4462–9. https://doi.org/10.1200/JCO.2012.41.9416.
54. Haioun C, Mounier N, Emile JF, et al. Rituximab versus observation after high-dose consolidative first-line chemotherapy with autologous stem-cell transplantation in patients with poor-risk diffuse large

B-cell lymphoma. Ann Oncol. 2009;20(12):1985–92. https://doi.org/10.1093/annonc/mdp237.
55. Ferreri AJM, Sassone M, Zaja F, et al. Lenalidomide maintenance in patients with relapsed diffuse large B-cell lymphoma who are not eligible for autologous stem cell transplantation: an open label, single-arm, multicentre phase 2 trial. Lancet Haematol. 2017;4(3):e137–46. https://doi.org/10.1016/S2352-3026(17)30016-9.
56. Van Den Neste E, Schmitz N, Mounier N, et al. Outcomes of diffuse large B-cell lymphoma patients relapsing after autologous stem cell transplantation: an analysis of patients included in the CORAL study. Bone Marrow Transplant. 2017;52(2):216–21. https://doi.org/10.1038/bmt.2016.213.
57. Wilson WH, Young RM, Schmitz R, et al. Targeting B cell receptor signaling with ibrutinib in diffuse large B cell lymphoma. Nat Med. 2015;21(8):922–6. https://doi.org/10.1038/nm.3884.
58. Epperla N, Fenske TS, Lazarus HM, Hamadani M. Post-autologous transplant maintenance therapies in lymphoid malignancies: are we there yet? Bone Marrow Transplant. 2015;50(11):1393–404. https://doi.org/10.1038/bmt.2015.184.
59. Kochenderfer JN, Dudley ME, Kassim SH, et al. Chemotherapy-refractory diffuse large B-cell lymphoma and indolent B-cell malignancies can be effectively treated with autologous T cells expressing an anti-CD19 chimeric antigen receptor. J Clin Oncol. 2015;33(6):540–9. https://doi.org/10.1200/JCO.2014.56.2025.
60. Brudno JN, Somerville RPT, Shi V, et al. Allogeneic T cells that express an anti-CD19 chimeric antigen receptor induce remissions of B-cell malignancies that progress after allogeneic hematopoietic stem-cell transplantation without causing graft-versus-host disease. J Clin Oncol. 2016;34(10):1112–21. https://doi.org/10.1200/JCO.2015.64.5929.
61. Goebeler M-E, Knop S, Viardot A, et al. Bispecific T-cell engager (BiTE) antibody construct blinatumomab for the treatment of patients with relapsed/refractory non-Hodgkin lymphoma: final results from a phase I study. J Clin Oncol. 2016;34(10):1104–11. https://doi.org/10.1200/JCO.2014.59.1586.
62. Viardot A, Goebeler M-E, Hess G, et al. Phase 2 study of the bispecific T-cell engager (BiTE) antibody blinatumomab in relapsed/refractory diffuse large B-cell lymphoma. Blood. 2016;127(11):1410–6. https://doi.org/10.1182/blood-2015-06-651380.

Burkitt Lymphoma

7

Kieron Dunleavy and Martine Chamuleau

7.1 Introduction

Burkitt lymphoma (BL) is a rare and highly aggressive B-cell lymphoma that was first described over 50 years ago by Denis Burkitt in African children [1]. His initial report identified Ugandan children with unusual jaw tumors in association with other specific anatomic sites. This first to be described "endemic" variant occurs in specific geographical areas and has a predilection for males between the ages of 4 and 7 years (Table 7.1). Sporadic BL, in contrast, affects children and young adults in all regions of the world and has no specific geographical distribution. Third, immunodeficiency-associated BL is associated with HIV infection. Over the recent years, with the advent of novel genomic technologies, we have made significant strides in elucidating BL biology. Many novel mutations that cooperate with *MYC* and have key roles in BL pathogenesis have been identified. While traditional standard approaches for this disease are highly toxic, there has been recent therapeutic progress in developing less toxic strategies that maintain the high cure rates of intensive standard treatments.

K. Dunleavy (✉)
George Washington University Cancer Center, Washington, DC, USA
e-mail: kdunleavy@mfa.gwu.edu

M. Chamuleau
VU University Medical Center, Amsterdam, Netherlands
e-mail: M.Chamuleau@vumc.nl

7.2 Pathology and Molecular Biology

One of the key biological characteristics of BL is a very high proliferation index approaching 100%, and this accounts for the "starry sky" appearance of the tumor (representing apoptotic tumor cells ingested by macrophages) that can be appreciated at low magnification under the microscope. BL is typically characterized by non-pleomorphic, intermediate size cells with basophilic cytoplasm that contains small vacuoles and round nuclei. The nuclear chromatin is granular with small nucleoli and frequent mitoses. BL is considered to be of germinal center B-cell origin, and cells typically express CD10, BCL6, CD20, CD79a, and CD45. The negative expression of terminal deoxynucleotidyl transferase (TdT) and BCL2 can help to distinguish BL from other diagnoses such as acute leukemia and diffuse large B-cell lymphoma. Epstein-Barr virus (EBV) expression varies according to the subtype of BL: it is detected in almost all cases of endemic BL and in 25–40% of other cases [2]. A pattern of EBV latency type 1 is typically observed with restricted EBV nuclear antigen 1 (EBNA1) expression. Many studies suggest

G. Lenz, G. Salles (eds.), *Aggressive Lymphomas*, Hematologic Malignancies,
https://doi.org/10.1007/978-3-030-00362-3_7

Table 7.1 Comparison of endemic, sporadic, and HIV-associated Burkitt lymphoma

	Endemic	Sporadic	HIV-associated
Epidemiology	Equatorial Africa and Papua, New Guinea. Geographic association with malaria	Worldwide	Worldwide
Incidence	5–10 cases per 100,000	2–3 cases per million	6 per 1000 AIDS cases
Age and gender	Malignancy of childhood Peak incidence: 4–7 years Male: female of 2:1	Malignancy of childhood and young adults Median age: 30 years Male: female of 2–3:1	Malignancy of adults Median age: 44 years. Associated with higher CD4 counts >100/mm^3
EBV association	100%	25–40%	25–40%
Genomics	*MYC* mutation 100%; *ID3* and/or *TCF3* mutations 40%; *CCND* mutations 1.8%	*MYC* mutation 100%; *ID3* and/or *TCF3* mutations 70%; *CCND* mutations 38%	*MYC* mutation 100%; *ID3* and/or *TCF3* mutations 67%; *CCND* mutations 67%
Clinical presentation	Jaw and facial bones in ≈ 50%. Also involves mesentery and gonads. Increased risk of CNS dissemination	Abdomen most common presentation often involving the ileocecal region. Other extranodal sites include bone marrow, ovaries, kidneys, and breasts. Increased risk of CNS dissemination	Nodal presentation most common with occasional bone marrow. Increased risk of CNS dissemination

evidence for an oncogenic role of EBV in the disease [3–5]. EBV contributes to genomic instability in endemic BL where cases are also linked to malaria prevalence with the incidence highest in people with high titers of *Plasmodium falciparum* [6–10].

BL cases harbor a *MYC* translocation, which is typically at 8q24 and results in deregulation of the *MYC* gene [11, 12]. In most (over 80%) cases, the translocation partner for *MYC* is the immunoglobulin heavy (IgH) chain locus on chromosome 14—in other cases, there is involvement of κ and λ light chain loci on chromosomes 2 and 22. The variation of *MYC* breakpoints that is appreciated when comparing sporadic and endemic BL suggests distinct oncogenic mechanisms of lymphomagenesis depending on the epidemiological variant of the disease [13, 14].

Over the past few years, RNA sequencing (RNA-seq) studies have identified novel mutations in addition to *MYC* in sporadic BL cases [15–18]. These studies have shown that 70% of cases have mutations in *TCF3* or its negative regulator *ID3*, which encodes a protein that blocks *TCF3* action (see Fig. 7.1). Additionally, approximately 38% of sporadic cases harbor a mutation in *CCND3*—this is

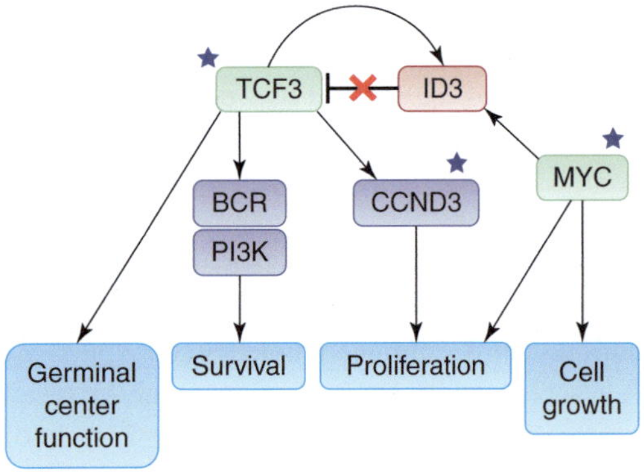

Fig. 7.1 Burkitt lymphoma frequently harbors mutations in ID3, TCF3, and CCND3 that activate the TCF3 pathway. The t(8:14) translocation present in BL dysregulates MYC. Cooperation of these two pathways plays a crucial role in BL, in which virtually all cells are proliferating, as evidenced by the expression of the cell cycle-related antigen Ki67. Adapted from Schmitz, Nature Genetics 2012 [19]

activated by *TCF3* and encodes cyclin D3, which is responsible for cell cycle progression. *TCF3* and/or *ID3* mutations also occur in the other BL variants (67% and 40% of HIV-associated and endemic cases, respectively)—the ongoing BL Genome Sequencing Project (BLGSP) is an international effort that aims to further interrogate and characterize the genomics of these different disease variants (https://ocg.cancer.gov/

programs/cgci/projects/burkitt-lymphoma). Studies that have used gene expression profiling (GEP) demonstrated that BL has a distinct molecular signature compared to other aggressive B-cell lymphomas, and this has germinal center B-cell derivation [20, 21]. The signature has high expression of c-*MYC* target and germinal center associated B-cell genes and low expression of MHC class 1 molecules and NF-kappa B target genes. In fact, in early GEP studies in BL, a subset of cases diagnosed as diffuse large B-cell lymphoma (DLBCL) by histologic criteria fell into the BL category, when GEP was applied. This is an important molecular distinction given that CHOP-based treatments that are standard in DLBCL do not have a high response rate in BL—therefore, GEP may be helpful in rare cases that would otherwise be diagnosed as DLBCL, if histologic criterial alone were used. GEP also identified cases that did not fit exactly into DLBCL or BL and had a molecular profile intermediate between both entities.

Recent studies have identified a subgroup of lymphomas that resemble BL by GEP, morphologically and clinically, but that lack the *MYC* translocation. These cases all display 11q alterations (gains and losses), leading to the provisional entity: *Burkitt-like lymphoma with 11q aberration* [22–24]. Future studies shall reveal whether this is a real separate entity of BL.

7.3 Clinical Presentation and Work-Up

BL has a variable clinical presentation that is dependent on the epidemiological variant as well as other factors. In endemic BL, involvement of the jaw and other facial sites commonly occurs; other extranodal sites that may be involved include the ileum and cecum, gonads, kidneys, and breasts. Jaw involvement rarely occurs in sporadic BL, and the ileocecal area is the most common site of involvement. In immunodeficiency-associated BL, sites of involvement that are common include the ileum and cecum, lymph nodes, and bone marrow. CNS involvement may occur at presentation with all variants of BL, particularly when there is advanced stage disease. CNS involvement is almost always leptomeningeal, and parenchymal brain involvement in BL is exceedingly rare. In patients with advanced-stage and bulky disease, tumor lysis syndrome (TLS) commonly develops typically after the institution of therapy (it may indeed occur before any treatment is started), and this needs to be anticipated and prophylaxis administered as appropriate.

The diagnosis of BL should be made by a hematopathologist, expert in the diagnosis of lymphoma as some cases are challenging diagnostically and difficult to distinguish from other aggressive B-cell lymphomas, especially diffuse large B-cell lymphomas that also can harbor a *MYC* translocation.

Routine hematology and biochemistry tests including lactate dehydrogenase (LDH) and uric acid should be performed as well as HIV and hepatitis B testing. Computed tomography (CT) imaging with or without positron-emission tomography (PET) should be done. A bone marrow biopsy is routine in all patients, and lumbar puncture with CSF analysis by cytology and flow cytometry should also be performed.

7.4 Staging and Prognostic Factors

No specific staging system and validated prognostic score has been developed for BL. Regarding staging in adult patients, the Ann Arbor classification is widely used. Identification of prognostic factors at diagnosis mostly relies on population-based studies due to lack of large clinical trials. These studies have identified numerous factors like age, black race, advanced stage, performance status, and elevated LDH [25–28]. Consequently, a prognostic score has not yet been validated, but most studies identify a low-risk category of BL characterized by normal LDH plus WHO performance status 0 or 1 plus Ann Arbor stage 1 or 2 plus no mass >7 cm (or 10 cm) [29] or no more than 2 extranodal localizations [30]. Some studies also take into account whether or not the tumor has been resected [31–33].

7.5 History of Burkitt Lymphoma Therapeutics

Historically, in early BL therapeutics, the high tumor proliferation rate of the disease and the risk of "kinetic" failures in between treatment cycles were considered to be key to address and overcome for curative therapy. Early strategies therefore were modeled on approaches that had been successful in children with ALL—these had used short-duration, dose-intensive, multi-agent regimens. Today's standard approaches therefore typically include multiple chemotherapy agents given in alternating cycles. Given the aggressiveness of "standard" BL approaches, treatment-related toxicity is a huge challenge, and while children and young adults can tolerate this, tolerance is much more difficult for older or immunosuppressed adults [34]. This difficulty in tolerating therapy led to the testing of risk-adaptive therapy, and while this has been somewhat helpful, there remains great room for improvement in BL therapeutics in the sense of developing less toxic approaches while maintaining traditional high cure rates [30]. The risk of developing tumor lysis syndrome (TLS) and CNS spread of disease are also important to consider. Many regimens, in an attempt to reduce the risk of TLS, employ a "pre-phase" where relatively low doses of chemotherapy drugs (typically cyclophosphamide) and prednisone are given. High-dose intravenous methotrexate and cytarabine (as well as intrathecal administration of these agents), both of which have CNS penetration, are frequently administered in an attempt to reduce CNS spread. Over the recent years, one important advance in BL therapeutics has been to eliminate prophylactic whole-brain radiation, and this of course has significantly reduced CNS toxicity. Some have questioned whether or not patients with low-risk BL require intrathecal therapy, and one study in patients with low-risk disease demonstrated a high cure rate and very low rate of CNS relapse without the use of this [33].

7.6 Current Treatment Approaches

Compared to DLBCL, BL is very rare in adults with a paucity of clinical trials performed. Therefore, the optimal approach to newly diagnosed patients is controversial, particularly in middle-aged and older adults where toxicity poses a significant challenge to successful therapeutic outcomes [35]. Many of the standard approaches that are used in adults today were initially developed in children, given that BL is much more common in pediatric populations (Table 7.2). An early risk-adapted strategy in children with BL and L3 ALL (LMB89) was developed by the Societe Francaise d'Oncologie Pediatrique (SOFP) group—in this approach, treatment was based on tumor burden and early response to chemotherapy [36]. Three risk groups (A, B, and C) were defined with group A receiving induction only; group B receiving pre-phase, induction, consolidation, and limited maintenance; and group C receiving extended maintenance and cranial irradiation in cases with involvement of the CNS. In groups B and C, if a CR was not achieved after the third or fourth induction-consolidation course, autologous stem cell transplant was performed. This strategy was very successful with 5-year event-free and overall survivals of 92%, and this led to testing of the strategy in adults with minor modifications—in 72 adult patients with a median age of 33 years, EFS and OS at 2 years were 65% and 70%, respectively [37]. The Berlin-Frankfurt-Munster (BFM) group developed approaches that reduced number of cycles based on risk stratification—the BFM 90 protocol continued to further refine risk stratification and to improve the outcome of patients who had an incomplete initial response with further treatment intensification. In their study, among 266 pediatric patients with BL, the overall EFS was 89% at 6 years [38].

CODOX-M/IVAC, which is commonly used today, was developed at the National Cancer Institute (NCI), and in initial studies, patients were risk-stratified according to their clinical

Table 7.2 Selected regimens for high-risk Burkitt lymphoma

Regimen	Pt No.	Histology	Median age years (range)	Stage (%)	CR (%)	EFS (%)	OS (%)
LMB 89 [36]	561	Burkitt B-ALL	8 (0.17–18)	III–IV 79%	97%	92% @ 5 years	92% @ 5 years
Modified LMB [37]	72	Burkitt B-ALL	33 (18–76)	III–IV 67%	72%	65% @ 2 years	70% @ 2 years
BFM 90 [38]	413	Burkitt B-ALL	9 (1.2–17.9)	III–IV 60%	N/A	89% @ 6 years	14 deaths
CODOX-M/ IVAC [39]	21 peds 20 adult	Burkitt B-ALL	12 (3–17) 25 (18–59)	III–IV 78%	95%	85% (peds) and 100% (adults) @ 2 years	2 deaths
CODOX-M/ IVAC [30]	52	Burkitt	35 (15–60)	III–IV 61%	77%	65% @ 2 years	73% @ 2 years
Hyper-CVAD [40]	26	Burkitt/B-ALL	58 (17–79)	N/A	81%	61% @ 3 years for DFS	49% @ 3 years
R-Hyper-CVAD [41]	31	Burkitt/B-ALL	46 (17–77)	N/A	86%	80% @ 3 years	89% @ 3 years
GMALL-B-ALL/ NHL 2002 [42]	363	Burkitt B-ALL	42 (16–85)	III–IV 71%	88%	PFS 75% @ 5 years	80% @ 5 years
DA-EPOCH-R [32]	19	Burkitt	25 (15–88)	III–IV 58%	N/A	FFP 95% @ 7 years	100% @ 7 years
SC-EPOCH-RR [32]	11	Burkitt HIV+	44 (24–60)	III–IV 82%	N/A	FFP 100% @ 6 years	90% @ 6 years
LMB +/– R [43]	260	Burkitt	N/A	III–IV 62%	N/A	EFS 75% vs. 62% (+R/–R) @ 3 years	83% vs. 70% (+R/–R) @ 3 years
AMC 048 [44] Modified R-CODOX-M/ IVAC	34	Burkitt HIV+	42 (19–55)	III–IV 74%	N/A	PFS 69% @ 1 year	69% @ 2 years
Modified R-CODOX-M/ IVAC	128	Burkitt HIV–	47 (IQR 31–59)	III–IV (62%)	N/A	EFS 75% @ 3 years	83% @ 3 years
RA-DA-EPOCH-R [35, 45]	112	Burkitt HIV– + HIV+	46 (19–86)	III–IV 69%	N/A	PFS 85% @ 3 years	85% @ 3 years

presentation and LDH [39]. All patients with either a single extra-abdominal mass <10 cm or completely resected abdominal disease with a normal LDH were considered to be low risk. All other patients were designated high risk. While low-risk patients received 3 cycles of CODOX-M (cyclophosphamide, doxorubicin, vincristine, methotrexate), high-risk patients received 4 cycles of alternating CODOX-M with IVAC (ifosfamide, cytarabine, and etoposide)—in 41 patients including 20 adults with a median age of 25 years, the event-free survival (EFS) was 92% at 2 years. Hematological toxicities were significant with sepsis occurring in 22% of cycles. Other groups confirmed the efficacy of this regimen although lower survival rates were observed. Mead and colleagues studied this approach in 52 adult patients with a median age of 35 years [30]. The overall EFS was 65% at 2 years and 83% and 59% for the low-risk and high-risk arms, respectively. A modified Magrath regimen has been tested in older adults and was effective and well tolerated. Hyper-CVAD was based on a modification of a regimen developed by Murphy et al. for pediatric

L3 ALL [40, 41]. Hyper-fractionated cyclophosphamide, vincristine, doxorubicin, and dexamethasone were alternated with methotrexate and cytarabine for a total of 8 cycles—in a study of 26 patients with BL and B-ALL (acute lymphoblastic lymphoma), the 3-year OS was 49% [40]. A later study combined the regimen with rituximab, and in 31 similar population patients, OS was 89% at 3 years [41]. While it has been explored in a number of studies, the role of consolidation autologous stem cell transplantation in BL is unclear with no convincing data that it is helpful.

Though "standard" strategies are highly effective in children and younger adults, in other populations, toxicity is excessive with these approaches, and new strategies are needed. Rituximab improves the cure rate in diffuse large B-cell lymphoma, and this prompted its testing in BL. In a recently published randomized study of 260 adults who received an LMB regimen with or without rituximab, at 38-month follow-up, the EFS was significantly higher in the group that received rituximab (75% vs. 62%; $p = 0.02$) [43]. In single-arm studies, when rituximab has been incorporated into "standard" intensive BL regimens, survival was superior compared to historical non-rituximab-containing arms [42].

The dose-adjusted EPOCH-R (etoposide, prednisone, vincristine, cyclophosphamide, doxorubicin, and rituximab) regimen is an intermediate intensity strategy that was tested in BL, due to its high efficacy in DLBCL, and the hypothesis that the high sensitivity of BL cells to genotoxic stress makes prolonged exposure time an important therapeutic strategy for optimizing tumor cell kill. An initial study testing the strategy in 30 patients with sporadic and immunodeficiency-associated BL demonstrated a freedom from progression exceeding 90%. To validate these results in a multicenter setting, a study is currently underway in which low-risk patients (all of stage I or II disease, normal LDH, ECOG performance status of 0–1, and mass size <7 cm) receive three cycles of therapy and high-risk (all other) patients receive six. A recent report of this study (which has finished accrual) in 112 patients demonstrated a PFS of 100% and 82% in low-risk and high-risk groups, respectively, at 34-month follow-up [45]. Older age or HIV status had an impact on outcome, and toxicity was low with very few patients developing tumor lysis syndrome. A multigroup randomized trial comparing DA-EPOCH-R versus R-CODOX-M/R-IVAC is currently recruiting in Europe.

7.7 Approach to Relapsed Burkitt Lymphoma

Treatment of BL in the relapsed or refractory setting is challenging and typically associated with very poor outcomes [46]. While some early-stage patients with relapse following limited treatment may still be curable, this is unlikely to be the case with advanced-stage patients who have received intensive treatment or are primary induction failures. The European Group for Blood and Marrow Transplantation (EBMT) in a retrospective review reported an OS of 37% at 3 years for patients with a chemosensitive relapse but only 7% for those with resistant disease following autologous SCT [47]. The ASBMT reported data on transplantation in 241 BL patients. For relapsed patient in second or later complete remission, 5-year OS was 44% for patients who received autologous SCT and 27% for those who received allogeneic SCT. For refractory patients 5-year OS was 22% for autologous and 12% for allogeneic stem cell transplantation recipients [48]. Although these data are retrospective and subject to selection bias, stem cell transplantation may be considered as a therapeutic strategy for a subgroup of patients.

7.8 HIV-Associated Burkitt Lymphoma

BL is not uncommon in the setting of HIV infection where it constitutes up to 20% of HIV-associated lymphomas and typically occurs with higher median CD4 counts than many other lymphomas that are encountered in the HIV setting. Offsetting historical reports, recent studies in HIV-associated BL report excellent outcomes for this population [44, 45, 49, 50].

HIV-associated BL presents in a similar fashion to sporadic BL and has variable association with EBV. As with middle-aged and older adults, standard full-dose BL regimens are generally considered too toxic for patients with HIV-associated BL, and as a result, less toxic modifications of approaches such as CODOX-M/IVAC-R have been investigated. Recently, the AIDS Malignancy Consortium (AMC) evaluated the outcome of 27 patients following modified CODOX-M/IVAC-rituximab and demonstrated a 1-year PFS of 69% [44]. DA-EPOCH-R is very well tolerated in this group of patients and associated with excellent outcomes—as mentioned previously, it is being investigated in a multicenter study, and an initial report demonstrated no inferiority in outcome in HIV-positive versus HIV-negative patients [35]. These recent experiences reinforce that HIV positivity should not be a negative prognostic factor in BL patients.

7.9 Future Directions and Conclusions

While pediatric patients and young adults with BL have an excellent outcome with "standard" BL regimens, high treatment toxicity is a significant issue, and future strategies should focus on reducing toxicity while maintaining very high cure rates. For most adults and immunosuppressed patients with the disease, some intermediate intensity approaches are much better tolerated, and as long as they do not compromise curability rates, they should be selected. While the role of *MYC* in BL has been recognized for some time, recent molecular insights have identified several novel genetic aberrations that have critical roles in lymphomagenesis and cooperate with *MYC*. *TCF3* and *ID3* which are rarely found in DLBCL are present in 70% of sporadic BL—additionally, the *CCND3* gene, which is activated by *TCF3* and interacts with *CDK6*, is mutated in a high percentage of BL cases. These novel genomic findings are a good rationale for investigating novel agents such as PI3 kinase inhibitors and inhibitors of *CDK6* as well as inhibitors of *MYC*. If novel agents can be incorporated into up-front BL regimens, they offer the possibility of optimal strategies with less reliance on very toxic agents. CAR T-cell anti-CD19 therapy, which is of course very effective in childhood ALL, is another very interesting approach and, given the biological similarity of BL and ALL, should be tested in relapsed/refractory BL [51].

References

1. Burkitt D. A sarcoma involving the jaws in African children. Br J Surg. 1958;46(197):218–23.
2. Kelly GL, Rickinson AB. Burkitt lymphoma: revisiting the pathogenesis of a virus-associated malignancy. Hematology Am Soc Hematol Educ Program. 2007:277–84.
3. Heslop HE. Biology and treatment of Epstein-Barr virus-associated non-Hodgkin lymphomas. Hematology Am Soc Hematol Educ Program. 2005:260–6.
4. Shimizu N, Tanabe-Tochikura A, Kuroiwa Y, Takada K. Isolation of Epstein-Barr virus (EBV)-negative cell clones from the EBV-positive Burkitt's lymphoma (BL) line Akata: malignant phenotypes of BL cells are dependent on EBV. J Virol. 1994;68(9):6069–73.
5. Komano J, Sugiura M, Takada K. Epstein-Barr virus contributes to the malignant phenotype and to apoptosis resistance in Burkitt's lymphoma cell line Akata. J Virol. 1998;72(11):9150–6.
6. Kamranvar SA, Gruhne B, Szeles A, Masucci MG. Epstein-Barr virus promotes genomic instability in Burkitt's lymphoma. Oncogene. 2007;26(35):5115–23.
7. Kelly GL, Milner AE, Baldwin GS, Bell AI, Rickinson AB. Three restricted forms of Epstein-Barr virus latency counteracting apoptosis in c-myc-expressing Burkitt lymphoma cells. Proc Natl Acad Sci U S A. 2006;103(40):14935–40.
8. Robbiani DF, Deroubaix S, Feldhahn N, Oliveira TY, Callen E, Wang Q, et al. Plasmodium infection promotes genomic instability and AID-dependent B cell lymphoma. Cell. 2015;162(4):727–37.
9. Rochford R, Cannon MJ, Moormann AM. Endemic Burkitt's lymphoma: a polymicrobial disease? Nat Rev Microbiol. 2005;3(2):182–7.
10. Chene A, Donati D, Orem J, Mbidde ER, Kironde F, Wahlgren M, et al. Endemic Burkitt's lymphoma as a polymicrobial disease: new insights on the interaction between Plasmodium falciparum and Epstein-Barr virus. Semin Cancer Biol. 2009;19(6):411–20.
11. Dalla-Favera R, Bregni M, Erikson J, Patterson D, Gallo RC, Croce CM. Human c-myc onc gene is located on the region of chromosome 8 that is translo-

cated in Burkitt lymphoma cells. Proc Natl Acad Sci U S A. 1982;79(24):7824–7.
12. Burotto M, Berkovits A, Dunleavy K. Double hit lymphoma: from biology to therapeutic implications. Expert Rev Hematol. 2016;9(7):669–78.
13. Lenze D, Leoncini L, Hummel M, Volinia S, Liu CG, Amato T, et al. The different epidemiologic subtypes of Burkitt lymphoma share a homogenous micro RNA profile distinct from diffuse large B-cell lymphoma. Leukemia. 2011;25(12):1869–76.
14. Piccaluga PP, De Falco G, Kustagi M, Gazzola A, Agostinelli C, Tripodo C, et al. Gene expression analysis uncovers similarity and differences among Burkitt lymphoma subtypes. Blood. 2011;117(13):3596–608.
15. Schmitz R, Young RM, Ceribelli M, Jhavar S, Xiao W, Zhang M, et al. Burkitt lymphoma pathogenesis and therapeutic targets from structural and functional genomics. Nature. 2012;490(7418):116–20.
16. Love C, Sun Z, Jima D, Li G, Zhang J, Miles R, et al. The genetic landscape of mutations in Burkitt lymphoma. Nat Genet. 2012;44(12):1321–5.
17. Richter J, Schlesner M, Hoffmann S, Kreuz M, Leich E, Burkhardt B, et al. Recurrent mutation of the ID3 gene in Burkitt lymphoma identified by integrated genome, exome and transcriptome sequencing. Nat Genet. 2012;44(12):1316–20.
18. Rohde M, Bonn BR, Zimmermann M, Lange J, Moricke A, Klapper W, et al. Relevance of ID3-TCF3-CCND3 pathway mutations in pediatric aggressive B-cell lymphoma treated according to the non-Hodgkin lymphoma Berlin-Frankfurt-Munster protocols. Haematologica. 2017;102(6):1091–8.
19. Campo E. New pathogenic mechanisms in Burkitt lymphoma. Nat Genet. 2012;44(12):1288–9.
20. Dave SS, Fu K, Wright GW, Lam LT, Kluin P, Boerma EJ, et al. Molecular diagnosis of Burkitt's lymphoma. N Engl J Med. 2006;354(23):2431–42.
21. Hummel M, Bentink S, Berger H, Klapper W, Wessendorf S, Barth TF, et al. A biologic definition of Burkitt's lymphoma from transcriptional and genomic profiling. N Engl J Med. 2006;354(23):2419–30.
22. Swerdlow SH, Campo E, Pileri SA, Harris NL, Stein H, Siebert R, et al. The 2016 revision of the World Health Organization classification of lymphoid neoplasms. Blood. 2016;127(20):2375–90.
23. Salaverria I, Martin-Guerrero I, Wagener R, Kreuz M, Kohler CW, Richter J, et al. A recurrent 11q aberration pattern characterizes a subset of MYC-negative high-grade B-cell lymphomas resembling Burkitt lymphoma. Blood. 2014;123(8):1187–98.
24. Ferreiro JF, Morscio J, Dierickx D, Marcelis L, Verhoef G, Vandenberghe P, et al. Post-transplant molecularly defined Burkitt lymphomas are frequently MYC-negative and characterized by the 11q-gain/loss pattern. Haematologica. 2015;100(7):e275–9.
25. Castillo JJ, Nadeem O. Improving the accuracy in prognosis for Burkitt lymphoma patients. Expert Rev Anticancer Ther. 2014;14(2):125–7.
26. Castillo JJ, Winer ES, Olszewski AJ. Population-based prognostic factors for survival in patients with Burkitt lymphoma: an analysis from the surveillance, epidemiology, and end results database. Cancer. 2013;119(20):3672–9.
27. Wasterlid T, Brown PN, Hagberg O, Hagberg H, Pedersen LM, D'Amore F, et al. Impact of chemotherapy regimen and rituximab in adult Burkitt lymphoma: a retrospective population-based study from the Nordic Lymphoma Group. Ann Oncol. 2013;24(7):1879–86.
28. Wasterlid T, Jonsson B, Hagberg H, Jerkeman M. Population based study of prognostic factors and treatment in adult Burkitt lymphoma: a Swedish Lymphoma Registry study. Leuk Lymphoma. 2011;52(11):2090–6.
29. Mead GM, Sydes MR, Walewski J, Grigg A, Hatton CS, Pescosta N, et al. An international evaluation of CODOX-M and CODOX-M alternating with IVAC in adult Burkitt's lymphoma: results of United Kingdom Lymphoma Group LY06 study. Ann Oncol. 2002;13(8):1264–74.
30. Mead GM, Barrans SL, Qian W, Walewski J, Radford JA, Wolf M, et al. A prospective clinicopathologic study of dose-modified CODOX-M/IVAC in patients with sporadic Burkitt lymphoma defined using cytogenetic and immunophenotypic criteria (MRC/NCRI LY10 trial). Blood. 2008;112(6):2248–60.
31. Barnes JA, Lacasce AS, Feng Y, Toomey CE, Neuberg D, Michaelson JS, et al. Evaluation of the addition of rituximab to CODOX-M/IVAC for Burkitt's lymphoma: a retrospective analysis. Ann Oncol. 2011;22(8):1859–64.
32. Dunleavy K, Pittaluga S, Shovlin M, Steinberg SM, Cole D, Grant C, et al. Low-intensity therapy in adults with Burkitt's lymphoma. N Engl J Med. 2013;369(20):1915–25.
33. Gerrard M, Cairo MS, Weston C, Auperin A, Pinkerton R, Lambilliote A, et al. Excellent survival following two courses of COPAD chemotherapy in children and adolescents with resected localized B-cell non-Hodgkin's lymphoma: results of the FAB/LMB 96 international study. Br J Haematol. 2008;141(6):840–7.
34. Corazzelli G, Frigeri F, Russo F, Frairia C, Arcamone M, Esposito G, et al. RD-CODOX-M/IVAC with rituximab and intrathecal liposomal cytarabine in adult Burkitt lymphoma and 'unclassifiable' highly aggressive B-cell lymphoma. Br J Haematol. 2012;156(2):234–44.
35. Dunleavy K, Little RF, Wilson WH. Update on Burkitt lymphoma. Hematol Oncol Clin North Am. 2016;30(6):1333–43.
36. Patte C, Auperin A, Michon J, Behrendt H, Leverger G, Frappaz D, et al. The Societe Francaise d'Oncologie Pediatrique LMB89 protocol: highly effective multiagent chemotherapy tailored to the tumor burden and initial response in 561 unselected children with B-cell lymphomas and L3 leukemia. Blood. 2001;97(11):3370–9.

37. Divine M, Casassus P, Koscielny S, Bosq J, Sebban C, Le Maignan C, et al. Burkitt lymphoma in adults: a prospective study of 72 patients treated with an adapted pediatric LMB protocol. Ann Oncol. 2005;16(12):1928–35.
38. Reiter A, Schrappe M, Tiemann M, Ludwig WD, Yakisan E, Zimmermann M, et al. Improved treatment results in childhood B-cell neoplasms with tailored intensification of therapy: a report of the Berlin-Frankfurt-Munster group trial NHL-BFM 90. Blood. 1999;94(10):3294–306.
39. Magrath I, Adde M, Shad A, Venzon D, Seibel N, Gootenberg J, et al. Adults and children with small non-cleaved-cell lymphoma have a similar excellent outcome when treated with the same chemotherapy regimen. J Clin Oncol Off J Am Soc Clin Oncol. 1996;14(3):925–34.
40. Thomas DA, Cortes J, O'Brien S, Pierce S, Faderl S, Albitar M, et al. Hyper-CVAD program in Burkitt's-type adult acute lymphoblastic leukemia. J Clin Oncol Off J Am Soc Clin Oncol. 1999;17(8):2461–70.
41. Thomas DA, Faderl S, O'Brien S, Bueso-Ramos C, Cortes J, Garcia-Manero G, et al. Chemoimmunotherapy with hyper-CVAD plus rituximab for the treatment of adult Burkitt and Burkitt-type lymphoma or acute lymphoblastic leukemia. Cancer. 2006;106(7):1569–80.
42. Hoelzer D, Walewski J, Dohner H, Viardot A, Hiddemann W, Spiekermann K, et al. Improved outcome of adult Burkitt lymphoma/leukemia with rituximab and chemotherapy: report of a large prospective multicenter trial. Blood. 2014;124(26):3870–9.
43. Ribrag V, Koscielny S, Bosq J, Leguay T, Casasnovas O, Fornecker LM, et al. Rituximab and dose-dense chemotherapy for adults with Burkitt's lymphoma: a randomised, controlled, open-label, phase 3 trial. Lancet. 2016;387(10036):2402–11.
44. Noy A, Lee JY, Cesarman E, Ambinder R, Baiocchi R, Reid E, et al. AMC 048: modified CODOX-M/IVAC-rituximab is safe and effective for HIV-associated Burkitt lymphoma. Blood. 2015;126(2):160–6.
45. Dunleavy K, Roschewski M, Abramson JS, Link B, Parekh S, Jagadeesh D, et al. Risk-adapted therapy in adults with Burkitt lymphoma: updated results of a multi-center prospective phase II study of DA-EPOCH-R. Hematol Oncol. 2017;35(S2):133–4.
46. Short NJ, Kantarjian HM, Ko H, Khoury JD, Ravandi F, Thomas DA, et al. Outcomes of adults with relapsed or refractory Burkitt and high-grade B-cell leukemia/lymphoma. Am J Hematol. 2017;92(6):E114–E7.
47. Sweetenham JW, Pearce R, Taghipour G, Blaise D, Gisselbrecht C, Goldstone AH. Adult Burkitt's and Burkitt-like non-Hodgkin's lymphoma—outcome for patients treated with high-dose therapy and autologous stem-cell transplantation in first remission or at relapse: results from the European Group for Blood and Marrow Transplantation. J Clin Oncol. 1996;14(9):2465–72.
48. Maramattom LV, Hari PN, Burns LJ, Carreras J, Arcese W, Cairo MS, et al. Autologous and allogeneic transplantation for burkitt lymphoma outcomes and changes in utilization: a report from the center for international blood and marrow transplant research. Biology Blood Marrow Transplant. 2013;19(2):173–9.
49. Little RF, Pittaluga S, Grant N, Steinberg SM, Kavlick MF, Mitsuya H, et al. Highly effective treatment of acquired immunodeficiency syndrome-related lymphoma with dose-adjusted EPOCH: impact of antiretroviral therapy suspension and tumor biology. Blood. 2003;101(12):4653–9.
50. Dunleavy K, Pittaluga S, Maeda LS, Advani R, Chen CC, Hessler J, et al. Dose-adjusted EPOCH-rituximab therapy in primary mediastinal B-cell lymphoma. N Engl J Med. 2013;368(15):1408–16.
51. Kochenderfer JN, Somerville RPT, Lu T, Shi V, Bot A, Rossi J, et al. Lymphoma remissions caused by anti-CD19 chimeric antigen receptor T cells are associated with high serum Interleukin-15 levels. J Clin Oncol. 2017;35(16):1803–13.

Human Immunodeficiency Virus-Related Lymphomas

8

Josep-Maria Ribera and Richard F. Little

8.1 Background

The acquired immunodeficiency syndrome (AIDS) was first described in 1981, in individuals with certain opportunistic infections (OI), Kaposi sarcoma, and central nervous system (CNS) lymphomas. Three years later the clinical spectrum of non-Hodgkin lymphomas (NHL) in the populations at risk of AIDS was first described [1, 2]. Since the introduction of combined antiretroviral therapy (cART) in the mid-1990s, the incidence of lymphomas, which formerly accounted for 2–3% of newly diagnosed AIDS patients, has decreased and outcomes have improved [3]. Simultaneously, a shift toward histologies that occur at higher CD4 lymphocyte counts, such as Burkitt lymphoma and classical Hodgkin lymphoma (cHL), was observed [4–7]. The increasing proportion of long-term survivors of lymphoma has raised the possibility of developing certain non-AIDS-defining solid tumors, especially those related to the lifestyle and viral infections in HIV-infected patients.

J.-M. Ribera (✉)
Clinical Hematology Department, ICO-Hospital Germans Trias i Pujol, Jose Carreras Research Institute, Badalona, Universitat Autònoma de Barcelona, Barcelona, Spain
e-mail: jribera@iconcologia.net

R. F. Little
Clinical Investigations Branch, Cancer Therapy Evaluation Program, National Cancer Institute, Bethesda, MD, USA
e-mail: Littler@mail.nih.gov

8.2 Epidemiology

The risk of lymphoid tumors in HIV disease is highly linked to the CD4+ T-cell count [8, 9]. The incidence of NHL has decreased approximately 80% in the cART era, with the greatest decrease occurring among those NHLs that develop in association with advanced immune depletion, such as AIDS-related primary CNS lymphoma [10]. The proposed explanation for this decline is the ability of cART to prevent depletion of CD4+ T-cells, thus decreasing the risk of such tumors. In contrast, those lymphomas that occur at higher CD4+ T-cell counts, such as Burkitt lymphoma, have not changed substantially in incidence since the introduction of cART [8]. The overall relative increase in risk for lymphoma still ranges between 10- and 20-fold higher than in the general population. This risk is similar to that for lymphomas arising in individual with immunosuppression of other origins. cHL incidence has increased since the introduction of cART, further illustrating the complex interaction of immune status with lymphoid malignancy [11]. cHL has 10- to 20-fold higher risk in comparison with the general population, but this increased risk is not

G. Lenz, G. Salles (eds.), *Aggressive Lymphomas*, Hematologic Malignancies,
https://doi.org/10.1007/978-3-030-00362-3_8

consistently observed across cHL subtypes, and there has been a shift over the cART era in subtype presentation. In the pre-cART era, mixed cellularity cHL accounted for the majority of cases. In the cART era, there has been a shift so that there is nearly equal presentation of mixed cellularity and nodular sclerosing cHL [12]. Lymphoma is currently the most frequent malignancy among HIV-infected individuals and a frequent neoplastic cause of death in these patients [13].

The diagnosis of AIDS precedes the onset of NHL in less than 50% of the patients, and the simultaneous diagnosis of NHL and HIV positivity is currently relatively frequent. The geographic distribution of NHL lymphomas is similar to the geographic spread of HIV infection, and the incidence is similar for all risk groups for HIV infection.

8.3 Pathogenesis

Although AIDS-related lymphomas are usually of B-cell origin as demonstrated by immunoglobulin heavy-chain gene rearrangement studies, they have also been shown to be oligoclonal, polyclonal, and monoclonal in origin. Although HIV is a risk factor for a variety of cancers, it does not appear to be directly implicated in lymphomagenesis. HIV indirectly creates an environment in which chronic antigen stimulation, cytokine dysregulation, and coinfection with oncogenic viruses, such as the Epstein-Barr virus (EBV), are involved, within the setting of genetic abnormalities and impaired immune surveillance. All these factors can lead to the emergence of monoclonal B cells. Impaired T-cell immunity toward EBV is strongly implicated in lymphomagenesis, especially in some aggressive lymphomas such as the immunoblastic and plasmablastic subtype [14, 15].

Infection by human herpesvirus 8 (HHV-8) or Kaposi sarcoma herpesvirus (KSHV) is frequently observed in HIV-infected patients with primary effusion lymphoma (PEL) [16], and the combined presence of EBV and HHV-8 appears to be unique to PEL [17]. Other lymphoproliferative disorders in HIV-infected patients involving HHV-8 include multicentric Castleman disease (MCD) and HHV8-positive plasmablastic lymphoma (PBL) [18].

8.4 Pathology

Traditionally, human immunodeficiency virus (HIV)-associated lymphomas have been categorized as follows: (1) aggressive B-cell lymphomas (diffuse large B-cell lymphoma [DLBCL], Burkitt lymphoma [BL], aggressive B-cell lymphoma with *MYC* and *BCL-2* and/or *BCL-6* rearrangements, PBL, and PEL), (2) primary central nervous system lymphoma (PCNSL), (3) classical HL, and (4) DLBCL arising in HHV-8-associated MCD [19]. The revised WHO classification of tumors is agnostic to HIV status [20]. Importantly, the updated classification is informed to some extent by molecular features relevant to treatment. For example, advances in treatment may soon include specific therapies according to DLBCL subtype. Definitive phase III clinical trials of lenalidomide and ibrutinib in activated B-cell subtype DLBCL are ongoing and may inform a new standard of care for this disease. Studies sponsored by the US National Cancer Institute to determine feasibility of combining these agents with chemotherapy in patients with HIV on cART are ongoing, positioning patients with these diseases to be availed of new therapeutics as defined by phase III trials in the background population.

DLBCL is still the most frequent NHL subtype. Most cases are of the germinal center variant assessed by immunohistochemistry methods [21, 22], whereas the frequency using digital multiplexed gene expression remains to be validated [23, 24]. Burkitt lymphoma (BL) is the second subtype in frequency and is similar to sporadic BL with variable association with EBV [25]. The high-grade B-cell lymphomas with *MYC* and *BCL-2* and/or *BCL-6* rearrangements (also known as dual hit or triple hit according to the presence of two or the three rearrangements) account for 5–10% of cases with DLBCL and are highly aggressive with poor response to standard therapies [26]. Primary DLBCL of the central nervous system (CNS) that are truly

AIDS-related occur at CD4+ T-cell levels of less than 50/mm^3, and essentially 100% are EBV positive [20, 27]. In the cART era, primary DLBCL in CNS are rarely seen. Among patients with over 100 CD4+ T-cell cells/mm^3, the occurrence of PCNSL in over 23,000 HIV-infected patients is not documented [6, 28].

PEL is a very aggressive malignancy, being first reported in the oral cavity of HIV-infected individuals. Subsequently, it has been shown to occur in other sites as well as in conjunction with other immunodeficient states. PEL comprises about 4% of all HIV-related NHL and usually involves patients with advanced immunosuppression, with a CD4 count less than 150 cells/mm^3 and a history of prior AIDS-defining illnesses. The immunophenotype of these lymphomas resembles that of plasma cells. More than 80% of cases are EBV positive, and approximately half have been shown to have the *MYC* translocation [29].

Lymphomas arising in HHV-8-associated MCD are very rare lymphomas and mainly occur in HIV-positive patients [30]. They are difficult to distinguish from PEL. Characteristically, they are HHV-8 positive but EBV negative, express IgMλ cytoplasmic immunoglobulin, and appear within the setting of MCD in the lymph nodes involved.

While not considered to be an AIDS-defining malignancy, cHL is increased in incidence in HIV-infected individuals and may surpass AIDS-NHL in frequency in some populations, especially in those with longer life expectancies and better immunological control with cART. In the pre-cART era, in contrast to non-immunosuppressed patients, HIV-related cHL was accompanied by EBV infection in close to 90% of cases, and the mixed cellularity or lymphocyte-depleted forms comprised a larger number of cases [31]. In populations where cART is widely available, these differences are much less pronounced [12].

8.5 Clinical Presentation, Diagnosis, and Staging

In the pre-cART era, the clinical setting of patients with AIDS-related lymphoma was very different from that of non-HIV patients and was characterized by advanced-stage disease and frequently extranodal involvement, including unusual sites. Currently the clinical picture resembles that of non-HIV-infected patients, especially for the lymphoma subtypes associated with improved CD4+ lymphocyte counts, although a trend to more disseminated disease and extranodal involvement still persists [32].

An excisional lymph node or tissue biopsy is required for the diagnosis of HIV-related lymphomas. Morphologic, cytogenetic, and molecular studies should be performed to obtain a high-precision diagnosis, and the biologic material should be stored for future studies. Assessment of EBV and HHV-8 virus in lymphoma cells is highly recommended. Diagnoses based exclusively on fine needle aspiration of tumor masses should be avoided. Certain confounding factors such as HIV-related reactive lymphadenopathy and an increased incidence of infections may make the interpretation of 18 F-fluorodeoxyglucose positron emission tomography (FDG-PET) scans more difficult than in the HIV-negative population, especially in patients with detectable HIV viral loads. Gadolinium-enhanced magnetic resonance imaging (MRI), ^{201}thallium single-photon emission computed tomography (^{201}Th-SPECT), or FDG-PET scan, combined with cytology, flow cytometry, and a polymerase chain reaction (PCR) method to detect EBV-DNA in cerebrospinal fluid (CSF), are helpful for the diagnosis of PCNSL and to differentiate between PCNSL and cerebral toxoplasmosis. Immediate definitive diagnosis with stereotactic biopsy, as is the standard of care in the non-HIV setting, is essential to optimize therapeutic outcome. In the pre-cART era, biopsy was delayed or even omitted in patients presenting with ring-enhancing brain lesions. A presumptive lymphoma diagnosis was made for those not responding to a short course of anti-toxoplasma treatment. This is no longer a justified practice.

The Ann Arbor/Cotswolds and the Lugano [33, 34] staging systems are commonly used for patients with NHL and HL. HIV viral load and CD4 lymphocyte count should be added to the usual procedures to assess the stage. Serologic studies for hepatitis B and C virus, cytomegalovirus, EBV, *Toxoplasma*, and varicella-zoster are also highly recommended. A detailed HIV history including assessment of prior opportunistic infections (OI), general immune function, antiretroviral treatment history, and HIV control should be obtained. Additionally, cardiac function should be assessed in selected cases with either a cardiac multigated acquisition (MUGA) scan or an echocardiogram before treatment planning.

8.6 Prognostic Factors

The prognosis of HIV-infected individuals with lymphoma is determined by patient-, lymphoma-, and HIV-specific factors [35]. The significance for each of these factors has varied over the last three decades due to changes in antiretroviral and lymphoma-directed therapy, improved supportive care, and a shift in the incidence and biology of lymphoma.

Since effective HIV control has become achievable, adequate lymphoma-directed therapy is possible in the contemporary cART era, and survival is now similar to that observed in immunocompetent patients. Hence, the International Prognostic Index (IPI) [36] and age-adjusted IPI have been extensively validated and remain reliable predictors of outcomes in HIV-related aggressive NHL. Similarly, the International Prognostic Score (IPS) [37] has shown prognostic relevance in HIV-associated cHL, although this prognostic significance was not observed in all studies. With regard to the impact of HIV-related factors on survival, low CD4 counts have been implicated as predictors of poor survival in several studies, while other reports have not found this association, especially in the cART era [38].

Composite scores including patient-, lymphoma-, and HIV-related factors have been developed. Of these, the combined AIDS-related lymphoma IPI (ARL-IPI) score for patients with DLBCL, which consists of prior history of AIDS, baseline CD4 count, and viral load, and the age-adjusted IPI is a better predictor of survival than the age-adjusted IPI alone [39]. Of note, in this analysis, the 5-year overall survival (OS) was 78% for the low-risk group, which is similar to outcomes described in HIV-negative patients with DLBCL. The prognostic value of other biologic parameters (e.g., germinal center vs. activated B-cell phenotype, EBV, or Bcl-2 expression) is less consistent and varies among the different studies.

Similarly, a composite score for HIV-related HL developed in six European countries includes two parameters independently associated with OS: CD4 counts <200 cells/mm^3 and IPS >2. A retrospective multicenter study of 229 advanced HIV-HL patients who had received ABVD plus cART showed CD4 cell counts <200/mm^3 to be an independent adverse prognostic factor for PFS and OS [40].

8.7 Treatment of HIV-Related Lymphomas

8.7.1 General Principles

In the cART era, the treatment of the specific subtypes of HIV-related lymphomas is similar or identical to that used for lymphomas arising in non- immunosuppressed patients, but the treatment recommendations are mostly based on evidence from phase II trials, retrospective series, or expert opinion [3, 41]. In addition, several specific aspects should be considered, being the concomitant antiretroviral therapy and the prophylaxis and eventual treatment of opportunistic infections (OI) the most relevant.

8.7.2 Diffuse Large B-Cell Lymphomas

Several phase II studies conducted in Europe and the USA have shown promising results with the combination of the anti-CD20 monoclonal antibody rituximab with chemotherapy schedules, such as CHOP (R-CHOP) [42] or infusional regimens such as CDE (cyclophosphamide, doxorubicin, and etoposide) (R-CDE) [43] or EPOCH (etoposide, prednisone, vincristine, cyclophosphamide, and doxorubicin) (R-EPOCH) [44].

Although the only phase III trial comparing CHOP vs. R-CHOP showed negative results for overall and progression-free survivals, the response was superior for R-CHOP [45]. The lack of survival benefit was attributed to the high treatment-related mortality of 36% for patients with a CD4 count <50 cells/mm^3 in the R-CHOP group and the lower than expected response rate in the whole group compared with that observed in other trials using R-CHOP. Despite these results, most contemporary trials use rituximab as part of the treatment, but some restrict its use in patients with CD4 counts <50 cells/mm^3. In the AMC034 trial, rituximab was given either consecutively with EPOCH or sequentially (weekly with six doses after completion of chemotherapy). In this "pick-the-winner" phase II trial, only the concurrent arm reached the predefined endpoint, with a CR rate of 73% (71% for DLBCL) versus only 55% in the sequential arm. With concurrent R-EPOCH, the 2-year OS reached 70%, similar to that achieved with R-CHOP or R-CDE regimens.

Based on the evidence from two-pooled clinical trials of 150 patients and a meta-analysis of pooled individual patient data for 1546 patients from 19 prospective clinical trials showing improved overall survival with the infusional EPOCH regimen and with rituximab, many experts and cooperative groups, especially in North America, have adapted six cycles of chemoimmunotherapy with R-EPOCH as their standard initial regimen for the treatment of HIV-positive patients with DLBCL [46]. However, there is no prospective randomized controlled trial comparing the R-EPOCH regimen to others, and in Europe the most used regimen is R-CHOP. Encouragingly, outcomes with initial therapy for HIV-DLBCL are close to those similarly treated for HIV-negative patients in the current era [47]. Of note, preliminary reports from the randomized CALGB phase III trial comparing dose-adjusted EPOCH-R and R-CHOP in the HIV-unrelated setting reported no difference in event-free survival [48, 49]. However, the dose adjustment in the HIV setting is substantially different compared to the phase III approach, limiting the ability to apply those results to the HIV setting.

Several areas of uncertainty remain unsolved due to lack of solid information: first, the treatment of patients in localized stages (I or II non-bulky), for which chemoimmunotherapy with six cycles of R-CHOP or R-EPOCH is generally preferred to three to four courses followed by radiotherapy; second, the use of rituximab in patients with a low CD4 count (<50/mm^3), in whom there are recent trends to use rituximab irrespective of the CD4 count, except in patients with history of prior or ongoing OI and a low likelihood of adequate HIV control with cART due to poor adherence; and third, the concurrent or sequential use of cART during chemotherapy. Possible benefits of concurrent cART include better HIV control leading to fewer infectious complications and AIDS-defining events [50], but these benefits could be counterbalanced by drug-drug interactions leading to either increased toxicities or possible underdosing, resulting in either the emergence of HIV or lymphoma resistance. Although there is no formal consensus, most groups tend to use the concurrent option, except if a short-term chemotherapy schedule is used. Given the availability of newer antiretroviral agents, such as the HIV integrase strand transfer inhibitors that have very little relevant drug-drug interactions, there is little reason to suspend cART while administering cancer chemotherapy, including with the DA-EPOCH-R regimen.

8.7.3 Burkitt Lymphoma

Prior to the advent of effective cART, all HIV NHL, including Burkitt lymphoma, were treated with CHOP-like therapy. Outcomes were dismal. The current therapy of BL in HIV-infected patients is similar or identical to that used in non-immunocompromised patients, based on specific short-term immunochemotherapy regimens. These regimens include rituximab combined with intensive chemotherapy schedules based on high-dose cyclophosphamide and methotrexate, among other cytotoxic drugs (e.g., hyper-CVAD, CODOX-M/IVAC, LMB86, B-ALL/NHL 2002, or BURKIMAB) [51–53]. Although the results are similar to those observed in BL arising in the general population (overall survival of 70–80%), the toxicity (especially mucositis and infections) is higher in HIV-infected patients [54].

In a very different approach from the intensive regimens mentioned above, the US National Cancer Institute has developed effective risk-adapted Burkitt lymphoma therapy based on the EPOCH-R regimen. For low-risk patients (defined as normal LDH, ECOG performance 1–2, stage I–II, and mass <7 cm), the "short-course EPOCH-RR" regimen has shown favorable results. This involves a short course of EPOCH (without dose adjustment: all patients receive a fixed dose of 750 mg of cyclophosphamide) with a double dose of rituximab [55]. Dunleavy et al. reported on 11 patients with HIV infection and BL (none presented CNS involvement) having an excellent OS at 73 months of 92%, which remains unchanged in further updates. In a larger expanded effort, the preliminary report at a median follow-up of 25 months of the first 77 patients of a US National Clinical Trials Network trial of risk-adapted DA-EPOCH-R showed progression-free survival of 87% and overall survival of 88% for all patients. There was no evidence that the 20 HIV+ patients outcome was different that the non-HIV patients [56]. The final results in over 100 patients are expected to be reported soon.

8.7.4 Aggressive B-Cell Lymphoma with MYC and BCL-2 and/or BCL-6 Rearrangements

There is limited experience on treatment of this poor-prognosis subgroup of patients in the HIV setting. The most reasonable option is to mimic the experience of non-immunocompromised patients, in whom the DA-EPOCH-R schedule seems to be the most promising immunochemotherapeutic approach [57].

8.7.5 Plasmablastic Lymphoma

Currently there is no standard of care with respect to chemotherapy in PBL in patients with HIV due to the rarity of the condition and to the fact that most studies have been retrospective in nature. In some studies, the DA-EPOCH regimen offered better results than CHOP, while in others the CODOX-M/IVAC was also superior than CHOP. In any case, the median survival of these patients is short, ranging between 5 and 17 months, making new therapeutic approaches necessary. New drugs such as vorinostat, bortezomib, or ibrutinib in combination with chemotherapy targeting the non-germinal phenotype and oncogenic viruses seem promising, and prolonged survival has been observed in individual cases or short series [58, 59].

8.7.6 Primary Effusion Lymphoma

The optimal treatment for HIV-PEL is undefined. Many patients with HIV-related PEL receive standard combination chemotherapy regimens such as CHOP, but the response is poor (50% CR and median overall survival of 6 months). The use of infusional regimens (CDE or EPOCH) or intensive regimens with high-dose methotrexate could provide better results. The benefit of autologous hematopoietic stem cell transplantation (HSCT) in patients in first CR is uncertain.

Antiviral medications targeting HHV-8 (e.g., valganciclovir, ganciclovir, or cidofovir) have been concomitantly used with chemotherapy in some cases, with long-term remissions having been reported. Other approaches are being preclinically evaluated. They include brentuximab vedotin, proteasome inhibitors, anti-endothelial vascular growth factor (VEGF), and other inhibitors of angiogenesis and HHV8 replication (valproate, HIV-protease inhibitors, nelfinavir, and ganciclovir).

8.7.7 Primary CNS Lymphoma

Profound immunosuppression (CD4 cells <50/ mm^3), EBV detection in lymphoma cells from virtually all patients, and high aggressive histology (frequently immunoblastic) are the hallmarks of this lymphoma and must be considered for treatment decision making [60]. The introduction of cART has not only led to a decline in the incidence of PCNSL but also a modest improvement in OS. However, outcomes remain dismal with few patients alive 2 years after diagnosis. Importantly, many patients who develop AIDS-PCNSL in the current era are previously undiagnosed and/or untreated for their HIV and can be salvaged immunologically. Since essentially 100% of AIDS-PCNSL are EBV+, immune recovery with cART and reconstitution of EBV-specific immunity may confer a therapeutic benefit in this setting. Therefore, rapid diagnosis of CNS lesions in HIV-infected patients is critical for optimal care. In the pre-cART era, there was an algorithm to begin anti-toxoplasmosis therapy and then to re-evaluate after 2 weeks of therapy. If the lesion worsened, it was presumed to be lymphoma. In the cART era, this approach should not be considered a reasonable medical practice.

The therapeutic approach recommended in immunocompetent patients with PCNSL includes upfront induction chemotherapy with high-dose methotrexate and cytarabine followed by consolidation with whole-brain radiotherapy or further chemotherapy with or without autologous HSCT. This treatment is not well defined in HIV-infected patients. A retrospective cohort of 13 patients treated with high-dose methotrexate-based therapy in whom HIV control was achieved with cART showed all patients free of lymphoma and high functional status with a median follow-up of 50 months [60, 61]. A trial of high-dose methotrexate with rituximab and cART is ongoing at the US NCI, with encouraging initial results [49]. Results reported using the combination of whole-brain radiotherapy and cART suggest poor long-term outcomes and late neurotoxicity (leukoencephalopathy) complicating around 20% of cases, suggesting chemotherapy approaches may be preferred. Importantly, HIV-related PCNSL can largely be prevented by early HIV diagnosis and treatment.

8.7.8 Classical Hodgkin Lymphoma

The ABVD (adriamycin, bleomycin, vinblastine, and dacarbazine) chemotherapy regimen with concurrent cART has been evaluated in retrospective studies in patients in advanced stages of HL, showing CR rates over 80% and EFS and OS probabilities of 75–85% [62, 63]. These results were similar to those achieved in HIV-negative patients [64]. The German HIV study group evaluated the incorporation of the BEACOPP regimen with concurrent cART to the treatment in patients with HIV-related HL. Patients with early favorable HL received two to four cycles of ABVD followed by involved-field radiation; patients with early unfavorable disease were treated with four cycles of BEACOPP baseline or four cycles of ABVD; and patients with advanced HIV-cHL received six to eight cycles of BEACOPP baseline. In patients with advanced HIV infection, BEACOPP was replaced by ABVD. The CR rate for patients with early favorable, early unfavorable, and advanced-stage cHL was 96%, 100%, and 86%, respectively, and no significant differences were observed in overall survival among the three (95.7%, 100%, and 86.8%, respectively) [65].

Taken together, a stage-adapted treatment approach is feasible and effective in HIV-related cHL. Two cycles of ABVD followed by 20 Gy involved-field (IF) radiotherapy (RT) can be regarded as standard treatment for early favorable cHL, while four cycles of ABVD followed by 30 Gy IF-RT may be considered the standard of care for patients with early-stage unfavorable cHL. For advanced stages, six cycles of ABVD or BEACOPP may be equally considered. However, ABVD is most commonly used for advanced HIV-cHL in many parts of the world.

There is limited data on interim PET scans in HIV-cHL, but recent data from a retrospective cohort study indicate a high negative predictive value of a PET scan performed after two to three cycles of ABVD [66]. In a prospective US intergroup trial of PET-2 response adapted therapy that included HIV-infected patients, the approach was feasible, and the outcomes did not appear to be different from that of the HIV-unrelated cases [67, 68]. Recent case studies indicate that brentuximab vedotin may also be useful in HIV-positive patients with relapsed HL, and a combination of brentuximab vedotin, doxorubicin, vinblastine, and dacarbazine is currently being investigated in a study by the AIDS Malignancy Consortium (AMC) (NCT 01771107). The AMC is also accruing patients with HIV-cHL to an NCI-sponsored trial using anti-programmed death 1 (PD1) agents (NCT 02408861).

Essential to the management of HIV-cHL is the absolute contraindication to use ritonavir and most other protease inhibitors as part of the cART regimen when vinblastine or brentuximab vedotin is used because of cyp3A4 interactions leading to severe neutropenia and neurotoxicity that can create inability to administer curative intent therapy [69].

8.7.9 Diffuse Large B-Cell Lymphoma in Patients with HHV-8 Multicentric Castleman Disease

The prognosis of MCD has dramatically improved in recent years, mainly due to the widespread use of cART and targeted therapies such as rituximab. This approach has markedly reduced the rate of progression to NHL [70]. These lymphomas are EBV unrelated, and IgM, lambda restricted. The spleen and lymph nodes are typically involved. Treatment for HHV-8 related DLBCL in these patients is poorly defined. Some cases may express CD30 providing a rationale for use of brentuximab vedotin therapeutically.

8.7.10 Treatment of Relapsed or Refractory HIV-Related Lymphomas

As most HIV-positive patients in the cART era can tolerate dose-intense multiagent regimens in first-line therapy, it seems recommendable to approach HIV-positive patients with relapsed or refractory DLBCL in a manner similar to immunocompetent patients. High-dose salvage regimens such as ICE (ifosfamide, carboplatin, etoposide), DHAP (dexamethasone, cytarabine, cisplatin), ESHAP (etoposide, dexamethasone, cytarabine, cisplatin), or GDP (gemcitabine, dexamethasone, cisplatin) in combination with rituximab appear to have similar efficacy and should be used for appropriate patients. Patients with chemosensitive disease who are transplant eligible should proceed to autologous hematopoietic stem cell transplantation (HSCT) [71–74]. In HIV-negative DLBCL, many new agents are under development, particularly inhibitors of the NF-kappa B pathway and B-cell receptor signaling, but experience in HIV-positive patients is lacking. The AMC in collaboration with the Cancer Therapy Evaluation Program at the US NCI is currently developing a study of ibrutinib in HIV-DLBCL.

Effective therapeutic options for patients with relapsed or refractory BL are limited, and the only reasonable option is to administer rescue immunochemotherapy followed immediately by autologous HSCT. The new approaches under development in HIV-negative individuals seem promising and will hopefully be translated to HIV-infected patients in the near future.

Patients with relapsed or refractory HIV-related cHL should be considered early for high-dose chemotherapy and autologous HSCT if chemosensitive relapse is achieved [71–74]. Peripheral blood stem cells can be effectively mobilized [75], and the results are similar to those shown in immunocompetent patients [71–76]. As mentioned previously immunotherapy approaches with brentuximab vedotin and anti-PD1 agents are being or will soon be incorporated in clinical trials in relapsed or refractory HIV-related cHL.

In HIV-infected patients with NHL and cHL submitted to high-dose therapy and autologous HSCT, adequate CD34+ cells are usually collected at the first mobilization attempt [75]. Tolerance to myeloablative chemotherapy is good, and engraftment kinetics is comparable to that of HIV-negative patients, also with similar regimen-related and infectious complications during the period of aplasia. The use of G-CSF as well as anti-infective prophylaxis is strongly recommended after transplant, with antibacterial, antifungal, and antiviral prophylaxis being advisable. Trimethoprim-sulfamethoxazole is used to prevent *Pneumocystis jirovecii* pneumonia but has to be withheld from the day of stem cell infusion until engraftment due to its known hematologic toxicity. Aerosolized pentamidine is a good option for this prophylaxis. Antiretroviral therapy is usually given along the HSCT program. The CD4+ cell count decreases after high-dose chemotherapy with the nadir at approximately 3–6 months after transplantation and subsequently recovers to pretransplant levels within the first year. The thymus-dependent pathway of T-cell reconstitution after autologous HSCT has been demonstrated to be as efficient as in HIV-uninfected individuals [74, 76].

Recent reports support allogeneic HSCT in HIV-infected persons as a standard of care when the underlying hematologic malignancy can benefit from this procedure [77, 78]. In one reported case, not only was leukemia cured, but there has been an inability to detect residual HIV infection, suggesting that the patient may even be cured by transplantation owing to a donor graft homozygous for a deletion 32 mutation in the CCR5 HIV co-receptor [77]. There are some special considerations in management. It is essential to have a multidisciplinary patient care team with expertise in antiretroviral therapy as well as in allogeneic HSCT. Patients will benefit from maintenance of cART throughout the transplant process, but special precaution must be taken with potential interactions with immunosuppressive and anti-infectious agents [78].

8.7.11 Antiretroviral and Supportive Therapy

Current literature is lacking for definitive clinical guidance on how best to combine cART and anticancer agents in patients with HIV and hematological malignancies [79, 80], and therefore until this information is available, communication among oncohematologists, infectious disease physicians, and pharmacologists is crucial to guide treatment decisions. Given that there is general consensus on the concurrent administration of cART and chemotherapy, the selection of the cART schedule is of paramount importance. The prior cART schedule, the sensitivity of the HIV strand, the possible coexistence of hepatitis B or C, and the type of chemotherapeutic and anti-infectious agents should be considered for choosing the most appropriate cART regimen. Although individualized cART is sometimes necessary, the most recommended schedule should include integrase inhibitors (raltegravir or dolutegravir) combined with nucleoside/nucleotide reverse transcriptase inhibitors such as lamivudine (3TC)/abacavir or emtricitabine (FTC)/tenofovir alafenamide (TAF). Most once-daily single-tablet formulations and the use of protease inhibitors and cobicistat should be avoided due to their frequent pharmacologic interactions, as well as disoproxil fumarate (TDF) if renal toxicity is expected. If there is coinfection with hepatitis B virus, the cART should preferentially include FTC/TAF or FTC/TDF as an alternative.

The general supportive measures used in non-immunocompromised patients with lymphomas such as prophylaxis and treatment of tumor lysis syndrome or infections during neutropenia and the use of colony-stimulating factors and transfusion, among others, are fully applicable to HIV-infected patients.

Primary and secondary anti-infectious prophylaxis should be administered according to the CD4+ counts and the previous history of OI. *Pneumocystis jirovecii* prophylaxis is recommended for all patients. Systematic prophylaxis against CMV is not recommended, but careful PCR monitoring of CMV blood levels should be performed in all patients with CD4+ counts lower than 100/mm^3, and preemptive therapy should be administered accordingly.

In the current era of HIV medicine, planning optimal cancer therapy requires that the HIV infection be evaluated as a comorbid condition and not as the primary disease. If the prospects for long-term successful management of the HIV infection are favorable, then cancer management can often proceed as it would for any patient with similar performance and malignant disease characteristics.

Acknowledgments Funded in part by grants PI10/01417 (FIS), RD12-0036-0029 from RTICC, Instituto Carlos III and RD14-SGR225(GRE), Generalitat de Catalunya.

References

1. Ziegler JL, Beckstead JA, Volberding PA, et al. Non-Hodgkin's lymphoma in 90 homosexual men. Relation to generalized lymphadenopathy and the acquired immunodeficiency syndrome. N Engl J Med. 1984;311:565–70.
2. Rabkin CS, Yellin F. Cancer incidence in a population with a high prevalence of infection with human immunodeficiency virus type 1. J Natl Cancer Inst. 1994;86:1711–6.
3. Dunleavy K, Wilson WH. How I treat HIV-associated lymphoma. Blood. 2012;119:3245–55.
4. Little RF, Wilson WH. Update on the pathogenesis, diagnosis, and therapy of AIDS-related lymphoma. Curr Infect Dis Rep. 2003;5:176–84.
5. Carbone A, Gloghini A. AIDS-related lymphomas: from pathogenesis to pathology. Br J Haematol. 2005;130:662–70.
6. Gopal S, Patel MR, Yanik EL, et al. Temporal trends in presentation and survival for HIV-associated lymphoma in the antiretroviral therapy era. J Natl Cancer Inst. 2013;105:1221–9.
7. Ingle SM, May MT, Gill MJ, et al. Impact of risk factors for specific causes of death in the first and subsequent years of antiretroviral therapy among HIV-infected patients. Clin Infect Dis. 2014;59:287–97.
8. Besson C, Goubar A, Gabarre J, et al. Changes in AIDS-related lymphoma since the era of highly active antiretroviral therapy. Blood. 2001;98:2339–44.
9. Engels EA, Pfeiffer RM, Goedert JJ, et al. Trends in cancer risk among people with AIDS in the United States 1980-2002. AIDS. 2006;20:1645–54.
10. Hernandez-Ramirez RU, Shiels MS, Dubrow R, Engels EA. Cancer risk in HIV-infected people in the USA from 1996 to 2012: a population-based, registry-linkage study. Lancet HIV. 2017;4:e495. https://doi.org/10.1016/S2352-3018(17)30125-X.
11. Gotti D, Danesi M, Calabresi A, et al. Clinical characteristics, incidence, and risk factors of HIV-related Hodgkin lymphoma in the era of combination antiretroviral therapy. AIDS Patient Care STDs. 2013;27:259–65.
12. Shiels MS, Koritzinsky EH, Clarke CA, Suneja G, Morton LM, Engels EA. Prevalence of HIV infection among U.S. Hodgkin lymphoma cases. Cancer Epidemiol Biomark Prev. 2014;23:274–81.
13. Lee JY, Dhakal I, Casper C, et al. Risk of cancer among commercially insured HIV-infected adults on antiretroviral therapy. J Cancer Epidemiol. 2016;2016:2138259.
14. Serraino D, Dal Maso L. Epidemiology. In: Henrich M, Barta SK, editors. HIV-associated hematological malignancies. New York: Springer; 2016. p. 27–38.
15. Carbone A, Volpi CC, Gualeni AV, Gloghini A. Epstein-Barr virus associated lymphomas in people with HIV. Curr Opin HIV AIDS. 2017;12:39–46.
16. Carbone A, Gloghini A, Caruso A, De Paoli P, Dolcetti R. The impact of EBV and HIV infection on the microenvironmental niche underlying Hodgkin lymphoma pathogenesis. Int J Cancer. 2017;140:1233–45.
17. Cesarman E, Chang Y, Moore PS, Said JW, Knowles DM. Kaposi's sarcoma-associated herpesvirus-like DNA sequences in AIDS-related body cavity-based lymphomas. N Engl J Med. 1995;332:1186–91.
18. Arora N, Gupta A, Sadeghi N. Primary effusion lymphoma: current concepts and management. Curr Opin Pulm Med. 2017;23:365–70.
19. Auten M, Kim AS, Bradley KT, Rosado FG. Human herpesvirus 8-related diseases: histopathologic diagnosis and disease mechanisms. Semin Diagn Pathol. 2017;34:371–6.
20. Swerdlow SH, Campo E, Pileri SA, et al. The 2016 revision of the World Health Organization classification of lymphoid neoplasms. Blood. 2016;127:2375–90.
21. Linke-Serinsöz E, Fend F, Quintanilla-Martinez L. Human immunodeficiency virus (HIV) and Epstein-Barr virus (EBV) related lymphomas, pathology view point. Semin Diagn Pathol. 2017;34:352–63.
22. Dunleavy K, Little RF, Pittaluga S, et al. The role of tumor histogenesis, FDG-PET, and short-course EPOCH with dose-dense rituximab (SC-EPOCH-RR) in HIV-associated diffuse large B-cell lymphoma. Blood. 2010;115:3017–24.
23. Xicoy B, Ribera J-M, Mate J-L, et al. Immunohistochemical expression profile and prognosis in patients with diffuse large B-cell lymphoma with or without human immunodeficiency virus infection. Leuk Lymphoma. 2010;51:2063–9.
24. Yoon N, Ahn S, Yong Yoo H, et al. Cell-of-origin of diffuse large B-cell lymphomas determined by the Lymph2Cx assay: better prognostic indicator than Hans algorithm. Oncotarget. 2017;8:22014–22.
25. Dunleavy K, Little RF, Wilson WH. Update on Burkitt lymphoma. Hematol Oncol Clin North Am. 2016;30:1333–43.
26. Staiger AM, Ziepert M, Horn H, et al. Clinical impact of the cell-of-origin classification and the MYC/BCL2 dual expresser status in diffuse large B-cell lymphoma treated within prospective clinical trials of the German high-grade non-Hodgkin's lymphoma study group. J Clin Oncol. 2017;35(22):2515–26.
27. Cinque P, Brytting M, Vago L, et al. Epstein-Barr virus DNA in cerebrospinal fluid from patients with AIDS-related primary lymphoma of the central nervous system. Lancet. 1993;342:398–401.
28. Karia SJ, McArdle DJT. AIDS-related primary CNS lymphoma. Lancet. 2017;389(10085):2238. https://doi.org/10.1016/S0140-6736(17)30056-9.
29. El-Fattah MA. Clinical characteristics and survival outcome of primary effusion lymphoma: a review of 105 patients. Hematol Oncol. 2016;35:878. https://doi.org/10.1002/hon.2372.

30. Gonzalez-Farre B, Martinez D, Lopez-Guerra M, et al. HHV8-related lymphoid proliferations: a broad spectrum of lesions from reactive lymphoid hyperplasia to overt lymphoma. Mod Pathol. 2017;30:745–60.
31. Hentrich M, Spina M, Montoto S. HIV-associated Hodgkin's lymphoma. In: Henrich M, Barta SK, editors. HIV-associated hematological malignancies. New York: Springer; 2016. p. 119–32.
32. Brunnberg U, Hentrich M, Hoffmann C, Wolf T, Hübel K. HIV-associated malignant lymphoma. Oncol Res Treat. 2017;40:82–7.
33. Cheson BD, Fisher RI, Barrington SF, et al. Recommendations for initial evaluation, staging, and response assessment of Hodgkin and non-Hodgkin lymphoma: the Lugano classification. J Clin Oncol. 2014;32:3059–68.
34. Cheson BD, Ansell S, Schwartz L, et al. Refinement of the Lugano classification lymphoma response criteria in the era of immunomodulatory therapy. Blood. 2016;128:2489–96.
35. Barta SK, Samuel MS, Xue X, et al. Changes in the influence of lymphoma- and HIV-specific factors on outcomes in AIDS-related non-Hodgkin lymphoma. Ann Oncol. 2015;26:958–66.
36. International Non-Hodgkin's Lymphoma Prognostic Factors Project. A predictive model for aggressive non-Hodgkin's lymphoma. N Engl J Med. 1993;329:987–94.
37. Hasenclever D, Diehl V. A prognostic score for advanced Hodgkin's disease. International prognostic factors project on advanced Hodgkin's disease. N Engl J Med. 1998;339:1506–14.
38. Xicoy B, Ribera JM, Miralles P, et al. Limited prognostic value of the international prognostic score in advanced stage human immunodeficiency virus infection-related Hodgkin lymphoma treated with the doxorubicin, bleomycin, vinblastine, and dacarbazine regimen. Leuk Lymphoma. 2009;50:1718–20.
39. Barta SK, Xue X, Wang D, et al. A new prognostic score for AIDS-related lymphomas in the rituximab-era. Haematologica. 2014;99:1731–7.
40. Castillo JJ, Bower M, Brühlmann J, et al. HIV-associated Hodgkin lymphoma in the cART Era Study Group. Prognostic factors for advanced-stage human immunodeficiency virus-associated classical Hodgkin lymphoma treated with doxorubicin, bleomycin, vinblastine, and dacarbazine plus combined antiretroviral therapy: a multi-institutional retrospective study. Cancer. 2015;121:423–31.
41. Wang CC, Kaplan LD. Clinical management of HIV-associated hematologic malignancies. Expert Rev Hematol. 2016;9:361–76.
42. Ribera JM, Oriol A, Morgades M, et al. Safety and efficacy of cyclophosphamide, adriamycin, vincristine, prednisone and rituximab in patients with human immunodeficiency virus-associated diffuse large B-cell lymphoma: results of a phase II trial. Br J Haematol. 2008;140:411–9.
43. Spina M, Jaeger U, Sparano JA, et al. Rituximab plus infusional cyclophosphamide, doxorubicin, and etoposide in HIV-associated non-Hodgkin lymphoma: pooled results from 3 phase 2 trials. Blood. 2005;105:1891–7.
44. Sparano JA, Lee JY, Kaplan LD, et al. Rituximab plus concurrent infusional EPOCH chemotherapy is highly effective in HIV-associated B-cell non-Hodgkin lymphoma. Blood. 2010;115:3008–16.
45. Kaplan LD, Lee JY, Ambinder RF, et al. Rituximab does not improve clinical outcome in a randomized phase 3 trial of CHOP with or without rituximab in patients with HIV-associated non-Hodgkin lymphoma: AIDS-Malignancies Consortium Trial 010. Blood. 2005;106:1538–43.
46. Barta SK, Xue X, Wang D, et al. Treatment factors affecting outcomes in HIV-associated non-Hodgkin lymphomas: a pooled analysis of 1546 patients. Blood. 2013;122:3251–62.
47. Barta SK, Lee JY, Kaplan LD, Noy A, Sparano JA. Pooled analysis of AIDS malignancy consortium trials evaluating rituximab plus CHOP or infusional EPOCH chemotherapy in HIV-associated non-Hodgkin lymphoma. Cancer. 2012;118:3977–83.
48. Wilson WH, Ho JS, Pitcher BN, et al. Phase III randomized study of R-CHOP versus DA-EPOCH-R and molecular analysis of untreated diffuse large B-cell lymphoma: CALGB/Alliance 50303. Blood. 2016;128:469; [abstract].
49. Uldrick T, et al. AIDS-associated Primary Central Nervous System Lymphoma (AIDS-PCNSL) treated with HAART and radiation-sparing therapy: The NCI HIV and AIDS Malignancy Branch experience, 2004-2011. CROI 19, 2012: Abstract R-129.
50. Borges ÁH, Neuhaus J, Babiker AG, et al. Immediate antiretroviral therapy reduces risk of infection-related cancer during early HIV infection. Clin Infect Dis. 2016;63:1668–76.
51. Ribera JM, Garcia O, Grande C, et al. Dose-intensive chemotherapy including rituximab in Burkitt's leukemia or lymphoma regardless of human immunodeficiency virus infection status: final results of a phase 2 study (Burkimab). Cancer. 2013;119:1660–8.
52. Noy A, Lee JY, Cesarman E, et al. AMC 048: modified CODOX-M/IVAC-rituximab is safe and effective for HIV-associated Burkitt lymphoma. Blood. 2015;126:160–6.
53. Alwan F, He A, Montoto S, et al. Adding rituximab to CODOX-M/IVAC chemotherapy in the treatment of HIV-associated Burkitt lymphoma is safe when used with concurrent combination antiretroviral therapy. AIDS. 2015;29:903–10.
54. Xicoy B, Ribera JM, Müller M, et al. Dose-intensive chemotherapy including rituximab is highly effective but toxic in human immunodeficiency virus-infected patients with Burkitt lymphoma/leukemia: parallel study of 81 patients. Leuk Lymphoma. 2014;55:2341–8.
55. Dunleavy K, Pittaluga S, Shovlin M, et al. Low-intensity therapy in adults with Burkitt's lymphoma. N Engl J Med. 2013;369:1915–25.

56. Dunleavy K, Noy A, Abramson JS, et al. Risk-adapted therapy in adults with Burkitt lymphoma: preliminary report of a multicenter prospective phase II study of DA-EPOCH-R. Blood. 2015;126:342; [abstract].
57. Dunleavy K. Aggressive B cell lymphoma: optimal therapy for MYC-positive, double-hit, and triple-hit DLBCL. Curr Treat Options in Oncol. 2015;16:58.
58. Castillo JJ, Reagan JL, Sikov WM, Winer ES. Bortezomib in combination with infusional dose-adjusted EPOCH for the treatment of plasmablastic lymphoma. Br J Haematol. 2015;169:352–5.
59. Castillo JJ, Bibas M, Miranda RN. The biology and treatment of plasmablastic lymphoma. Blood. 2015;125:2323–30.
60. Barta SK, Joshi J, Mounier N, et al. Central nervous system involvement in AIDS-related lymphomas. Br J Haematol. 2016;173:857–66.
61. Gupta NK, Nolan A, Omuro A, et al. Long-term survival in AIDS-related primary central nervous system lymphoma. Neuro-Oncology. 2017;19:99–108.
62. Xicoy B, Ribera JM, Miralles P, et al. Results of treatment with doxorubicin, bleomycin, vinblastine and dacarbazine and highly active antiretroviral therapy in advanced stage, human immunodeficiency virus-related Hodgkin's lymphoma. Haematologica. 2007;92:191–8.
63. Montoto S, Shaw K, Okosun J, et al. HIV status does not influence outcome in patients with classical Hodgkin lymphoma treated with chemotherapy using doxorubicin, bleomycin, vinblastine, and dacarbazine in the highly active antiretroviral therapy era. J Clin Oncol. 2012;30:4111–6.
64. Sorigué M, García O, Tapia G, et al. HIV-infection has no prognostic impact on advanced-stage Hodgkin lymphoma. AIDS. 2017;31:1445–9.
65. Hentrich M, Berger M, Wyen C, et al. Stage-adapted treatment of HIV-associated Hodgkin lymphoma: results of a prospective multicenter study. J Clin Oncol. 2012;30:4117–23.
66. Okosun J, Warbey V, Shaw K, et al. Interim fluoro-2-deoxy-D-glucose-PET predicts response and progression-free survival in patients with Hodgkin lymphoma and HIV infection. AIDS. 2012;26:861–5.
67. Danilov AV, Li H, Press OW, et al. Feasibility of interim PET-adapted therapy in HIV-positive patients with advanced Hodgkin lymphoma (HL): sub-analysis of SWOG S0816 phase 2 trial. Blood. 2015;126:1498; [abstract].
68. Pres OW, Li H, Schöder H, et al. US intergroup trial of response-adapted therapy for stage III to IV Hodgkin lymphoma using early interim fluorodeoxyglucose–positron emission tomography imaging: Southwest Oncology Group S0816. J Clin Oncol. 2016;34:2020–7.
69. Ezzat HM, Cheung MC, Hicks LK, et al. Incidence, predictors and significance of severe toxicity in patients with human immunodeficiency virus-associated Hodgkin lymphoma. Leuk Lymphoma. 2012;53:2390–6.
70. Gerard L, Michot JM, Burcheri S, et al. Rituximab decreases the risk of lymphoma in patients with HIV-associated multicentric Castleman disease. Blood. 2012;119:2228–33.
71. Diez-Martin JL, Balsalobre P, Re A, et al. Comparable survival between HIV+ and HIV− non-Hodgkin and Hodgkin lymphoma patients undergoing autologous peripheral blood stem cell transplantation. Blood. 2009;113:6011–4.
72. Balsalobre P, Diez-Martin JL, Re A, et al. Autologous stem-cell transplantation in patients with HIV-related lymphoma. J Clin Oncol. 2009;27:2192–8.
73. Johnston C, Harrington R, Jain R, Schiffer J, Kiem HP, Woolfrey A. Safety and efficacy of combination antiretroviral therapy in human immunodeficiency virus-infected adults undergoing autologous or allogeneic hematopoietic cell transplantation for hematologic malignancies. Biol Blood Marrow Transplant. 2016;22:149–56.
74. Alvarnas JC, Le Rademacher J, Wang Y, et al. Autologous hematopoietic cell transplantation for HIV-related lymphoma: results of the (BMT CTN) 0803/(AMC) 071 trial. Blood. 2016;128:1050–8.
75. Re A, Cattaneo C, Skert C, et al. Cooperative European Group on AIDS and Tumors. Stem cell mobilization in HIV seropositive patients with lymphoma. Haematologica. 2013;98:1762–8.
76. Re A, Krishnan A, Hentrich M, et al. Autologous stem cell transplantation. In: Henrich M, Barta SK, editors. HIV-associated hematological malignancies. New York: Springer; 2016. p. 153–64.
77. Hutter G, Nowak D, Mossner M, et al. Long-term control of HIV by CCR5 Delta32/Delta32 stem-cell transplantation. N Engl J Med. 2009;360:692–8.
78. Ambinder RF, Kanakry JA, Durand C. Allogeneic stem cell transplantation. In: Henrich M, Barta SK, editors. HIV-associated hematological malignancies. New York: Springer; 2016. p. 165–72.
79. Rudek MA, Flexner C, Ambinder RF. Use of antineoplastic agents in patients with cancer who have HIV/AIDS. Lancet Oncol. 2011;12:905–12.
80. Torres HA, Rallapalli V, Saxena A, et al. Efficacy and safety of antiretrovirals in HIV-infected patients with cancer. Clin Microbiol Infect. 2014;20:O672–9.

Primary CNS Lymphoma

9

Agnieszka Korfel

9.1 Epidemiology

PCNSL accounts for 2–4% of intracranial neoplasms and 4–6% of extranodal lymphomas [1]. Median age at diagnosis is 65 years, and immunosuppression is the only risk factor identified thus far. While an increasing incidence had been found in the 1980s and 1990s, the incidence of PCNSL in young patients has decreased thereafter, but it is still growing in elderly patients without other clear risk factors [2].

9.2 Clinical Presentation

Symptoms are usually rapidly evolving, reflecting the aggressive behavior of the tumor. Patients most frequently present with cognitive dysfunction, psychomotor slowing, disorientation, and neurological focal symptoms. Headache, seizures, cranial nerves palsies, and symptoms of increased intracranial pressure are less frequent. Radicular symptoms and back pain are indicative of spinal cord localization, which however is very rare. Blurred vision and floaters are typical for patients with ocular involvement (=vitreoretinal lymphoma) [3].

A. Korfel (✉)
Department of Hematology, Oncology, and Tumor Immunology, Charite Universitätsmedizin Berlin, Berlin, Germany
e-mail: agnieszka.korfel@charite.de

9.3 Diagnostic Work-Up

9.3.1 Initial Imaging

Contrast-enhanced MRI of the brain is the diagnostic method of choice when PCNSL is suspected. PCNSL lesions in the immunocompetent typically present as solitary rather than multiple brain masses, hypo- or isointense on T1-weighted MR imaging, with an intense and relatively homogenous contrast enhancement and only moderate edema. The location is usually in the cerebral hemispheres, followed by the basal ganglia, thalamus, and corpus callosum. Nearly all lesions abut either the ependyma or the pia. Necrosis and peripheral ringlike enhancement are uncommon in the immunocompetent and typically seen in immunosuppressed patients (Fig. 9.1) [4–6].

The highly cellular nature of PCNSL contributes to the restricted diffusion of water on diffusion-weighted imaging (DWI) in approximately 90% of cases [7–9]. On MR spectroscopy, elevation of lipid and choline levels is typical [9, 10]. PCNSL has only mildly increased blood volume (rCBV) on perfusion imaging and a characteristic perfusion time-intensity curve, which may overshoot the baseline because of gadolinium leakage with T1 effects [7, 10]. ^{18}F-FDG PET readily shows the expected hypermetabolism of PCNSL before and after therapy [11, 12].

G. Lenz, G. Salles (eds.), *Aggressive Lymphomas*, Hematologic Malignancies,
https://doi.org/10.1007/978-3-030-00362-3_9

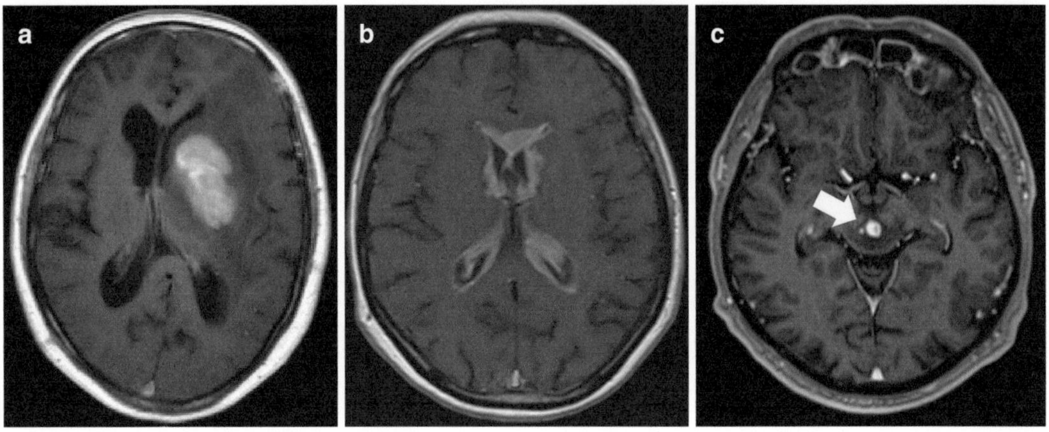

Fig. 9.1 Primary CNS lymphoma on contrast-enhanced MRI: (**a**) typical appearance in an immunocompetent patient, (**b**) patient with meningeal involvement, (**c**) patient with renal transplant and chronic immunosuppression

9.3.2 Diagnosis Making/Pathologic Findings

Diagnosis of PCNSL requires histopathological confirmation before treatment. The biopsy should be performed using stereotactic or navigation-guided needle biopsy [13]. Patients with immunocompromising conditions including HIV infection with suggestive radiographic findings represent an exception where the proof of Epstein-Barr virus (EBV) in the CSF is being considered sufficient to make diagnosis of PCNSL without tissue biopsy [14]. If clinically possible, steroids should be avoided before biopsy due to their lymphocytotoxic effect. For patients pretreated with steroids showing tumor regression, re-biopsy is recommended as soon as serial MRI indicates tumor regrowth [13].

PCNSL morphologically and phenotypically usually corresponds to diffuse large B-cell lymphoma (DLBCL), whereas low-grade B-cell lymphoma, Burkitt lymphoma, high-grade T-cell lymphoma, and NK/T-cell lymphoma are much less frequent [15]. Microscopically, PCNSL is a highly cellular neoplasm composed of large lymphoid cells with a characteristic angiocentric arrangement. Isolated tumor cells diffusely infiltrate brain parenchyma and are associated with reactive astrogliosis and microglial infiltration. Mitotic figures and apoptotic bodies are frequently seen. Immunohistochemically, tumor cells express B-cell markers, such as CD20, CD79a, CD19, CD22, and PXA5, as well as BCL6 (60–80%), MUM1/IRF4 (90%), BCL2, and cell surface immunoglobulins IgM and IgD with light chain restriction.

9.3.3 CSF Diagnostics

The diagnostic yield of routine CSF analysis such as conventional cytomorphology, flow cytometry, and monoclonality assessment by polymerase chain reaction (PCR) is low due to low frequency of CSF involvement in PCNSL of approx. 10% [16, 17]. Several additional potential diagnostic markers for PCNSL in the CSF have been described, including particular microRNA (miRNA), CXC chemokine ligand 13 (CXCL-13), interleukin 10, neopterin, osteopontin, and others [18–22]. A validation in independent patient populations is required before their use in routine practice can be recommended.

9.3.4 Ophthalmologic Evaluation

Ocular involvement (vitreoretinal lymphoma) can occur prior to brain manifestations, simultaneously with brain lesions (approx. 10% of patients) or at relapse. Many patients remain asymptomatic. In patients with ocular involvement, slit lamp examination typically reveals vitreous cellular infiltration (lymphoma and inflammatory cells) and/or subretinal tumor cell infiltrates on fundoscopy. A vitrectomy or even chorioretinal biopsy is often needed for definitive diagnosis, whereas an anterior chamber puncture carries a lower diagnostic yield. Pathologic diagnosis is often difficult due to predominance of inflammatory cells and relative paucity of lymphoma cells. A high interleukin 10/interleukin 6 ratio (>1) in the vitreous is regarded indicative of lymphoma [23, 24].

9.3.5 Additional Diagnostic Work-Up

A thorough patient history should be obtained with specific emphasis on immunocompromising conditions including therapy with immunosuppressive drugs. Blood testing should include an HIV test, serum LDH as a prognostic factor [25], and testing for hepatitis, since this may be reactivated under chemotherapy or immunotherapy. Physical examination of all peripheral lymph node regions and the testes; a CT of the neck, chest, abdomen, and pelvis; and bone marrow biopsy are recommended to differentiate PCNSL from systemic lymphoma with CNS involvement (secondary CNS lymphoma).

9.4 Standard of Care in First Line

9.4.1 Local Therapies

PCNSL is considered a whole-brain disease. Thus, surgical resection has generally not been regarded part of therapy or even deemed harmful given the risk of irreversible neurological deficits after surgery. However, in a secondary analysis of a randomized phase III trial [26] in the subset of patients with a single lesion, a significant benefit for both progression-free survival (PFS) and overall survival (OS) was found for patients with (sub)total resection of visible lesions as compared to those with biopsy only [27]. Based on these findings, tumor resection before chemotherapy can be considered in the treatment of single lesions amenable to resection, though this approach remains controversial and is not yet part of the generally accepted standard of care.

With whole-brain radiotherapy (WBRT) alone, a high response rate but very rarely long-term control can be obtained. The median with WBRT alone is 12–16 months [28]. WBRT as the only therapy should thus be offered only to patients who cannot tolerate systemic chemotherapy.

9.4.2 Choice of Initial Chemotherapy

Systemic blood-brain barrier-crossing chemotherapy is a treatment of choice in PCNSL. While there is no standard treatment universally accepted, a consensus exists on the status of high-dose methotrexate (HDMTX) as the most important drug in the treatment of PCNSL. However, there is a great deal of variability in HDMTX dose and schedule used. It is generally accepted that doses ≥ 3 g/m^2 and infusion times of a few hours (rather than 24 h) should be used to reliably achieve cytotoxic levels in the CSF [29].

With HDMTX monochemotherapy, complete response (CR) rates of 15% and 18% were achieved in two studies [30, 31], whereas a higher CR rate of 52% was reported in a third study using much more HDMTX courses [32].

HDMTX-based polychemotherapy is generally regarded more effective than HDMTX alone. In the only randomized phase II study with 79 patients comparing HDMTX alone to HDMTX combined with high-dose cytarabine (HDAraC), in both arms followed by WBRT, a significantly higher CR rate (primary end point) was found for the combination: 46% versus 18% (p = 0.006); 3-year overall survival (OS) was 46% versus 32% (p = 0.07), respectively [30].

In a more recent randomized trial, 219 patients <70 years were randomized to the combination of HDMTX and HDAraC (group A), HDMTX and HDAraC plus rituximab (group B), and HDMTX and HDAraC plus both thiotepa and rituximab (group C, MATRix) [33]. A significantly higher CR rate was found with MATRix of

49% as compared to 23% in arm A and 30% in arm B (the trial was not prospectively designed to test the benefit of addition of rituximab or thiotepa to HDMTX and HDAraC).

Besides these two randomized trials, only non-comparative trials using different HDMTX-based combinations have been published with CR rates between 27 and 69% (Table 9.1).

Summarizing the results, 4–6 courses of HDMTX ($\geq$3 g/m^2)-based chemotherapy (with HDAraC, thiotepa, ifosfamide, or temozolomide) can be recommended for initial treatment of PCNSL patients able to tolerate it. Although rituximab is added to chemotherapy at most centers, its contribution in this setting is not clear.

9.4.3 Choice of Consolidating Therapy

Consolidating of HDMTX-based primary chemotherapy by WBRT was a standard therapy for PCNSL until 1990s. This, although quite effective with a 2-year OS of approx. 65%, was associated with a high risk of delayed neurotoxicity, particularly in elderly patients [34].

The role of WBRT for consolidation after HDMTX-based primary chemotherapy was evaluated in a randomized phase III trial (G-PCNSL-SG1). Patients randomized to radiation received HDMTX-based chemotherapy followed by immediate WBRT (30 fractions of 1.5 Gy each). Patients randomized to chemotherapy alone received no further therapy if they had achieved CR and second-line chemotherapy with HDAraC if they had not. Patients treated with WBRT had a benefit in terms of PFS, 15.5 vs. 9.9 months ($p = 0.04$), but no significant difference in OS, with a median OS of 32.1 months with WBRT and 34.4 months without WBRT ($p = 0.94$) [26]. These results were confirmed in a long-term analysis of this study with a median follow-up of 82 months [40]. Moreover, quality of life (QoL) and cognition were better conserved in the arm without early WBRT [41]. This is in accordance with other analyses of delayed CNS toxicity in long-term PCNSL survivors, showing that patients who received WBRT had significant impairments across most cognitive domains, interfering with QoL, while those treated with chemotherapy alone had significantly higher scores in neuropsychometric testing [42, 43].

The comparison of WBRT versus high-dose chemotherapy followed by autologous stem cell transplantation (HD-ASCT) for consolidation was the object of a second randomization in the randomized phase II trial mentioned above [39] with the combination of BCNU + carmustine as high-dose regimen. No significant difference in 2-year PFS was found with 80% versus 70%, respectively.

Consolidation with non-cross-resistant conventional chemotherapy (HDAraC + etoposide) was tested in a non-comparative trial with 44 patients up to 76 years with a promising 2-year PFS of 57% and 4-year OS of 65% [37].

In summary, consolidation of HDMTX-based initial chemotherapy with HD-ASCT (e.g., BCNU + thiotepa) or non-cross-resistant conventional chemotherapy (HDAraC + etoposide) is currently being considered optimal first-line treatment for PCNSL. Standard-dose WBRT for consolidation is associated with higher risk of delayed CNS toxicity and should be avoided (Fig. 9.2).

9.4.4 Role of Intrathecal Therapy

In retrospective analyses, no advantage of adding intrathecal chemotherapy to HDMTX-based systemic chemotherapy was found. However, in a non-comparative study combining an intensive systemic chemotherapy with HDMTX, HDAraC, vincristine, alkylating agents, and dexamethasone and intensive intraventricular chemotherapy via Ommaya reservoir, very promising results with a median event-free survival (EFS) of 21 months and a median OS of 50 months were reached [44, 45]. Moreover, in none of the long-term survivors, cognitive impairment was found on neuropsychological testing [44].

In a head-to-head comparison of induction with HDMTX, ifosfamide, and rituximab followed by either HDAraC/thiotepa and HD-ASCT (BCNU/thiotepa) or continuation with conventional

Table 9.1 Large prospective studies with high-dose methotrexate-based induction chemotherapy followed by different consolidations

Reference	*n*	Age: median (range), y	Induction	RR (CR/PR) after induction, %	Consolidation	2-y PFS, %	2-y OS, %
[34]	102	56.5 (n.r.)	5 × MVP + MTX intraventricularly	94 (58/36)	WBRT 45 Gy, HDAraC	n.r.	64
[35]	52	51 (21–65)	2 × MBVP	73 (33/40)	WBRT 40 Gy	n.r.	69
[30][a]	79	58 59 (18–75)	Arm A: 4 × HDMTX Arm B: 4 × HDMTX + HDAraC	40 (18/22) 69 (46/23)	WBRT	21 (3-y PFS) 38 (3-y PFS)	32 (3-y OS) 46 (3-y OS)
[26][a]	523	63 (18–85)	6 × HDMTX ± ifosfamide	54 (35/19)	Arm RT: WBRT 45 Gy Arm no RT: none (CR pts) or HDAraC (no CR pts)	ITT ($n = 411$): 44 ITT ($n = 411$): 31	ITT: 58 ITT: 57
[36]	52	60 (30–79)	5–7 × R-MPV	83 (69/14)	WBRT 23.4 Gy (CR pts) or 45 Gy (non CR pts)	77	90
[37]	44	61 (12–76)	4 × MT	77 (66/11)	2 × VP16 + HDAraC	57	65 (4-y OS)
[38]	79	56 (IQR 51–62)	5 × HDMTX + HDAraC + R + TT	91 (27/64)	HD-ASCT (BCNU/TT)	70	80
[33, 39][a]	219	58 (IQR 50–64) 57 (IQR 53–62) 57 (IQR 53–62)	Arm A: 4 × HDMTX + HDAraC Arm B: 4 × HDMTX + HDAraC + R Arm C: 4 × HDMTX + HDAraC + R + TT (MATRix)	54 (23/31) 73 (30/43) 86 (49/37)	WBRT versus HD-ASCT (BCNU/TT)	36 46 61	42 56 69

CR complete remission, *BCNU* carmustine, *Gy* gray, *HDAraC* high-dose cytarabine, *HD-ASCT* high-dose chemotherapy followed by autologous stem cell transplantation, *HDMTX* high-dose methotrexate, *ITT* intent to treat population ($n = 411$), *MBVP* high-dose methotrexate, teniposide, carmustine, prednisolone, *MT* high-dose methotrexate, temozolomide, *MVP* high-dose methotrexate, vincristine, procarbazine, *MTX* methotrexate, *n* number, *n.r.* not reported, *OS* overall survival, *PFS* progression-free survival, *PR* partial remission, *pts* patients, *IQR* interquartile interval, *R* rituximab, *RR* overall response rate, *T* temozolomide, *TT* thiotepa, *VP16* etoposide, *WBRT* whole-brain radiotherapy, *y* years

[a]Randomized study

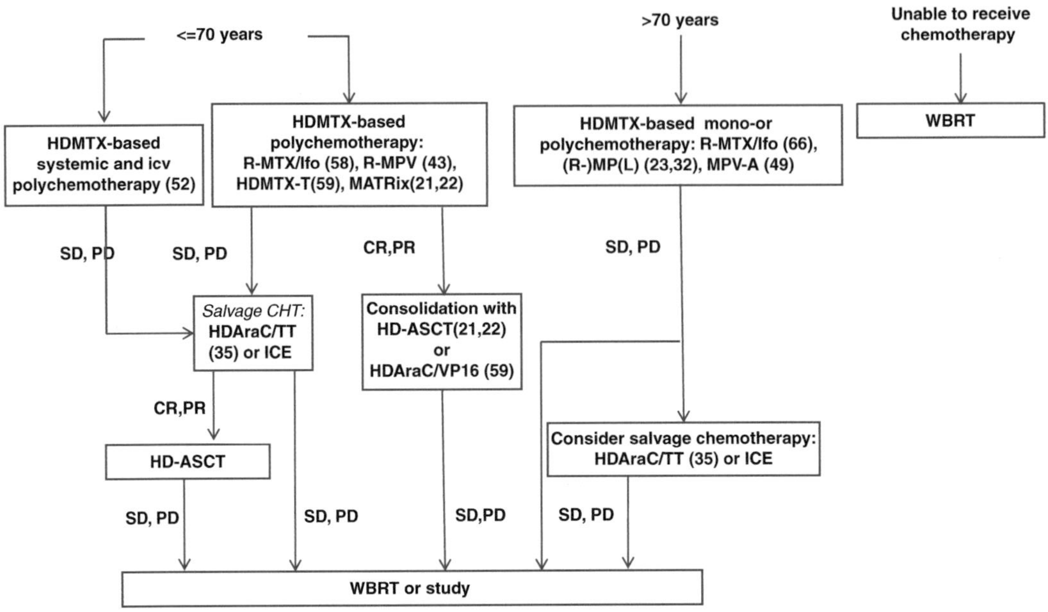

Fig. 9.2 Therapy recommendations. *CR* complete remission, *HDMTX* high-dose methotrexate, *HD-ASCT* high-dose chemotherapy followed by stem cell transplantation, *ICE* ifosfamide, carboplatin, etoposide, *ivc* intraventricularly, *PR* partial remission, *SD* stable disease, *PD* progressive disease, *WBRT* whole-brain radiotherapy

HDMTX- and HDAraC-based chemotherapy combined with intensive intraventricular chemotherapy, no significant outcome difference between the two groups was found [46].

Based on these results, HDMTX- and HDAraC-based chemotherapy combined with intensive intraventricular chemotherapy can be considered an alternative to the induction-consolidation concept described above (Fig. 9.2). However, the reservoir should be used with caution to prevent its infection.

9.4.5 Elderly Patients

Older age is the major negative prognostic factor in PCNSL, being associated both with reduced survival and increased risk of neurotoxicity.

In trials designed for elderly patients with PCNSL using HDMTX-based polychemotherapy alone, response rates of approximately 50% to >90% and 1-year PFS of 40–50% were reported with substantial acute toxicity and high rate of treatment discontinuation in some of them (Table 9.2). In the only randomized phase II study for elderly patients, 98 patients >60 years were treated with MPV-A (HDMTX, procarbazine, vincristine, HDAraC) or MT (HDMTX with temozolomide). Response rates and toxicity were comparable, but median OS was 31 versus 14 months [51]; however, the trial was not powered for a direct comparison, and the differences did not reach statistical significance.

Elderly patients may benefit from maintenance therapy. This is suggested by a phase II study, in which 66 patients were treated with a dose-adjusted HDMTX- and HDAraC-based protocol combined with liposomal AraC intrathecally; those between 66 and 75 years ($n = 27$) additionally received a maintenance therapy with temozolomide for 1 year or until progression [53]. The outcome of elderly patients was comparable with that of the younger patients, probably reflecting the benefit of maintenance therapy.

In summary, HDMTX is feasible in elderly PCNSL patients without serious comorbidities and most likely produces a better outcome than WBRT alone, which should be reserved for

Table 9.2 Studies in elderly patients

Reference	*n*	Age: median (range), y	Protocol	RR (CR/PR), %	1-y PFS, %	1-y OS, %	Death on therapy, %
[47][a]	50	72 (60–81)	MPL[b] + MTX + AraC i.th.	48 (42/6)	40	52	2
[48][a]	30	70 (57–79)	MPL[b]	70 (44/26)	Median 5.9	Median 15.4	7
[49]	31	74 (70–85)	HDMTX	97 (60/37)	Median 7.1	Median 37.1	–
[50][a]	35	65 (60–70)	HDMTX, vindesine, idarubicin	51 (17/34)	Median 13	Median 19	11
[51][a,c]	98	73 (60–85)	MT versus MPV-A	71 (45/26) 82 (62/20)	36 36	2y OS: 14 2y OS: 31	10 6
[52][a]	112	73 (66–85)	R-MPL[b] or R-MP, maintenance with P	50 (36/14)	46	57	9

AraC cytarabine, *CR* complete remission, *HDMTX* high-dose methotrexate, *i.th.* intrathecally, *MP* high-dose methotrexate, procarbazine, *MPL* high-dose methotrexate, lomustine, procarbazine, *MPV-A* high-dose methotrexate, procarbazine, vincristine, *HDAraC* high-dose cytarabine, *MT* high-dose methotrexate, temozolomide, *MTX* high-dose methotrexate, *OS* overall survival, *P* procarbazine, *PFS* progression-free survival, *PR* partial remission, *R* rituximab, *RR* overall response rate, *y* years

[a]Prospective study

[b]Protocol used in [47] differed from that used in [48, 52]

[c]Randomized study

patients not able to receive chemotherapy. To minimize the risk of late neurotoxicity, WBRT should be avoided (Fig. 9.2).

9.4.6 Treatment of Immunosuppressed Patients

Patients with chronic drug-induced immunosuppression (for treatment of autoimmune disorders or following organ transplantation) currently represent the major at-risk population for the development of PCNSL. The so-called post-transplantation lymphoproliferative disorders (PTLD) are B-cell lymphomas developed on the basis of B-cell proliferation stimulated by EBV infection. In patients on long-term immunosuppressive drugs diagnosed with PCNSL, reduction of immunosuppression is usually performed to allow the immune system to reconstitute. In HIV-positive patients with PCNSL, reconstitution of the immune system can be achieved with highly active antiretroviral therapy which has been shown to prolong survival [54]. In the largest retrospective analysis of 84 patients with PTLD-PCNSL, immunosuppressive medications were reduced in 93% of patients. Additional primary therapies in this patient group included HDMTX in 48%, HDAraC in 33%, WBRT in 24%, and/or rituximab in 44%. The ORR was 60%, however, with a treatment-related mortality of 13%; 3-year PFS was 32% and 3-year OS 43% [55]. These findings suggest that patients with immunosuppression-caused PCNSL can be treated similarly to immunocompetent patients, however, with higher risk of serious infectious complications.

9.5 Salvage Treatment

Relapse is frequent in PCNSL even after intensive initial therapy and is almost always localized in the CNS. Moreover, PCNSL shows a continuing tendency to recur with longer follow-up. Patients generally benefit from salvage therapy after failure to primary treatment if not in a severely compromised condition. Choice of salvage treatment should be driven by a patient's age, performance status, prior therapy, and duration of previous response. Salvage chemotherapy is generally preferred over WBRT, particularly in patients with good performance status and response to previous chemotherapy. Rechallenge with HDMTX is a reasonable option for patients who experienced a long-term remission after primary HDMTX therapy [56, 57].

Numerous chemotherapy/immunotherapy approaches to recurrent PNCSL have been evaluated, utilizing agents such as topotecan, rituximab, temozolomide with or without concurrent rituximab, bendamustine, HDAraC, ifosfamide- and/or etoposide-based polychemotherapy, and yttrium 90-labeled ibritumomab tiuxetan [58–65]. The median PFS figures were uniformly short at 2–5 months.

A phase II study with the mTOR inhibitor temsirolimus is the first completed prospective trial of a targeted agent in PCNSL [66]. A relatively high overall response rate (primary end point) of 54% was seen; however, median PFS was only 2.6 months.

For younger patients who are able to tolerate intensive therapy, HD-ASCT can be considered. In the two prospective trials published thus far [67, 68], median patients' age 52 and 57 years, HDAraC-based induction followed by thiotepa-based high-dose regimen was used. The 2-year PFS was 43% and 46% and the 2-year OS 45% and 46%, respectively; however, there were 10% treatment-related deaths.

WBRT is a very effective salvage treatment with response rates of 60–79% in refractory and relapsed patients and median OS of 10.9–16 months after progression/relapse [69, 70]. Due to higher risk of late neurotoxicity as compared to second-line chemotherapy, WBRT should be offered to patients who will unlikely tolerate chemotherapy and those in whom salvage chemotherapies have failed.

References

1. Dolecek TA, Propp JM, Stroup NE, et al. CBTRUS statistical report: primary brain and central nervous system tumors diagnosed in the United States in 2005-2009. Neuro Oncol. 2012;14(Suppl 5):v1–49.
2. O'Neill BP, Decker PA, Tieu C, et al. The changing incidence of primary central nervous system lymphoma is driven primarily by the changing incidence in young and middle-aged men and differs from time trends in systemic diffuse large B-cell non-Hodgkin's lymphoma. Am J Hematol. 2013;88(12):997–1000.
3. Korfel A, Schlegel U. Diagnosis and treatment of primary CNS lymphoma. Nat Rev Neurol. 2013;9(6):317–27.
4. Haldorsen IS, Espeland A, Larsson EM. Central nervous system lymphoma: characteristic findings on traditional and advanced imaging. AJNR Am J Neuroradiol. 2011;32(6):984–92.
5. Kuker W, Nagele T, Korfel A, et al. Primary central nervous system lymphomas (PCNSL): MRI features at presentation in 100 patients. J Neurooncol. 2005;72(2):169–77.
6. Yap KK, Sutherland T, Liew E, et al. Magnetic resonance features of primary central nervous system lymphoma in the immunocompetent patient: a pictorial essay. J Med Imaging Radiat Oncol. 2012;56(2):179–86.
7. Calli C, Kitis O, Yunten N, et al. Perfusion and diffusion MR imaging in enhancing malignant cerebral tumors. Eur J Radiol. 2006;58(3):394–403.
8. Toh CH, Castillo M, Wong AM, et al. Primary cerebral lymphoma and glioblastoma multiforme: differences in diffusion characteristics evaluated with diffusion tensor imaging. AJNR Am J Neuroradiol. 2008;29(3):471–5.
9. Zacharia TT, Law M, Naidich TP, et al. Central nervous system lymphoma characterization by diffusion-weighted imaging and MR spectroscopy. J Neuroimaging. 2008;18(4):411–7.
10. Harting I, Hartmann M, Jost G, et al. Differentiating primary central nervous system lymphoma from glioma in humans using localised proton magnetic resonance spectroscopy. Neurosci Lett. 2003;342(3):163–6.
11. Kawai N, Miyake K, Yamamoto Y, et al. 18F-FDG PET in the diagnosis and treatment of primary central nervous system lymphoma. Biomed Res Int. 2013;2013:247152.
12. Palmedo H, Urbach H, Bender H, et al. FDG-PET in immunocompetent patients with primary central nervous system lymphoma: correlation with MRI and clinical follow-up. Eur J Nucl Med Mol Imaging. 2006;33(2):164–8.
13. Hoang-Xuan K, Bessell E, Bromberg J, et al. Diagnosis and treatment of primary CNS lymphoma in immunocompetent patients: guidelines from the European Association for Neuro-Oncology. Lancet Oncol. 2015;16(7):e322–32.
14. Cinque P, et al. Epstein-Barr virus DNA in cerebrospinal fluid from patients with AIDS-related primary lymphomas of the central nervous system. Lancet. 1993;342:398–401.
15. Deckert M, Engert A, Brück W, et al. Modern concepts in the biology, diagnosis, differential diagnosis and treatment of primary central nervous system lymphoma. Leukemia. 2011;25(12):1797–807.
16. Korfel A, Weller M, Martus P, et al. Prognostic impact of meningeal dissemination in primary CNS lymphoma (PCNSL): experience from the G-PCNSL-SG1 trial. Ann Oncol. 2012;23(9):2374–80.
17. Schroers R, Baraniskin A, Heute C, et al. Diagnosis of leptomeningeal disease in diffuse large B-cell lymphomas of the central nervous system by flow

cytometry and cytopathology. Eur J Haematol. 2010;85(6):520–8.
18. Baraniskin A, Kuhnhenn J, Schlegel U, et al. Identification of microRNAs in the cerebrospinal fluid as marker for primary diffuse large B-cell lymphoma of the central nervous system. Blood. 2011;117(11):3140–6.
19. Fischer L, Korfel A, Pfeiffer S, et al. CXCL13 and CXCL12 in central nervous system lymphoma patients. Clin Cancer Res. 2009;15(19):5968–73.
20. Rubenstein JL, Wong VS, Kadoch C, et al. CXCL13 plus interleukin 10 is highly specific for the diagnosis of CNS lymphoma. Blood. 2013;121(23):4740–8.
21. Strehlow F, Bauer S, Martus P, et al. Osteopontin in cerebrospinal fluid as diagnostic biomarker for central nervous system lymphoma. J Neurooncol. 2016;129(1):165–71.
22. Viaccoz A, Ducray F, Tholance Y, et al. CSF neopterin level as a diagnostic marker in primary central nervous system lymphoma. Neuro Oncol. 2015;17(11):1497–503.
23. Chan CC, Rubenstein JL, Coupland SE, et al. Primary vitreoretinal lymphoma: a report from an International Primary Central Nervous System Lymphoma Collaborative Group symposium. Oncologist. 2011;16(11):1589–99.
24. Grimm SA, McCannel CA, Omuro AM, et al. Primary CNS lymphoma with intraocular involvement: International PCNSL Collaborative Group Report. Neurology. 2008;71(17):1355–60.
25. Ferreri AJ, Blay JY, Reni M, et al. Prognostic scoring system for primary CNS lymphomas: the International Extranodal Lymphoma Study Group experience. J Clin Oncol. 2003;21(2):266–72.
26. Thiel E, Korfel A, Martus P, et al. High-dose methotrexate with or without whole brain radiotherapy for primary CNS lymphoma (G-PCNSL-SG-1): a phase 3, randomised, non-inferiority trial. Lancet Oncol. 2010;11(11):1036–47.
27. Weller M, Martus P, Roth P, et al. Surgery for primary CNS lymphoma? Challenging a paradigm. Neuro Oncol. 2012;14(12):1481–4.
28. Nelson DF, Martz KL, Bonner H, et al. Non-Hodgkin's lymphoma of the brain: can high dose, large volume radiation therapy improve survival? Report on a prospective trial by the radiation oncology group (RTOG): RTOG 8315. Int J Radiat Oncol Biol Phys. 1992;23:9–17.
29. Borsi JD, Moe PJ. A comparative study on the pharmacokinetics of methotrexate in a dose range of 0.5 g to 33.6 g/m2 in children with acute lymphoblastic leukemia. Cancer. 1987;60(1):5–13.
30. Ferreri AJ, Reni M, Foppoli M, et al. High-dose cytarabine plus high-dose methotrexate versus high-dose methotrexate alone in patients with primary CNS lymphoma: a randomised phase 2 trial. Lancet. 2009;374(9700):1512–20.
31. Herrlinger U, Schabet M, Brugger W, et al. German Cancer Society Neuro-Oncology Working Group NOA-03 multicenter trial of single-agent high-dose methotrexate for primary central nervous system lymphoma. Ann Neurol. 2002;51(2):247–52.
32. Batchelor T, Carson K, O'Neill A, et al. Treatment of primary CNS lymphoma with methotrexate and deferred radiotherapy: a report of NABTT 96-07. J Clin Oncol. 2003;21(6):1044–9.
33. Ferreri AJ, Cwynarski K, Pulczynski E, et al. Chemoimmunotherapy with methotrexate, cytarabine, thiotepa, and rituximab (MATRix regimen) in patients with primary CNS lymphoma: results of the first randomisation of the International Extranodal Lymphoma Study Group-32 (IELSG32) phase 2 trial. Lancet Haematol. 2016;3(5):e217–27.
34. DeAngelis LM, Seiferheld W, Schold SC, et al. Combination chemotherapy and radiotherapy for primary central nervous system lymphoma: Radiation Therapy Oncology Group Study 93-10. J Clin Oncol. 2002;20(24):4643.
35. Poortmans PM, Kluin-Nelemans HC, Haaxma-Reiche H, et al. High-dose methotrexate-based chemotherapy followed by consolidating radiotherapy in non-AIDS-related primary central nervous system lymphoma: European Organization for Research and Treatment of Cancer Lymphoma Group Phase II Trial 20962. J Clin Oncol. 2003;21(24):4483–8.
36. Morris PG, Correa DD, Yahalom J, et al. Rituximab, methotrexate, procarbazine, and vincristine followed by consolidation reduced-dose whole-brain radiotherapy and cytarabine in newly diagnosed primary CNS lymphoma: final results and long-term outcome. J Clin Oncol. 2013;31(31):3971–9.
37. Rubenstein JL, Hsi ED, Johnson JL, et al. Intensive chemotherapy and immunotherapy in patients with newly diagnosed primary CNS lymphoma: CALGB 50202 (Alliance 50202). J Clin Oncol. 2013;31(25):3061–8.
38. Illerhaus G, Kasenda B, Ihorst G, et al. High-dose chemotherapy with autologous haemopoietic stem cell transplantation for newly diagnosed primary CNS lymphoma: a prospective, single-arm, phase 2 trial. Lancet Haematol. 2016;3(8):e388–97.
39. Ferreri A, Cwynarski K, Pulczynski E, et al. Effects on survival and neurocognitive functions of whole-brain radiotherapy (WBRT) and autologous stem cell transplantation (ASCT) as consolidation options after high-dose methotrexate-based chemoimmunotherapy in patients with newly diagnosed primary CNS lymphoma (PCNSL): results of the second randomization of the IELSG32 trial. Blood. 2016;128:511.
40. Korfel A, Thiel E, Martus P, et al. Randomized phase III study of whole-brain radiotherapy for primary CNS lymphoma. Neurology. 2015;84(12):1242–8.
41. Herrlinger U, Schäfer N, Fimmers R, et al. Early whole brain radiotherapy in primary CNS lymphoma: negative impact on quality of life in the randomized G-PCNSL-SG1 trial. J Cancer Res Clin Oncol. 2017;143(9):1815–21.

42. Correa DD, DeAngelis LM, Shi W, et al. Cognitive functions in survivors of primary central nervous system lymphoma. Neurology. 2004;62(4):548–55.
43. Doolittle ND, Korfel A, Lubow MA, et al. Long-term cognitive function, neuroimaging, and quality of life in primary CNS lymphoma. Neurology. 2013;81(1):84–92.
44. Juergens A, Pels H, Rogowski S, et al. Long-term survival with favorable cognitive outcome after chemotherapy in primary central nervous system lymphoma. Ann Neurol. 2010;67:182–1899.
45. Pels H, Schmidt-Wolf IG, Glasmacher A, et al. Primary central nervous system lymphoma: results of a pilot and phase II study of systemic and intraventricular chemotherapy with deferred radiotherapy. J Clin Oncol. 2003;21(24):4489–95.
46. Rieger L, Schlegel U, Le Coutre P, et al. A head-to-head comparison of two different high dose methotrexate (HDMTX)—and high dose cytarabin (HDAraC)-based chemotherapy regimens in younger patients with primary central nervous system lymphoma (PCNSL). Oral presentation at WFNOS 2017 Meeting, 5th Quadrennial Meeting of the World Federation of Neuro-Oncology Societies, May 4–7, 2017, Zurich, Switzerland.
47. Hoang-Xuan K, Taillandier L, Chinot O, et al. Chemotherapy alone as initial treatment for primary CNS lymphoma in patients older than 60 years: a multicenter phase II study (26952) of the European Organization for Research and Treatment of Cancer Brain Tumor Group. J Clin Oncol. 2003;21(14):2726–31.
48. Illerhaus G, Marks R, Müller F, et al. High-dose methotrexate combined with procarbazine and CCNU for primary CNS lymphoma in the elderly: results of a prospective pilot and phase II study. Ann Oncol. 2009;20(2):319–25.
49. Zhu JJ, Gerstner ER, Engler DA, et al. High-dose methotrexate for elderly patients with primary CNS lymphoma. Neuro Oncol. 2009;11(2):211–5.
50. Olivier G, Clavert A, Lacotte-Thierry L. A phase 1 dose escalation study of idarubicin combined with methotrexate, vindesine, and prednisolone for untreated elderly patients with primary central nervous system lymphoma. The GOELAMS LCP 99 trial. Am J Hematol. 2014;89(11):1024–9.
51. Omuro A, Chinot O, Taillandier L, et al. Methotrexate and temozolomide versus methotrexate, procarbazine, vincristine, and cytarabine for primary CNS lymphoma in an elderly population: an intergroup ANOCEF-GOELAMS randomised phase 2 trial. Lancet Haematol. 2015;2(6):e251–9.
52. Fritsch K, Kasenda B, Schorb E, et al. High-dose methotrexate-based immuno-chemotherapy for elderly primary CNS lymphoma patients (PRIMAIN study). Leukemia. 2017;31(4):846–52.
53. Pulczynski EJ, Kuittinen O, Erlanson M, et al. Successful change of treatment strategy in elderly patients with primary central nervous system lymphoma by de-escalating induction and introducing temozolomide maintenance: results from a phase II study by the Nordic Lymphoma Group. Haematologica. 2015;100(4):534–40.
54. Skiest DJ, Crosby C. Survival is prolonged by highly active antiretroviral therapy in AIDS patients with primary central nervous system lymphoma. AIDS. 2003;17(12):1787–93.
55. Evens AM, Choquet S, Kroll-Desrosiers AR, et al. Primary CNS posttransplant lymphoproliferative disease (PTLD): an international report of 84 cases in the modern era. Am J Transplant. 2013;13(6): 1512–22.
56. Pentsova E, Deangelis LM, Omuro A. Methotrexate re-challenge for recurrent primary central nervous system lymphoma. J Neurooncol. 2014;117(1):161–5.
57. Plotkin SR, Betensky RA, Hochberg FH, et al. Treatment of relapsed central nervous system lymphoma with high-dose methotrexate. Clin Cancer Res. 2004;10(17):5643–6.
58. Arellano-Rodrigo E, Lopez-Guillermo A, Bessell EM, et al. Salvage treatment with etoposide (VP-16), ifosfamide and cytarabine (Ara-C) for patients with recurrent primary central nervous system lymphoma. Eur J Haematol. 2003;70(4):219–24.
59. Chamberlain MC. Salvage therapy with bendamustine for methotrexate refractory recurrent primary CNS lymphoma: a retrospective case series. J Neurooncol. 2014;118(1):155–62.
60. Chamberlain MC. High-dose cytarabine salvage therapy for recurrent primary CNS lymphoma. J Neurooncol. 2016;126(3):545–50.
61. Enting RH, Demopoulos A, DeAngelis LM, et al. Salvage therapy for primary CNS lymphoma with a combination of rituximab and temozolomide. Neurology. 2004;63(5):901–3.
62. Fischer L, Thiel E, Klasen HA, et al. Prospective trial on topotecan salvage therapy in primary CNS lymphoma. Ann Oncol. 2006;17(7):1141–5.
63. Maza S, Kiewe P, Munz DL, et al. First report on a prospective trial with yttrium-90-labeled ibritumomab tiuxetan (Zevalin) in primary CNS lymphoma. Neuro Oncol. 2009;11(4):423–9.
64. Nayak L, Abrey LE, Drappatz J, et al. Multicenter phase II study of rituximab and temozolomide in recurrent primary central nervous system lymphoma. Leuk Lymphoma. 2013;54(1):58–61.
65. Reni M, Zaja F, Mason W, et al. Temozolomide as salvage treatment in primary brain lymphomas. Br J Cancer. 2007;96(6):864–7.
66. Korfel A, Schlegel U, Herrlinger U, et al. Phase II trial of temsirolimus for relapsed/refractory primary CNS lymphoma. J Clin Oncol. 2016;34(15):1757–63.
67. Kasenda B, Ihorst G, Schroers R, et al. High-dose chemotherapy with autologous hematopoietic stem cell support for relapsed or refractory primary CNS lymphoma—a prospective multicentre trial by the German Cooperative PCNSL Study Group. Leukemia. 2017;31(12):2623–9.

68. Soussain C, Hoang-Xuan K, Taillandier L, et al. Intensive chemotherapy followed by hematopoietic stem-cell rescue for refractory and recurrent primary CNS and intraocular lymphoma: Societe Francaise de Greffe de Moelle Osseuse-Therapie Cellulaire. J Clin Oncol. 2008;26(15):2512–8.
69. Hottinger AF, DeAngelis LM, Yahalom J, et al. Salvage whole brain radiotherapy for recurrent or refractory primary CNS lymphoma. Neurology. 2007;69(11):1178–82.
70. Nguyen PL, Chakravarti A, Finkelstein DM, et al. Results of whole-brain radiation as salvage of methotrexate failure for immunocompetent patients with primary CNS lymphoma. J Clin Oncol. 2005;23(7):1507–13.

Extranodal Localization of Aggressive Lymphoma

10

Jeremy S. Abramson
and Armando López-Guillermo

10.1 Introduction

Aggressive lymphomas with primary extranodal origin can be found in virtually all extranodal sites [1–6]. In fact, no less than 25% of diffuse large B-cell lymphomas (DLBCLs) primarily arise in a site other than a lymph node or lymphoid organ [7]. There are some discrepancies in the definition of primary extranodal lymphoma that may contribute to the wide range in the incidence described for these cases [6, 8–11]. Whereas the situation is clear for localized lymphomas isolated to a single extranodal location, secondary extranodal involvement by a systemic lymphoma cannot always be ruled out in advanced stage disease. Although definitions have varied, for practical terms lymphomas with a dominant extranodal component and only minimal nodal disease can be considered primary extranodal [6, 8]. Secondary lymphoid organs such as the spleen and Waldeyer's ring, including the tonsils, are typically not considered extranodal sites.

In addition to primary extranodal cases, extranodal involvement is common in typical nodal lymphomas, with around one half of diffuse large B-cell lymphoma (DLBCL) patients showing one extranodal site and 20% two or more. The latter is considered a poor risk parameter in the majority of prognostic scores for aggressive lymphomas, including the International Prognostic Index (IPI) [12–15]. Additionally, DLBCL arising in immunocompromised patients, including HIV+ and posttransplant [16, 17], constitutes distinct biologic subsets with frequently extranodal localization, including the central nervous system (CNS); these lymphomas are reviewed in detail in Chaps. 8 and 9.

The distribution of extranodal sites in aggressive lymphoma is very heterogeneous. The gastrointestinal (GI) tract is the most frequent extranodal site, particularly the stomach, followed by the skin, bone, and CNS. Other sites are rare but include the liver, lungs, and genitourinary organs [4–8, 11]. Within aggressive lymphomas, certain cytogenetic abnormalities increase the likelihood of extranodal involvement. Cases with a MYC translocation, especially in concert with a BCL2 and/or BCL6 rearrangement (so-called double- or triple-hit lymphoma), often involves extranodal locations, including the CNS [18–20].

Staging of primary extranodal DLBCL is similar to nodal DLBCL [21–23], including a PET/CT scan as per the Lugano criteria [23]. Nevertheless, some sites require specific techniques, such as MRI for CNS lymphomas or

J. S. Abramson (✉)
Massachusetts General Hospital Cancer Center, Boston, MA, USA
e-mail: jabramson@mgh.harvard.edu

A. López-Guillermo
Hospital Clínic, IDIBAPS, Barcelona, Spain
e-mail: alopezg@clinic.cat

G. Lenz, G. Salles (eds.), *Aggressive Lymphomas*, Hematologic Malignancies,
https://doi.org/10.1007/978-3-030-00362-3_10

endoscopies with or without endoscopic ultrasound for GI cases. Primary extranodal DLBCL limited to a single extranodal location is considered stage IE or IIE in the setting of local nodal extension only. If extranodal involvement occurs in the setting of either diffuse nodal or additional extranodal sites, then the stage is IV [4, 5, 23].

The aim of this chapter is to review the unique characteristics and treatment approach for patients with the most common primary extranodal aggressive lymphomas. Most correspond to DLBCL, but other histologies, including mantle-cell lymphomas (MCL), Burkitt lymphomas (BL), and peripheral T-cell lymphomas (PTCL), will be also covered. Overall, treatment depends primarily on the histology and, therefore, immunochemotherapy; usually the standard regimen R-CHOP (rituximab, cyclophosphamide, adriamycin, vincristine, and prednisone) is the gold standard in most DLBCL cases, irrespective of the nodal or extranodal origin [24]. Nevertheless, some specific consideration should be mentioned for each subtype for the most frequent extranodal sites, including the GI tract, bone, breast, testis and ovary, skin, and primary mediastinal. CNS lymphomas are addressed separately in Chap. 10.

10.2 Gastrointestinal (GI) Lymphomas

GI lymphomas represent 30–40% of all extranodal cases and 5–20% of all non-Hodgkin lymphomas [1, 25, 26]. The stomach is the most frequently involved organ, followed by the small intestine and colon [1, 6, 25, 26]. DLBCL is the predominant histology, representing 60% of gastric and 70% of intestinal lymphomas [27]. Other aggressive histologies include BL (5% of cases) and MCL (5% of cases, in most cases showing the characteristic multiple lymphomatous polyposis) [26].

Patients with aggressive GI lymphomas may present with abdominal pain, dyspepsia, nausea and vomiting, obstruction, or GI hemorrhage. The diagnosis is determined by tissue biopsy, usually obtained in the course of an endoscopic evaluation [7]. Routine staging includes a full body PET/CT scan, as in other aggressive lymphomas; as well as endoscopy (esophagogastroduodenoscopy or colonoscopy), sometimes combined with endoscopic ultrasound which may provide additonal information on depth of invasion and local nodal extension. Notably, aggressive gastric lymphomas, even with bulky presentation, frequently are localized, with no infiltration of any other organ outside GI and regional lymph nodes [6].

10.2.1 Gastric Lymphomas

As already indicated, the stomach is the most frequently involved GI site. DLBCL represents the vast majority of cases, but concomitant MALT lymphoma can also be seen in approximately half of the cases [29]. These cases are often seen in association with *H. pylori* infection, which should be checked in all patients at diagnosis, and may present with symptoms of gastric ulceration including pain or bleeding.

R-CHOP remains the gold-standard treatment for gastric DLBCL [1, 24–30]. Nevertheless, some aspects, including the role of surgery or radiotherapy, and the eradication of *Helicobacter pylori* (HP) deserve further discussion. Prior to the development of effective chemotherapy, surgery with total or partial gastrectomy was considered the standard treatment. Currently, however, the role of surgery is marginal, except in the setting of severe but unusual complications including perforation or refractory hemorrhage [31, 32]. Local therapy with involved field radiotherapy (IF-RT) has also been used but is not considered appropriate monotherapy in gastric lymphomas, even for localized disease, since the risk of relapse is much higher without systemic therapy. Radiation can be considered as local consolidation after chemotherapy, where combined modality does appear to reduce the rate of local relapse but without improvement in overall survival [33]. Notably, this trial was in the pre-rituximab era and no experience has been published in patients receiving chemoimmunotherapy. *H. pylori* eradication must also be considered in *H. pylori*-positive aggressive gastric lymphomas, as is the gold standard for gastric MALT lymphomas, usually as the only treatment modality. In *H. pylori*-positive DLBCL, however, *H. pylori* eradication is usually considered an adjunct to standard immunochemotherapy. Interestingly, *H. pylori* eradication alone has been preliminarily investigated in gastric DLBCL [34–37]. Two clinical trials have shown high CR rates (63–69%) in de novo limited-stage gastric *H. pylori*-positive DLBCL, as well as in patients with DLBCL arising from *H. pylori*-positive MALT lymphoma (CR rate 56%) [35, 36, 38]. These intriguing data warrant further evaluation but do not presently support antibiotic therapy alone in *H. pylori*-positive DLBCL patients who can tolerate chemoimmunotherapy.

10.2.2 Intestinal Lymphomas

Intestinal lymphomas are the second in frequency within the GI tract. Most cases are DLBCL, although BL, MCL, and PTCL (especially enteropathy-associated T-cell lymphoma) are also seen. MCL is associated with a characteristic syndrome of multiple lymphomatous polyposis, which may be asymptomatic or be associated with discomfort or bleeding.

Diagnosis of intestyinal lymphomas may be made endoscopically, but surgery may also have a role in the diagnosis of intestinal lymphoma (laparoscopy or open surgery with bowel resection) as well as in dealing with complications of the lymphoma itself or sequelae of treatment, including perforation, hemorrhage, or obstruction [39, 40]. R-CHOP is the standard for intestinal DLBCL. The risk of complications is higher than for gastric cases, about 20–30% of cases, and so patients must be followed closely and counseled accordingly.

MCL involvement is usually secondary in the setting of extensive systemic disease and should be treated with the standard approach of this type (chemoimmunotherapy including cytarabine followed by intensification with autologous stem cell transplantation for young fit patients) [41]. At present, the systematic investigation of gastric and colonic involvement by means of endoscopies is not formally recommended for all patients with MCL, since the finding of infiltration does not substantially change prognosis or treatment in this disease which is virtually always advanced stage at the time of diagnosis [42].

Sporadic BL, the predominant subtype seen in Western countries, often presents as a bulky abdominal mass, with the ileocecal area being the most frequently involved location [43]. HIV-associated Burkitt lymphoma will usually present at advanced stage with extensive involvement of virtually any extranodal location [44]. Curative treatment of BL is typically with intensive multi-agent chemotherapy and rituximab. Dose-adjusted EPOCH-R is emerging as a less intensive and highly effective alternative, particularly in older or less fit patients [45].

Finally, primary intestinal T-cell lymphoma is usually diagnosed as enteropathy-associated T-cell lymphoma and occurs in patients with underlying celiac disease [46]. The small intestine is the most commonly involved location, and patients typically present with abdominal pain and diarrhea and may have malabsorption with anorexia, fatigue, and malnutrition. The diagnosis is usually made via endoscopic biopsy. Less commonly, a primary intestinal T-cell lymphoma can occur in the absence of underlying celiac disease, known as intestinal T-cell lymphoma NOS, and also follows an aggressive clinical course. Although localized in the bowel, the prognosis of patients with primary intestinal T-cell lymphomas is generally unfavorable, with a median OS of less than 1 year in multiple series [47]. CHOP-like therapy remains the most popular approach, followed by consolidation with autologous or allogeneic stem cell transplantation in younger patients with a favorable performance status [47–49].

10.3 Primary Bone Lymphoma

Lymphomas primarily arising in bone represent about 5% of extranodal lymphomas and 5% of bone cancers. Histologically, 70–80% are DLBCL, although other histologies are possible, including BL and anaplastic large-cell lymphomas (ALCL), among others [50–53]. Symptoms are usually local, including pain (80–90% of the cases), presence of tumor mass, or pathologic fractures. Osteolysis, hypercalcemia, or spinal cord compression is possible but infrequent. Three forms of presentation are described: a single bone lesion, a polyostotic location with multiple bone lesions, and disseminated lesions in the setting of secondary bone infiltration of a systemic lymphoma [50, 51].

The diagnosis is by means of a bone biopsy. Fine needle aspiration is not sufficient to reach the correct diagnosis and characterization of the lymphoma, so diagnosis usually needs a core needle or surgical biopsy. Plain radiographs are nonspecific, so CT scans or magnetic resonance imaging (MRI) is often employed to define the local extension as well as the cortical invasion and destruction. PET/CT is the standard modality for staging, as for any other DLBCL, with the PET component being particularly important as bone involvement by DLBCL may not sufficiently distort cortical anatomy sufficiently to be obvious on CT alone. PET is also critical in the restaging setting where FDG-avidity is necessary to distinguish active lymphoma from posttreatment sclerotic change [54]. Notably, low-level FDG-avidity posttreatment is common in primary DLBCL of bone due to low-level avidity within sites of bone remodeling following therapy and may need to be followed with serial imaging to insure resolution. Staging is performed with the Lugano criteria where a single bony location is classified as stage IE and mutifocal bone disease classified as stage IV [11]. Patients with localized primary bone DLBCL (stage IE) typically have an excellent outcome, and the usefulness of the IPI may be lower in this subset relative to other DLBCLs [50]. The International Extranodal Lymphoma Study Group (IELSG) found that younger age, normal LDH, good performance status, combined modality therapy, and higher radiation dose predicted particularly favorable outcome [50, 51, 55]. R-CHOP followed by consolidative radiation therapy should therefore be considered the preferred therapy in limited-stage DLBCL of bone if the site is amenable to radiation therapy with an acceptable toxicity profile. For advanced stage disease, R-CHOP remains the cornerstone of therapy for six complete cycles [24, 30]. Data from the German High Grade Lymphoma Study Group has suggested that radiation consolidation to bony sites adds value even in advanced stage disease with an improvement in event-free survival, though without a statistical improvement in OS [56]. Further analysis is required to understand if patients in a complete metabolic remission by PET scan garner benefit from consolidation following chemoimmunotherapy or whether the value of radiation may be limited to PR patients.

10.4 Primary Mediastinal B-Cell Lymphoma

Primary mediastinal B-cell lymphoma (PMBCL) is a distinct clinical and biological variant of DLBCL derived from thymic B cells. Transcriptional profiling has shown that PMBCL shares overlapping molecular features with the nodular sclerosis variant of classical Hodgkin lymphoma (NSHL), including activation of the nuclear factor-kappa B (NF-kB) pathway and Janus kinase/signal transduction and activator of transcription (JAK/STAT) signaling [57–59]. Amplification of the 9p24.1 locus containing JAK2 as well as PD-1 ligands further promotes JAK/STAT activation and immune escape, respectively.

Biologic similarities with NSHL may be reflected histologically as well with the diffuse proliferation of malignant lymphocytes separated by compartmentalizing fibrosis [60]. The malignant cells are often pleomorphic, and Reed-Sternberg-like variants may be observed. Unlike the classical Hodgkin lymphoma, the pan B-cell markers CD19, CD20, CD22, and CD79a are expressed in PMBCL, though surface immunoglobulin is typically absent. Most cases will also express CD23 and CD30, though the latter is usually dim and heterogeneous in contrast to NSHL where it is bright and uniform. Most cases will express PD-L1 and PD-L2, reflecting the underlying amplification of the 9p24.1 genetic locus.

Clinically, PMBCL occurs in younger patients than typical DLBCL NOS with a median age of approximately 35 years. There is a slight female predominance, and three quarters of patients will present with bulky mediastinal disease. Mediastinal tumors may be locally invasive of midline mediastinal structures, the lungs, pericardium, and chest wall, and can result in superior vena cava syndrome as well as pleural or pericardial effusions. Despite the locally invasive nature, advanced stage disease is uncommon, occurring in only approximately 20% of cases at diagnosis. When disease does occur outside of the mediastinum, disseminated nodal or bone marrow involvement is markedly less common than visceral metastatic disease.

Prior to the introduction of rituximab, the traditional CHOP regimen had been associated with a higher failure rate than would be expected in a large-cell lymphoma occurring predominantly in young people with limited-stage disease. Retrospective analyses of more intensive regimens such as MACOP-B (methotrexate, doxorubicin, cyclophosphamide, vincristine, prednisone, and bleomycin) and VACOP-B (etoposide, doxorubicin, cyclophosphamide, vincristine, prednisone, and bleomycin) appeared superior to CHOP [61–63]. The majority of patients in historic series also received consolidative mediastinal radiation, which was associated with an improved progression-free survival compared to patients treated with radiation alone [61, 62]. In the modern era, rituximab added to CHOP may not obviate the deficits of CHOP alone. A retrospective analysis of 63 PMBCL patients treated with R-CHOP reported a 21% incidence of primary induction failure and a 5-year PFS of 68% [64]. Adverse prognostic factors in this analysis included advanced stage disease, older age, and increased age-adjusted IPI score. As in the pre-rituximab era, the majority (77%) of R-CHOP-treated patients received consolidative mediastinal radiation. A subset analysis of 87 patients with PMBCL treated in the prospective Mabthera International Trial (MInT) of CHOP-like chemotherapy with or without rituximab found a benefit for rituximab plus chemotherapy compared to chemotherapy alone [65]. The 3-year event-free survival for patients treated with R-CHOP was excellent at 78%, though notably the trial was limited to patients under the age of 60 with no more than one IPI risk factor, so 92% of subjects had limited-stage disease and the vast majority of high-risk patients who may have fared poorly were excluded. As with prior series, over 70% of subjects also required consolidative radiation therapy. The failure rate with R-CHOP, particularly in high-risk patients, as well as the long-term potential side effects of radiation therapy including secondary malignancies, heart disease, lung disease, and thyroid dysfunction or cancer, prompted further investigation of more intensive regimens combined with rituximab. Dose-adjusted EPOCH-R was evaluated in a phase II study from the National Cancer Institute which included 51 patients with PMBCL treated with 6 cycles of DA-EPOCH-R and no planned radiation therapy. The 5-year event-free survival was 97%; only two patients required radiation treatment, and no patient experienced relapse [66]. These data suggest that DA-EPOCH-R carries a low rate of primary induction failure, appears to obviate the need for irradiation in most patients, and has resulted in a widespread adoption of this treatment as initial therapy in PMBCL.

Though most patients with PMBCL will be cured with frontline chemo-immunotherapy, a significant minority will have primary refractory disease or relapse after achieving initial remission. Most treatment failures occur early—either during initial treatment or within 1 year of completing therapy—and relapses greater than 18 months from completing frontline therapy in this disease are rare. Relapsed and refractory PMBCL is a challenging disease as patients are often resistant to second-line therapy as well. The current approach to relapsed or refractory PMBCL is identical to DLBCL whereby second-line chemoimmunotherapy is administered, and patients with chemosensitive disease then proceed to high-dose chemotherapy with autologous stem cell transplantation. Unfortunately, PMBCL patients do not fare as well with this traditional salvage approach as other patients with DLBCL [67, 68]. A retrospective analysis of patients with relapsed PMBCL compared to DLBCL NOS found lower rates of overall response to second-line therapy (25% versus 48%) and worse overall survival at 2 years (15% versus 34%) [68]. Novel therapies are therefore needed for these high-risk patients at relapse. Expression of CD30 in the majority of tumors prompted investigation of brentuximab vedotin, a CD30-directed antibody drug conjugate, which is highly effective and FDA approved for treatment of relapsed classical Hodgkin lymphoma, a biologic cousin of PMBCL. Unfortunately, the results of a phase II study in relapsed PMBCL were disappointing with objective responses observed in only 2 of 15 treated patients in a phase II study, both partial responses, prompting early closure of the trial [69]. More appealing has been targeting the amplified PD-L1 and PD-L2 with immune checkpoint inhibitors, as has also proven effective in relapsed classical Hodgkin lymphoma. A prospective phase II study of the PD-1 inhibitor pembrolizumab included 17 evaluable patients with PMBCL and showed responses in 7 of 17 patients (41%) [70]. The median duration of remission had not been reached at a median follow-up of 11 months, suggesting that many of these responses may prove durable. Finally, anti-CD19 CAR T-cells have shown the ability to induce complete and durable remissions in a significant proportion of patients with chemorefractory PMBCL and are now considered the standard therapy in this extremely high-risk indication after failure of 2 or more prior lines of therapy [71, 72].

10.5 Testicular Lymphomas

Primary testicular lymphoma (PTL) accounts for less than 5% of all testicular tumors and only 1–2% of all non-Hodgkin lymphomas. The vast majority of cases (approximately 90%) are DLBCL, though rarely other histologies can involve the testis, including extranodal marginal zone lymphoma, BL, MCL, extranodal NK/T-cell lymphoma, peripheral T-cell lymphoma, and ALCL. This chapter will focus on primary DLBCL of the testis. PTL occurs at a median age in the late 60s and is the most common testicular malignancy in men over the age of 60 [73, 74]. The most common clinical presentation is with a painless unilateral testicular mass, and systemic "B" symptoms are uncommon. Three quarters of patients present with limited (Ann Arbor stages I–II) disease, with the remaining quarter presenting at advanced stage. Stage I patients have isolated testicular involvement, while stage II patients will also have involvement of the retroperitoneal nodes. Similar to PMBCL, when PTL presents at advanced stage, it has a predilection for extranodal locations, particularly the CNS and the contralateral testis. These sites are also common locations of relapse after initial therapy, with nearly a third of relapses involving the CNS [74, 75], most commonly the brain parenchyma. Interestingly, relapses in the CNS may occur as late as 10 years after initial treatment.

Diagnosis of PTL is typically made via orchiectomy. The tumor cells express pan B-cell markers CD19, CD20, and CD79A and are usually positive for BCL-2. Cell of origin, as determined either by gene expression profiling or immunohistochemistry, is the activated B-cell (ABC) subtype in the vast majority of cases. Activating MYD88 mutations are found in 70–86% of cases, often in association with a concomitant activating CD79B mutation [76, 77]. Deletions of the HLA loci are common, as are gains of chromosome 19q13 [78]. Copy number gains of 9p24.1, resulting in increased expression of PD-L1 and PD-L2, are also observed in the majority of cases and may have therapeutic relevance [77].

All patients with PTL require systemic therapy as the relapse rate after orchiectomy alone is approximately 80% with a median overall survival of 1 year [74, 75]. In a multicenter retrospective analysis of PTL by the International Extranodal Lymphoma Study Group (IELSG), the 5-year overall survival for the entire population was 48%, but patients treated with combination chemotherapy (prior to rituximab), intrathecal chemotherapy, and prophylactic scrotal radiation had the best outcome with a 3-year overall survival of 88%. This led to a phase II clinical trial by the IELSG-evaluating R-CHOP, intrathecal methotrexate, and prophylactic scrotal radiation in 53 patients with limited-stage PTL and resulted in a 5-year PFS and OS of 74% and 85%, respectively [79]. This study did have three CNS relapses, one of which was in the brain parenchyma. Whether intrathecal methotrexate represents the optimal method of CNS prophylaxis, however, remains unknown. The majority of CNS recurrences of PTL occur within the brain parenchyma, which is unlikely to be successfully reached by intrathecal therapy alone. Further, intrathecal injections via lumbar puncture yield highly variable concentrations within the cerebral ventricles, with many patients not achieving therapeutic concentrations [80]. This has led some to employ systemic methotrexate for CNS prophylaxis in patients at high risk for CNS relapse of DLBCL, as it can be safely and effectively combined with R-CHOP, usually administered at a dose of 3–3.5 g/m^2 on day 15 of the 21-day R-CHOP cycle [81]. Whether systemic or intrathecal prophylaxis is preferable remains uncertain at this time, and so either modality can be considered appropriate. Certainly, optimal initial therapy of PTL should include orchiectomy, R-CHOP with incorporation of CNS prophylaxis (either intrathecal or systemic), and prophylactic scrotal radiotherapy.

Relapsed PTL is treated similar to other cases of relapsed DLBCL where second-line chemotherapy followed by high-dose chemotherapy with autologous stem cell transplant remains the treatment of choice for transplant-eligible patients with chemosensitive relapsed disease. Several biologically targeted therapies are also commercially available with biologic and clinical rationale in relapsed PTL. Both lenalidomide and ibrutinib have shown activity in relapsed DLBCL, particularly the ABC subtype which comprises most cases of PTL [82, 83]. Ibrutinib appears to have particularly encouraging activity within ABC DLBCLs which harbor mutations of both MYD88 and CD79B, a mutational pattern enriched within PTL, making this a potentially appealing therapy for chemorefractory disease. Amplification and expression of PD-1 ligands in the majority of PTLs also raise the prospect of PD-1/PD-L1 inhibitors in this disease, and preliminary evidence of efficacy has been demonstrated in a small number of patients [84]. Encouragingly, lenalidomide, ibrutinib, and PD-1 inhibitors have all shown activity in CNS lymphomas, which is of great relevance in this DLBCL subtype. Further data regarding the proper use and sequencing of these novel agents is needed.

10.6 Breast Lymphoma

Lymphomas localized to the breast represent about 2% of extranodal lymphomas and less than 1% of breast malignancies [85, 86]. DLBCL is the most frequent aggressive histology, although other types, including BL, may be seen. Of note, indolent lymphomas, particularly MALT, often appear in the breast and are managed akin to other localized indolent lymphomas. Primary breast DLBCL is biologically different from other sites. The mutational profile mostly involves the NF-kB signaling pathway, with a high frequency of *PIM1* mutations [87].

Primary breast lymphoma typically presents with a mass that is clinically suspicious of a breast carcinoma [88–90]. Local symptoms are frequent, whereas general manifestations are rare in localized cases. Surgical or core needle biopsy is mandatory for diagnosis as fine needle aspiration is insufficiently diagnostic. According to the largest retrospective study by the IELSG [90], primary DLBCL of the breast has some substantial differences with respect to standard nodal DLBCLs including (1) high risk of contralateral breast involvement, (2) relapse tendency in other extranodal sites, and (3) risk of CNS involvement or relapse (although this latter point remains controversial in the modern era). Based on the IELSG data, treatment with CHOP and radiation produced a median PFS and OS of 5.5 and 8 years, respectively, in the pre-rituximab era. More recent data suggest that IF-RT still adds significant therapeutic benefits receiving chemoimmunotherapy [91]. Although not demonstrated in a specific trial, the addition of rituximab is likely to be beneficial, so R-CHOP is the current standard of care [9]. Whether increased CNS risk persists in the rituximab era is unclear as it has not emerged as a discrete risk factor on multivariable analyses in DLBCL. Attention should be paid to other risk factors, and CNS prophylaxis considered in patients with high-risk IPI scores, but insufficient data exists to recommend routine inclusion in low-risk patients with stage IE disease treated with combined modality therapy. Breast involvement in Burkitt lymphoma is common and should be managed similar to other Burkitt lymphomas with intensive regimens that include CNS prophylaxis.

10.7 Primary Cutaneous Lymphoma

The skin is a common site of lymphoma involvement, most frequently of T-cell origin (about 80%), including mycosis fungoides and primary cutaneous anaplastic large-cell lymphoma, usually presenting at early stage and managed by dermatologists. Among cutaneous B-cell lymphomas, most are indolent histologies such as MALT and primary cutaneous follicle center lymphomas, but a small percentage are DLBCL. Among the latter, primary cutaneous DLBCL leg-type is an aggressive lymphoma frequently seen in elderly women and appearing on the legs as the name implies. These lymphomas are of ABC origin and are characterized by an aggressive clinical course with subsequent relapse in extra-cutaneous sites in more than 50% of cases [92]. The outcome is generally unfavorable, with 5-year OS of about 50%. Treatment is with standard R-CHOP [93, 94], but novel approaches targeting the ABC subtype, such as with the inclusion of lenalidomide or ibrutinib, warrant investigation. The role of IF-RT is not well established, but given the relatively poor outcome with immunochemotherapy alone, radiation consolidation should be strongly considered for limited-stage disease.

10.8 Extranodal Aggressive Lymphoma in Other Locations

Aggressive extranodal lymphomas can arise in virtually any other extranodal site, but there is no sufficient data to classify them presently as discrete diseases with unique management recommendations. So DLBCLs occurring primarily within the lung, liver, kidney, adrenal gland, ovary, uterus, or other extranodal locations are typically treated with R-CHOP as with typical cases of DLBCL [24, 30]. Consolidative radiation therapy is not routinely employed in most visceral DLBCLs given the concern for organ toxicity, and the encouraging efficacy of R-CHOP alone, but should be considered on a case-by-case basis dependent on location, field size, and response to chemoimmunotherapy. Whether these discrete locations are independently associated with risk of CNS relapse remains controversial without consistent results observed in multivariable analyses in the modern era. Involvement of the kidney or adrenal gland has been fairly consistent and should warrant CNS prophylaxis in eligible patients [95]. Other extranodal locations should be assessed in the context of their overall disease burden and additional risk factors for CNS dissemination such as IPI score and translocation status of *MYC* and *BCL2* [96].

References

1. Freeman C, Berg JW, Cutler SJ. Occurrence and prognosis of extranodal lymphomas. Cancer. 1972;29:252–60.
2. Norris HJ, Jensen RD. Relative frequency of ovarian neoplasms in children and adolescents. Cancer. 1972;30:713–9.
3. Konje JC, Otolorin EO, Odukoya OA, et al. Burkitts lymphoma of the ovary in Nigerian adults—a 27-year review. Afr J Med Med Sci. 1989;18:301–5.
4. Zucca E, Roggero E, Bertoni F, et al. Primary extranodal non-Hodgkin's lymphomas. Part 1: gastrointes-

tinal, cutaneous and genitourinary lymphomas. Ann Oncol. 1997;8:727–37.
5. Zucca E, Roggero E, Bertoni F, et al. Primary extranodal non-Hodgkin's lymphomas. Part 2: head and neck, central nervous system and other less common sites. Ann Oncol. 1999;10:1023–33.
6. Lopez-Guillermo A, Colomo L, Jimenez M, et al. Diffuse large B-cell lymphoma: clinical and biological characterization and outcome according to the nodal or extranodal primary origin. J Clin Oncol. 2005;23:2797–804.
7. Swerdlow SH, Campo E, Harris NL, Jaffe ES, Pileri SA, Stein H, Thiele J, Arber DA, Hasserjian RP, Le Beau MM, Orazi A, Siebert R, editors. WHO classification of tumours of haematopoietic and lymphoid tissues. Lyon: International Agency for Research on Cancer; 2017.
8. d'Amore F, Christensen BE, Brincker H, et al. Clinicopathological features and prognostic factors in extranodal non-Hodgkin's lymphomas. Danish LYFO Study Group. Eur J Cancer. 1991;27:1201–8.
9. Groves FD, Linet MS, Travis LB, et al. Cancer surveillance series: non-Hodgkin's lymphoma incidence by histologic subtype in the United States from 1978 through 1995. J Natl Cancer Inst. 2000;92:1240–51.
10. Müller AM, Ihorst G, Mertelsmann R, et al. Epidemiology of non-Hodgkin's lymphomas (NHL): trends, geographic distribution, and aetiology. Ann Hematol. 2005;84:1–12.
11. Vannata B, Zucca E. Primary extranodal B-cell lymphoma: current concepts and treatment strategies. Chin Clin Oncol. 2015;4:10–27.
12. The International Non-Hodgkin's Lymphoma Prognostic Factors Project. A predictive model for aggressive non-Hodgkin's lymphoma. N Engl J Med. 1993;329:987–94.
13. Sehn LH, Berry B, Chhanabhai M, Fitzgerald C, et al. The revised International Prognostic Index (R-IPI) is a better predictor of outcome than the standard IPI for patients with diffuse large B-cell lymphoma treated with R-CHOP. Blood. 2007;109:1857–61.
14. Zhou Z, Sehn LH, Rademaker AW, et al. An enhanced International Prognostic Index (NCCN-IPI) for patients with diffuse large B-cell lymphoma treated in the rituximab era. Blood. 2014;123:837–42.
15. Montalbán C, Díaz-López A, Dlouhy I, et al. Validation of the NCCN-IPI for diffuse large B-cell lymphoma (DLBCL): the addition of β2-microglobulin yields a more accurate GELTAMO-IPI. Br J Haematol. 2017;176:918–28.
16. Besson C, Lancar R, Prevot S, et al. Outcomes for HIV-associated diffuse large B-cell lymphoma in the modern combined antiretroviral therapy era. AIDS. 2017;31:2493–501.
17. Al Mansour Z, Nelson BP, Evens AM. Post-transplant lymphoproliferative disease (PTLD): risk factors, diagnosis, and current treatment strategies. Curr Hematol Malig Rep. 2013;8:173–83.
18. Copie-Bergman C, Gaulard P, Leroy K, et al. Immunofluorescence in situ hybridization index predicts survival in patients with diffuse large B-cell lymphoma treated with R-CHOP: a GELA study. J Clin Oncol. 2009;27:5573–9.
19. Hu S, Xu-Monette ZY, Tzankov A, et al. MYC/BCL2 protein coexpression contributes to the inferior survival of activated B-cell subtype of diffuse large B-cell lymphoma and demonstrates high-risk gene expression signatures: a report from the International DLBCL Rituximab-CHOP Consortium Program. Blood. 2013;121:4021–31.
20. Friedberg JW. How I treat double-hit lymphoma. Blood. 2017;130:590–6.
21. Cheson BD, Horning SJ, Coiffier B, et al. Report of an international workshop to standardize response criteria for non-Hodgkin's lymphomas. NCI Sponsored International Working Group. J Clin Oncol. 1999;17:1244–53.
22. Cheson BD, Pfistner B, Juweid ME, et al. Revised response criteria for malignant lymphoma. J Clin Oncol. 2007;25:579–86.
23. Cheson BD, Fisher RI, Barrington SF, et al. Recommendations for initial evaluation, staging, and response assessment of Hodgkin and non-Hodgkin lymphoma: the Lugano classification. J Clin Oncol. 2014;32:3059–62.
24. Tilly H, Gomes da Silva M, Vitolo U, et al. Diffuse large B-cell lymphoma (DLBCL): ESMO clinical practice guidelines for diagnosis, treatment and follow-up. Ann Oncol. 2015;26(Suppl 5):v116–25.
25. d'Amore F, Brincker H, Gronbaek K, et al. Non-Hodgkin's lymphoma of the gastrointestinal tract: a population-based analysis of incidence, geographic distribution, clinicopathologic presentation features, and prognosis. Danish Lymphoma Study Group. J Clin Oncol. 1994;12:1673–84.
26. Kock P, del Valle F, Berdel WE, et al. Primary gastrointestinal non-Hodgkin's lymphoma: I. Anatomic and histologic distribution, clinical features, and survival data of 371 patients registered by the German Multicenter Study GIT NHL 01/92. J Clin Oncol. 2001;19:3861–73.
27. Howell JM, Auer-Grzesiak I, Zhang J, et al. Increasing incidence rates, distribution and histological characteristics of primary gastrointestinal non-Hodgkin's lymphoma in a North American population. Can J Gastroenterol. 2012;26:452–6.
28. Song MK, Chung JS, Shin HJ, et al. Prognostic value of metabolic tumor volume on PET/CT in primary gastrointestinal diffuse large B cell lymphoma. Cancer Sci. 2012;103:477–82.
29. Ferreri A, Freschi M, Dell'Oro S, et al. Prognostic significance of the histopathologic recognition of low- and high-grade components in stages I-II B-cell gastric lymphomas. Am J Surg Pathol. 2001;25:95–102.
30. Ghielmini M, Vitolo U, Kimby E, et al. ESMO guidelines consensus conference on malignant lymphomas 2011 part I: diffuse large B-cell lymphoma (DLBCL), follicular lymphoma (FL), and chronic lymphocytic leukemia (CLL). Ann Oncol. 2013;24:561–76.

31. Dickson BC, Serra S, Chetty R. Primary gastrointestinal tract lymphoma: diagnosis and management of common neoplasm. Expert Rev Anticancer Ther. 2006;6:1609–28.
32. Ikoma N, Badgwell BD, Mansfield PF. Multimodality treatment of gastric lymphoma. Surg Clin North Am. 2017;97:405–20.
33. Martinelli G, Gigli F, Calabrese L, et al. Early stage gastric diffuse large B-cell lymphomas: results of a randomized trial comparing chemotherapy alone versus chemotherapy + involved field radiotherapy (IELSG 4). Leuk Lymphoma. 2009;50:925–31.
34. Chen LT, Lin JT, Shyu RY, et al. Prospective study of helicobacter pylori eradication therapy in stage I(E) high-grade mucosa-associated lymphoid tissue lymphoma of the stomach. J Clin Oncol. 2001;19:4245–51.
35. Ferreri AJ, Govi S, Raderer M, et al. Helicobacter pylori eradication as exclusive treatment for limited-stage gastric diffuse large B-cell lymphoma: results of a multicenter phase 2 trial. Blood. 2012;120:3858–60.
36. Kuo SH, Yeh KH, Wu M, et al. Helicobacter pylori eradication therapy is effective in the treatment of early stage H pylori-positive gastric diffuse large B-cell lymphomas. Blood. 2012;119:4838–44.
37. Cuccurullo R, Govi S, Ferreri AJ. De-escalating therapy in gastric aggressive lymphoma. World J Gastroenterol. 2014;20:8993–7.
38. Kuo SH. Helicobacter pylori-related diffuse large B-cell lymphoma of the stomach: a distinct entity with lower aggressiveness and higher chemosensitivity. Blood Cancer J. 2014;4:e220.
39. Cortelazzo S, Rossi A, Oldani F, et al. The modified International Prognostic Index can predict the outcome of localized primary intestinal lymphoma of both extranodal marginal zone B-cell and diffuse large B-cell histologies. Br J Haematol. 2002;118:218–28.
40. Ibrahim EM, Ezzat AA, El-Weshi AN, et al. Primary intestinal diffuse large B-cell non-Hodgkin's lymphoma: clinical features, management, and prognosis of 66 patients. Ann Oncol. 2001;12:53–8.
41. Dreyling M. Mantle cell lymphoma: biology, clinical presentation, and therapeutic approaches. Am Soc Clin Oncol Educ Book. 2014:191–8.
42. Shannon EM, MacQueen IT, Miller JM, et al. Management of primary gastrointestinal non-Hodgkin lymphomas: a population-based survival analysis. J Gastrointest Surg. 2016;20:1141–9.
43. Dunleavy K, Little RF, Wilson WH. Update on Burkitt lymphoma. Hematol Oncol Clin North Am. 2016;30:1333–43.
44. Kaplan LD. HIV-associated lymphoma. Best Pract Res Clin Haematol. 2012;25:101–17.
45. Hoelzer D. Dose-adjusted EPOCH-R for Burkitt lymphoma. Clin Adv Hematol Oncol. 2014;12:777–9.
46. Foss FM, Zinzani PL, Vose JM, et al. Peripheral T-cell lymphoma. Blood. 2011;117:6756–67.
47. Armitage JO. The aggressive peripheral T-cell lymphomas: 2017. Am J Hematol. 2017;92:706–15.
48. Ondrejka S, Jagadeesh D. Enteropathy-associated T-cell lymphoma. Curr Hematol Malig Rep. 2016;11:504–13.
49. Nijeboer P, Malamut G, Mulder CJ, et al. Enteropathy-associated T-cell lymphoma: improving treatment strategies. Dig Dis. 2015;33:231–5.
50. Messina C, Ferreri AJ, Govi S, et al. Clinical features, management and prognosis of multifocal primary bone lymphoma: a retrospective study of the International Extranodal Lymphoma Study Group (the IELSG 14 study). Br J Haematol. 2014;164:834–40.
51. Bruno Ventre M, Ferreri AJ, Gospodarowicz M, et al. Clinical features, management, and prognosis of an international series of 161 patients with limited-stage diffuse large B-cell lymphoma of the bone (the IELSG-14 study). Oncologist. 2014;19:291–8.
52. Horsman JM, Thomas J, Hough R, et al. Primary bone lymphoma: a retrospective analysis. Int J Oncol. 2006;28:1571–5.
53. Beal K, Allen L, Yahalom J. Primary bone lymphoma: treatment results and prognostic factors with long-term, follow-up of 82 patients. Cancer. 2006;106:2652–6.
54. Seam P, Juweid ME, Cheson BD. The role of FDG-PET scans in patients with lymphoma. Blood. 2007;110:3507–16.
55. Govi S, Christie D, Messina C, et al. The clinical features, management and prognostic effects of pathological fractures in a multicenter series of 373 patients with diffuse large B-cell lymphoma of the bone. Ann Oncol. 2014;25:176–81.
56. Held G, Zeynalova S, Murawski N, et al. Impact of rituximab and radiotherapy on outcome of patients with aggressive B-cell lymphoma and skeletal involvement. J Clin Oncol. 2013;31:4115–22.
57. Rosenwald A, Wright G, Leroy K, et al. Molecular diagnosis of primary mediastinal B cell lymphoma identifies a clinically favorable subgroup of diffuse large B cell lymphoma related to Hodgkin lymphoma. J Exp Med. 2003;198:851–62.
58. Savage KJ, Monti S, Kutok JL, et al. The molecular signature of mediastinal large B-cell lymphoma differs from that of other diffuse large B-cell lymphomas and shares features with classical Hodgkin lymphoma. Blood. 2003;102:3871–9.
59. Green MR, Monti S, Rodig SJ, et al. Integrative analysis reveals selective 9p24.1 amplification, increased PD-1 ligand expression, and further induction via JAK2 in nodular sclerosing Hodgkin lymphoma and primary mediastinal large B-cell lymphoma. Blood. 2010;116:3268–77.
60. Gaulard P, Harris NL, Pileri SA, et al. Primary mediastinal (thymic) large B-cell lymphoma. In: Swerdlow SH, Campo E, Harris NL, et al., editors. WHO classification of tumours of haematopoietic and lymphoid tissues. 4th ed. (revised) ed. Lyon: International Agency for Research on Cancer; 2017. p. 314–6.
61. Todeschini G, Secchi S, Morra E, et al. Primary mediastinal large B-cell lymphoma (PMLBCL): long-term results from a retrospective multicentre Italian

experience in 138 patients treated with CHOP or MACOP-B/VACOP-B. Br J Cancer. 2004;90:372–6.
62. Zinzani PL, Martelli M, Magagnoli M, et al. Treatment and clinical management of primary mediastinal large B-cell lymphoma with sclerosis: MACOP-B regimen and mediastinal radiotherapy monitored by (67)gallium scan in 50 patients. Blood. 1999;94:3289–93.
63. Savage KJ, Al-Rajhi N, Voss N, et al. Favorable outcome of primary mediastinal large B-cell lymphoma in a single institution: the British Columbia experience. Ann Oncol. 2006;17:123–30.
64. Soumerai JD, Hellmann MD, Feng Y, et al. Treatment of primary mediastinal B-cell lymphoma with rituximab, cyclophosphamide, doxorubicin, vincristine and prednisone is associated with a high rate of primary refractory disease. Leuk Lymphoma. 2014;55:538–43.
65. Rieger M, Osterborg A, Pettengell R, et al. Primary mediastinal B-cell lymphoma treated with CHOP-like chemotherapy with or without rituximab: results of the Mabthera International Trial Group Study. Ann Oncol. 2011;22:664–70.
66. Dunleavy K, Pittaluga S, Maeda LS, et al. Dose-adjusted EPOCH-rituximab therapy in primary mediastinal B-cell lymphoma. N Engl J Med. 2013;368:1408–16.
67. Lazzarino M, Orlandi E, Paulli M, et al. Treatment outcome and prognostic factors for primary mediastinal (thymic) B-cell lymphoma: a multicenter study of 106 patients. J Clin Oncol. 1997;15:1646–53.
68. Kuruvilla J, Pintilie M, Tsang R, Nagy T, Keating A, Crump M. Salvage chemotherapy and autologous stem cell transplantation are inferior for relapsed or refractory primary mediastinal large B-cell lymphoma compared with diffuse large B-cell lymphoma. Leuk Lymphoma. 2008;49:1329–36.
69. Zinzani PL, Pellegrini C, Chiappella A, et al. Brentuximab vedotin in relapsed primary mediastinal large B-cell lymphoma: results from a phase 2 clinical trial. Blood. 2017;129:2328–30.
70. Zinzani PL, Ribrag V, Moskowitz CH, et al. Safety and tolerability of pembrolizumab in patients with relapsed/refractory primary mediastinal large B-cell lymphoma. Blood. 2017;130:267–70.
71. Kochenderfer JN, Dudley ME, Kassim SH, et al. Chemotherapy-refractory diffuse large B-cell lymphoma and indolent B-cell malignancies can be effectively treated with autologous T cells expressing an anti-CD19 chimeric antigen receptor. J Clin Oncol. 2015;33:540–9.
72. Neelapu SS, Locke FL, Bartlett NL, et al. Axicabtagene ciloleucel CAR T-cell therapy in refractory large B-cell lymphoma. N Engl J Med. 2017;377:2531–44.
73. Gundrum JD, Mathiason MA, Moore DB, Go RS. Primary testicular diffuse large B-cell lymphoma: a population-based study on the incidence, natural history, and survival comparison with primary nodal counterpart before and after the introduction of rituximab. J Clin Oncol. 2009;27:5227–32.
74. Zucca E, Conconi A, Mughal TI, et al. Patterns of outcome and prognostic factors in primary large-cell lymphoma of the testis in a survey by the International Extranodal Lymphoma Study Group. J Clin Oncol. 2003;21:20–7.
75. Fonseca R, Habermann TM, Colgan JP, et al. Testicular lymphoma is associated with a high incidence of extranodal recurrence. Cancer. 2000;88:154–61.
76. Kraan W, Horlings HM, van Keimpema M, et al. High prevalence of oncogenic MYD88 and CD79B mutations in diffuse large B-cell lymphomas presenting at immune-privileged sites. Blood Cancer J. 2013;3:e139.
77. Chapuy B, Roemer MG, Stewart C, et al. Targetable genetic features of primary testicular and primary central nervous system lymphomas. Blood. 2016;127:869–81.
78. Booman M, Szuhai K, Rosenwald A, et al. Genomic alterations and gene expression in primary diffuse large B-cell lymphomas of immune-privileged sites: the importance of apoptosis and immunomodulatory pathways. J Pathol. 2008;216:209–17.
79. Vitolo U, Chiappella A, Ferreri AJ, et al. First-line treatment for primary testicular diffuse large B-cell lymphoma with rituximab-CHOP, CNS prophylaxis, and contralateral testis irradiation: final results of an international phase II trial. J Clin Oncol. 2011;29:2766–72.
80. Shapiro WR, Young DF, Mehta BM. Methotrexate: distribution in cerebrospinal fluid after intravenous, ventricular and lumbar injections. N Engl J Med. 1975;293:161–6.
81. Abramson JS, Hellmann M, Barnes JA, et al. Intravenous methotrexate as central nervous system (CNS) prophylaxis is associated with a low risk of CNS recurrence in high-risk patients with diffuse large B-cell lymphoma. Cancer. 2010;116:4283–90.
82. Hernandez-Ilizaliturri FJ, Deeb G, Zinzani PL, et al. Higher response to lenalidomide in relapsed/refractory diffuse large B-cell lymphoma in nongerminal center B-cell-like than in germinal center B-cell-like phenotype. Cancer. 2011;117:5058–66.
83. Wilson WH, Young RM, Schmitz R, et al. Targeting B cell receptor signaling with ibrutinib in diffuse large B cell lymphoma. Nat Med. 2015;21:922–6.
84. Nayak L, Iwamoto FM, LaCasce A, et al. PD-1 blockade with nivolumab in relapsed/refractory primary central nervous system and testicular lymphoma. Blood. 2017;129:3071–3.
85. Cheah CY, Campbell BA, Seymour JF. Primary breast lymphoma. Cancer Treat Rev. 2014;40:900–8.
86. Jia Y, Sun C, Liu Z, et al. Primary breast diffuse large B-cell lymphoma: a population-based study from 1975 to 2014. Oncotarget. 2017;9:3956–67.
87. Franco F, González-Rincón J, Lavernia J, et al. Mutational profile of primary breast diffuse large B-cell lymphoma. Oncotarget. 2017;8:102888–97.
88. Avilés A, delgado S, Nambo MJ, et al. Primary breast lymphoma: results of a controlled clinical trial. Oncology. 2005;69:256–60.

89. Lin Y, Guo XM, Shen KW, et al. Primary breast lymphoma: long-term treatment outcome and prognosis. Leuk Lymphoma. 2006;47:2102–9.
90. Ryan G, Martinelli G, Kuper-Hommel M, et al. Primary diffuse large B-cell lymphoma of the breast: prognostic factors and outcomes of a study by the International Extranodal Lymphoma Study Group. Ann Oncol. 2008;19:233–41.
91. Liu PP, Wang KF, Jin JT, et al. Role of radiation therapy in primary breast diffuse large B-cell lymphoma in the rituximab era: a SEER database analysis. Cancer Med. 2018;7:1845–51.
92. Willemze R, Vergier B, Duncan LM. Primary cutaneous diffuse large B-cell lymphoma, leg type. In: Swerdlow SH, Campo E, Harris NL, Jaffe ES, Pileri SA, Stein H, Thiele J, Arber DA, Hasserjian RP, MM LB, Orazi A, Siebert R, editors. WHO classification of tumours of haematopoietic and lymphoid tissues. Lyon: International Agency for Research on Cancer; 2017. p. 303–4.
93. Hamilton SN, Wai ES, Tan K, et al. Treatment and outcomes in patients with primary cutaneous B-cell lymphoma: the BC Cancer Agency experience. Int J Radiat Oncol Biol Phys. 2013;87:719–25.
94. Grange F, Joly P, Barbe C, et al. Improvement of survival in patients with primary cutaneous diffuse large B-cell lymphoma, leg type, in France. JAMA Dermatol. 2014;150:535–41.
95. Schmitz N, Zeynalova S, Nickelsen M, et al. CNS International Prognostic Index: a risk model for CNS relapse in patients with diffuse large B-cell lymphoma treated with R-CHOP. J Clin Oncol. 2016;34:3150–6.
96. Rosenthal A, Younes A. High grade B-cell lymphoma with rearrangements of MYC and BCL2 and/or BCL6: double hit and triple hit lymphomas and double expressing lymphoma. Blood Rev. 2017;31:37–42.

CD20-Negative Aggressive Lymphomas

11

Jorge J. Castillo

11.1 Introduction

Diffuse large B-cell lymphoma (DLBCL) is the most common non-Hodgkin lymphoma, accounting for approximately 30% of the cases. The addition of the anti-CD20 monoclonal antibody rituximab to combination chemotherapy has increased response and survival rates in patients with DLBCL in randomized studies [1, 2]. A small proportion of DLBCL show marked plasma cell differentiation with loss of CD20 expression.

In general, patients diagnosed with CD20-negative DLBCL tend to have extranodal involvement, a more aggressive clinical course, resistance to chemotherapy, and a poor prognosis. The use of rituximab has not been of benefit in these cases. Given its rarity, most of the available evidence in CD20-negative DLBCL consists of case reports and small case series. Due to lack of prospective data, there are no standards of care for these patients.

In this chapter, we review the most common variants of CD20-negative DLBCL including plasmablastic lymphoma (PBL), primary effusion lymphoma (PEL), large B-cell lymphoma arising in HHV-8-associated multicentric Castleman disease (MCD), and anaplastic lymphoma kinase (ALK)-positive DLBCL. This is an evolving field, and patients with CD20-negative DLBCL not meeting criteria for the ones mentioned above have been described [3–5]. These cases of CD20-negative DLBCL are beyond the scope of this review.

11.2 Plasmablastic Lymphoma

Delecluse et al. first described PBL as a separate entity in 1997 [6]. This report included 16 patients, 15 were HIV-positive, who presented with aggressive lesions located primarily in the oral cavity. These patients had a high rate of relapse resulting in poor survival. PBL was then included within the group of B-cell malignancies more commonly seen in HIV-infected individuals [7].

Morphologically, the malignant cells have round to oval shape with abundant cytoplasm, eccentric nucleus, prominent nucleolus, and a perinuclear hof [7]. The background is usually composed by small lymphocytes, mitotic figures, and tingible body macrophages that can impart a starry-sky pattern. Immunophenotypically, the malignant PBL cells express plasma cell markers such as CD38, CD138, or multiple myeloma 1/interferon regulatory factor 4 protein (MUM1/IRF4) but do not express CD20. The proliferation index is usually high with Ki67 > 80%. Recently,

J. J. Castillo (✉)
Division of Hematologic Malignancies, Dana-Farber Cancer Institute, Harvard Medical School, Boston, MA, USA
e-mail: jorgej_castillo@dfci.harvard.edu

G. Lenz, G. Salles (eds.), *Aggressive Lymphomas*, Hematologic Malignancies,
https://doi.org/10.1007/978-3-030-00362-3_11

novel markers such as BLIMP1 and XBP1 have been identified [8]. A representative profile of PBL is shown in Fig. 11.1. The cell of origin in PBL is thought to be the plasmablast, an activated B-cell that has already undergone the germinal center reaction but has not yet fully matured into a plasma cell. PBL is sometimes difficult to distinguish from plasmablastic myeloma [9], especially in the setting of immunodeficiency. However, the presence of monoclonal paraproteinemia and/or skeletal lytic lesions favors a diagnosis of myeloma.

MYC gene rearrangements and Epstein-Barr virus (EBV)-encoded RNA (EBER) expression are common molecular markers present in PBL. EBER has been reported in approximately

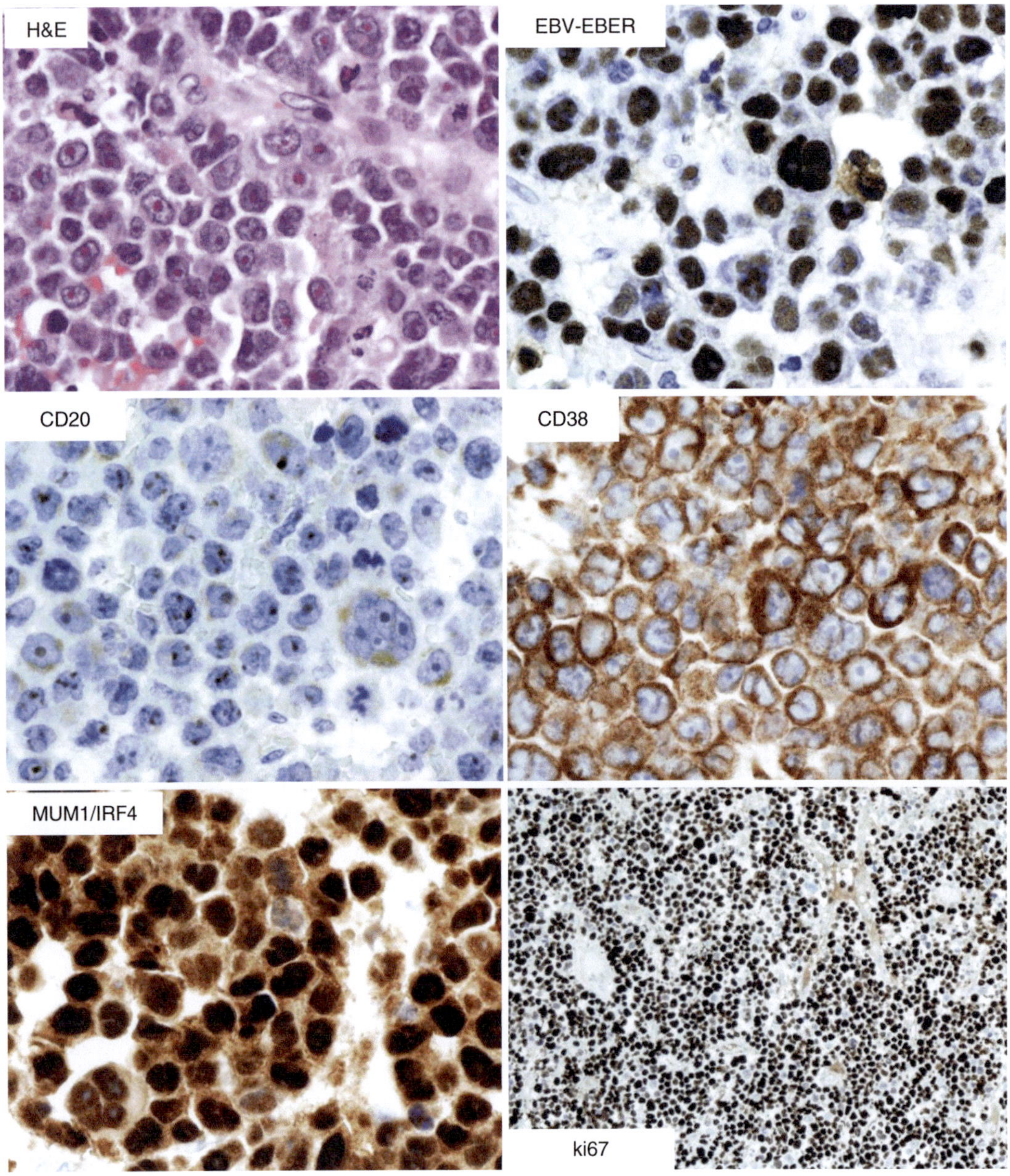

Fig. 11.1 Representative case of plasmablastic lymphoma

80% of cases with HIV-positive PBL and suggests a role of EBV in the pathogenesis of PBL [10]. *MYC* gene rearrangements can be seen in approximately 40% of cases of HIV-positive PBL and have been associated with a worse prognosis [11]. A study has suggested that EBV-positive PBL cases are more likely to carry *MYC* gene rearrangements than EBV-negative cases [12].

A systematic review of the literature that included 112 HIV-positive patients with PBL showed a median age at presentation of 38 years with a male predominance, with a median time from HIV infection to PBL diagnosis of 5 years [13]. Approximately 50% of the patients presented with stage III or IV disease and 50% with primary site of involvement in the oral cavity. Approximately 75% of the patients received some type of combination chemotherapy, most commonly cyclophosphamide, doxorubicin, vincristine, and prednisone (CHOP) with an overall response rate (ORR) of 72%. These findings have been confirmed by a more recent meta-analysis on approximately 300 patients with PBL [14].

A later systematic review identified 76 HIV-negative patients with a pathological diagnosis of PBL [15]. The median age at diagnosis was 57 years with a male-to-female ratio of 1.7:1. Advanced-stage disease was seen in 60% of the cases with 90% presenting with extranodal involvement. The most common sites of involvement were the oral cavity and the gastrointestinal tract. Approximately 50% of the patients received treatment with CHOP. The ORR was 66%. Another study showed that approximately 30% of HIV-negative PBL patients had some form of immunosuppression such as posttransplantation, concurrent malignancy, or autoimmune disorders [16].

A study comparing 157 HIV-positive and 71 HIV-negative PBL patients showed that HIV-positive PBL patients were younger with more pronounced male predominance and higher proportion of oral cavity involvement [10]. There were no differences in stage distribution, bone marrow involvement, or presence of B symptoms. Of note, HIV-positive patients experienced higher rates of ORR to chemotherapy (81% vs. 56%). CR rates were 52% and 41% for HIV-positive and HIV-negative PBL patients, respectively.

The prognosis of patients with PBL remains poor. Systematic reviews have reported median OS times that have ranged between 9 and 15 months [14, 15]. More recently, a multicenter study on 50 HIV-positive PBL patients treated in the highly active antiretroviral therapy (HAART) era reported a median OS of 12 months [11]. Other smaller case series in PBL patients treated in the ART era have shown median OS ranging between 5 and 12 months [17, 18]. An Italian study has shown better outcomes in PBL patients with 3-year OS of 67% [19]. The reasons for this difference are unclear although the patients in the Italian study had shorter HIV diagnosis to PBL diagnosis time and presented with median CD4+ count >200 cells/mm^3.

Comparative studies between HIV-negative and HIV-positive PBL patients showed that HIV-negative status might be associated with worse survival, but results are inconsistent [10, 14]. Advanced-stage and poor performance status have shown to be indicators of worse prognosis in PBL [11, 18]. Hence, the use of the International Prognostic Index (IPI) score should be appropriate in PBL [11, 18, 19]. The association of EBV expression and outcomes in PBL is unclear [14, 18]. CD4+ counts <200 cells/mm^3 might be associated with shorter progression-free survival (PFS) time [11, 18]. More recently, the presence of *MYC* gene rearrangements has shown to be associated with worse OS [11, 14]. In patients with HIV-positive PBL who are treated with chemotherapy, the attainment of CR has been associated with longer survival [11, 20]. In the HIV-negative setting, concurrent immunosuppression has been associated with a worse outcome [16].

Current guidelines recommend against the use of CHOP, as it is considered inadequate therapy [21]. This recommendation is reasonable given the poor outcomes seen in patients with PBL. However, studies evaluating survival benefits in HIV-positive PBL patients treated with regimens more intensive than CHOP have failed to show survival benefits [11, 20]. Based on consensus opinion, regimens such as dose-adjusted infusional etoposide, vincristine, and doxorubicin along with bolus cyclophosphamide and prednisone (EPOCH), cyclophosphamide, vincristine, doxorubicin, methotrexate alternating with ifosfamide, etoposide, cytarabine (CODOX-M/IVAC), or hyperfractionated cyclophosphamide, vincristine, doxorubicin, and dexamethasone alternating with methotrexate and cytarabine (hyperCVAD) are appropriate for PBL therapy. These regimens could include the administration of intrathecal agents to minimize the risk of central nervous system (CNS) involvement by PBL. In HIV-infected patients, initiation or optimization of HAART is highly recommended and should be directed by an infectious disease specialist. Finally, for the small portion of PBL cases that express CD20, rituximab should be considered in addition to chemotherapy. The EPOCH regimen is being evaluated prospectively in high-risk DLBCL patients, which could include PBL patients (NCT01092182).

High-dose chemotherapy followed by autologous stem cell support (ASCT) can be an option in patients with PBL. This topic has been recently reviewed [22]. Based on case reports and small case series, ASCT does have limited value in the relapsed setting. However, the use of ASCT as consolidation after achieving CR to frontline treatment (CR1) might be associated with longer OS times [19, 22]. A case series on nine HIV-negative PBL patients suggested longer OS time in patients who received ASCT in first remission [16]. There are no reports on the use of allogeneic SCT in PBL patients.

The poor results observed with current available treatments warrant the identification of novel agents for PBL patients. Given the plasmacytic nature of PBL, the use of anti-myeloma agents appears reasonable. The proteasome inhibitor bortezomib alone and in combination with chemotherapy has been used with limited efficacy in patients with relapsed PBL [23–25]. Recently, the combination of bortezomib and chemotherapy has been tried with success in the frontline treatment of patients with HIV-positive and HIV-negative PBL [26–28]. In a few case reports, the immunomodulatory drug lenalidomide induced a temporary response in relapsed PBL [23, 29, 30]. CD30 expression has been reported in approximately 30% of PBL cases [12, 31]. Recently, a case report described the antitumor activity of brentuximab vedotin in a patient with CD30-expressing relapsed PBL [32].

There is an almost universal expression of CD38 by PBL cells, and about 50% of PBL patients carry MYC gene rearrangements, providing potential treatment options. Daratumumab is a monoclonal antibody that targets CD38, which is a membrane glycoprotein expressed by B-cells, T-cell, NK-cell, and plasma cells. The FDA has approved daratumumab for the treatment of multiple myeloma. However, no reports on the use of daratumumab in PBL have been published. The *MYC* gene regulates multiple cellular functions influencing cell division, metabolic adaptation, and survival [33]. The *MYC* gene itself is not easily targetable, as it lacks a ligand-binding domain. *MYC* transcription depends on the assembly of complexes called bromodomains. BRD4 is a member of the bromodomain and extraterminal (BET) subfamily of human bromodomain proteins and seems to be an important factor for *MYC*-dependent transcription [34]. BET inhibition has shown to downregulate *MYC* transcription and to induce a genome-wide downregulation of *MYC*-dependent target genes [35]. Furthermore, BET inhibition has induced cell cycle arrest and cell senescence in cellular and animal myeloma models. Finally, recent studies have shown that EBV-positive lymphoma cells express PD-L1 and that PD-1 blockade inhibits their growth and survival [36, 37], providing the rationale on trying the monoclonal antibodies nivolumab or pembrolizumab in PBL. Nivolumab is FDA approved for the treatment of melanoma, non-small cell lung cancer, head and neck cancer, renal cell carcinoma, and Hodgkin lymphoma. Pembrolizumab is FDA approved for melanoma, non-small cell lung cancer, head and neck cancer, and Hodgkin lymphoma.

11.3 Primary Effusion Lymphoma

PEL is an aggressive lymphoma that affects body cavities without detectable tumor masses in the setting of HIV infection. It was recognized as a new entity in 2001 [38]. The Kaposi sarcoma-associated herpesvirus, also known as human herpesvirus 8 (HHV-8), is universally present in PEL tumor cells [38].

Knowles and colleagues reported the first case of PEL in an HIV-infected patient in 1989 [39]. Later, in 1995, Cesarman and colleagues reported on a case series, in which seven out of eight HIV-positive patients presented with malignant pleural effusions. B-cell lineage was demonstrated by clonal rearrangement, as flow cytometry was unable to show typical CD20 expression. DNA analysis found sequences of HHV-8 and EBV genome in the neoplastic cells. The survival was short with poor tolerance to chemotherapy [40].

The diagnosis of PEL is based on morphologic, immunophenotypic, and molecular analysis of the affected tissue along with demonstration of viral infection by HHV-8. As effusion fluid is universally present, the diagnosis is made on cell blocks or cytospin samples. Morphologically, PEL cells are large with variable nuclear size and form, with prominent nucleoli. Sometimes PEL cells can resemble plasmablasts, or large immunoblasts with eccentric nuclei containing nuclear hof, or anaplastic cells with large polygonal cells with pleomorphic nuclei [38].

Immunophenotypic studies in PEL malignant cells reveal a "null" lymphocyte phenotype with expression of CD45 but no expression of CD19 or CD20. PEL cells can express markers of lymphocyte activation such as CD30, CD38, CD71, and HLA-DR and the plasma cell-related antigens CD138 and MUM-1/IRF4 [41]. In addition, PEL cells are negative for Bcl-6 and for anaplastic lymphoma kinase 1 (ALK-1), and the Ki-67 index is usually high. A representative case of PEL is shown in Fig. 11.2.

Recurrent chromosome translocations of *BCL2*, *BCL6*, and *MYC*, typically present in other B-cell lymphomas, are absent in PEL [42, 43]. Gene expression profile demonstrated that PEL cells have features of immunoblasts and plasma

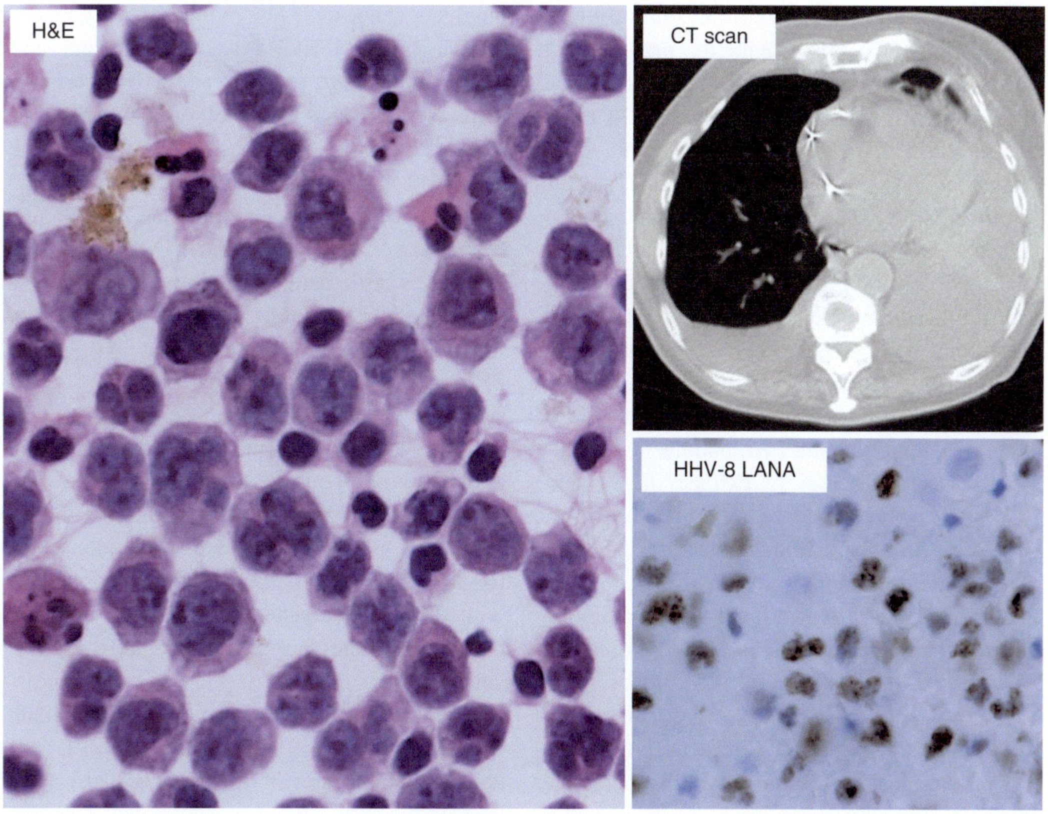

Fig. 11.2 Representative case of primary effusion lymphoma

cells. In addition, immunoglobulin gene rearrangements and somatic hypermutation are present in PEL. These findings suggest that the cell of origin in PEL is a post-germinal B-cell that has undergone plasma cell differentiation [44]. Array-based comparative genomic hybridization (CGH) studies showed gain and losses of several chromosomes including chromosomes 1, 5, 11, 12, and 17q, among other abnormalities [45].

HHV-8 plays an important role on promoting PEL. It is also useful to differentiate from other lymphomas complicated by effusions, which are consistently negative for HHV-8 infection [41]. The immunohistochemical staining for HHV-8 latent nuclear antigen 1 (LANA-1) is the standard assay performed. Although not standardized, detection of HHV-8 viral load by quantitative PCR could be useful, and its prognostic significance is still under investigation [44, 46]. Detection of EBV occurs in approximately 70% of cases using EBER in situ hybridization [41].

Cases of PEL have also been observed in the setting of post solid organ transplant and in debilitated elderly patients with chronic comorbidities [47]. Commonly, these patients present with other AIDS-associated diseases such as KS and MCD due to the association with HHV-8 infection in addition with severe immunosuppression caused by HIV [40, 48]. In general, PEL is characterized by the presence of malignant pleural, pericardial, or peritoneal effusions without evident mass or tumor. Due to the effects of malignant fluid accumulation, patients can experience chest pain, progressive dyspnea, abdominal distension, or constitutional symptoms. The pleural space is the most commonly affected (70% of cases). By definition, all PEL patients have stage IV disease [49]. Cases of extracavitary (solid) PEL with no evidence of malignant effusions have been described. Extracavitary PEL is morphologically and genetically identical to classic PEL [50]. The gastrointestinal tract is commonly affected, but there are also reports of involvement of the skin, lungs, lymph nodes, and CNS. Extracavitary PEL cases are also universally associated with HHV-8 infection [51, 52].

The prognosis of PEL is generally poor with few patients being cured from the disease. The 1-year survival rate is less than 40% [53, 54]. The multivariate analysis showed that poor performance status and no HAART at diagnosis were independent predictors of poor OS. The impact of HAART on PEL prognosis is similar to other AIDS-associated lymphomas [54, 55]. The number of body cavities involved in PEL seems to be prognostic, with more than one cavity associated with poorer prognosis. Isolated pericardial involvement appears to correlate with longer survival [56]. Integrating the number and type of body cavities into a prognostic score specific for PEL might warrant further investigation. The IPI score has not been validated in PEL to date. CD4 count and HHV-8 viral load at diagnosis were not prognostic of worse outcomes, although some studies suggest that the HHV-8 viral load might correlate with survival in HHV-8-associated lymphoproliferative disorders, including MCD [57].

There is no standard treatment for PEL. Response rates with CHOP are approximately 40% with a median OS of 6 months [53]. Other regimens such as doxorubicin, cyclophosphamide, vindesine, bleomycin, and prednisone (ACVBP) and CHOP plus methotrexate have been administered to PEL patients with variable response rates [54, 58]. Methotrexate should be used with caution as it could accumulate in effusions and lead to increased toxicity [54]. Dose-adjusted EPOCH has been reported in individual cases as well [59]. Recently, EPOCH has been associated with better outcomes than CHOP in patients with HIV-associated lymphomas [60]. Initiation of HAART is essential at HIV-infected PEL patients. In some cases, prolonged remissions and lymphoma regression have been reported with HAART alone [54, 61]. The experience of autologous or allogeneic SCT in PEL is limited to case reports, and consideration for the procedure should be based on individual cases [62, 63]. Provided the poor prognosis associated with PEL, SCT constitutes an attractive option, but larger studies are needed to assess efficacy and toxicity.

The constitutive activation of the NF-kB pathway appears critical for survival of PEL cells [64], and inhibition of the NF-kB pathway by bortezomib induced apoptosis in PEL cell lines

[65]. Despite these promising findings, the activity of bortezomib has been modest [66]. However, it appears that combination therapy could be promising [67]. There is limited preclinical and clinical data supporting the use of lenalidomide in PEL [68, 69]. CD30 is frequently expressed in PEL cells, and targeting with the conjugated monoclonal antibody anti-CD30 brentuximab vedotin improved the survival of a xenograft mouse PEL model by inhibiting proliferation and causing arrest in G2/M cell cycle phase [70]. PEL cells express CD38, making daratumumab an interesting, commercially available treatment options. Immunotherapy has emerged as a potential target for B-cell malignancies. Programed cell death ligand-1 (PD-L1) is an attractive target in PEL, as approximately 50% of HHV-8-associated PEL cases express PD-L1 [71]. Another interesting therapeutic option is NOTCH1 inhibitors. NOTCH1 expression has been demonstrated in almost 80% of PEL cells [72]. Other agents of interest in PEL are the PI3K/AKT/mTOR inhibitors and histone deacetylase inhibitors, which have shown preclinical activity [67, 73].

11.4 Large B-Cell Lymphoma Arising in HHV-8-Associated Multicentric Castleman Disease

Dupin and colleagues reported the first cases of this rare condition [74]. The authors described patients with HHV-8-associated MCD that later developed "plasmablastic" lymphoma. Most of these patients died within months of MCD diagnosis and some within weeks of overt lymphoma diagnosis.

Patients with HIV and MCD have a 15-fold greater risk of developing lymphoma than the general HIV-positive population [75]. Specific lymphoma types associated with HHV-8 infection are cavitary and extracavitary PEL and large B-cell lymphomas with plasmablastic differentiation arising in HHV-8-associated MCD [74–76]. While PEL shows typically hypermutated Ig and dim expression of surface and cytoplasmic immunoglobulin, large B-cell lymphomas in MCD show unmutated Ig and expression of IgM and λ chain restriction suggesting HHV-8-positive plasmablasts as the cell of origin [76]. However, the molecular events leading from polyclonal HHV-8-positive plasmablastic expansions in MCD to monoclonal HHV-8-positive large cell lymphoma are unknown.

Large B-cell lymphoma arising in HHV-8-associated MCD is histopathologically defined by large confluent sheets of plasmablasts with HHV-8 expression [77]. These blasts are not coinfected with EBV, show cytoplasmic IgM with λ chain restriction, and have a phenotypic profile characterized by loss of B-cell markers such as CD20 and PAX-5, and acquisition of phenotypic profile of plasma cells such as upregulation of MUM-1/IRF-4, PRDM-1/BLIMP-1, and surface markers such as CD38 [8, 75, 78]. A representative case of large B-cell lymphoma arising from HHV-8-associated MCD is shown in Fig. 11.3.

The histopathological differences between overt lymphoma and the so-called plasmablastic microlymphoma are not well defined, and the latter might represent an intermediate step in the progression from MCD to large B-cell lymphoma. While MCD is polyclonal in nature and overt lymphoma is monoclonal, plasmablastic microlymphomas in the lymph node have been found monoclonal in only two of eight cases with subsequent development of lymphoma in one. However, another case with associated polyclonal microlymphoma also developed overt lymphoma [76]. A similar picture is found in three cases reported as severe MCD with polyclonal IgMλ plasmablastic lymphocytosis successfully treated with combined chemotherapy [79].

MCD is a distinct type of lymphoproliferative disorder associated with IL-6 dysregulation [75]. Clinically, patients may have systemic symptoms such as fever, night sweats, polyclonal hypergammaglobulinemia, and cytopenias. HHV-8 infection is commonly associated with MCD in patients infected with HIV and also in some HIV-negative patients [80]. HHV-8 replicates in immunoblasts and plasmablasts and signals the

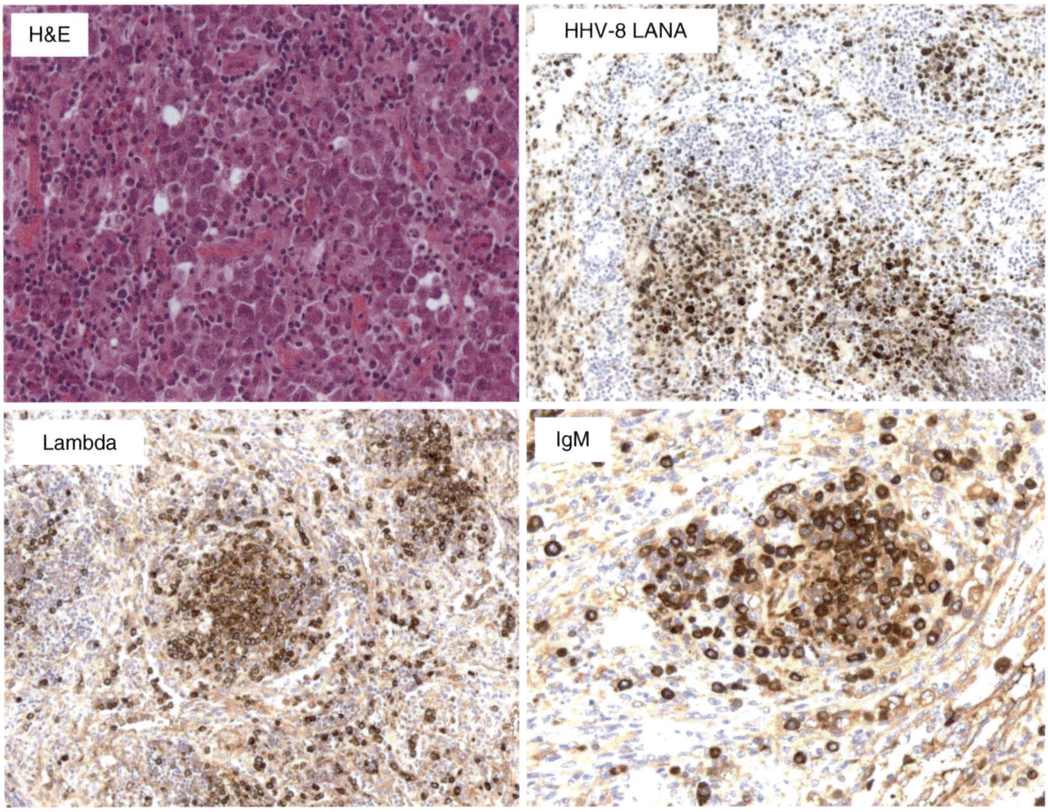

Fig. 11.3 Representative case of a large B-cell lymphoma arising from HHV-8-associated multicentric Castleman disease

release of viral-derived and human-derived IL-6 and other inflammatory cytokines [81], which induce B-cell and plasma cell proliferation and angiogenesis, and an acute phase reaction [82]. B-cell proliferation leads to the accumulation in the lymph nodes of clusters of HHV-8+, IgM+, λ chain restricted but polyclonal plasmablasts [74, 83]. These plasmablasts were found to be polyclonal/multiclonal in nature when Ig clonality analyses were performed and do not fulfill the current histopathological criteria to be considered DLBCL.

The outcome of patients with HHV-8-associated MCD is poor and is measured within few to several months from the development of MCD [74, 75]. The median OS is shorter (several weeks) in patients who develop overt lymphoma and extremely poor (few weeks) in cases of leukemic phase. Patients with so-called plasmablastic microscopic lymphomas should be treated as high-risk MCD [76, 79, 84]. Given the definite risk of developing overt lymphoma in patients with HHV-8-positive MCD, control of HHV8-positive MCD is the primary step for lymphoma prevention.

Rituximab, alone or in combination with chemotherapy, has significant activity in both HIV-negative and HIV-positive MCD. In HIV-positive patients, it has been evaluated in observational and retrospective analysis showing higher response rates and longer response duration than chemotherapy [60]. In one prospective study, the incidence of lymphoma was significantly reduced (>90% reduction) in patients receiving rituximab [85]. For most HIV-positive, HHV-8-positive patients with MCD, a combination of ganciclovir plus rituximab with etoposide added for aggressive/high-risk disease is suggested. In patients with uncontrolled HIV infection defined by low CD4 counts and/or high HIV viral load and/or active KS, HAART should be included. Treatment with rituximab alone or rituximab plus combination chemotherapy such as CHOP or EPOCH can be given at time of relapse or if the patient is refractory to initial therapy.

Agents to consider in the relapsed setting are bortezomib, lenalidomide, and the anti-IL-6 monoclonal antibody siltuximab. In xenograft mouse model of HHV-8-positive PEL, bortezomib induced apoptosis and lytic reactivation of HHV-8 in lymphoma cells [86]. Siltuximab has shown to be safe and efficacious in a randomized study in patients with HIV-negative, HHV-8-negative MCD [87, 88]. Finally, there are case reports supporting the use of lenalidomide in MCD [89, 90].

11.5 ALK+ Diffuse Large B-Cell Lymphoma

ALK is a receptor tyrosine kinase originally described at the breakpoint of the t(2;5) translocation observed in patients with anaplastic large cell lymphoma (ALCL) [91]. ALK+ DLBCL is a rare subtype of DLBCL. In contrast with ALCL, ALK+ DLBCL is commonly associated with t(2;17) in which the ALK gene is juxtaposed to the clathrin (CLTC) gene. Delsol and colleagues originally described seven patients with ALK+ DLBCL [92]. Since then, no more than 100 cases of ALK+ DLBCL have been reported in the literature [93–95].

Pathologically, ALK+ DLBCL is comprised of monomorphic large immunoblastic or plasmablastic cells, containing large central nucleoli that tend to invade the lymphatic sinuses. The cells exhibit a high proliferative index, perhaps related to MYC overexpression. In contrast to ALCL, ALK+ DLBCL does not express CD30 [92]. The immunophenotype of ALK+ DLBCL is characterized by the expression of CD138, CD38, EMA, and cytoplasmic immunoglobulin and the absence of CD20 expression [92]. In addition, ALK+ DLBCL expresses other plasma cell differentiation antigens such as BLIMP1 and XBP1 [93]. The t(2;17) is the most common cytogenetic abnormality observed in ALK+ DLBCL and leads to the expression of the CLTC-ALK fusion gene. However, other chromosomal rearrangements involving the ALK gene had been described such as the t(2;5) (NMP-ALK) [96]. Of interest, ALK+ DLBCL does not seem to carry MYC translocations [97, 98]. A representative case of ALK+ DLBCL is shown in Fig. 11.4.

The precise mechanism(s) by which ALK fusion genes induce the oncological transformation of lymphoid cells are unclear. However, laboratory studies suggest that NPM-ALK and to a lesser degree CLTC-ALK activate the signal transducer and activator of transcription (STAT) family proteins, specifically STAT3 and STAT5 [99–101]. Studies have shown that STAT3 activation was induced by the NPM-ALK fusion gene and was necessary for NPM-ALK lymphomagenesis. STAT3 and STAT5 activation is associated with the upregulation of anti-apoptotic proteins [102]. In addition, STAT3 activation observed in ALK+ DLBCL results in the upregulation of BLIMP1 and c-MYC accounting for the plasmacytic differentiation and increase in cell proliferation observed, respectively [98].

Clinically, there is a male predominance, pediatric and adult patients can be affected, and it appears there is no relation with viral infections [103]. Patients present with advanced-stage disease in 60% of the cases and with bone marrow involvement in 25%. In a retrospective study on 38 patients, the survival rates were poor with a 5-year OS of 25%. Half of the patients died within the first year following diagnosis. It seems that patients with early-stage disease may have a better prognosis with an estimated 5-year OS of 50%.

ALK+ DLBCL has poor clinical outcomes despite current available therapy that includes systemic multi-agent chemotherapy. Targeted agents against CD20 or CD30 are unlikely to produce clinical benefit in ALK+ DLBCL given the lack of expression of these surface receptors. The current management of patients with ALK+ DLBCL consists on the administration of systemic chemotherapy using regimens commonly used for other subtypes of DLBCL in the first-line or second-line setting. However, given the poor clinical results observed with this approach

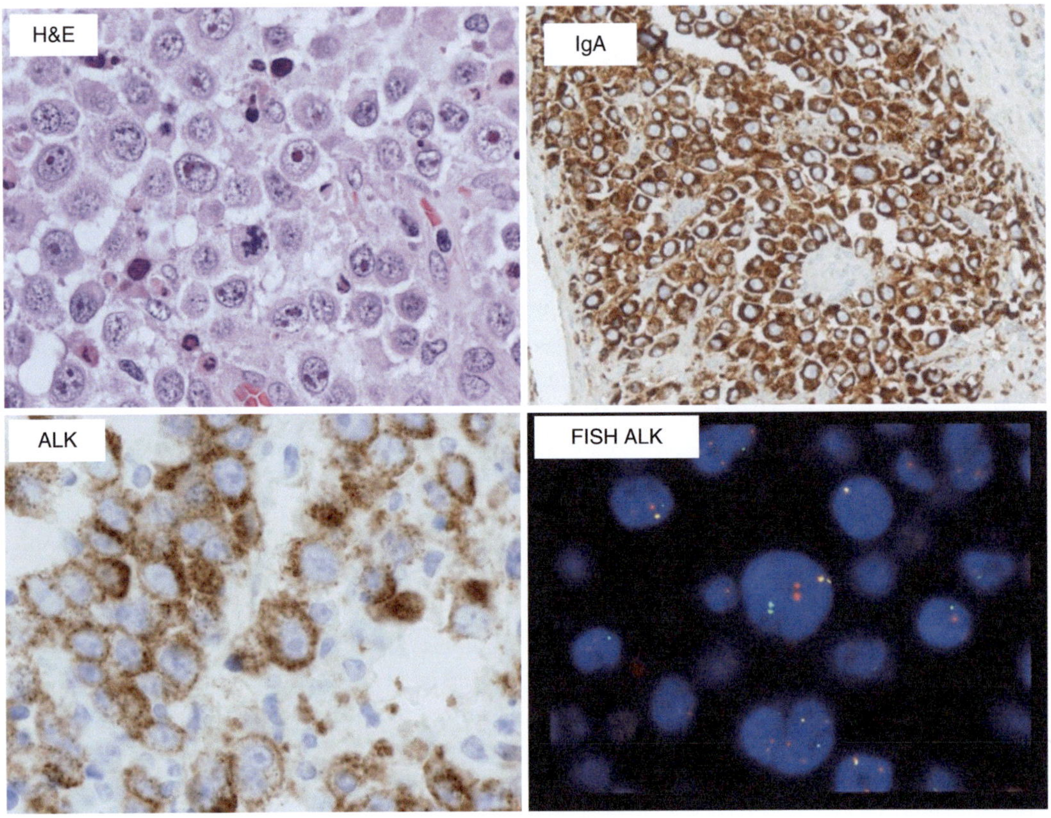

Fig. 11.4 Representative case of ALK+ diffuse large B-cell lymphoma

with median OS ranging from 10 to 20 months, there is a need to develop novel therapeutic approaches.

Crizotinib is the only ALK inhibitor approved by the FDA for the treatment of ALK+ non-small cell lung cancer and relapsed ALK+ ALCL. Anecdotal case reports had described the clinical use of crizotinib in ALK+ relapsed/refractory DLBCL. Wass et al. reported significant antitumor activity in a refractory ALK+ DLBCL patient treated with crizotinib single agent. However, the patient experienced a very short duration of response [104]. Preclinical studies have suggested that pharmacological inhibition of STAT3 or CLTC-ALK fusion protein results in antitumor activity against lymphoma cell lines or lymphoma xenograft murine models [105, 106]. Given CD38 expression by ALK+ DLBCL cells, daratumumab could also be an attractive therapeutic option.

11.6 Conclusion

CD20-negative lymphomas are rare, and they pose a significant diagnostic challenge given their atypical morphology. Additionally, CD20-negative lymphomas are associated with clinical courses characterized by primary chemoresistance, early relapse, and the obvious lack of benefit from anti-CD20 therapy. Furthermore, the survival of patients with CD20-negative lymphomas is measured in several months to a few years. Despite recent advances in the biology of CD20-negative DLBCL, several questions remain unanswered. It is interesting to see that these conditions, with exception of ALK+ DLBCL, occur mainly in immunosuppressed patients with chronic viral infections. Given the rarity associated with these conditions, therapeutic standards of care have not been established. It is encouraging to see clinical data showing that novel agents such as bortezomib, lenalidomide, and brentuximab vedotin have activity in some of these patients. Given overexpression of CD38, PD-L1, and PD-1 in CD20-negative DLBCL, novel agents such as daratumumab, nivolumab, and pembrolizumab can prove to be helpful in treating these patients. Similarly, the use of BET inhibitors could be of value in *MYC*-positive lymphomas. Finally, crizotinib should be evaluated in patients with ALK+ DLBCL. However, given the aggressive nature of CD20-negative DLBCL, it is unlikely that molecular or targeted agents used alone would induce durable responses or be curative. In that sense, the combination of novel agents with chemotherapy such as CHOP or dose-adjusted EPOCH might be reasonable. The answers to these questions should come from well-designed multicenter prospective studies.

References

1. Feugier P, Van Hoof A, Sebban C, et al. Long-term results of the R-CHOP study in the treatment of elderly patients with diffuse large B-cell lymphoma: a study by the Groupe d'Etude des Lymphomes de l'Adulte. J Clin Oncol. 2005;23:4117–26.
2. Pfreundschuh M, Kuhnt E, Trumper L, et al. CHOP-like chemotherapy with or without rituximab in young patients with good-prognosis diffuse large-B-cell lymphoma: 6-year results of an open-label randomised study of the MabThera International Trial (MInT) Group. Lancet Oncol. 2011;12:1013–22.
3. Garg M, Lee BE, McGarry K, et al. CD20-negative diffuse large B-cell lymphoma presenting with lactic acidosis. Am J Hematol. 2015;90:E49–50.
4. Gaur S, Padilla O, Nahleh Z. Clinical features and prognosis of CD20 negative aggressive B-cell non-Hodgkins lymphoma. Lymphoma. 2013;2013:290585.
5. Li YJ, Li ZM, Rao HL, et al. CD20-negative de novo diffuse large B-cell lymphoma in HIV-negative patients: a matched case-control analysis in a single institution. J Transl Med. 2012;10:84.
6. Delecluse HJ, Anagnostopoulos I, Dallenbach F, et al. Plasmablastic lymphomas of the oral cavity: a new entity associated with the human immunodeficiency virus infection. Blood. 1997;89:1413–20.
7. Campo E, Stein H, Harris NL. Plasmablastic lymphoma. In: Swerdlow SH, Campo E, Harris NL, et al., editors. WHO classification of tumours of the haematopoietic and lymphoid tissues. Revised 4th ed. Lyon: IARC; 2017. p. 321–2.
8. Montes-Moreno S, Gonzalez-Medina AR, Rodriguez-Pinilla SM, et al. Aggressive large B-cell lymphoma with plasma cell differentiation: immunohistochemical characterization of plasmablastic lymphoma and diffuse large B-cell lymphoma with partial plasmablastic phenotype. Haematologica. 2010;95:1342–9.
9. Vega F, Chang CC, Medeiros LJ, et al. Plasmablastic lymphomas and plasmablastic plasma cell myelomas have nearly identical immunophenotypic profiles. Mod Pathol. 2005;18:806–15.
10. Castillo JJ, Winer ES, Stachurski D, et al. Clinical and pathological differences between human immunodeficiency virus-positive and human immunodeficiency virus-negative patients with plasmablastic lymphoma. Leuk Lymphoma. 2010;51:2047–53.
11. Castillo JJ, Furman M, Beltran BE, et al. Human immunodeficiency virus-associated plasmablastic lymphoma: poor prognosis in the era of highly active antiretroviral therapy. Cancer. 2012;118:5270–7.
12. Valera A, Balague O, Colomo L, et al. IG/MYC rearrangements are the main cytogenetic alteration in plasmablastic lymphomas. Am J Surg Pathol. 2010;34:1686–94.
13. Castillo J, Pantanowitz L, Dezube BJ. HIV-associated plasmablastic lymphoma: lessons learned from 112 published cases. Am J Hematol. 2008;83:804–9.
14. Morscio J, Dierickx D, Nijs J, et al. Clinicopathologic comparison of plasmablastic lymphoma in HIV-positive, immunocompetent, and posttransplant patients: single-center series of 25 cases and meta-analysis of 277 reported cases. Am J Surg Pathol. 2014;38:875–86.
15. Castillo JJ, Winer ES, Stachurski D, et al. HIV-negative plasmablastic lymphoma: not in the mouth. Clin Lymphoma Myeloma Leuk. 2011;11:185–9.
16. Liu JJ, Zhang L, Ayala E, et al. Human immunodeficiency virus (HIV)-negative plasmablastic lymphoma: a single institutional experience and literature review. Leuk Res. 2011;35:1571–7.
17. Noy A, Chadburn A, Lensing SY, Moore P. Plasmablastic lymphoma is curable the HAART era. A 10 year retrospective by the AIDS Malignancy Consortium (AMC). Leuk Lymphoma. 2013;122:1801.
18. Schommers P, Wyen C, Hentrich M, et al. Poor outcome of HIV-infected patients with plasmablastic lymphoma: results from the German AIDS-related lymphoma cohort study. AIDS. 2013;27:842–5.
19. Cattaneo C, Re A, Ungari M, et al. Plasmablastic lymphoma among human immunodeficiency virus-positive patients: results of a single center's experience. Leuk Lymphoma. 2015;56:267–9.
20. Castillo JJ, Winer ES, Stachurski D, et al. Prognostic factors in chemotherapy-treated patients with HIV-associated plasmablastic lymphoma. Oncologist. 2010;15:293–9.
21. NCCN guidelines version 3.2017. AIDS-related B-cell lymphomas. AIDS-4. http://www.nccn.org/professionals/physician_gls/pdf/nhl.pdf. Accessed 30 May 2017.
22. Al-Malki MM, Castillo JJ, Sloan JM, Re A. Hematopoietic cell transplantation for plasma-

blastic lymphoma: a review. Biol Blood Marrow Transplant. 2014;20:1877–84.
23. Bibas M, Grisetti S, Alba L, et al. Patient with HIV-associated plasmablastic lymphoma responding to bortezomib alone and in combination with dexamethasone, gemcitabine, oxaliplatin, cytarabine, and pegfilgrastim chemotherapy and lenalidomide alone. J Clin Oncol. 2010;28:e704–8.
24. Dasanu CA, Bauer F, Codreanu I, et al. Plasmablastic haemato-lymphoid neoplasm with a complex genetic signature of Burkitt lymphoma responding to bortezomib. Hematol Oncol. 2013;31:164–6.
25. Yan M, Dong Z, Zhao F, et al. CD20-positive plasmablastic lymphoma with excellent response to bortezomib combined with rituximab. Eur J Haematol. 2014;93:77–80.
26. Castillo JJ, Reagan JL, Sikov WM, Winer ES. Bortezomib in combination with infusional dose-adjusted EPOCH for the treatment of plasmablastic lymphoma. Br J Haematol. 2015;169:352–5.
27. Fedele PL, Gregory GP, Gilbertson M, et al. Infusional dose-adjusted epoch plus bortezomib for the treatment of plasmablastic lymphoma. Ann Hematol. 2016;95:667–8.
28. Fernandez-Alvarez R, Gonzalez-Rodriguez AP, Rubio-Castro A, et al. Bortezomib plus CHOP for the treatment of HIV-associated plasmablastic lymphoma: clinical experience in three patients. Leuk Lymphoma. 2016;57(2):463–6.
29. Carras S, Regny C, Peoc'h M, et al. Dramatic efficacy of low dose lenalidomide as single agent in a patient with refractory gastric non-human immunodeficiency virus-associated plasmablastic lymphoma. Leuk Lymphoma. 2015;56:2986–8.
30. Schmit JM, DeLaune J, Norkin M, Grosbach A. A case of plasmablastic lymphoma achieving complete response and durable remission after lenalidomide-based therapy. Oncol Res Treat. 2017;40:46–8.
31. Colomo L, Loong F, Rives S, et al. Diffuse large B-cell lymphomas with plasmablastic differentiation represent a heterogeneous group of disease entities. Am J Surg Pathol. 2004;28:736–47.
32. Holderness BM, Malhotra S, Levy NB, Danilov AV. Brentuximab vedotin demonstrates activity in a patient with plasmablastic lymphoma arising from a background of chronic lymphocytic leukemia. J Clin Oncol. 2013;31:e197–9.
33. Beroukhim R, Mermel CH, Porter D, et al. The landscape of somatic copy-number alteration across human cancers. Nature. 2010;463:899–905.
34. Rahl PB, Lin CY, Seila AC, et al. c-Myc regulates transcriptional pause release. Cell. 2010;141:432–45.
35. Delmore JE, Issa GC, Lemieux ME, et al. BET bromodomain inhibition as a therapeutic strategy to target c-Myc. Cell. 2011;146:904–17.
36. Guo L, Bodo J, Durkin L, Hsi ED. Evaluation of PD1/PDL1 expression and their clinicopathologic association in EBV-associated lymphoproliferative disorders in nonimmunosuppressed patients. Appl Immunohistochem Mol Morphol. 2017; Epub ahead of print.
37. Kim SJ, Hyeon J, Cho I, Ko YH, Kim WS. Comparison of efficacy of pembrolizumab between Epstein-Barr virus–positive and –negative relapsed or refractory non-Hodgkin lymphomas. Cancer Res Treat. 2018; Epub ahead of print.
38. Said J, Cesarman E. Primary effusion lymphoma. In: Swerdlow SH, Campo E, Harris NL, et al., editors. WHO classification of tumours of haematopoietic and lmyphoid tissues. Revised 4th ed. Lyon: IARC; 2017. p. 323–4.
39. Knowles DM, Inghirami G, Ubriaco A, Dalla-Favera R. Molecular genetic analysis of three AIDS-associated neoplasms of uncertain lineage demonstrates their B-cell derivation and the possible pathogenetic role of the Epstein-Barr virus. Blood. 1989;73:792–9.
40. Cesarman E, Chang Y, Moore PS, et al. Kaposi's sarcoma-associated herpesvirus-like DNA sequences in AIDS-related body-cavity-based lymphomas. N Engl J Med. 1995;332:1186–91.
41. Said J, Cesarman E. Primary effusion lymphoma. In: Swerdlow S, Campo E, Harris N, et al., editors. WHO classification of tumours of haematopoietic and lymphoid tissues. 4th ed. Lyon: IARC; 2008. p. 260–1.
42. Wilson KS, McKenna RW, Kroft SH, et al. Primary effusion lymphomas exhibit complex and recurrent cytogenetic abnormalities. Br J Haematol. 2002;116:113–21.
43. Boulanger E, Agbalika F, Maarek O, et al. A clinical, molecular and cytogenetic study of 12 cases of human herpesvirus 8 associated primary effusion lymphoma in HIV-infected patients. Hematol J. 2001;2:172–9.
44. Kim Y, Park CJ, Roh J, Huh J. Current concepts in primary effusion lymphoma and other effusion-based lymphomas. Korean J Pathol. 2014;48:81–90.
45. Luan SL, Boulanger E, Ye H, et al. Primary effusion lymphoma: genomic profiling revealed amplification of SELPLG and CORO1C encoding for proteins important for cell migration. J Pathol. 2010;222:166–79.
46. Gantt S, Casper C. Human herpesvirus 8-associated neoplasms: the roles of viral replication and antiviral treatment. Curr Opin Infect Dis. 2011;24:295–301.
47. Shi Y, Hou Y, Hu Q, et al. A rare case of HHV-8-positive/HIV-negative/EBV-negative primary effusion lymphoma in a renal transplant recipient. Cytopathology. 2012;23:137–9.
48. Matsumoto Y, Nomura K, Ueda K, et al. Human herpesvirus 8-negative malignant effusion lymphoma: a distinct clinical entity and successful treatment with rituximab. Leuk Lymphoma. 2005;46:415–9.
49. Kaplan LD. Human herpesvirus-8: Kaposi sarcoma, multicentric Castleman disease, and primary effusion lymphoma. Hematology Am Soc Hematol Educ Program. 2013;2013:103–8.
50. Carbone A, Gloghini A, Vaccher E, et al. Kaposi's sarcoma-associated herpesvirus/human herpesvirus type 8-positive solid lymphomas: a tissue-based

variant of primary effusion lymphoma. J Mol Diagn. 2005;7:17–27.
51. Chadburn A, Hyjek E, Mathew S, et al. KSHV-positive solid lymphomas represent an extra-cavitary variant of primary effusion lymphoma. Am J Surg Pathol. 2004;28:1401–16.
52. Pan ZG, Zhang QY, Lu ZB, et al. Extracavitary KSHV-associated large B-cell lymphoma: a distinct entity or a subtype of primary effusion lymphoma? Study of 9 cases and review of an additional 43 cases. Am J Surg Pathol. 2012;36:1129–40.
53. Simonelli C, Spina M, Cinelli R, et al. Clinical features and outcome of primary effusion lymphoma in HIV-infected patients: a single-institution study. J Clin Oncol. 2003;21:3948–54.
54. Boulanger E, Gerard L, Gabarre J, et al. Prognostic factors and outcome of human herpesvirus 8-associated primary effusion lymphoma in patients with AIDS. J Clin Oncol. 2005;23:4372–80.
55. Lim ST, Karim R, Nathwani BN, et al. AIDS-related Burkitt's lymphoma versus diffuse large-cell lymphoma in the pre-highly active antiretroviral therapy (HAART) and HAART eras: significant differences in survival with standard chemotherapy. J Clin Oncol. 2005;23:4430–8.
56. Castillo JJ, Shum H, Lahijani M, et al. Prognosis in primary effusion lymphoma is associated with the number of body cavities involved. Leuk Lymphoma. 2012;53:2378–82.
57. Simonelli C, Tedeschi R, Gloghini A, et al. Characterization of immunologic and virological parameters in HIV-infected patients with primary effusion lymphoma during antiblastic therapy and highly active antiretroviral therapy. Clin Infect Dis. 2005;40:1022–7.
58. Boulanger E, Daniel MT, Agbalika F, Oksenhendler E. Combined chemotherapy including high-dose methotrexate in KSHV/HHV8-associated primary effusion lymphoma. Am J Hematol. 2003;73:143–8.
59. El-Ayass W, Yu EM, Karcher DS, Aragon-Ching JB. Complete response to EPOCH in a patient with HIV and extracavitary primary effusion lymphoma involving the colon: a case report and review of literature. Clin Lymphoma Myeloma Leuk. 2012;12:144–7.
60. Barta SK, Lee JY, Kaplan LD, et al. Pooled analysis of AIDS malignancy consortium trials evaluating rituximab plus CHOP or infusional EPOCH chemotherapy in HIV-associated non-Hodgkin lymphoma. Cancer. 2012;118:3977–83.
61. Ripamonti D, Marini B, Rambaldi A, Suter F. Treatment of primary effusion lymphoma with highly active antiviral therapy in the setting of HIV infection. AIDS. 2008;22:1236–7.
62. Won JH, Han SH, Bae SB, et al. Successful eradication of relapsed primary effusion lymphoma with high-dose chemotherapy and autologous stem cell transplantation in a patient seronegative for human immunodeficiency virus. Int J Hematol. 2006;83:328–30.
63. Bryant A, Milliken S. Successful reduced-intensity conditioning allogeneic HSCT for HIV-related primary effusion lymphoma. Biol Blood Marrow Transplant. 2008;14:601–2.
64. Keller SA, Schattner EJ, Cesarman E. Inhibition of NF-kappaB induces apoptosis of KSHV-infected primary effusion lymphoma cells. Blood. 2000;96:2537–42.
65. An J, Sun Y, Fisher M, Rettig MB. Antitumor effects of bortezomib (PS-341) on primary effusion lymphomas. Leukemia. 2004;18:1699–704.
66. Boulanger E, Meignin V, Oksenhendler E. Bortezomib (PS-341) in patients with human herpesvirus 8-associated primary effusion lymphoma. Br J Haematol. 2008;141:559–61.
67. Bhatt S, Ashlock BM, Toomey NL, et al. Efficacious proteasome/HDAC inhibitor combination therapy for primary effusion lymphoma. J Clin Invest. 2013;123:2616–28.
68. Antar A, El Hajj H, Jabbour M, et al. Primary effusion lymphoma in an elderly patient effectively treated by lenalidomide: case report and review of literature. Blood Cancer J. 2014;4:e190.
69. Davis DA, Mishra S, Anagho HA, et al. Restoration of immune surface molecules in Kaposi sarcoma-associated herpesvirus infected cells by lenalidomide and pomalidomide. Oncotarget. 2017;8:50342–58.
70. Bhatt S, Ashlock BM, Natkunam Y, et al. CD30 targeting with brentuximab vedotin: a novel therapeutic approach to primary effusion lymphoma. Blood. 2013;122:1233–42.
71. Chen BJ, Chapuy B, Ouyang J, et al. PD-L1 expression is characteristic of a subset of aggressive B-cell lymphomas and virus-associated malignancies. Clin Cancer Res. 2013;19:3462–73.
72. Wang HY, Fuda FS, Chen W, Karandikar NJ. Notch1 in primary effusion lymphoma: a clinicopathological study. Mod Pathol. 2010;23:773–80.
73. Granato M, Rizzello C, Gilardini Montani MS, et al. Quercetin induces apoptosis and autophagy in primary effusion lymphoma cells by inhibiting PI3K/AKT/mTOR and STAT3 signaling pathways. J Nutr Biochem. 2017;41:124–36.
74. Dupin N, Diss TL, Kellam P, et al. HHV-8 is associated with a plasmablastic variant of Castleman disease that is linked to HHV-8-positive plasmablastic lymphoma. Blood. 2000;95:1406–12.
75. Oksenhendler E, Boulanger E, Galicier L, et al. High incidence of Kaposi sarcoma-associated herpesvirus-related non-Hodgkin lymphoma in patients with HIV infection and multicentric Castleman disease. Blood. 2002;99:2331–6.
76. Du MQ, Liu H, Diss TC, et al. Kaposi sarcoma-associated herpesvirus infects monotypic (IgM lambda) but polyclonal naive B cells in Castleman disease and associated lymphoproliferative disorders. Blood. 2001;97:2130–6.
77. Issacson P, Campo E, Harris NL. Large B-cell lymphoma arising in HHV8-associated multicentric Castlemans disease. In: Swerdlow S, Campo

E, Harris N, et al., editors. WHO classification of tumours of haematopoietic and lymphoid tissues. 4th ed. Lyon: IARC; 2008. p. 258–9.
78. Montes-Moreno S, Montalban C, Piris MA. Large B-cell lymphomas with plasmablastic differentiation: a biological and therapeutic challenge. Leuk Lymphoma. 2012;53:185–94.
79. Oksenhendler E, Boutboul D, Beldjord K, et al. Human herpesvirus 8+ polyclonal IgMlambda B-cell lymphocytosis mimicking plasmablastic leukemia/lymphoma in HIV-infected patients. Eur J Haematol. 2013;91:497–503.
80. Suda T, Katano H, Delsol G, et al. HHV-8 infection status of AIDS-unrelated and AIDS-associated multicentric Castleman's disease. Pathol Int. 2001;51:671–9.
81. Cronin DM, Warnke RA. Castleman disease: an update on classification and the spectrum of associated lesions. Adv Anat Pathol. 2009;16:236–46.
82. Kishimoto T. IL-6: from its discovery to clinical applications. Int Immunol. 2010;22:347–52.
83. Hsi ED, Lorsbach RB, Fend F, Dogan A. Plasmablastic lymphoma and related disorders. Am J Clin Pathol. 2011;136:183–94.
84. Pagni F, Bosisio FM, Sala E, et al. The plasmablasts in Castleman disease. Am J Clin Pathol. 2013;139:555–9.
85. Gerard L, Michot JM, Burcheri S, et al. Rituximab decreases the risk of lymphoma in patients with HIV-associated multicentric Castleman disease. Blood. 2012;119:2228–33.
86. Sarosiek KA, Cavallin LE, Bhatt S, et al. Efficacy of bortezomib in a direct xenograft model of primary effusion lymphoma. Proc Natl Acad Sci U S A. 2010;107:13069–74.
87. Fajgenbaum DC, van Rhee F, Nabel CS. HHV-8-negative, idiopathic multicentric Castleman disease: novel insights into biology, pathogenesis, and therapy. Blood. 2014;123:2924–33.
88. van Rhee F, Wong RS, Munshi N, et al. Siltuximab for multicentric Castleman's disease: a randomised, double-blind, placebo-controlled trial. Lancet Oncol. 2014;15:966–74.
89. Szturz P, Adam Z, Rehak Z, et al. Salvage lenalidomide in four rare oncological diseases. Tumori. 2013;99:e251–6.
90. Zhou X, Wei J, Lou Y, et al. Salvage therapy with lenalidomide containing regimen for relapsed/refractory Castleman disease: a report of three cases. Front Med. 2017;11:287–92.
91. Rimokh R, Magaud JP, Berger F, et al. A translocation involving a specific breakpoint (q35) on chromosome 5 is characteristic of anaplastic large cell lymphoma ('Ki-1 lymphoma'). Br J Haematol. 1989;71:31–6.
92. Delsol G, Lamant L, Mariame B, et al. A new subtype of large B-cell lymphoma expressing the ALK kinase and lacking the 2;5 translocation. Blood. 1997;89:1483–90.
93. Momose S, Tamaru J, Kishi H, et al. Hyperactivated STAT3 in ALK-positive diffuse large B-cell lymphoma with clathrin-ALK fusion. Hum Pathol. 2009;40:75–82.
94. Beltran B, Castillo J, Salas R, et al. ALK-positive diffuse large B-cell lymphoma: report of four cases and review of the literature. J Hematol Oncol. 2009;2:11.
95. Sachdev R, Goel S, Gupta S, Sood N. Anaplastic lymphoma kinase (ALK) positive diffuse large B cell lymphoma in a 20 year old: a rare entity. Indian J Pathol Microbiol. 2014;57:157–8.
96. Stachurski D, Miron PM, Al-Homsi S, et al. Anaplastic lymphoma kinase-positive diffuse large B-cell lymphoma with a complex karyotype and cryptic 3′ ALK gene insertion to chromosome 4 q22-24. Hum Pathol. 2007;38:940–5.
97. Ott G, Rosenwald A, Campo E. Understanding MYC-driven aggressive B-cell lymphomas: pathogenesis and classification. Hematology Am Soc Hematol Educ Program. 2013;2013:575–83.
98. Valera A, Colomo L, Martinez A, et al. ALK-positive large B-cell lymphomas express a terminal B-cell differentiation program and activated STAT3 but lack MYC rearrangements. Mod Pathol. 2013;26:1329–37.
99. Nieborowska-Skorska M, Slupianek A, Xue L, et al. Role of signal transducer and activator of transcription 5 in nucleophosmin/anaplastic lymphoma kinase-mediated malignant transformation of lymphoid cells. Cancer Res. 2001;61:6517–23.
100. Zamo A, Chiarle R, Piva R, et al. Anaplastic lymphoma kinase (ALK) activates Stat3 and protects hematopoietic cells from cell death. Oncogene. 2002;21:1038–47.
101. Zhang Q, Wang HY, Liu X, Wasik MA. STAT5A is epigenetically silenced by the tyrosine kinase NPM1-ALK and acts as a tumor suppressor by reciprocally inhibiting NPM1-ALK expression. Nat Med. 2007;13:1341–8.
102. Bai RY, Ouyang T, Miething C, et al. Nucleophosmin-anaplastic lymphoma kinase associated with anaplastic large-cell lymphoma activates the phosphatidylinositol 3-kinase/Akt antiapoptotic signaling pathway. Blood. 2000;96:4319–27.
103. Laurent C, Do C, Gascoyne RD, et al. Anaplastic lymphoma kinase-positive diffuse large B-cell lymphoma: a rare clinicopathologic entity with poor prognosis. J Clin Oncol. 2009;27:4211–6.
104. Wass M, Behlendorf T, Schadlich B, et al. Crizotinib in refractory ALK-positive diffuse large B-cell lymphoma: a case report with a short-term response. Eur J Haematol. 2014;92:268–70.
105. Cerchietti L, Damm-Welk C, Vater I, et al. Inhibition of anaplastic lymphoma kinase (ALK) activity provides a therapeutic approach for CLTC-ALK-positive human diffuse large B cell lymphomas. PLoS One. 2011;6:e18436.
106. Amin HM, McDonnell TJ, Ma Y, et al. Selective inhibition of STAT3 induces apoptosis and G(1) cell cycle arrest in ALK-positive anaplastic large cell lymphoma. Oncogene. 2004;23:5426–34.

Standard of Care in T-Cell Lymphoma

12

Alessandro Broccoli, Dai Chihara,
Michelle A. Fanale, and Pier Luigi Zinzani

12.1 Introduction

Peripheral T-cell non-Hodgkin lymphoma (PTCL) is a heterogeneous group of mature T-cell neoplasms generally associated with a poor prognosis and displaying a wide geographical heterogeneity. They account for 5–10% of all aggressive lymphoma in Europe and in the United States, whereas they tend to be much more represented (up to roughly 20%) in Asia, where some peculiar forms of disease (like neoplasms of the NK-/T-cell origin) are prevalent [1–5].

PTCL have a nodal origin in most of cases, although extranodal non-cutaneous entities do exist, described by their tissue tropism. The 2016 revision of the World Health Organization classification of lymphoid neoplasms underscores several new insights into the complexity of PTCL, which emerge from molecular and genetic studies that point out many specific molecular signatures helpful in distinguishing among different entities, albeit displaying similarities in terms of morphology and immunophenotype [4, 6]. Aggressive PTCLs with nodal presentations include three main categories: nodal T-cell lymphoma with T-follicular helper (TFH) phenotype, which is a broad category which comprises the entire spectrum of nodal lymphoma displaying a TFH phenotype and includes angioimmunoblastic T-cell lymphoma (AITL), follicular T-cell lymphoma, and other nodal PTCL with a TFH phenotype; anaplastic large cell lymphoma (ALCL), either with or without the expression of the anaplastic lymphoma kinase (ALK), which clearly distinguishes two separated entities in terms of prognostic implications (ALK^- ALCL is no longer regarded as a provisional entity in the 2016 classification); and peripheral T-cell lymphoma, not otherwise specified (PTCL-NOS), a category that still shows extreme cytological and phenotypic heterogeneity, in which fall all the T-cell lymphoma that cannot be further classified into any other of the existing classifiers [7]. A unique form of ALK^- ALCL, which arises in association with saline and silicone-filled breast implants and clinically presents with the accumulation of seroma fluid at the interface between the implant itself and the surrounding fibrous capsule, is now a provisional entity termed breast implant-associated ALCL [8]. Among the entities with a prevalent non-cutaneous extranodal

A. Broccoli · P. L. Zinzani (✉)
Institute of Hematology "L. e A. Seràgnoli"—University of Bologna, Bologna, Italy
e-mail: alessandro.broccoli@studio.unibo.it; pierluigi.zinzani@unibo.it

D. Chihara
Department of Internal Medicine, The University of New Mexico, Albuquerque, NM, USA
e-mail: dchihara-kob@umin.ac.jp

M. A. Fanale
Department of Lymphoma/Myeloma, The University of Texas M.D. Anderson Cancer Center, Houston, TX, USA
e-mail: mfanale@mdanderson.org

G. Lenz, G. Salles (eds.), *Aggressive Lymphomas*, Hematologic Malignancies,
https://doi.org/10.1007/978-3-030-00362-3_12

involvement and an aggressive behavior are enteropathy-associated T-cell lymphoma (EATL), formerly defined as EATL type I, typically associated with celiac disease and of αβ origin, clearly distinguished by monomorphic epitheliotropic intestinal T-cell lymphoma (formerly known as EATL type II, now a separated provisional entity); hepatosplenic T-cell lymphoma of γδ origin (HSTCL); subcutaneous panniculitis-like T-cell lymphoma (SPTCL); and extranodal NK-/T-cell lymphoma (ENKL), nasal type [4].

Despite clinical, morphological, phenotypic, and molecular differences, the management of these aggressive diseases is substantially the same for all the nodal entities: an initial systemic chemotherapy and a prompt evaluation of which patient is suitable for an up-front consolidation by means of an autologous stem cell transplantation are nowadays a widely accepted standard of treatment. Peculiar entities—like low International Prognostic Index (IPI, see below) ALK^+ ALCL, ALK^- breast implant-associated ALCL, EATL, SPTCL, or ENKL—may take advantage of specifically designed strategies, based on their clinical course and their reduced tendency to spread to distant organs or nodes and which take into account the specific tropism to an organ or tissue and their sensitivity to some specific cytostatic drugs [9].

The aim of this chapter is to review the current clinical management of aggressive T-cell lymphoma, moving from disease diagnosis, initial staging, and available prognostic tools up to the discussion of the first-line therapy and the adopted strategies for relapsed and refractory disease, with a focus on newly available single agents and innovative combinations.

12.2 Clinical Presentation of Aggressive T-Cell Lymphoma

Subtypes with a prevalent nodal expression—PTCL-NOS, ALCL (either in the ALK^+ or ALK^- forms), and nodal T-cell lymphoma with T-follicular helper (TFH) phenotype (including AITL)—involve adult patients (median age at presentation variable between 60 and 65 years) with male predominance. The key feature of these diseases is generalized lymphadenopathy, with the involvement of both superficial and abdominal nodal stations, although any extranodal organ or tissue may be concomitantly affected: the skin (particularly in AITL), the liver, the spleen, and the gastrointestinal tract are among the most involved sites of disease. Hepatic and splenic enlargements are clinical hallmarks of HSTCL, which is characterized by parenchymal infiltration (including bone marrow involvement in more than 70% of cases) without forming growing and coalescent nodal masses.

Advanced stage (Ann Arbor stage III/IV) at presentation is a constant for these disease entities; B symptoms are reported in 50–70% of cases, and bone marrow infiltration is documented in 10–30% of patients. A significant proportion of patients display poor performance status at disease onset, and many of them have their clinical conditions worsening during treatment, thus being unable to undergo intensive chemotherapy or myeloablative conditioning: this is one of the major determinants of the dismal prognosis of this category of lymphoma.

Autoimmune phenomena may be associated with certain disease entities. Autoimmune markers, such as rheumatoid factor, circulating immunocomplexes, and anti-smooth muscle antibodies, may be detected in 30–50% of AITL patients, and Coombs-positive hemolytic anemia may complicate up to one-third of cases [10]. Autoimmune or immune-mediated disease, such as Crohn's disease, is concomitantly observed with HSTCL, which also correlates with the immunosuppressive regimens chronically administered after solid organ transplantation.

Signs and symptoms of PTCL with extranodal manifestations strictly depend on the involved organ or tissue. EATL may be associated with abdominal discomfort and pain at onset, along with fatigue and anorexia. Reappearance of malabsorption in a patient with a history of celiac disease favorably responding to a gluten-free diet or, alternatively, the sudden onset of gluten-insensitive severe malabsorption in an otherwise healthy individual can be key symptoms of disease at its onset. Acute abdominal symptoms, like perforation, obstruction, and hemorrhage, require an urgent treatment and surgical intervention with bowel resection in most of cases, as a result of disease penetration into the intestinal wall. The jejunum is the mostly affected site, although any segment can be involved. When multiple segments of the small intestine have been involved, it is likely that the disease has disseminated to nearby and distant organs (mesenteric nodes, liver, spleen, lungs, and bone marrow).

SPTCL presents with solitary or multiple nodules or plaques on the lower extremities, more rarely involving the trunk and the upper limbs. Lesions may mimic an abscess but do not resolve after surgical incision. Systemic symptoms, including fever, fatigue, and weight loss, can be present at onset. Hemophagocytic syndrome may complicate the clinical picture in some rare cases, and it is associated with a highly aggressive clinical course.

ENKL, in its nasal form, arises in the nasal cavity and invades the nasopharynx, paranasal sinus, orbits, oral cavity, and palate, usually with bone erosions, ulceration, and destructive behavior, although remaining confined to the facial district in most of cases (stages I and II). On the contrary, extranasal ENKL is an aggressive systemic disease, with the involvement of multiple anatomical sites (stages III and IV) such as skin, gastrointestinal tract, testis, lung, eye, and soft tissues (the same to which the nasal type of the disease tends to disseminate), along with systemic symptoms, lactate dehydrogenase (LDH) elevation, and poor performance status.

12.3 Diagnosis and Staging

12.3.1 Establishing the Diagnosis

The diagnosis of PTCL is always established on the biopsy of the involved tissue, which is mainly represented by a lymph node. However, virtually any extranodal site may be the target for biopsy target for biopsy: the liver, small intestine, and skin are among the mostly involved extralymphatic tissues [11, 12]. Fine needle aspiration is not sufficient to correctly establish the diagnosis. The review of all slides and of formalin-fixed paraffin-embedded tissue by a pathologist with expertise in T-cell lymphoma is always encouraged: hematopathologists are able to apply the WHO classification to diagnose a PTCL, although with heterogeneous agreement on diagnosis depending on the specific disease entity they are looking at [5]. Diagnostic accuracy is very good for ALCL, ALK-positive, but agreement is lost in case of other lymphoma subtypes, with a rate of concordance inferior to 75% for the most common subtype, PTCL-NOS.

Molecular studies may be helpful under certain circumstances to clarify or refine the diagnosis: at present, however, no molecular markers specifically dictate treatment decisions. The sole demonstration of T-cell clonality through the assessment of T-cell receptor rearrangement alone is not sufficient for diagnosis, as this may be seen also with reactive and inflammatory processes.

Physical examination, including the evaluation of the Waldeyer's ring, nasopharynx, node-bearing areas, liver, and spleen, along with thoracic auscultation and a full skin inspection, is mandatory at disease onset. Patient's evaluation is completed by full history taking, mainly focusing on lymphoma-related symptoms (recent weight loss, fever, night sweats), and by the assessment of performance status. A complete blood count with differential counts and a comprehensive metabolic panel, including LDH measurement, is also required at baseline, even for prognostic assessment. Reticulocytes and bilirubin (complete and fractionated) are useful markers in case of suspect hemolysis, which may be associated with some PTCL cases (mainly AITL). Direct Coombs test is also necessary to rule out the diagnosis of autoimmune hemolytic anemia [10].

12.3.2 Staging Procedures

Like nodal B-cell lymphoma, PTCL are staged according to the Ann Arbor staging system. Computed tomography (CT) scan of the neck, chest, abdomen, and pelvis with contrast and a bone marrow trephine biopsy are requested to accomplish a thorough disease staging [12].

12.3.3 Role of PET Scan

^{18}F-fluorodeoxyglucose (FDG) PET scan is not mandatory for disease staging, although it has proven to be helpful in detecting FDG-avid nodal or extranodal lesions that can be missed by a CT scan evaluation. Nevertheless, PET is able to change the disease stage in no more than 5% of patients at diagnosis as compared to CT [13], and this change does not translate into any treatment modification: systemic chemotherapy in nodal PTCL, in fact, is generally used regardless of tumor extent and disease stage at presentation. It should be noted, however, that PET positivity found at the end of induction treatment and in patients who have received autologous stem cell transplantation (autoSCT) is a strong predictor of reduced survival [14]. Maximum standard uptake values in patients with PTCL are lower than in aggressive B-cell counterparts and usually less pronounced for extranodal lesions than for lymph node localizations of the disease.

12.4 Prognosis

The International Prognostic Index (IPI), although specifically designed for aggressive B-cell lymphoma, is also the mainstay of the prognostic stratification of patients with PTCL and can be determined using clinically derived variables. Similarly to B-cell counterparts, it inversely correlates with survival rates, although overall survival (OS) for each category is lower if compared to diffuse large B-cell lymphoma. Lower IPI scores (0/1 prognostic factors) correlate with a 5-year OS ranging from 90% for ALK-positive ALCL to less than 30% for EATL and extranasal NK-/T-cell lymphoma; on the contrary, patients with four/five risk factors display significantly dismal figures, with a 5-year OS of 25–33% for ALK-positive ALCL and AITL and less than 10% for all the other nodal and extranodal subtypes [5]. Newer scores have been developed to better describe the outcome of specific subtypes of T-cell lymphoma (Table 12.1): the Prognostic Index for PTCL-NOS (PIT, [15]), the modified PIT (m-PIT, [16]), and a prognostic index derived from the International T-cell Lymphoma Project (ITCLP, [17]) are descriptive of populations of PTCL-NOS patients treated with a cyclophosphamide, doxorubicin, vincristine, and prednisone (CHOP) approach, whereas the prognostic index for AITL (PIA) has predicted OS more reliably than IPI in patients with AITL [18]. The stratification of patients into lower- and higher-risk categories, however, does not necessarily translate into a different management: at least 60–70% of lower-risk patients, in fact, are likely to relapse within the first 5 years; thus a less aggressive initial approach seems not to be justified (Table 12.2).

Table 12.1 Variables used in the calculation of relevant prognostic scores

	IPI	PIT	m-PIT	ITCLP	PIA
Age (>60 years)	•	•	•	•	•
ECOG (>1)	•	•	•	•	
ECOG (>2)					•
LDH (elevated values)	•	•	•		
Ann Arbor stage (III–IV)	•				
Extranodal involvement (≥2 sites)	•				•
Bone marrow involvement		•			
Platelet count (<150,000/mm^3)				•	•
Ki-67 (≥80%)			•		
B symptoms					•
Context	All T-cell lymphoma	PTCL-NOS			AITL

ECOG Eastern Cooperative Oncology Group, *LDH* lactate dehydrogenase

Table 12.2 Prognosis of aggressive PTCL according to the most widely used prognostic scores

		5-year OS (%)		5-year FFS (%)		
Disease	Score	Low score	High score	Low score	High score	Reference
PTCL-NOS	IPI	50	11	36	9	Weisenburger et al. [19]
	PIT	50	11	34	8	
AITL	IPI	56	25	34	16	Federico et al. [18]
	PIA	44	24	28	15	
ALK^+ ALCL	IPI	90	33	80	25	Savage et al. [20]
ALK^- ALCL		74	13	62	13	
ENKL, nasal	IPI	57	0	53	0	Au et al. [21]
ENKL, extranasal		17	20	21	20	
EATL	[a]	20		4–17		Delabie et al. [22], Ellin et al. [3][b]
HSTCL	[a]	0–43		0–20		Vose et al. [5], Ellin et al. [3][b]
SPTCL	[a]	60		30–40		Vose et al. [5], Ellin et al. [3][b]

OS overall survival, *FFS*, failure-free survival. See text for disease and prognostic score abbreviations. "Low score" means score 0/1 for IPI, score 0 (group 1) for PIT, and score 0/1 for PIA. "High score" means score 4/5 for IPI, score 3/4 (group 4) for PIT, and score ≥ 2 for PIA. Data are from the International Peripheral T-cell and Natural Killer/T-cell Lymphoma Study ([5] and related articles for specific subtypes) and mostly rely on anthracycline-treated patients during induction. Data from the Swedish Lymphoma Registry [3] integrate prognostic figures for rarer entities

[a]IPI (or any other prognostic score) not relevant for prognostic stratification of patients

[b]Data in this publication refer to progression-free rather than failure-free survival

12.5 First-Line Treatment Approach

12.5.1 Induction Regimens

The main goal of first-line treatment should be the achievement of a deep remission, which allows a timely application of a consolidative autologous stem cell transplantation (autoSCT), where appropriate, and enhances the opportunity to gain a good control of the disease in the long term.

The treatment strategies most widely adopted in aggressive PTCL are derived from the experience acquired in B-cell aggressive lymphoma: this is generally true for PTCL with a predominantly nodal presentation, whereas disease entities with an exquisitely extranodal involvement or a particular aggressiveness may be managed differently (this will be discussed separately below). It should be noted, however, that PTCL are biologically and clinically different from B-cell counterparts and this may explain the significant prognostic gap existing between lymphoma of B- and T-cell origin when the same (or at least very similar) approaches are applied.

Anthracycline-based regimens are considered the current standard of care in induction treatment of PTCL patients, as demonstrated in several reported experiences in which the cyclophosphamide, doxorubicin, vincristine, and prednisone (CHOP) combination was adopted in a proportion of patients variable from 60 to 85% [5, 23, 24] (Table 12.2). Patients with ALCL respond better to CHOP in comparison to other PTCL subtypes. The overall response rates (ORR) range from 70 to 80% for ALK^- ALCL patients, with complete response (CR) rates up to 50% of the cases. On the contrary, ALK^+ ALCL patients respond to first-line CHOP in up to 90% of cases. Nevertheless, nearly 40% of patients with ALK^+ disease and roughly 60% of those with ALK^- disease fail to maintain their response over time with only first-line induction [20, 25]. The role of anthracycline-containing regimens is however much more debated in patients affected by AITL and PTCL-NOS [7, 10]. On the one hand, it should be noted that according to the International Peripheral T-cell and Natural Killer/T-cell Lymphoma Study, the CR rate observed in patients receiving an anthracycline-based induction was 61% for AITL patients [18] and 56% for PTCL-NOS patients

[19], however without any significant survival advantage for those receiving anthracyclines if compared to patients treated with anthracycline-free schedules [5]. On the other, different data sets provide the evidence that anthracycline-containing regimens are associated with improved OS and PFS in all patients affected by PTCL, particularly in those with both AITL and PTCL-NOS subtypes, and that the benefit is reinforced by first-line consolidation with autoSCT, as discussed below [26]. A 30-month improvement in median OS was observed in PTCL patients treated with anthracyclines over those who were not, which was the consequence of a 13% increase in 2-year PFS documented in anthracycline-treated patients.

Much more disappointing results have been achieved in patients affected by extranodal disease subtypes, like EATL [22], HSTCL, SPTCL, and ENKL [21], which nowadays still represent a clearly unmet medical need [9]: alternative treatment strategies are urgently required.

More intensive chemotherapy regimens have not proven to be more effective than CHOP: the only phase III randomized study in which an induction schedule including etoposide, ifosfamide, cisplatin, alternating with doxorubicin, bleomycin, vinblastine, and dacarbazine (VIP-rABVD) was tested against CHOP (given every 21 days) did not show any superiority of the former regimen in terms of event-free survival (EFS), thus confirming CHOP as the reference standard for PTCL patients [27]. There is some evidence that the addition of etoposide to CHOP can be more effective than CHOP alone, at least in PTCL-NOS and ALCL patients: the CHOEP regimen, given either every 14 or 21 days, improved response and EFS rates in young patients with normal LDH levels (3-year EFS was 70.5% after CHOEP and 51.0% after CHOP, $P = 0.004$), although 3-year OS did not significantly differ between the two groups [28]. Attempts to improve outcomes in younger patients by escalating doses of any of the drugs included in CHOEP have failed. In addition, CHOEP failed to enhance clinical outcomes in patients older than 60 years, for whom CHOP should remain the standard first-line approach.

12.5.2 Frontline Consolidation with Autologous Transplantation

Patients responding to first-line treatment generally display a short duration of remission and a high risk of relapse: for this reason, a frontline consolidation with autoSCT has been considered a valid therapeutic opportunity for patients achieving at least a partial response (PR) to induction, in particular for those with intermediate to high IPI score and with histologies other than ALK^+ ALCL. However, no randomized trials have specifically clarified whether up-front autoSCT should be regarded superior to conventional chemotherapy [23].

Two prospective Italian phase II studies, involving 62 patients with advanced stage PTCL, demonstrated a high CR rate (89%) after frontline autoSCT, with a 12-year OS and disease-free survival (DFS) of 34% and 55%, respectively [29]. A Spanish study enrolling 41 PTCL treated up-front with intensified CHOP alternated with an etoposide, cisplatin, cytarabine, and prednisone (ESHAP) regimen documented that 51% of the 24 transplanted patients were in CR after autoSCT, with 4-year OS and PFS of 39% and 30%, respectively, for the intention-to-treat population [30]. These more disappointing results may be due to the fact that this study excluded ALK^+ ALCL patients, whereas the former Italian studies did not.

Reimer et al. reported the results of a prospective multicenter trial in which 83 patients were treated with 6–8 CHOP cycles followed by mobilizing chemotherapy and total body irradiation + cyclophosphamide myeloablative conditioning, with the rescue of autologous stem cells: 55 patients were transplanted, with an intention-to-treat CR rate of 58% and an estimated 3-year OS of 48%, which increased to 71% if the only cohort of transplanted patient was considered [31]. ALK^+ ALCL patients were again excluded from the study. Recently published results regarding an extension and update of this trial (involving 111 patients, 68% of whom received autoSCT) confirmed a 59% of CR after myeloablative conditioning, with 5-year OS, DFS, and

PFS rates of 44%, 54%, and 39%, respectively, for the entire patient population [32].

The Nordic Lymphoma Group applied a CHOEP induction strategy (given every 14 days), although omitting etoposide in patients over 60 years, in 160 PTCL patients (again excluding ALK+ ALCL). The fifth or sixth cycle was used as a mobilizing therapy, while the up-front autoSCT was conditioned by carmustine, etoposide, cytarabine, and melphalan (or high-dose cyclophosphamide). The reported CR rate was 51%; the 5-year OS and PFS were 51% and 44% for the entire patient population, respectively [33].

These trials indicate that autoSCT consolidation is able to offer a chance of long-term survival in PTCL patients: nevertheless, it should be noted that a substantial proportion of patients (16–41%) had evidence of disease progression during induction or immediately before transplantation, thus precluding an effective consolidation in a relevant proportion of cases.

12.5.3 Management of Peculiar Disease Subtypes

If on the one hand the management of the most frequent nodal entities relies on a multiagent-based induction followed by autologous stem cell transplantation, if possible and indicated, some specific entities may be managed differently, based on their overall prognosis and on their tendency to disseminate. The management of some peculiar disease subtypes is briefly discussed.

Low-risk ALK+ ALCL (IPI 0/1). Given the overall better prognosis of this disease entity, stem cell transplant is not often considered as part of initial therapy in this category of patients [25]. In particular, those with low IPI score (and more in general those whose IPI score is lower than 3, according to some authors, [11]) may take advantage of an anthracycline-containing induction (either CHOP or CHOEP, as discussed above), without the need of consolidation with autoSCT. Of note, the most relevant trials of autoSCT in PTCL have excluded ALK+ ALCL patients; therefore no definitive conclusions may be drawn for this category of patients regarding the role of autoSCT.

ALK− breast implant-associated ALCL. Complete surgical excision, which consists of removal of the implant, total capsulectomy, and complete removal of any associated mass with negative margins upon pathological evaluation, is recommended in any patients presenting both with effusion and with tumor masses [34]. Systemic chemotherapy alone is regarded as an insufficient treatment strategy, unless applied after surgical resection: at least 30% of patients undergoing chemotherapy showed unsatisfactory responses or progressed in a recently published series of 87 patients with breast implant-associated ALCL, whereas only 4% of patients had recurrence or progression when treated by complete resection of the implant, tumor tissue, and fibrous capsule [34]. Better OS and PFS rates were described for patients undergoing complete surgical excision if compared to those who received chemotherapy, radiotherapy, or just a limited surgical approach (partial capsulectomy, implant removal or replacement, excisional biopsy of capsule or tumor mass). Multiagent chemotherapy is justified in patients with a tumor mass presentation at onset rather than with effusion only, as they are thought to display a more aggressive clinical behavior, as well as in those whose disease disseminates to nearby and distant nodes; however, any systemic approach should be necessarily preceded by a radical surgical resection [35].

EATL. Patients with EATL display one of the poorest prognoses among all patients with PTCL, with a 5-year OS and progression-free survival (PFS) of only 20% and 4%, respectively, even in case of favorable IPI score. An initial surgical approach is rather common in EATL patients, as many of them show acute abdominal symptoms (bowel perforation, hemorrhage, obstruction) requiring prompt intervention. An intensified induction with ifosfamide, vincristine, etoposide, and methotrexate (IVE/MTX), followed by autologous stem cell transplantation, has demonstrated better outcomes in terms of OS and PFS (60% and 52% at 5 years, respectively) if compared with historical controls receiving standard anthracycline-containing inductions [36]. Nevertheless, overall toxicity is not negligible, and most of patients are unable to tolerate this aggressive approach or fail to proceed to autoSCT consolidation because of poor performance status after surgery, rapid disease progression, or clinical decay.

SPTCL. Radiation therapy (20–30 Gy), possibly preceded by reductive surgery, should be recommended in patients with localized lesions. Multiple, noncontiguous lesions may be treated with pulse steroids (prednisone or equivalents), at the dose of 0.6–0.7 mg/kg/day × 10 days/month [37]. Systemic chemotherapy with gemcitabine or multiagent chemotherapy (CHOP, CHOP-like) is advisable in case of systemic dissemination or progressive disease [38].

ENKL, nasal type. Management strictly depends on stage at presentation and local versus distant disease spread. Patients with localized ENKL, which indicates a lymphoma that involves the nose and nasal sinuses, may benefit of external radiation therapy (at a dose of at least 50 Gy), which is sometimes the only required treatment. In a recently published cooperative study from Japan [39], concurrent systemic chemotherapy has also been administered in nearly three-quarters of patients, with the dexamethasone, etoposide, ifosfamide, and carboplatin (DeVIC) regimen being the most widely used. Patients with primary disease localization other than nose and nasal sinuses rarely show localized disease and require systemic multiagent approaches. ENKL has proved to be particularly sensitive to L-asparaginase, which has been incorporated in several induction schemes, like SMILE (dexamethasone, methotrexate, ifosfamide, L-asparaginase, etoposide), which produced higher response rates (79% of ORR, with 45% of CR) if compared to standard anthracycline-containing inductions [40]. Toxicity is however severe, and this regimen should be applied with a careful supportive treatment. An asparaginase-containing regimen, the GELOX (gemcitabine, L-asparaginase, oxaliplatin), has also been applied with concomitant radiotherapy in localized stage ENKL, yielding an ORR of 96%, with at least 74% of patients achieving a CR [41].

12.6 Relapsed and Refractory PTCL

The survival outcome of patients with PTCL who experience relapse or progression following first-line treatment is generally very poor. British Columbia Cancer Agency (BCCA) analyzed 153 patients with relapsed/refractory PTCL diagnosed between 1976 and 2010 and showed that the median PFS and OS after the first recurrence or disease progression were only 3.1 and 5.5 months, respectively, without stem cell transplant [42]. Among patients who relapsed, 91 patients (59%) received systemic chemotherapy, and patients who received chemotherapy after progression/relapse did not have significantly improved survival compared to whom did not with a median PFS and OS of only 3.7 and 6.5 months, respectively. Although the survival outcome was generally very poor, small amounts of patients survived relatively long period without transplant with 3-year OS of 18%. In patients who responded to first-line therapy, normal LDH, good performance status, and one or less extranodal involvement upon relapse were good prognostic factors [42]. There was no significant difference in PFS and OS after first recurrence or disease progression by PTCL subtypes.

The MD Anderson Cancer Center has also assessed the survival outcome of patients with PTCL-NOS and AITL diagnosed between 1999 and 2015 who experienced disease progression or relapse after first-line and subsequent therapy [43]. Within 321 patients who were newly diagnosed with PTCL-NOS (n = 180) or AITL (n = 141), 240 patients (135 PTCL-NOS, 105 AITL) experienced progression/relapse with a median follow-up duration of 52 months. The median PFS and OS after first progression/relapse for patients who did not proceed to stem cell transplantation were 4.0 months (95%CI, 3.1–4.7 months) and 9.2 months (95%CI, 6.9–11.8 months), respectively. With the subsequent relapses, PFS and OS became shorter and shorter, and PFS after second relapse were only 2.5 months and 2.9 months in PTCL-NOS and AITL, respectively. Although with approvals of new drugs for relapsed/refractory PTCL such as pralatrexate and romidepsin, there was no improvement in PFS and OS by the time of recurrence during this period (1999–2004, 2005–2009, and 2010–2015). Patients who underwent either autologous or allogeneic transplant had longer survival with 5-year OS rates after salvage autologous and allogeneic transplant of 32% and 52%, respectively; the 5-year OS rate for patients who did not undergo transplant was 10%.

The patients with ALCL who experienced disease progression or relapse after first-line were analyzed separately [44]. A total of 176 patients (74 ALK^+ ALCL, 102 ALK^- ALCL) diagnosed between 1999 and 2014 were retrospectively analyzed. With a median follow-up of 64 months, 111 patients (38 ALK^+ ALCL, 73 ALK^- ALCL) experienced progression/relapse after the first-line therapy. The median PFS following first progression/relapse in patients with ALK^+ ALCL and ALK^- ALCL were 5.2 and 3.0 months, respectively. The median OS following second-line therapy in patients with ALK^+ ALCL and ALK^- ALCL were 47.3 and 10.8 months, respectively. Interestingly, there were no significant differences in PFS following second-line treatment between ALK^+ ALCL and ALK^- ALCL. Patients who experienced recurrent or refractory disease had a poor outcome, with less than 20% long-term disease control rate; however, there seems to be an improvement by newer treatment strategies for relapsed/refractory disease.

12.7 Management of Relapsed and Refractory PTCL

12.7.1 Conventional Chemotherapy

Commonly used traditional salvage chemotherapy regimens for relapsed/refractory PTCL are platinum-containing regimens, such as ifosfamide, carboplatin, and etoposide (ICE); dexamethasone, high-dose Ara-C, and cisplatin (DHAP); and etoposide, methylprednisolone, high-dose Ara-C, and cisplatin (ESHAP), or gemcitabine-based regimens such as gemcitabine, dexamethasone, and cisplatin (GDP) and gemcitabine, dexamethasone, and oxaliplatin (GemOx). There is no big randomized trial comparing conventional salvage chemotherapy at this point, and all abovementioned regimens are considered reasonable options (https://www.nccn.org/professionals/physician_gls/pdf/t-cell.pdf).

The ORR with ICE ranges from 20 to 70% with 5-year PFS rate of 29% in PTCL from the largest study [45–47]. Hematologic toxicities are the main side effects with about 30% of patients who develop grade 3/4 thrombocytopenia. The ORR with DHAP and ESHAP were 55% and 64%, respectively, in patients with different histologies [48, 49]. DHAP in combination with alemtuzumab was evaluated in relapsed/refractory PTCL and showed remarkable response in PTCL-NOS, with an ORR of 86% and 43% CR, although with very small number of patients [50]. Modified ESHAP regimen, which includes carboplatin instead of cisplatin, showed an ORR of 32% with 18% of CR in patients with relapsed/refractory PTCL [51]. Hematologic toxicities and renal toxicities were the main side effects for both DHAP and ESHAP which were observed in 30–50% and about 20% of cases, respectively.

GDP in relapsed/refractory lymphoma was first evaluated in a phase I study with 22 patients including 5 patients with PTCL [52]. Among five PTCL patients, one achieved a CR and one achieved a PR. Recently, two studies evaluated GDP in patients with relapsed/refractory PTCL. In one study, 25 patients were evaluated for response, and the ORR was 72% with 48% of CR [53]. The median PFS was 9.3 months. GDP was generally well tolerated, with grade 3/4 neutropenia and thrombocytopenia observed in 16% and 13% of cycles, respectively. The other study included 25 patients with relapsed/refractory PTCL-NOS, and the ORR was 64% with 20% of CR [54]. The median PFS was 5.4 months, but patients who responded to GDP had median duration of response of 10.3 months. GemOx was evaluated in 24 elderly (age $\geq$ 60) patients with relapsed/refractory PTCL [55]. The ORR was 38% with 8% of CR after three cycles of GemOx. The median PFS was 10 months. Grade 3/4 neutropenia and thrombocytopenia were observed in 51% and 33% of all delivered courses, respectively.

As described, survival outcome of patients with relapsed/refractory PTCL is usually dismal if stem cell transplant is not an option. Thus, these combination salvage chemotherapies are commonly offered for patients who are to undergo stem cell transplant after such salvage therapy considering higher toxicities. For those who are not transplant candidates, single-agent chemotherapy such as gemcitabine or other novel therapeutic options can be good options.

Phase II studies have evaluated single-agent gemcitabine in T-cell lymphoma, including mycosis fungoides [56–58]. Gemcitabine, given at the dose of 1200 mg/m^2, was administered on days 1, 8, and 15 of a 28-day schedule for 3–6 cycles. In the largest trial evaluating 20 patients with relapsed/refractory PTCL-NOS, ORR was 55% with 30% of CR [58]. Treatment was fairly well tolerated with no grade 3/4 hematologic toxicities observed.

12.7.2 New Approaches

Since 2009, the US Food and Drug Administration (FDA) approved four drugs with novel mechanisms of action for the treatment of patients with recurrent PTCL, including pralatrexate in 2009, brentuximab vedotin (BV) for anaplastic large cell lymphoma in 2011, romidepsin in 2011, and belinostat in 2014.

Pralatrexate, the first drug approved for patients with relapsed/refractory PTCL, is an inhibitor of dihydrofolate reductase, showing more than tenfold higher cytotoxic effect than methotrexate. A pivotal phase II study (PROPEL trial) enrolled 115 patients with relapsed/refractory PTCL. Pralatrexate was given intravenously at 30 mg/m^2/week for 6 weeks followed by 1 week rest (7-week cycles). The ORR was 29% with CR rate of 11%, and 63% of response were observed during first cycle [59]. Of note, 25% of patients who were refractory to prior treatment responded to pralatrexate. When response rates were analyzed based on histology, the ORR of patients with PTCL-NOS ($n = 59$), AITL ($n = 13$), and ALCL ($n = 17$) were 31%, 8%, and 29%, respectively, showing a very low response rate to AITL. The median PFS was 3.5 months in all patients and 10.1 months in responding patients. Severe mucositis (grade 3/4 in 22%) often led to dose delays or interruption. Grade 3/4 thrombocytopenia was observed in 33% of patients.

Histone deacetylase (HDAC) inhibitors are epigenetic modulating agents that keep histones acetylated, leading to differentiation and/or apoptosis in transformed cells. Studies have shown that epigenetic regulation plays an important role in the pathogenesis of PTCL [60], and epigenetic therapies using HDAC inhibitors have shown activity in PTCL. There are two FDA-approved HDAC inhibitors for relapsed/refractory PTCL which are romidepsin and belinostat.

Romidepsin was approved for the treatment of cutaneous T-cell lymphoma in 2009 and for the treatment of relapsed/refractory PTCL in 2011, supported by two phase II trials. The first trial enrolled 47 patients with relapsed/refractory PTCL, and romidepsin was administered intravenously on days 1, 8, and 15 of a 28-day cycle with a starting dose of 14 mg/m^2 [61]. Median number of cycles given was 3 (range, 1–57). The ORR was 38% with CR rate of 18%. Responses were seen even after prior stem cell transplant, and the median duration of response was 8.9 month. Next larger phase II study ($n = 130$) in relapsed/refractory PTCL showed ORR of 25% with CR rate of 15% [62]. Even in patients who were refractory to prior treatment, CR was seen in 18% of patients. There was no significant difference in response by histologic subtypes. The median PFS was 4 months; however, it should be noted that responses were frequently durable and the median duration of response was 28 months [63]. Hematologic toxicities were the most common adverse events, with grade 3/4 thrombocytopenia and neutropenia observed in 24 and 20%, respectively. Several clinical trials are ongoing to evaluate romidepsin combination regimens with chemotherapy or new drugs. A phase I study of romidepsin in combination with ICE was started at the MD Anderson Cancer Center, and preliminary results were reported [64]. Within the 14 patients available for the response evaluation at the time of analysis, the ORR was 78% with a CR rate of 64%. However, this treatment was also associated with higher rate of hematologic toxicities, and grade 3/4 thrombocytopenia, grade 3/4 neutropenia, and grade 3 anemia occurred in 95%, 84%, and 73% of the cycles, respectively.

Belinostat was the second FDA-approved HDAC inhibitor for treatment of relapsed/refractory PTCL, based on the result of a phase II study (BELIEF trial) [65]. Belinostat 1000 mg/m^2 was administered intravenously on days 1–5 every 21 days. The study enrolled patients with PTCL after a failure of one or more prior systemic therapies. Among the 129 patients enrolled, the ORR was 26% with a CR rate of 10%. The median PFS was only 1.6 months; however the median duration of response was 13.6 months, and the median duration of response was not reached in patients who achieved a CR. Compared to romidepsin, belinostat had less hematologic toxicities, with grade 3/4 thrombocytopenia and neutropenia observed in 7% and 6% of cases, respectively.

BV is an intravenously administered antibody-drug conjugate that consists of the CD30-specific monoclonal antibody conjugated with monomethyl auristatin E by a linker peptide. Binding of the antibody-drug conjugate to CD30 on the cell surface causes internalization of the drug by endocytosis. The drug subsequently travels to the lysosome, causing cell cycle arrest and apoptotic death. BV was studied for the treatment of relapsed/refractory systemic ALCL. In a pivotal phase II study in patients with relapsed/refractory systemic ALCL, BV 1.8 mg/kg was administered intravenously every 3 weeks [66]. The ORR was 86% with a CR rate of 57%, and median time to response was 5.9 weeks. Grade $\geq$ 3 adverse events included neutropenia (21%), thrombocytopenia (14%), peripheral sensory neuropathy (12%), and anemia (7%). Long-term follow-up data were presented in December 2016 and showed durable remission in majority of patients [67]. With a median follow-up of 71.4 months, the 5-year OS and PFS for all the enrolled patients were 60% and 39%, respectively. Median duration of response in patients who achieved a CR was not reached, and 16 patients (8 of them received consolidation transplant) remained in remission without starting any new therapy. In a retrospective study from the MD Anderson Cancer Center [44], patients who received BV at some point during treatment after first-line therapy had significantly longer OS than those who did not (median OS after first progression or relapse: 49.9 vs. 9.6 months). In patients with ALCL who had previously responded to BV and experienced a recurrence after discontinuation of this therapy, retreatment with BV was very frequently effective [68]. In the reported study, response was observed in seven of eight patients (88%) with a CR in five patients (63%) by retreatment. Median duration of response was 12.3 months (range, 6.6–28.0+ months). BV has also been evaluated as a bridging agent to allogeneic transplantation in 24 patients with CD30$^+$ lymphoma refractory to at least two lines of chemotherapy or to autoSCT [69]. In this study, among the five enrolled patients with ALCL, three achieved a CR after four doses of BV and two of them had undergone allogeneic stem cell transplantation (alloSCT). BV is a very effective treatment for relapsed/refractory ALCL; however, once disease progresses on BV, the reported median OS after BV failure was only 3 months with a 2-year OS of 30% [70], indicating a high unmet need for new treatment strategies for patients with BV refractory ALCL disease.

Based on this high efficacy, BV was evaluated in first-line treatment in patients with CD30-positive PTCL [71]. The phase I study of BV (sequential or in combination) in combination of CHOP or CHP (CHOP without vincristine) showed very promising results with manageable toxicities. Of note, the ORR was 100% with CR rate of 84% in 19 patients with ALCL who received BV plus CHP as combination therapy. Long-term follow-up data with a median follow-up of 52 months showed high durable remission, with 4-year PFS and OS rates of 52% and 80%, respectively [72]. Given these very promising results, a phase III study comparing BV plus CHP vs. CHOP for first-line treatment in patients with CD30-positive PTCL (ECHELON-2) is ongoing and has completed enrolment, awaiting for final results (NCT 01777152, [73]).

BV was also investigated in a rather small number of patients with other PTCL expressing CD30 [74]. In PTCL-NOS, the ORR was 33% with a CR rate of 14%, and median PFS was 7.6 months. The ORR in AITL patients was 54% with a CR rate of 38%, and median PFS was 5.5 months. Interestingly, there was no correlation between immunohistochemical CD30 expression and clinical response.

Several other agents are also evaluated in patients with relapsed refractory PTCL. Bendamustine is nitrogen mustard, consisting of chloroethylamine, an alkylating group, attached to a benzimidazole ring, a purine analog. In a phase II study (BENTLY trial) of 60 patients with relapsed PTCL or cutaneous T-cell lymphoma, bendamustine at the dose of 120 mg/m^2 was administered on days 1 through 2 every 3 weeks for six cycles. Although 33% of patients could not receive more than 3 cycles mainly due to disease progression, the ORR was 50% with a CR rate of 28% [75]. Median PFS was 3.6 months. The median duration of response was 3.5 months, with 30% of responses lasting greater than 6 months. Grade 3/4 neutropenia and thrombocytopenia were seen in 30% and 24% of patients, respectively.

Lenalidomide is an immunomodulatory drug and showed activity to relapsed/refractory PTCL [76–78]. Lenalidomide, at the dose of 25 mg, was given on days 1–21 of each 28-days cycle. A phase II study evaluating lenalidomide monotherapy to PTCL enrolled 29 patients with relapsed/refractory disease: the ORR was 29% with median duration of response of 5 months [77]. Another phase II study focusing on patients with PTCL-NOS showed an ORR of 30% [78]. In a multicenter phase II trial with 54 patients conducted in France, the ORR was 22% with CR rate of 11% [76]. Nonsignificant slightly higher response was seen in patients with AITL with the ORR of 31%. The median PFS and the median duration of response were 2.5 and 3.6 months, respectively. The most common side effects were hematologic toxicities, with grade 3/4 thrombocytopenia and neutropenia observed in 20% and 15% of patients, respectively.

Mogamulizumab is a defucosylated anti-CC chemokine receptor 4 (CCR4) antibody which was initially developed for the treatment of adult T-cell leukemia/lymphoma (ATLL). In a phase II study of 28 patients with relapsed $CCR4^+$ ATLL, single-agent mogamulizumab showed an ORR of 50% with a CR rate of 31%. Median PFS was 5.2 months [79]. Since CCR4 is also expressed in various proportions of PTCL, mogamulizumab was evaluated in patient with $CCR4^+$ relapsed PTCL or cutaneous T-cell lymphoma: among the 38 patient treated, the ORR was 35% with a CR rate of 14%. Median PFS in responders was 5.5 months [80].

Alisertib is an Aurora A kinase inhibitor, which functions as a serine/threonine kinase regulating G2-M transition and centrosome separation during mitosis. Alisertib showed promising response in PTCL in a phase II study including aggressive lymphoma. In this trial, patients received alisertib 50 mg twice daily for 7 days every 21 days. Within 48 patients with relapsed/refractory non-Hodgkin lymphoma treated with alisertib in this trial, 8 had PTCL, and the ORR was 50% [81]. The treatment was associated with substantial hematologic toxicities with grade 3/4 neutropenia and thrombocytopenia seen in 63% and 33% of patients, respectively. In another phase II trial focused on PTCL and mycosis fungoides which enrolled 37 patients, alisertib showed an ORR of 33% in PTCL [82]. Based on these promising results, a phase III multicentre trial (LUMIERE trial) was conducted comparing alisertib to investigator's choice single-agent drug (pralatrexate, gemcitabine, or romidepsin) in relapsed/refractory PTCL. Overall, 238 pts were randomized across 27 countries (120 received alisertib, 118 comparator). ORR with alisertib versus comparator was 33% versus 43%, including 16% versus 25% CR, with no significant differences between the two arms. With a median follow-up of around 9 months, median PFS was 3.7 months and 3.4 months in alisertib and comparator, respectively, and again without significant difference [83]. Based on these results, the trial was discontinued, however, still waiting for final results.

12.7.3 New Combinations

The response rate in relapsed/refractory setting is not satisfactory except for BV for ALCL, and thus currently many clinical trials are evaluating novel combinations to improve outcomes. Romidepsin in combination with alisertib was evaluated in phase I trial, and one in three patients with PTCL enrolled in the study achieved a CR (NCT01897012) [84]. Romidepsin in combination with pralatrexate showed remarkable response rates in relapsed/refractory PTCL in phase I study (NCT01947140) [85]. The ORR was 77% (10/13 patients) with a CR rate of 31%, and the median duration of response was 6.6 months. Romidepsin with lenalidomide was also evaluated in phase I/II trial, and it showed 50% response (5/10 patients) in PTCL (NCT01755975) [86]. These are early phase studies with premature data and further investigations are warranted.

12.8 Hematopoietic Stem Cell Transplant for Relapsed and Refractory Disease

The benefit of autoSCT in patients with relapsed/refractory disease was initially reported rather disappointing, with 5-year PFS after autoSCT being 10–30% [87–90]: therefore, it has been relatively discouraged to consider autoSCT in relapsed/refractory patients. However, more recent data suggest that there is no significant difference in survival outcome (at least in short term) by autoSCT and alloSCT [43]. In a retrospective analysis from the MD Anderson Cancer Center, 76 patients with PTCL underwent autoSCT ($n = 41$) or alloSCT ($n = 35$) in relapsed/refractory disease [87]. The 4-year OS rates were 50% and 36% for autoSCT and alloSCT patients with chemosensitive disease, respectively, and there was no statistical difference. Response prior to SCT is a significant factor to predict survival outcome [87, 91], and thus patients who achieve a CR to salvage chemotherapy would be good candidate for autoSCT consolidation, particularly if there is no option for alloSCT. While the most commonly used high-dose regimen is the combination of carmustine, etoposide, cytarabine, and melphalan (BEAM), alternative conditioning regimens may improve outcomes. Currently, a phase II trial to evaluate romidepsin maintenance therapy after autoSCT is ongoing (NCT01908777).

AlloSCT has shown significant graft-versus-lymphoma effect including response to donor lymphocyte infusion, and thus it may provide effective disease control in relapsed/refractory PTCL [92–97]. The French group has reported the outcome of 77 patients who received alloSCT: the 5-year transplant-related mortality (TRM) was 33%, and the 5-year OS and PFS were 57% and 53%, respectively [96]. In this study, the majority of patients received myeloablative conditioning regimen, and relatively high TRM was a concern. Recently, reduced-intensity conditioning regimen (RIC) is becoming a more standard approach. A phase II study of RIC with alloSCT in 17 patients with relapsed/refractory PTCL showed 3-year OS and PFS rates of 81% and 64%, respectively, with low TRM (6% in 2 years) [92]. The Fred Hutchinson Cancer Center has reported on 17 patients with relapsed/refractory PTCL who underwent RIC alloSCT [97]. The 3-year OS and PFS were 59% and 53%, respectively, with a 3-year TRM of 19%. In a Japanese study, 354 patients (PTCL-NOS, $n = 200$; AITL, $n = 77$; ALCL, $n = 77$) who received alloSCT were retrospectively analyzed [98]. The 3-year TRM rates and the 3-year OS rates in younger patients (16–49 years of age) who received myeloablative regimen were 22% and 43%, and those who received reduced-intensity conditioning regimen (RIC) were 14% and 56%, respectively, suggesting that RIC is a good option even for younger patients.

12.9 Conclusion

PTCL are a group of biologically and clinically heterogeneous disease, and their classification is still evolving. First-line anthracycline-containing regimens, mainly CHOP or CHOEP, are at present the accepted and most widely applied standard of care, although the best first-line approach is yet to be defined. AutoSCT is regarded as part of the first-line approach, to be performed after induction in transplant-eligible patients. Nevertheless, only a minority of patients could receive transplantation at the right time, mainly because of disease progression during treatment or refractoriness to induction.

Several new drugs are active in relapsed and refractory patients: these drugs are able to induce high OR rates and CR rates, although response durations are limited over time, thus without a significant impact on survival rates. Whether these drugs can be safely and efficiently combined with CHOP or CHOEP in newer first-line regimens to improve the efficacy of standard induction regimens is under investigation.

Allogeneic transplantation in patients achieving a remission after salvage treatment may at present offer the possibility of long-term disease control or even a cure, due to a well-acknowledged graft-versus-lymphoma effect.

References

1. Adams SV, Newcomb PA, Shustov AR. Racial patterns of peripheral T-cell lymphoma incidence and survival in the United States. J Clin Oncol. 2016;34:963–71.
2. Chihara D, Ito H, Matsuda T, Shibata A, Katsumi A, Nakamura S, et al. Differences in incidence and trends of haematological malignancies in Japan and the United States. Br J Haematol. 2014a;164:536–45.
3. Ellin F, Landström J, Jerkeman M, Relander T. Real-world data on prognostic factors and treatment in peripheral T-cell lymphomas: a study from the Swedish Lymphoma Registry. Blood. 2014;124:1570–7.
4. Swerdlow SH, Campo E, Pileri SA, Harris NL, Stein H, Siebert R, et al. The 2016 revision of the World Health Organization classification of lymphoid neoplasms. Blood. 2016;127:2375–90.
5. Vose J, Armitage J, Weisenburger D. International T-Cell Lymphoma Project. International peripheral T-cell and natural killer/T-cell lymphoma study: pathology findings and clinical outcomes. J Clin Oncol. 2008;26:4124–30.
6. Iqbal J, Wright G, Wang C, Rosenwald A, Gascoyne RD, Weisenburger DD, et al. Gene expression signatures delineate biological and prognostic subgroups in peripheral T-cell lymphoma. Blood. 2014;123:2915–23.
7. Broccoli A, Zinzani PL. Peripheral T-cell lymphoma, not otherwise specified. Blood. 2017a;129:1103–12.
8. Thompson PA, Lade S, Webster H, Ryan G, Prince HM. Effusion-associated anaplastic large cell lymphoma of the breast: time for it to be defined as a distinct clinico-pathological entity. Haematologica. 2010;95:1977–9.
9. Ansell S. How to select the frontline treatment for a patient with peripheral T-cell lymphoma. Leuk Lymphoma. 2016;57:783–8.
10. Broccoli A, Zinzani PL. Angioimmunoblastic T-cell lymphoma. Hematol Oncol Clin North Am. 2017b;31:223–38.
11. Corradini P, Marchetti M, Barosi G, Billio A, Gallamini A, Pileri S, et al. SIE-SIES-GITMO guidelines for the management of adult peripheral T- and NK-cell lymphomas, excluding mature T-cell leukaemias. Ann Oncol. 2014;25:2339–50.
12. d'Amore F, Gaulard P, Trümper L, Corradini P, Kim WS, Specht L, et al. Peripheral T-cell lymphomas: ESMO clinical practice guidelines for diagnosis, treatment and follow-up. Ann Oncol. 2015;26(Suppl. 5):v108–15.
13. Casulo C, Schöder H, Feeney J, Lim R, Maragulia J, Zelenetz AD, et al. ^{18}F-fluorodeoxyglucose positron emission tomography in the staging and prognosis of T cell lymphoma. Leuk Lymphoma. 2013;54:2163–7.
14. Tomita N, Hattori Y, Fujisawa S, Hashimoto C, Taguchi J, Takasaki H, et al. Post-therapy ^{18}F-fluorodeoxyglucose positron emission tomography for predicting outcome in patients with peripheral T cell lymphoma. Ann Hematol. 2015;94:431–6.
15. Gallamini A, Stelitano C, Calvi R, Bellei M, Mattei D, Vitolo U, et al. Peripheral T-cell lymphoma unspecified (PTCL-U): a new prognostic model from a retrospective multicentric clinical study. Blood. 2004;103:2474–9.
16. Went P, Agostinelli C, Gallamini A, Piccaluga PP, Ascani S, Sabattini E, et al. Marker expression in peripheral T-cell lymphoma: a proposed clinical-pathologic prognostic score. J Clin Oncol. 2006;24:2472–9.
17. Vose JM. International peripheral T-cell lymphoma (PTCL) clinical and pathologic review project: poor outcome by prognostic indices and lack of efficacy with anthracyclines. Blood. 2005;106:811.
18. Federico M, Rudiger T, Bellei M, Nathwani BN, Luminari S, Coiffier B, et al. Clinicopathologic characteristics of angioimmunoblastic T-cell lymphoma: analysis of the International Peripheral T-cell lymphoma project. J Clin Oncol. 2012;31:240–6.
19. Weisenburger DD, Savage KJ, Harris NL, Gascoyne RD, Jaffe ES, MacLennan KA, et al. Peripheral T-cell lymphoma, not otherwise specified: a report of 340 cases from the International Peripheral T-cell Lymphoma Project. Blood. 2011;117:3402–8.
20. Savage KJ, Harris NL, Vose JM, Ullrich F, Jaffe ES, Connors JM, et al. ALK- anaplastic large-cell lymphoma is clinically and immunophenotypically different from both ALK+ ALCL and peripheral T-cell lymphoma, not otherwise specified: report from the

International Peripheral T-Cell Lymphoma Project. Blood. 2008;111:5496–504.
21. Au WY, Weisenburger DD, Intraqumtornchai T, Nakamura S, Kim WS, Sng I, et al. Clinical differences between nasal and extranasal natural killer/T-cell lymphoma: a study of 136 cases from the International Peripheral T-Cell Lymphoma Project. Blood. 2009;113:3931–7.
22. Delabie J, Holte H, Vose JM, Ullrich F, Jaffe ES, Savage KJ, et al. Enteropathy-associated T-cell lymphoma: clinical and histological findings from the international peripheral T-cell lymphoma project. Blood. 2011;118:148–55.
23. Abramson JS, Feldman T, Kroll-Desrosiers AR, Muffly LS, Winer E, Flowers CR, et al. Peripheral T-cell lymphomas in a large US multicentre cohort: prognostication in the modern era including impact of frontline therapy. Ann Oncol. 2014;25:2211–7.
24. Savage KJ, Chhanabhai M, Gascoyne RD, Connors JM. Characterization of peripheral T-cell lymphomas in a single North American institution by the WHO classification. Ann Oncol. 2004;15:1467–75.
25. Chihara D, Fanale MA. Management of anaplastic large cell lymphoma. Hematol Oncol Clin North Am. 2017;31:209–22.
26. Briski R, Feldman AL, Bailey NG, Lim MS, Ristow K, Habermann TM, et al. The role of front-line anthracycline-containing chemotherapy regimens in peripheral T-cell lymphomas. Blood Cancer J. 2014;4:e214.
27. Simon A, Peoch M, Casassus P, Deconinck E, Colombat P, Desablens B, et al. Upfront VIP-reinforced-ABVD (VIP-rABVD) is not superior to CHOP/21 in newly diagnosed peripheral T cell lymphoma. Results of the randomized phase III trial GOELAMS-LTP95. Br J Haematol. 2010;151:159–66.
28. Schmitz N, Trümper L, Ziepert M, Nickelsen M, Ho AD, Metzner B, et al. Treatment and prognosis of mature T-cell and NK-cell lymphoma: an analysis of patients with T-cell lymphoma treated in studies of the German High-Grade Non-Hodgkin Lymphoma Study Group. Blood. 2010;116:3418–25.
29. Corradini P, Tarella C, Zallio F, Dodero A, Zanni M, Valagussa P, et al. Long-term follow-up of patients with peripheral T-cell lymphomas treated up-front with high-dose chemotherapy followed by autologous stem cell transplantation. Leukemia. 2006;20:1533–8.
30. Mercadal S, Briones J, Xicoy B, et al. Intensive chemotherapy (high-dose CHOP/ESHAP regimen) followed by autologous stem-cell transplantation in previously untreated patients with peripheral T-cell lymphoma. Ann Oncol. 2008;19(5):958–63.
31. Reimer P, Rüdiger T, Geissinger E, Weissinger F, Nerl C, Schmitz N, et al. Autologous stem-cell transplantation as first-line therapy in peripheral T-cell lymphomas: results of a prospective multicentre study. J Clin Oncol. 2009;27:106–13.
32. Wilhelm M, Smetak M, Reimer P, Geissinger E, Ruediger T, Metzner B, et al. First-line therapy of peripheral T-cell lymphoma: extension and long-term follow-up of a study investigating the role of autologous stem cell transplantation. Blood Cancer J. 2016;6:e452.
33. d'Amore F, Relander T, Lauritzsen GF, Jantunen E, Hagberg H, Anderson H, et al. Up-front autologous stem-cell transplantation in peripheral T-cell lymphoma: NLG-T-01. J Clin Oncol. 2012;30:3093–9.
34. Clemens MW, Medeiros J, Butler CE, Hunt KK, Fanale MA, Horwitz S, et al. Complete surgical excision is essential for the management of patients with breast implant-associated anaplastic large-cell lymphoma. J Clin Oncol. 2016;34:160–8.
35. Miranda RN, Aladily TN, Prince HM, Kanagal-Shamanna R, de Jong D, Fayad LE, et al. Breast implant-associated anaplastic large-cell lymphoma: long-term follow-up of 60 patients. J Clin Oncol. 2014;32:114–20.
36. Sieniawski M, Angamuthu N, Boyd K, Chasty R, Davies J, Forsyth P, et al. Evaluation of enteropathy-associated T-cell lymphoma comparing standard therapies with a novel regimen including autologous stem cell transplantation. Blood. 2010;115:3664–70.
37. Jang MS, Baek JW, Kang DY, Kang JS, Suh KS, Kim ST. Subcutaneous panniculitis-like T-cell lymphoma: successful treatment with systemic steroid alone. J Dermatol. 2012;39:96–9.
38. Willemze R, Jansen PM, Cerroni L, Berti E, Santucci M, Assaf C, et al. Subcutaneous panniculitis-like T-cell lymphoma: definition, classification, and prognostic factors: an EORTC Cutaneous Lymphoma Group Study of 83 cases. Blood. 2008;111:838–45.
39. Yamaguchi M, Suzuki R, Oguchi M, Asano M, Amaki J, Akiba T, et al. Treatments and outcomes of patients with extranodal natural killer/T-cell lymphoma diagnosed between 2000 and 2013: a cooperative study in Japan. J Clin Oncol. 2017;35:32–9.
40. Yamaguchi M, Kwong YL, Kim WS, Maeda Y, Hashimoto C, Suh C, et al. Phase II study of SMILE chemotherapy for newly diagnosed stage IV, relapsed, or refractory extranodal natural killer (NK)/T-cell lymphoma, nasal type: the NK-cell tumor study group study. J Clin Oncol. 2011;29:4410–6.
41. Wang L, Wang Z, Chen X, Li YJ, Wang KF, Xia YF, et al. First-line combination of gemcitabine, oxaliplatin, and L-asparaginase (GELOX) followed by involved-field radiation therapy for patients with stage IE/IIE extranodal natural killer/T-cell lymphoma. Cancer. 2013;119:348–55.
42. Mak V, Hamm J, Chhanabhai M, Shenkier T, Klasa R, Sehn LH, et al. Survival of patients with peripheral T-cell lymphoma after first relapse or progression: spectrum of disease and rare long-term survivors. J Clin Oncol. 2013;31:1970–6.
43. Chihara D, Fanale MA, Miranda RN, Noorani M, Westin JR, Nastoupil LJ, et al. The survival outcome of patients with relapsed/refractory peripheral T-cell lymphoma-not otherwise specified and angioimmunoblastic T-cell lymphoma. Br J Haematol. 2017;176:750–8.

44. Chihara D, Fanale M, Noorani M, Westin JR, Nastoupil L, Hagemeister F, et al. The survival outcome of the patients with relapsed/refractory anaplastic large-cell lymphoma. Blood. 2015;126:2738.
45. Mikesch JH, Kuhlmann M, Demant A, Krug U, Thoennissen GB, Schmidt E, et al. DexaBEAM versus ICE salvage regimen prior to autologous transplantation for relapsed or refractory aggressive peripheral T cell lymphoma: a retrospective evaluation of parallel patient cohorts of one center. Ann Hematol. 2013;92:1041–8.
46. Moskowitz CH, Bertino JR, Glassman JR, Hedrick EE, Hunte S, Coady-Lyons N, et al. Ifosfamide, carboplatin, and etoposide: a highly effective cytoreduction and peripheral-blood progenitor-cell mobilization regimen for transplant-eligible patients with non-Hodgkin's lymphoma. J Clin Oncol. 1999;17:3776–85.
47. Zelenetz AD, Hamlin P, Kewalramani T, Yahalom J, Nimer S, Moskowitz CH. Ifosfamide, carboplatin, etoposide (ICE)-based second-line chemotherapy for the management of relapsed and refractory aggressive non-Hodgkin's lymphoma. Ann Oncol. 2003;14(Suppl. 1):i5–i10.
48. Velasquez WS, Cabanillas F, Salvador P, McLaughlin P, Fridrik M, Tucker S, et al. Effective salvage therapy for lymphoma with cisplatin in combination with high-dose Ara-C and dexamethasone (DHAP). Blood. 1988;71:117–22.
49. Velasquez WS, McLaughlin P, Tucker S, Hagemeister FB, Swan F, Rodriguez MA, et al. ESHAP—an effective chemotherapy regimen in refractory and relapsing lymphoma: a 4-year follow-up study. J Clin Oncol. 1994;12:1169–76.
50. Kim SJ, Kim K, Kim BS, Suh C, Huh J, Ko YH, et al. Alemtuzumab and DHAP (A-DHAP) is effective for relapsed peripheral T-cell lymphoma, unspecified: interim results of a phase II prospective study. Ann Oncol. 2009;20:390–2.
51. Kogure Y, Yoshimi A, Ueda K, Nannya Y, Ichikawa M, Nakamura F, et al. Modified ESHAP regimen for relapsed/refractory T cell lymphoma: a retrospective analysis. Ann Hematol. 2015;94:989–94.
52. Emmanouilides C, Colovos C, Pinter-Brown L, Hernandez L, Schiller G, Territo M, et al. Pilot study of fixed-infusion rate gemcitabine with cisplatin and dexamethasone in patients with relapsed or refractory lymphoma. Clin Lymphoma. 2004;5:45–9.
53. Park BB, Kim WS, Suh C, Shin DY, Kim JA, Kim HG, et al. Salvage chemotherapy of gemcitabine, dexamethasone, and cisplatin (GDP) for patients with relapsed or refractory peripheral T-cell lymphomas: a consortium for improving survival of lymphoma (CISL) trial. Ann Hematol. 2015;94:1845–51.
54. Qi F, Dong M, He X, Li Y, Wang W, Liu P, et al. Gemcitabine, dexamethasone, and cisplatin (GDP) as salvage chemotherapy for patients with relapsed or refractory peripheral T cell lymphoma-not otherwise specified. Ann Hematol. 2017;96:245–51.
55. Yao YY, Tang Y, Zhu Q, Zhuang Y, Cheng YM, Wang L, et al. Gemcitabine, oxaliplatin and dexamethasone as salvage treatment for elderly patients with refractory and relapsed peripheral T-cell lymphoma. Leuk Lymphoma. 2013;54:1194–200.
56. Sallah S, Wan JY, Nguyen NP. Treatment of refractory T-cell malignancies using gemcitabine. Br J Haematol. 2001;113:185–7.
57. Zinzani PL, Magagnoli M, Bendandi M, Orcioni GF, Gherlinzoni F, Albertini P, et al. Therapy with gemcitabine in pretreated peripheral T-cell lymphoma patients. Ann Oncol. 1998;9:1351–3.
58. Zinzani PL, Venturini F, Stefoni V, Fina M, Pellegrini C, Derenzini E, et al. Gemcitabine as single agent in pretreated T-cell lymphoma patients: evaluation of the long-term outcome. Ann Oncol. 2010;21:860–3.
59. O'Connor OA, Pro B, Pinter-Brown L, Bartlett N, Popplewell L, Coiffier B, et al. Pralatrexate in patients with relapsed or refractory peripheral T-cell lymphoma: results from the pivotal PROPEL study. J Clin Oncol. 2011;29:1182–9.
60. Piekarz RL, Robey RW, Zhan Z, Kayastha G, Sayah A, Abdeldaim AH, et al. T-cell lymphoma as a model for the use of histone deacetylase inhibitors in cancer therapy: impact of depsipeptide on molecular markers, therapeutic targets, and mechanisms of resistance. Blood. 2004;103:4636–43.
61. Piekarz RL, Frye R, Prince HM, Kirschbaum MH, Zain J, Allen SL, et al. Phase 2 trial of romidepsin in patients with peripheral T-cell lymphoma. Blood. 2011;117:5827–34.
62. Coiffier B, Pro B, Prince HM, Foss F, Sokol L, Greenwood M, et al. Results from a pivotal, open-label, phase II study of romidepsin in relapsed or refractory peripheral T-cell lymphoma after prior systemic therapy. J Clin Oncol. 2012;30:631–6.
63. Coiffier B, Pro B, Prince HM, Foss F, Sokol L, Greenwood M, et al. Romidepsin for the treatment of relapsed/refractory peripheral T-cell lymphoma: pivotal study update demonstrates durable responses. J Hematol Oncol. 2014;7:11.
64. Chihara D, Oki Y, Fayad L, Wesson E, Ruben C, Horowitz SB, et al. Phase I study of romidepsin in combination with ICE (ifosfamide, carboplatin and etoposide) in patients with relapsed or refractory peripheral T-cell lymphoma. Blood. 2014b; 124:1748.
65. O'Connor OA, Horwitz S, Masszi T, Van Hoof A, Brown P, Doorduijn J, et al. Belinostat in Patients With Relapsed or Refractory Peripheral T-Cell Lymphoma: results of the Pivotal Phase II BELIEF (CLN-19) Study. J Clin Oncol. 2015a;33:2492–9.
66. Pro B, Advani R, Brice P, Bartlett NL, Rosenblatt JD, Illidge T, et al. Brentuximab vedotin (SGN-35) in patients with relapsed or refractory systemic anaplastic large-cell lymphoma: results of a phase II study. J Clin Oncol. 2012;30:2190–6.
67. Pro B, Advani RH, Brice P, Bartlett NL, Rosenblatt JD, Illidge T, et al. Five-year survival data from a pivotal phase 2 study of brentuximab vedotin in patients

with relapsed or refractory systemic anaplastic large cell lymphoma. Blood. 2016;128:4144.
68. Bartlett NL, Chen R, Fanale MA, Brice P, Gopal A, Smith SE, et al. Retreatment with brentuximab vedotin in patients with CD30-positive hematologic malignancies. J Hematol Oncol. 2014;7:24.
69. Gibb A, Jones C, Bloor A, Kulkarni S, Illidge T, Linton K, et al. Brentuximab vedotin in refractory CD30+ lymphomas: a bridge to allogeneic transplantation in approximately one quarter of patients treated on a Named Patient Programme at a single UK center. Haematologica. 2013;98:611–4.
70. Oki Y, Feldman T, Chihara D, Fanale MA, Connors JM, Wong S, et al. Prognostic factors in patients with relapsed or refractory systemic anaplastic large T-cell lymphoma (ALCL) receiving brentuximab vedotin and outcome after treatment failure. Hematol Oncol. 2017;35(Suppl S2):252.
71. Fanale MA, Horwitz SM, Forero-Torres A, Bartlett NL, Advani RH, Pro B, et al. Brentuximab vedotin in the front-line treatment of patients with CD30+ peripheral T-cell lymphomas: results of a phase I study. J Clin Oncol. 2014;32:3137–43.
72. Fanale MA, Horwitz SM, Forero-Torres A, Bartlett NL, Advani RH, Pro B, et al. Four-year survival and durability results of brentuximab vedotin in combination with CHP in the frontline treatment of patients with CD30-expressing peripheral T-cell lymphomas. Blood. 2016;128:2993.
73. O'Connor OA, Pro B, Illidge T, Trumper LH, Larsen EK, Kennedy DA. Phase 3 trial of brentuximab vedotin and CHP versus CHOP in the frontline treatment of patients (pts) with CD30+ mature T-cell lymphomas (MTCL). J Clin Oncol. 2014;32(Suppl 15):TPS8612.
74. Horwitz SM, Advani RH, Bartlett NL, Jacobsen ED, Sharman JP, O'Connor OA, et al. Objective responses in relapsed T-cell lymphomas with single agent brentuximab vedotin. Blood. 2014;123:3095–100.
75. Damaj G, Gressin R, Bouabdallah K, Cartron G, Choufi B, Gyan E, et al. Results from a prospective, open-label, phase II trial of bendamustine in refractory or relapsed T-cell lymphomas: the BENTLEY trial. J Clin Oncol. 2013;31:104–10.
76. Morschhauser F, Fitoussi O, Haioun C, Thieblemont C, Quach H, Delarue R, et al. A phase 2, multicentre, single-arm, open-label study to evaluate the safety and efficacy of single-agent lenalidomide (Revlimid) in subjects with relapsed or refractory peripheral T-cell non-Hodgkin lymphoma: the EXPECT trial. Eur J Cancer. 2013;49:2869–76.
77. Toumishey E, Prasad A, Dueck G, Chua N, Finch D, Johnston J, et al. Final report of a phase 2 clinical trial of lenalidomide monotherapy for patients with T-cell lymphoma. Cancer. 2015;121:716–23.
78. Zinzani PL, Pellegrini C, Broccoli A, Stefoni V, Gandolfi L, Quirini F, et al. Lenalidomide monotherapy for relapsed/refractory peripheral T-cell lymphoma not otherwise specified. Leuk Lymphoma. 2011;52:1585–8.
79. Ishida T, Joh T, Uike N, Yamamoto K, Utsunomiya A, Yoshida S, et al. Defucosylated anti-CCR4 monoclonal antibody (KW-0761) for relapsed adult T-cell leukemia-lymphoma: a multicenter phase II study. J Clin Oncol. 2012;30:837–42.
80. Ogura M, Ishida T, Hatake K, Taniwaki M, Ando K, Tobinai K, et al. Multicenter phase II study of mogamulizumab (KW-0761), a defucosylated anti-cc chemokine receptor 4 antibody, in patients with relapsed peripheral T-cell lymphoma and cutaneous T-cell lymphoma. J Clin Oncol. 2014;32:1157–63.
81. Friedberg JW, Mahadevan D, Cebula E, Persky D, Lossos I, Agarwal AB, et al. Phase II study of alisertib, a selective Aurora A kinase inhibitor, in relapsed and refractory aggressive B- and T-cell non-Hodgkin lymphomas. J Clin Oncol. 2014;32:44–50.
82. Barr PM, Li H, Spier C, Mahadevan D, LeBlanc M, Ul Haq M, et al. Phase II intergroup trial of alisertib in relapsed and refractory peripheral T-cell lymphoma and transformed mycosis fungoides: SWOG 1108. J Clin Oncol. 2015;33:2399–404.
83. O'Connor OA, Ozcan M, Jacobsen E, Vidal JMR, Trotman J, Demeter J. First multicenter, randomized phase 3 study in patients (pts) with relapsed/refractory (R/R) peripheral T-cell lymphoma (PTCL): alisertib (MLN8237) versus investigator's choice (Lumiere trial; NCT01482962). Blood. 2015b;126:341.
84. Fanale MA, Wang Z, Ma W, Oki Y, Hagemeister FB, Fayad LE, et al. Gene expression profiling for molecular features of response in a phase I trial of alisertib plus romidepsin for relapsed/refractory aggressive B- and T-cell lymphomas. Blood. 2015; 126:2705.
85. Amengual JE, Lichtenstein R, Rojas C, Sawas A, Deng C, Lichtenstien E, et al. The pralatrexate—romidepsin doublet: a well tolerated and highly effective combination for patients with relapsed or refractory peripheral T-cell lymphoma. Blood. 2016;128:1824.
86. Mehta-Shah N, Lunning MA, Boruchov AM, Ruan J, Nair S, Lynch P, et al. A phase I/II trial of the combination of romidepsin and lenalidomide in patients with relapsed/refractory lymphoma and myeloma: activity in T-cell lymphoma. J Clin Oncol. 2015;33(Suppl 15):8521.
87. Beitinjaneh A, Saliba RM, Medeiros LJ, Turturro F, Rondon G, Korbling M, et al. Comparison of survival in patients with T cell lymphoma after autologous and allogeneic stem cell transplantation as a frontline strategy or in relapsed disease. Biol Blood Marrow Transplant. 2015;21:855–9.
88. Chen AI, McMillan A, Negrin RS, Horning SJ, Laport GG. Long-term results of autologous hematopoietic cell transplantation for peripheral T cell lymphoma: the Stanford experience. Biol Blood Marrow Transplant. 2008;14:741–7.
89. Jantunen E, Wiklund T, Juvonen E, Putkonen M, Lehtinen T, Kuittinen O, et al. Autologous stem cell transplantation in adult patients with peripheral T-cell lymphoma: a nation-wide survey. Bone Marrow Transplant. 2004;33:405–10.

90. Smith SD, Bolwell BJ, Rybicki LA, Brown S, Dean R, Kalaycio M, et al. Autologous hematopoietic stem cell transplantation in peripheral T-cell lymphoma using a uniform high-dose regimen. Bone Marrow Transplant. 2007;40:239–43.
91. Kim MK, Kim S, Lee SS, Sym SJ, Lee DH, Jang S, et al. High-dose chemotherapy and autologous stem cell transplantation for peripheral T-cell lymphoma: complete response at transplant predicts survival. Ann Hematol. 2007;86:435–42.
92. Corradini P, Dodero A, Zallio F, Caracciolo D, Casini M, Bregni M, et al. Graft-versus-lymphoma effect in relapsed peripheral T-cell non-Hodgkin's lymphomas after reduced-intensity conditioning followed by allogeneic transplantation of hematopoietic cells. J Clin Oncol. 2004;22:2172–6.
93. Dodero A, Spina F, Narni F, Patriarca F, Cavattoni I, Benedetti F, et al. Allogeneic transplantation following a reduced-intensity conditioning regimen in relapsed/refractory peripheral T-cell lymphomas: long-term remissions and response to donor lymphocyte infusions support the role of a graft-versus-lymphoma effect. Leukemia. 2012;26:520–6.
94. Kim SW, Yoon SS, Suzuki R, Matsuno Y, Yi HG, Yoshida T, et al. Comparison of outcomes between autologous and allogeneic hematopoietic stem cell transplantation for peripheral T-cell lymphomas with central review of pathology. Leukemia. 2013;27:1394–7.
95. Jacobsen ED, Kim HT, Ho VT, Cutler CS, Koreth J, Fisher DC, et al. A large single-center experience with allogeneic stem-cell transplantation for peripheral T-cell non-Hodgkin lymphoma and advanced mycosis fungoides/Sezary syndrome. Ann Oncol. 2011;22:1608–13.
96. Le Gouill S, Milpied N, Buzyn A, De Latour RP, Vernant JP, Mohty M, et al. Graft-versus-lymphoma effect for aggressive T-cell lymphomas in adults: a study by the Societe Francaise de Greffe de Moelle et de Therapie Cellulaire. J Clin Oncol. 2008;26:2264–71.
97. Shustov AR, Gooley TA, Sandmaier BM, Shizuru J, Sorror ML, Sahebi F, et al. Allogeneic haematopoietic cell transplantation after nonmyeloablative conditioning in patients with T-cell and natural killer-cell lymphomas. Br J Haematol. 2010;150:170–8.
98. Aoki K, Suzuki R, Chihara D, Suzuki T, Kim S-W, Fukuda T, et al. Reduced-intensity conditioning of allogeneic transplantation for nodal peripheral T-cell lymphomas. Blood. 2014;124:2585.

Aggressive Lymphoma in Children and Adolescents

13

Birte Wistinghausen and Birgit Burkhardt

13.1 Introduction

Non-Hodgkin lymphomas (NHL) account for 7% of childhood malignancies between the ages of 0 and 19 according to SEERS data from 2010 to 2014. NHL are rare in early childhood with an incidence of 7.3/10^6 children/year in the 1–4-year age group. By adolescence, the annual incidence rises with 14/10^6 children in the 10–14-year age range and 18.3/10^6 children in the 15–19-year age group. In addition, lymphoblastic leukemia accounts for another 20% of childhood cancers making malignancies of lymphatic origin the largest group of childhood cancers.

The vast majority of childhood NHL are high grade. This chapter will focus on the most commonly seen childhood NHL: Burkitt lymphoma (BL) and Burkitt leukemia (B-AL), diffuse large B-cell lymphoma (DLBCL), lymphoblastic lymphoma (LBL), and anaplastic large cell lymphoma (ALCL). In addition, posttransplant lymphoproliferative disease (PTLD), the most common childhood lymphoproliferation, will be discussed.

B. Wistinghausen
Pediatric Hematology-Oncology, Mount Sinai Hospital, New York, NY, USA
e-mail: BWISTINGHA@childrensnational.org

B. Burkhardt (✉)
Department of Pediatric Hematology and Oncology, University of Münster, Münster, Germany
e-mail: birgit.burkhardt@ukmuenster.de

13.2 Mature Aggressive B-Cell Lymphoma

13.2.1 Introduction

Mature aggressive B-cell non-Hodgkin lymphoma (B-NHL) accounts for about 60% of non-Hodgkin lymphoma (NHL) among children and adolescents [1, 2]. The main subtypes include Burkitt lymphoma (BL), Burkitt leukemia or FAB L3 leukemia (B-AL), and diffuse large B-cell lymphoma (DLBCL). Prospective cooperative studies have contributed significantly to the current understanding as well as to the success in treating pediatric aggressive B-NHL. Combination chemotherapy, refined by incorporation of new active agents, succeeded in overall survival of 90% in childhood and adolescent B-NHL/B-AL [3, 4].

13.2.2 Epidemiology and Clinical Presentation

In contrast to the adult population, in which the incidence of indolent lymphomas increases with increasing age, the vast majority of pediatric cases of B-NHL are aggressive lymphoma. In children under the age of 14 years, aggressive B-cell NHL account for approximately 60% of all NHL, with most of them being either Burkitt lymphoma/leukemia (BL/B-AL) in about three

G. Lenz, G. Salles (eds.), *Aggressive Lymphomas*, Hematologic Malignancies,
https://doi.org/10.1007/978-3-030-00362-3_13

quarters of pediatric B-NHL or diffuse large B-cell lymphoma (DLBCL) in the remaining patients [2, 5]. Small percentages account for less common entities such as primary mediastinal large B-cell lymphoma, pediatric follicular lymphoma, pediatric nodal marginal zone lymphoma, and intermediate lymphoma between BL and DLBCL or intermediate between DLBCL and Hodgkin lymphoma. In adolescents aged 15–19 years, the proportion of the histological subtypes changes with DLBCL becoming more frequent than BL/B-AL [6]. This trend continues in the age group above 20 years, in which BL/B-AL account for no more than 5% of B-NHL.

Patients with BL/B-AL are predominantly male (>4:1) with a median age of about 9 years [2]. Frequent manifestations are abdominal and cervical lymph nodes and the tonsils. About a quarter of patients are diagnosed with bone marrow involvement and 5–10% with central nervous system (CNS) involvement. In contrast, in DLBCL, the median age at presentation is 11–12 years, and the sex ratio showed a moderate trend toward males (1.7:1). CNS and/or bone marrow involvement is rarely observed in DLBCL patients. In large patient series of aggressive B-NHL, stage I, II, III, IV, and B-AL were diagnosed in approximately 10%, 15–25%, 40–50%, 5–10%, and 15–25% of patients, respectively. In BL, the majority of patients with overt CNS are diagnosed by the detection of FAB L3 blasts in the CSF [7]. In contrast, intracranial masses are the most frequent CNS manifestation in DLBCL. For both subgroups, the diagnosis of CNS disease remains a parameter associated with poor prognosis [8]. Primary CNS lymphoma without systemic disease is rarely diagnosed in children and adolescents and suspected to be associated with inherited or acquired immunodeficiency [9, 10].

13.2.3 Pathology and Molecular Characterization

Classification of B-NHL is performed according to the *WHO Classification of Tumours of Haematopoietic and Lymphoid Tissues* of 2008 and updated in 2016 [11, 12]. Histopathological distinction of the several subtypes of mature aggressive B-cell malignancies can be challenging. With respect to the distinction of DLBCL, typical and atypical BL, agreement among expert hematopathologists has been reported to be about 50% of cases [13]. Therefore several studies have addressed the issue of diagnosing and distinguishing specific B-cell malignancies by molecular profiling, and two groups defined molecular classifier to distinguish BL from DLBCL [14, 15]. In most pediatric treatment protocols, all aggressive mature B-NHL are eligible and treated in the same way. In contrast, several study groups for adult patients use CHOP (cyclophosphamide, doxorubicin, vincristine, prednisolone) or variants for the treatment of DLBCL and methotrexate (MTX)-based protocols or others for BL. Therefore, the correct distinction of the histological subtype might be crucial for those patients.

Burkitt lymphoma and Burkitt leukemia are the most common subtypes of NHL in children but rare NHL subtypes among adult patients. Whether there are biological differences between pediatric and adult BL is unsolved today [16, 17]. BL is composed of monomorphic, small, non-cleaved cells with round nuclei, clumped chromatin, and basophilic cytoplasm. A high uniform proliferation index is seen, with the Ki-67 positivity approaching 100%. BL usually express surface immunoglobulins and B-cell markers such as CD19, CD20, and CD22. BL is negative for TdT and BCL2. The unifying attribute of BL on the molecular level is the juxtaposition of the *c-Myc* oncogene next to one of the immunoglobulin gene loci by the translocation t(8;14)(q24;q32) in 70–80% of cases and the less common translocations t(2;8)(p12;q24) and t(8;22)(q24;q11) in 10–15% [18]. This results in activation of the *MYC* (proto-)oncogene by the immunoglobulin gene enhancer. In addition to the c-MYC activation, recent studies identified the inhibitor of DNA3 (*ID3*) to be one of the most frequently altered genes in BL. *ID3* mutations are thought to diminish inhibitory control on transcription factor 3 (*TCF3*) resulting in increased cell proliferation. Notably *TCF3* was also found to be mutated in BL. Thus *ID3/TCF3* pathway alterations, which are hardly ever found in DLBCL, seem to be unique BL features [19–22]. Focused on uniformly diagnosed *cMYC* rearranged pediatric and adolescent Burkitt lymphoma/leukemia, the frequency of *ID3-TCF3-CCND3* pathway alterations is more than 88% and therefore higher than in adult populations [23]. *ID3* and *CCND3* mutations are associated with more advanced stages of the disease, and the pathway may represent a highly relevant second hit of Burkitt lymphoma pathogenesis, especially in children and adolescents.

In DLBCL the nuclei are usually more than twice the size of normal lymphocytes. They express pan-B-cell antigens, including CD19, CD20, CD22, and CD79a, with or without surface immunoglobulin. Most express CD10 and BCL6 and approximately 40% express BCL2. However, breaks or translocations in *BCL2* and *BCL6* are rare in pediatric DLBCL. Among DLBCL, different biological subtypes were reported several years ago [24–26]. Two reproducible subtypes are identified by gene expression profiling with lymphoma cells corresponding to germinal center B-cell-like (GCB) cells in about 50% of cases and DLBCL corresponding to activated B-cell-like (ABC) cells in about 30% of patients. The remaining cases represent different small heterogeneous subgroups of DLBCL. The distinction between GCB and ABC was demonstrated using gene expression analysis to immunophenotyping by Hans et al. in 2004, and since then, algorithms were refined by other groups with ongoing progress [27, 28]. In 2006, Oschlies et al. reported a distinct dominance of the GCB type in children and adolescents with 83% of analyzed cases [29]. However the small proportion of children diagnosed with ABC DLBCL did not show an inferior outcome. More recently gene expression profiling using NanoString technology to identify molecular DLBCL subtypes is applied successfully for pediatric and adolescent populations and confirms the rarity of the ABC subtype of DLBCL in this age group and the lack of association with outcome [30]. In an attempt to further specify GCB lymphoma, Salaverria et al. described chromosomal translocations juxtaposing the *IRF4* oncogene next to one of the immunoglobulin (IG) loci [31]. It was shown that these translocations predominantly occur in children, adolescents, and young adults and less frequent in adults. In addition to the predominance of the favorable GCB phenotype, pediatric DLBCL are characterized by moderate to high proliferation rates, increased c-Myc protein expression, and decreased Bcl2 protein expression when compared to adult DLBCL [32]. As these are molecular characteristics resembling Burkitt characteristics, it has been speculated that DLCBL and BL share more molecular characteristics in pediatric than in adult patient series.

13.2.4 Staging and Treatment of Mature Aggressive B-Cell Lymphoma

Standard diagnostics in children usually follows pediatric treatment protocols (e.g., Children's Oncology Group (COG), French-American-British Lymphomes Malins B (FAB-LMB), NHL-Berlin-Frankfurt-Münster (BFM)). The diagnosis of mature aggressive B-NHL needs to be confirmed either by cytomorphology and flow cytometry of malignant effusions or by biopsy and immunohistochemistry of a lymphoma manifestation. The confirmation of the diagnosis by a central reference laboratory should be intended whenever possible. Standard diagnostics include differential blood count, coagulation, clinical chemistry including serum lactate dehydrogenase (LDH), bone marrow (BM) and cerebrospinal fluid (CSF) evaluation, and virus serology according to local standards, often including EBV, CMV, VZV, and hepatitis serology and imaging. Routine imaging in pediatric patients comprises ultrasound of the abdomen, testes, and lymph nodes, a chest x-ray, and magnetic resonance imaging (MRI) of the CNS in case of (sub)-cranial manifestation or neurologic symptoms. In addition MRI of involved sites is recommended, at least in case of doubt after ultrasound imaging. In order to limit the radiation exposure in children and adolescents, computed tomography (CT) scans are not routine procedures of staging. However, there might be individual courses in which CT scans are preferred over MRI, e.g., in critically ill small children who would require sedation for MRI. The role of positron emission tomography (PET) is not systematically analyzed and validated in pediatric and adolescent patients with B-NHL and therefore not part of routine staging except for clinical trials. Staging in children and adolescents is performed according to the St. Jude classification [33] and the recently introduced revised classification system, the International Paediatric Non-Hodgkin Lymphoma Staging System (IPNHLSS) that allows more precise documentation of extranodal dissemination and advanced diagnostic and imaging methods [34].

13.2.5 Frontline Therapy

The treatment for pediatric BL and DLBCL patients is identical and results in favorable outcome. Patients are stratified into different risk groups using stratification criteria that reflect the individual risk of the patient to suffer a relapse. The criteria vary over the time and between the treatment groups but are mainly based on the stage of the disease, the resection status, the status of BM and/or CNS involvement, and the initial serum LDH level which has been shown to reflect the tumor load [35–37]. In addition, the response to treatment is used in some protocols [38–41]. The International Prognostic Index (IPI) which has been shown to serve as a prognostic parameter in adult B-NHL patients is rarely used for the pediatric and adolescent population [42].

Risk-adapted therapy of current common backbones consists of short, dose-intense courses of chemotherapy including steroids, vincristine, high-dose methotrexate, cyclophosphamide, doxorubicin, cytarabine and high-dose cytarabine, etoposide, and intrathecal chemotherapy. The number of courses and the dose of cytostatic agents are adapted to the risk group of the patient. Patients with limited disease receive two to four courses with excellent results as summarized in Table 13.1. For patients with intermediate stages of disease and intermediate risk, the treatment consists of an intermediate number and intensity of courses. The results of current trials are summarized in Table 13.2. Common criteria for the definition of patients with advanced disease and need of intense treatment are CNS involvement, bone marrow involvement, and high tumor burden as indicated by the LDH level. For those patients the dose of methotrexate and the number

Table 13.1 Treatment results in patients with limited disease

Protocol	No of pts	Risk group	Treatment	Events	Outcome (95% CI)	Reference
LMB 89	52	A	A: 2 courses COPAD, no IT injections	A: 1 event	A: 5 year OS 100% EFS 98% (90–100%)	Patte et al., Blood, 2001 [38]
FAB-LMB 96	132	A	2 courses COPAD, no IT injections	3 events	4 year OS 99% (96–100%), 4 year EFS 98% (94–99%)	Gerrard et al., BJH, 2008 [43]
NHL-BFM95	48	R1	R1: courses A and B	R1: 2 events	R1: EFS 94 ± 4%	Woessmann et al., Blood, 2005 [35]
AIEOP LNH92	13	R1	2 cycles A and B		OS 100% EFS 100%	Pillon et al., Cancer, 2004 [41]
JACLS NHL 98	13	A	8-day courses of steroids, vincristine, CPM, pirarubicin, and triple-drug IT therapy	No events or toxic deaths	A: 6 year OS and 6 year EFS 100%	Fujita et al.; Leuk Lymph, 2011 [37]
TCCSG NHL-B9604	3	A	3 steroid courses, VCR, CPM, HD-MTX, Ara-C, etoposide, double-drug IT	1 relapse	A: OS 100% EFS 66.7 ± 27.2%	Kikuchi et al., Leuk Lymph, 2008 [44]

Table 13.2 Treatment results in patients with intermediate stage of disease

Protocol	No of pts	Risk group	Treatment	Events	Outcome (95% CI)	Reference
LMB 89	B: 386	B	B: 2 courses COPAD, 2 courses CYM, and 1 course maintenance	B: 54 events	B: 5 year OS 94% (91–96) and 5 year EFS 92% (89–95%)	Patte et al., Blood, 2001 [38]
FAB-LMB96	657 random	B	COP, COPADM1, COPADM2, CYM, CYM, ±M1	52 events after randomization equally distributed	4 year EFS: 91–93% according to random. arm	Patte et al., Blood, 2007 [39]
NHL-BFM95	R2: 233 R3: 82	R2/R3	R2: prephase, A; B, A, B randomization to MTX-24 h or MTX-4 h with 1 g/m^2 R3: prephase, AA, BB, CC, AA, BB	R2: 13 events R3: 12 events	R2:EFS 94 ± 2% R3: 3 year EFS 85 ± 4%	Woessmann et al., Blood, 2005 [35]
AIEOP LNH92	R2: 54	R2	4 cycles of repeated AA and BB	5 relapse	R2: OS 94% EFS 87 ± 9%	Pillon et al., Cancer, 2004 [41]
JACLS NHL 98	B: 17 C: 21	B and C	8-day courses of steroids, vincristine, CPM, HD-MTX, Ara-C, pirarubicin, and triple-drug IT therapy	B: no events or toxic deaths C: 5 relapses	B: 6 year OS and 6 year EFS 100% C: OS 85 ± 8% 6 year EFS 75 ± 10%	Fujita et al., Leuk Lymph, 2011 [37]
TCCSG NHL-B9604	B: 25 C: 46	B and C	6 courses of steroids, VCR/VDS, CPM, HD-MTX, Ara-C, epirubicin, etoposide triple-/double-drug IT	B: 1 relapse C: 10 events with 7 progresses/relapse, 2 second malignancy, 1 TRM	B: OS 100% EFS 95.8 ± 4.1% C: OS 87 ± 5% EFS 78 ± 6%	Kikuchi et al., Leuk Lymph, 2008 [44]

of intrathecal administrations for CNS-directed therapy are increased in all protocols. The results of recent published trials are summarized in Table 13.3.

13.2.6 Treatment Strategies at Relapse

In Burkitt lymphoma/leukemia, relapses occur early during frontline treatment or shortly after the end of treatment. Relapses more than 1 year after initial diagnosis are rare and suspicious for a second disease rather than relapse. Comparative molecular analyses of the B-cell receptor gene rearrangement are recommended in those cases to clarify the molecular relation of the tumors. Sites of relapse are often the initial manifestations combined with bone marrow and/or CNS involvement. In DLBCL relapses can occur later than in BL/B-AL and often involve the initial sites. At the time of relapse, lymphoma manifestations often respond to relapse treatment but tend to regrow as soon as the bone marrow recovers from treatment after each course. For that reason dose-intense treatment without interruptions is crucial to prevent multiple progressions during relapse treatment. Recently reported data from different study groups underline the impact of high-dose treatment followed by hematopoietic stem cell transplantation. Only individual patients can survive without transplant. However the optimal re-induction treatment as well as the conditioning regimen as well as the optimal graft are under discussion. The Société Française des Cancers de l'Enfant (SFCE) reported 67 relapsed B-NHL among 1322 patients, diagnosed between 1989 and 2007, including 57 BL/B-AL,

Table 13.3 Treatment results in patients with advanced disease

Protocol	No of pts	Risk group	Treatment	Events	Outcome	Reference
LMB89	123	C	COP, COPADM1, COPADM2, CYVE, CYVE, m1, m2, m3, m4	Group C: 20 events	5 year OS 85% (78–90%) 5 year EFS 84% (77–90%)	Patte et al., Blood, 2001 [38]
FAB-LMB96	190 random.	C	COP, COPADM1, COPADM2, CYVE, CYVE, m1, m2, m3, m4; randomized trial	49 pts with events, 42 pts died	4 year OS: 79 ± 3% 4 year EFS 82 ± 3%; differences according to arms	Cairo et al., Blood, 2007 [40]
NHL-BFM95	142 (40 CNS+)	R4	Prephase, AA BB, CC, AA, BB, CC Randomization to MTX-24 h or MTX-4 h with 5 g/m^2	R4: 27 events CNS+: 12 events	R4: 3 year EFS 81 ± 3% CNS+: 3 year EFS 69 ± 7%	Woessmann et al., Blood, 2005 [35]
AIEOP LNH92	77	R3	4 cycles of repeated AA and BB; CC in case of residual disease	R3: 9 progresses/relapse Grade 3/4 infection n = 14 with 5 deaths	R3: OS 84% EFS 75 ± 10%	Pillon et al., Cancer, 2004 [41]
JACLS NHL-98	18	D	8-day courses of steroids, vincristine, CPM, HD-MTX, Ara-C, pirarubicin, etoposide, and triple-drug IT	D: 6 events with 4 relapses and 2 TRM	D: OS 77 ± 10% 6 year EFS 66 ± 11%	Fujita et al., Leuk Lymph, 2011 [37]
TCCSG NHL-B9604	17	D	7 courses of steroids, VCR/VDS, CPM, HD-MTX, Ara-C, epirubicin, etoposide, triple-/double-drug IT	D: 2 progressive disease/relapse, 1 TRM	D: OS 82 ± 9% EFS 82 ± 9%	Kikuchi et al., Leuk Lymph, 2008 [44]

6 DLBCL, and 4 primary mediastinal B-cell lymphoma [45]. Forty-one patients underwent high-dose chemotherapy with autologous (n = 33) or allogeneic (n = 8) HSCT. The 5-year survival rate is 30%. The probability of survival was 70% for the 10 patients with DLBCL and PMLBL histology compared to 23% for the 57 BL/B-AL and not further specified B-NHL. For those patients who underwent HSCT, there was no difference in outcome according to type of transplant. The British Children's Cancer Study Group (CCSG) reported a retrospective analysis of 33 pediatric B-NHL patients who suffered progression or relapse [46]. Interestingly, histology of DLBCL was more frequent than BL in that series. Sixteen patients had consolidation followed by autologous stem cell transplant (SCT), and four had allogeneic SCT. Nine out of the total 33 patients survived, and all 9 had either autologous or allogeneic SCT. As a consequence from that analysis, intensive re-induction with two cycles of CYVE and ICE (ifosfamide, carboplatin, and etoposide) along with four doses rituximab is recommended in the CCSG. For those patients who achieve CR, autologous SCT is recommended. A retrospective analysis in the United States obtaining data on patients undergoing SCT from the statistical center of the Center for International Blood and Marrow Transplant Research (CIBMTR) included 41 refractory or recurrent BL (n = 41) and 52 DLBCL patients [47]. The 5-year EFS were similar after allogeneic and autologous SCT for DLBCL (50% vs. 52%) and BL (31% vs. 27%). The Japanese study

group reported 33 refractory or relapsed B-NHL patients [48]. After a median follow-up period of 48 months, the 4-year OS for these patients was about 20%. Among the 17 patients achieving complete or partial remission, 4 of 5 patients who underwent SCT and 3 of the 12 patients who did not receive SCT were alive without disease progression. Data from the NHL-BFM group support the idea that autologous SCT might be adequate for DLBCL, while outcome for Burkitt relapses is poor in any way but superior with allogeneic SCT [49]. New treatment modalities are urgently needed for relapsed B-NHL patients.

13.2.7 Ongoing Trials, Novel and Targeted Therapies

One of the challenges of B-NHL and B-AL treatment in pediatric and adolescent patients today and in the upcoming years is the integration of new drugs. Driven by the relevance of B-NHL in adult patients, several substances are under investigation or recently licensed for adult patients. Given the current legislation, all these substances need to be tested in pediatric populations. However, the different distribution of histological NHL subtypes, the favorable results with current regimen, and the unknown profile of acute and long-term toxicities in children and adolescents prohibit the inclusion of these new substances in frontline treatment. Attempts to investigate the impact of the drugs in relapsed pediatric B-NHL patients are limited by the low absolute number of patients available for such trials. The delay in the availability of new drugs for pediatric B-NHL patients can be illustrated by rituximab, a monoclonal anti-CD20 antibody which was licensed for B-NHL treatment in adults in the mid-1990s. The first series of pediatric patients was reported by Griffin et al. in 2009 presenting the results of rituximab combined to standard salvage chemotherapy including ifosfamide, carboplatin, and etoposide (ICE) in 20 pediatric patients with relapsed and refractory B-NHL or B-AL. Objective response was noted in 60% of patients. Although hematological toxicities were common, only one patient was removed from the study due to prolonged myelosuppression [50]. First observations on the feasibility of adding rituximab to a modified NHL-BFM90 protocol in pediatric patients with advanced-stage mature B-NHL were reported by Samochatova et al. few years later. The major differences from the original BFM protocol were the dose reduction of methotrexate from 5000 to 1000 mg/m^2 in the first two courses and the addition of 375 mg/m^2 rituximab to each of the first four courses of therapy. Eighty-three newly diagnosed Burkitt or DLBCL lymphoma patients with stage III to IV were included. Complete remission was achieved in 77 (93%) patients; 2 patients relapsed, and 2 patients developed secondary malignancies. The 5-year OS was 82% ± 8% [51]. In parallel two other trials investigated rituximab in the frontline therapy of newly diagnosed patients: The NHL-BFM group conducted a phase II trial with an upfront window of one-dose rituximab monotherapy 5 days before the start of standard chemotherapy [52]. The aim of the study was to evaluate the single-agent activity of rituximab in newly diagnosed pediatric CD20-positive B-NHL/B-AL. One hundred thirty-six patients were enrolled and treated on day 1 with rituximab at 375 mg/m^2. The response rate to rituximab treatment was 41% with response in 36 of 87 evaluable patients. Three of the 87 patients suffered a relapse. According to the statistical plan of the study, an acceptable response rate was defined as 65%. As the measured response rate was only 41%, for subsequently enrolled 64 patients, the dose of rituximab was increased to 700 mg/m^2 as a single dose 5 days before the start of standard chemotherapy [53]. The toxicity profile of the increased rituximab dose did not differ from the lower dose. Although outcome was not a primary objective of this rituximab trial, EFS rates at 2 years were 96% and 97% for rituximab responders and non-responders and thus superior compared to EFS at 3 years of 89% in the trial NHL-BFM 95 with standard chemotherapy without rituximab [35]. And in parallel the COG conducted a study to assess safety, toxicity, and pharmacokinetics of the addition of rituximab to frontline FAB-based chemotherapy in children and adolescents with advanced-stage

B-NHL [54–60]. Patients stratified according to risk (intermediate group B, $n = 48$; high group C, $n = 42$) received two doses of rituximab at the beginning of each COPADM courses and one dose at the beginning of each consolidation courses resulting in a total of six rituximab doses. The study or parts of the study were reported on different occasions and showed feasibility of the addition of rituximab as well as increased outcome compared to historical controls treated without rituximab, although the trial was not powered for that analysis like the NHL-BFM trial. In response to those results, a transatlantic international cooperation of study groups agreed to perform the randomized trial Inter-B-NHL 2010 for advanced-stage B-NHL/B-AL based on the LMB/FAB regimen with six doses of rituximab in the experimental arm randomized against standard treatment without rituximab (NCT01516580). The trial stopped the randomization early and closed the standard arm without rituximab because of lower frequency of relapsed in the experimental arm.

In contrast to adults, data regarding the impact of rituximab on immune reconstitution in children are limited and vary [61]. While some report decreased immunoglobulin levels that remain within the normal range, others report hypogammaglobulinemia with immunoglobulin concentrations that fell below the age-adjusted values or even requires substitution. To learn more about the relevance of these observations, the NHL-BFM group together with the Scandinavian NOPHO group started the trial B-NHL 2013 with EFS with immune reconstitution as primary endpoints. In low-risk patients, the hypothesis is tested whether rituximab can substitute anthracyclines, while in advanced B-NHL/B-AL, it is tested whether rituximab can increase EFS. Of note this investigator initiated trial starts recruiting 20 years after licensing of rituximab for adults.

13.2.8 Conclusion

Standard chemotherapy regimen are available for pediatric and adolescents with mature aggressive B-NHL and B-AL resulting in favorable survival rates of 80–95%. There are three major aspects of further research and optimization. First, current research improved understanding of lymphoma biology and revealed distinct molecular and histological subtypes for whom the best treatment has to be identified. Second, the available regimens need to be optimized in the sense of reducing toxicity and prevention of relapse. Detailed understanding of the value of the available cytostatic agents and new drugs might offer opportunities. And third, effective treatment regimen for refractory and relapsed B-NHL and B-AL needs to be established as well as the definition of patients who qualify for allo-SCT and who are adequately treated with autologous SCT. As current re-induction regimens failed, new regimens need to be designed.

13.3 Lymphoblastic Lymphoma

13.3.1 Introduction

Lymphoblastic lymphoma (LBL) accounts for about 25–35% of NHL in childhood and adolescence [2]. Although the event-free survival and overall survival for pediatric LBL patients substantially increased during the last decades, the prognosis of relapsed patients remains poor [62]. On the other hand, the intensive treatment regimens are accompanied by high toxicity with considerable mortality, morbidity, and late squeal. Ongoing and future efforts therefore focus on systemic treatment optimization for pediatric and adolescent LBL patients with the prevention of low-risk patients from overtreatment and with well-balanced treatment intensification of high-risk patients. Progress in the understanding of the pathogenesis of the disease as well as the identification of patients prone to an increased risk of refractory disease or adverse events is an essential step to achieve these aims.

13.3.2 Epidemiology and Clinical Presentation

Among pediatric and adolescent LBL patients, about 70–80% are diagnosed with a T-cell lymphoblastic lymphoma (T-LBL), 20–25% with a precursor B-cell lymphoblastic lymphoma (pB-LBL), and rare cases with mixed lineage or not further classifiable immunophenotype [2, 63]. The median age of diagnosis is not significantly different in pB-LBL (8 years) and T-LBL (8.8 years) [2]. There is no difference in gender distribution in pB-LBL, while in T-LBL males are 2.5 times as often affected than girls [2]. The vast majority of T-LBL patients presents with a mediastinal tumor of the arising from the thymus frequently accompanied with pleural or pericardial effusions. Other manifestations are lymphadenopathy. The presence of a predominantly anterior mediastinal mass can cause respiratory symptoms from coughing, stridor, dyspnea, edema, and elevated jugular venous pressure to acute respiratory distress. About 15–20% of patients exhibit bone marrow infiltration. Less than 5% show central nervous system (CNS) involvement. The most frequent sites of involvement in pB-LBL are the lymph nodes, skin, soft tissue, and bone [64, 65]. Compared to T-LBL, these patients are more likely to present with limited-stage disease. However, the proportion of patients with bone marrow involvement is about 30–40% and thus higher in pB-LBL compared to T-LBL [2, 64]. CNS affection was detected in about 5%. Depending on the site of manifestation, the symptoms vary.

13.3.3 Pathology

The diagnosis of LBL can be assured by cytomorphological and flow cytometry analysis of malignant effusion or by histological and immunohistochemical analysis of paraffin embedded biopsies. If the diagnosis is based on flow cytometry, the criteria agreed upon by the European Group for Immunophenotyping of Leukemias are frequently used [66], whereas histologic diagnosis after tumor biopsy is based on the criteria by the WHO classification [11].

Lymphoblastic lymphomas of precursor B-cell lineage express B-cell markers CD19, CD79a, CD22, and/or PAX5. They also stain positive for TdT and HLA-DR. Lymphomas of the common ALL type stain positive for CD10. Pre-B-LBL can be identified by their positivity for cytoplasmic IgM and no expression of surface immunoglobulin. Early B-cell lymphoma is defined as lymphoma morphologically FAB L1 or L2, but surface immunoglobulin is identified by flow cytometry. These patients should be treated as having lymphoblastic lymphoma.

T-LBL is cytoplasmic or membrane-bound CD3 and mostly TdT positive and is further subclassified referring to the stage of differentiation of T-lymphoblasts on their passage through the thymus [67]. In addition to TdT, the most specific markers to indicate the precursor nature of T-lymphoblasts are CD99, CD34, and CD1a. For the histopathological diagnosis of LBL, the WHO criteria are widely accepted. Interestingly, the EGIL criteria and the WHO criteria are not identical, although the WHO guidelines for lineage determination and subtyping of precursor cell neoplasm are mainly derived from flow cytometry analyses of ALL. In consequence, the WHO guidelines are not directly transferable to the histopathological procedures necessary to diagnose LBL as discussed by Oschlies and colleagues [67]. Based on the analysis of 188 patients with LBL, an algorithm for immunohistochemical staining was developed to address the problem of challenging morphologic and immunophenotypical variants. Accordingly, the diagnosis of LBL requires typical morphology, confirmation of precursor cell immunophenotype, detailed lineage definition, and subtyping by additional staining and/or genetic analysis. TdT expression has been identified as the best marker for determining the precursor cell nature of a lymphoma. In TdT-negative lymphoma with typical lymphoblastic morphology, either expression of CD1a or CD34, coexpression of CD79a and CD3, or coexpression of CD4 and CD8 can be used to determine the precursor cell nature of lymphoma.

The Children's Oncology Group reported immunophenotypic characteristics of T-lymphoblastic lymphoma in children and adolescents [68]. The immunophenotypic profile of 180 children and adolescents with newly diagnosed T-LBL enrolled in the COG trial 5971 was analyzed by flow cytometry and/or immunohistochemistry. Diagnostically useful immunophenotypic features of T-LBL were identified as well as distinct immunophenotypic subgroups. None of these were statistically related to event-free or overall survival. Smock et al. reported that a majority of LBL samples expressed MIB1 (59%) and cMYC (77%) in greater than 50% of analyzed cells by immunohistochemistry [69]. It is to discuss if the cMyc overexpression is due to NOTCH-signaling perturbation or if other NOTCH-independent mechanisms are involved.

Recently it has been recognized that a very early stage of differentiation may be seen in about 10–15% of cases of T-ALL, termed early T-precursor acute lymphoblastic leukemia (ETP-ALL), defined as having expression of T-cell antigens CD7 and low-level CD5 (and occasionally cytoplasmic CD3) but lacking expression of CD1a, CD4, and CD8. There is expression of CD34 as well as at least one myeloid-related antigen such as CD117, CD33, or CD13 [70, 71], and it has also been described in T-LBL [68]. This phenotype is associated with increased AML-type mutations rather than T-ALL/LBL-associated *NOTCH* mutations [72]. ETP-ALL was originally described as a higher-risk disease due to increased induction failures, but more recent data does not show significant differences in outcomes with current therapies [73].

In addition, the WHO classification of 2008 introduced the entity of "acute leukemias of ambiguous lineage" (ALAL) [11]. Interestingly, this disease is not only seen as leukemic manifestation but also as lymphoma without or only limited bone marrow infiltration. The international pathology panel of the trial EURO-LB 02 reported 7% cases of mixed phenotype acute leukemia (MPAL) among 188 LBL patients [67]. The number of cases is too small to allow standard treatment recommendation. Ongoing analyses of histologic and immunophenotypic characteristics of LBL could complement current criteria to identify biological LBL subgroups with distinct chemosensitivity.

13.3.4 Prognostic Factors and Genetic and Molecular Alterations

It is agreed that prognostic parameters are most urgently needed for pediatric LBL patients to prevent overtreatment and subsequent acute and long-term toxicities as, e.g., osteonecrosis in low-risk patients. And on the other hand, prognostic parameters identifying high-risk patients allowing subsequent treatment intensification to prevent often fatal relapses are highly warranted [74]. Concerning the prognostic relevance of clinical characteristics, several parameters had been tested as, e.g., age, sex, stage, presence of mediastinal mass, and level of serum lactate dehydrogenase [74]. Tubergen et al. reported an unfavorable prognosis for children older than 14 years based on the results of the trial CCG502 [75]. Analysis of the outcome of T-LBL patients treated within different NHL-BFM trials revealed a lower pEFS in adolescent females compared to males with comparable clinical characteristics [6]. Based on the COG pilot trial, Abromowitch et al. identified CNS involvement as prognostic factor, although the case numbers were low [76]. Analysis of the EORTC 58881 trial led to the identification of response to therapy as a prognostic factor [77]. Non-response after 7 days of prephase with prednisolone and one intrathecal injection with MTX was associated with very poor outcome. Other groups have not confirmed these data so far.

In the trials NHL-BFM 90, NHL-BFM 95, and EURO-LB 02, patients were stratified according to stage. Patients with limited stage I/II disease did not receive re-induction treatment protocol II. Outcome analysis of the trial EURO-LB 02 supported stage of disease as stratification criterion for pB-LBL resulting in favorable pEFS for pB-LBL with limited disease representing almost half of pB-LBL patients [78]. However, for pB-LBL patients with advanced stage III/IV disease, pEFS and cumulative incidence of relapse were poor even with intensified treatment including protocol II. In T-LBL it is well known that the number of patients with limited stage I/II disease is very low. Therefore stage of disease is an insufficient parameter to identify low-risk T-LBL patients potentially available for treatment de-escalation. In the trial EURO-LB 02, only 8 out of 233 T-LBL patients (3%) were diagnosed with stage

I/II disease. Importantly, there was no relevant difference in pEFS for T-LBL stage III compared to stage IV disease.

13.3.4.1 Genetic Characterization and Genetic Markers

Although it is subject of discussion if T-ALL and T-LBL are separate diseases [79–81], they share a range of genetic alterations. Due to the recombination processes of T-cell receptor rearrangement, the T-cell receptor (TCR) genes are predisposed to recombination with oncogenes or genes involved in thymocyte development through chromosomal translocations. These recurrent translocations are found in 50% of pediatric T-ALLs. The prevalence of these translocations in pediatric T-LBL is not exactly known. The current literature shows that most cytogenetic abnormalities reported in T-LBL have been reported earlier in T-ALL [80–83].

More recent molecular studies suggest candidate genes of prognostic relevance for T-LBL. It is well known that mutations in *NOTCH1* and/or *FBXW7* at hotspots within the genes are observed in ca. 50% of pediatric T-ALL patients and are reported to be associated with an improved treatment response or outcome [84, 85]. Concerning pediatric T-LBL patients, five studies are published reporting the results of *NOTCH1* and/or *FBXW7* mutation analyses in 116, 54, 14, 11, and 9 cases, respectively [80, 86–89]. In the larger series, *NOTCH1* and/or *FBXW7* mutations are associated with a favorable response to treatment and/or outcome. The prognostic effect of activating NOTCH1 mutations might be influenced by the applied treatment.

In descriptive retrospective analyses of pediatric T-LBL patients, loss of heterozygosity at chromosomal region 6q14-24 (LOH6q) is shown to be highly significantly associated with adverse outcome and increased risk of relapse [82, 86, 90]. Within a total of 217 analyzed patients, pEFS at 5 years is 86 ± 3% for LOH6q-negative patients compared to 27 ± 9% in LOH6q-positive patients ($p < 0.0001$).

Mutations in the tumor suppressor *PTEN* have been observed in different types of solid and hematological malignancies. Some studies report an association of these mutations with unfavorable outcome of patients. Concerning pediatric T-LBL, one report of the NHL-BFM study group reports a significant association of *PTEN* mutations with adverse outcome of analyzed patients [91]. Within a clinically well-described cohort of 114 pediatric patients, *PTEN* mutations are detected in 15% of cases and identified as poor prognostic marker with pEFS at 5 years of 82 ± 4 for non-mutated versus 59 ± 12% for *PTEN* mutated cases ($p = 0.014$). Although biological data suggest that any *PTEN* mutations lead to hyperactivated PI3K-AKT signaling, the prognostic impact is weaker when other PI3K-AKT pathway mutations are included in the analysis, indicating that the negative prognostic impact mostly depended on *PTEN* mutations. It is hence hypothesized that *PTEN* controls resistance to therapy by PI3K-AKT-independent signaling. Outcomes of patients with heterozygous or homozygous/biallelic *PTEN* mutations are similar, suggesting that *PTEN* acts as haploinsufficient tumor suppressor in pediatric T-LBL. It is reported that the expression of *PTEN* was transcriptionally repressed by active NOTCH1 in, e.g., T-ALL cell lines but also normal mouse thymocytes [92, 93]. This suggests a synergistic effect of both mutations in *NOTCH1* and *PTEN*, but investigation of the prognostic impact of a combination of both genetic markers in the analyzed cohort of patients treated according to NHL-BFM regimens revealed the opposite: the unfavorable prognostic effect of *PTEN* mutations seems to be abrogated by the favorable prognostic *NOTCH1* mutations, as this group of patients presented with a pEFS of 91 ± 9% [91]. Similar associations and interactions of *NOTCH1* and *PTEN* mutations with outcome have recently been described in pediatric T-ALL treated with BFM-type regimens [94]. In contrast to these findings, pediatric T-ALL patients treated according to DCOG and COALL regimens without *NOTCH1* and *PTEN* mutations showed a significantly lower cumulative incidence of relapse at 5 years compared with the rest of the cohort [95].

Absence of biallelic T-cell receptor gene gamma (TRG) locus deletion (ABD), which is characteristic for early thymocyte precursors before V(D)J recombination, correlates statistically significant with the failure of induction chemotherapy of pediatric T-ALL patients but also poorer outcomes [96, 97]. For pediatric T-LBL, ABD is observed in a small subgroup of 4 out of 54 patients (7%) treated according to NHL-BFM 95 or EURO-LB 02 regimen [87]. All four patients had mutations in *NOTCH1* and/or *FBXW7*. ABD was in this cohort associated with a poor pEFS of 0% compared to 80 ± 6% for non-ABD patients ($p = 0.01$).

13.3.4.2 Minimal Disseminated (MDD) and Minimal Residual Disease (MRD)

Risk stratification in T-ALL is primarily based on microscopic and submicroscopic evaluation of blasts in the peripheral blood and bone marrow using either quantitative PCR-based patient-specific TCR gene rearrangements or flow cytometric analysis. Both methods were extended to pediatric T-LBL samples for MDD evaluation [98, 99]. The study by Coustan-Smith et al. revealed that flow cytometric analysis of blood samples provided sensitive detection of disseminated T-LBL, allowing for screening of blast clearance during therapy. Their analysis predicted inferior outcomes for stage IV disease with the treatment applied and could distinguish patients with disease dissemination among the stage II/III disease [99]. In a more recent study conducted by the Italian AIEOP study group, the prognostic value of MDD analyzed by multiparametric flow cytometry (FCM) in bone marrow and peripheral blood samples was evaluated in a cohort of 65 children affected by T- and B-lineage lymphoblastic lymphoma. MDD was detected in 49% (32/65) of BM samples, whereas only 21% (14/65) were positive at standard morphological evaluation. Using an MDD cutoff level of 3% by FCM, 5-year EFS is 60% for patients with MDD >3% LBL cells versus 83% for the remaining patients ($p = 0.04$) [100]. Prospective trials are needed to evaluate the role of MDD and MRD evaluation in pediatric T-LBL as prognostic markers.

13.3.4.3 Perspective

With the new and rapidly evolving next-generation sequencing technology, genome-wide profiling studies have enabled to study not just gene mutations using whole genome sequencing and whole exome sequencing but also have allowed study of genome organization using chromatin conformation capture techniques that allow for screening for rare chromosomal rearrangements and translocation events in small subpopulations of cells. In addition the epigenetic signature of T-LBL is currently unknown but may add relevant pathogenetic insights. Mutations in genes regulating epigenetic pathways are one of the key regulators of malignant transformation of hematopoietic progenitor cells by modifications of DNA and histones that regulate gene expression. DNA methylation, in particular hypermethylation of the promoter regions, is a recurrent mechanism of gene silencing in several cancers [101, 102] and is associated with aggressive phenotypes and poor prognosis.

13.3.5 Staging and Treatment of Lymphoblastic Lymphoma

Staging of newly diagnosed patients includes complete medical history, physical examination, and lumbar puncture with cerebrospinal fluid (CSF) cytology, bone marrow aspirate, and possible bone marrow biopsy. Laboratories include a full and differential blood count, assessment of kidney and liver function, electrolytes, and LDH level. Imaging procedures include abdominal ultrasound and ultrasound of lymph nodes as well as testicular ultrasound in case of male patients. Imaging procedures may be extended with magnetic resonance imaging (MRI) or computerized tomography (CT). Fluorodeoxyglucose (FDG) positron emission tomography (PET) CT/MRI scanning is now more frequently used for routine staging in LBL patients, but published data is limited [103–107], and the role of FDG-PET-CT/MRI in the management remains to be evaluated. To date, the St. Jude NHL staging classification was applied to pediatric patients with NHL [33]. Recently, a revised classification system, the International Paediatric Non-Hodgkin Lymphoma Staging System (IPNHLSS) that allows more precise documentation of extranodal dissemination and advanced diagnostic and imaging methods [34], has been introduced.

13.3.6 Frontline Therapy

With ALL-type treatment regimens, outcome of pediatric T-LBL patients has improved with event-free survival rates of 75–90. The results are summarized in Table 13.4. Current protocols are mostly derived from either the LSA2L2-regimen that was established in the United States (Memorial Sloan Kettering Cancer Center) or the NHL-BFM protocol based on the ALL-BFM strategy [110, 119–121]. During the last few decades, almost all subsequently developed treatment regimens are based on one of these pioneer protocols that represent major achievements in the therapy of pediatric LBL. There is limited data regarding Asian pediatric LBL patients with few studies published [122–124]. Results of a retrospective Chinese cohort study on pediatric T-LBL patients treated with one of three treatment protocols revealed outcomes in the range of 64% for all patients. However, patient numbers were small [125]. Recently, data on 136 analyzed Japanese pediatric LBL patients with advanced

Table 13.4 Summary of treatment results of recent clinical trials for children and adolescents with lymphoblastic lymphoma

Trial	Age	Stage	Treatment	No. pts.	pEFS	Reference
LMT81	9 years (0.9–16)	I–IV	Mod. LSA2-L2	84	75 ± 3%	Patte et al. 1992 [108]
CCG502	9 years (0.5–19)	I–IV	Mod. LSA2-L2 vs. ADCOMP	143 138	74% 64%	Tubergen et al. 1995 [75]
	10 years (5–15)	III/IV	L-Asp – vs. L-Asp +	83 84	64 ± 6% 78 ± 5%	Amylon et al. 1999 [109]
NHL-BFM90	9 years (1–16)	I–IV	ALL-BFM	105	90%	Reiter et al. 2000 [110]
NHL-BFM95	8 years (0.2–19)	III/IV	ALL-BFM	169	78 ± 3%	Burkhardt et al. 2006 [111]
EORTC58881	8 years (0–16)	I–IV	ALL-BFM	119	78 ± 3%	Uyttebroeck et al. 2008 [77]
COG Pilot	n.d.	III/IV	Mod. LSA2-L2	85	78 ± 5%	Abromowitch et al. 2008 [112]
COG A5971	10 years	III/IV	NHL-BFM95 MTX w/o HD-MTX intensification w/o intensification	257 (all)	85 ± 4% 83 ± 4% 83 ± 4% 83 ± 4%	Abromowitch et al. 2008 (Abstract) [76]
LNH92	8 years (0–<16)	I–IV	Mod. LSA2-L2	55	69 ± 6%	Pillon et al.2009 [113]
St. Jude 13	n.d.	III//V	T-ALL	41	83%	Sandlund et al. 2009 [114]
POG 9404	50% < 10 years	III//V	Mod. DFCI ALL with HD-MTX w/o HD-MTX	137 66 71	 82 ± 5% 88 ± 4%	Asselin et al. 2011 [115]
A 5971	>12 months	I–II	CCG-BFM	56	90%	Termuhlen et al. 2012 [116]
EURO-LB 02	0–<21 years	I–IV	NHL/ALL-BFM 90 dexa (10 mg/m^2) vs. pred (60 mg/m^2)	319 (all) 98 88	81 ± 2% 84 ± 4 (dexa) 84 ± 4% (pred)	Reiter et al. 2012 [78]
EORTC58951	n.d.		Mod. BFM 90 dexa (6 mg/m^2) vs. pred (60 mg/m^2)	 37 37	85% 89 ± 5% (pred) 81 ± 6% (dexa)	Uyttebroeck et al. 2012 (Abstract) [117]
SFOP LMT96	10.5 years		Mod. BFM	79	85%	Bergeron et al. 2015 [118]

disease were published [126] confirming by univariate analysis results of a previous Japanese report that showed an inferior outcome of T-LBL patients presenting with stage III compared to stage IV [123].

In contrast to ALL treatment regimens, the only parameter for risk group stratification for patients with LBL is the stage of disease at diagnosis which groups into treatment for limited (stage I and II) and advanced stages of disease (stage III and IV). Published EFS for patients with limited-stage disease range from 73 ± 8% (LMT81) to 100% (LNH92). These results may be achievable with relevant dose reductions, as indicated by the trial NHL-BFM 90, which administered no re-induction for patients with limited disease [110]. Treatment durations for patients with limited disease ranged from 12 to 24 months.

To improve CNS-directed treatment, several protocol modifications of MTX administration are evaluated. The French LMT81 trial modified the LSA2L2 protocol by addition of ten courses of high-dose MTX (HD-MTX) with a resultant EFS of 75% [108]. The US trial POG 9404 analyzed the effectiveness of a Dana-Farber backbone therapy with or without addition of HD-MTX in T-ALL and T-LBL patients. In T-LBL patients, in contrast to T-ALL patients, there were no significant differences in EFS in the two arms [115]. In addition the COG trial A5971 tested a COG BFM-type regimen with different schedules of CNS-directed treatment where HD-MTX without additional intrathecal MTX in maintenance was randomized against an intensified intrathecal MTX (IT-MTX) treatment arm without HD-MTX for CNS prophylaxis. Each treatment arm was randomized with or without early intensification. There were no significant differences in EFS, and the authors concluded that either IT-MTX or HD-MTX effectively prevented CNS relapse [127]. A recent presentation reported the Capizzi methotrexate combined with BFM protocols in 58 LBL patients. CNS-directed treatment was mainly based on frequent intrathecal injections. The EFS was reported to be of 90.8% [128].

13.3.7 Treatment Strategies at Relapse

Relapsed lymphoblastic lymphoma (LBL) is still at dismal outcome, with survival rates of 10–30%. In a Japanese cohort, the incidence of relapse/progression was 18%, with 48 cases among 260 LBL patients diagnosed between 1996 and 2004. Among 19 patients who underwent allogeneic SCT, 6 suffered relapse, and 3 died of treatment-related mortality (TRM), while 10 survived without further progression. Among the six patients who had undergone autologous SCT, four suffered relapse and died, while two survived [129]. The Center for International Blood and Marrow Transplant Research of North America summarized 53 pediatric LBL patients who received HSCT between 1990 and 2005. EFS for 39 patients treated with allo-SCT was 40% compared with 4% in the 14 patients who underwent autologous SCT [130]. The EORTC focused on LBL of B-cell phenotype and reported a 15% relapse/progression rate of 8 patients out of 53 diagnosed between 1989 and 2008. All these eight patients died, seven after allogeneic HSCT, five of disease progression, and three of TRM [64]. The NHL-BFM group reported a relapse rate of 10%, with 34 LBL relapses among 324 LBL patients, diagnosed between 1990 and 2003. Among 13 patients who received allo-SCT, 5 survived, 6 suffered relapse, and 2 died of TRM. Two patients underwent autologous SCT, and both died of disease progression [131]. Overall, available data in relapsed LBL show that patients without high-dose treatment followed by autologous (auto) or allogeneic (allo) hematopoietic stem cell transplantation (SCT) have almost no chance of cure. Concerning the ongoing discussion whether auto- or allo-SCT is superior, the available data indicate a trend for higher TRM but also higher probability of disease-free survival after allogeneic SCT compared to autologous SCT. However the absolute numbers of cases in the literature are too small to draw conclusions.

13.3.8 Novel and Targeted Therapies

Survival rates in relapsed pediatric T-LBL patients are poor, and due to toxicity, there are few possibilities for salvage therapies. New targeted, less toxic drugs would be an opportunity for additional treatment in these patients. Nelarabine, a nucleoside analogue, was FDA approved after publication of two phase II trials in pediatric and adult patients with relapsed or refractory T-ALL or T-LBL. Complete remission was achieved in 5/39 pediatric patients. Neurologic toxicity has been observed and was dose-limiting [132]. The COG AALL00P2 trial assessed the safety of nelarabine administration within a NHL-BFM 86 chemotherapy backbone in pediatric T-ALL patients [133]. The subsequent COG phase III study, AALL0434, is designed to show the safe addition of nelarabine to a COG-augmented BFM-type regimen [134]. Further trials to evaluate the benefit of nelarabine in pediatric patients with T-LBL and, even more importantly, identification and implementation of additional new drugs for high-risk, refractory, or relapsed pediatric T-LBL are needed. A current review on pediatric T-ALL summarizes several potential drugs of interest targeting pathways like Notch, PI3K-Akt-mTOR, JAK/STAT, and MAPK pathways, the cell cycle regulation, the proteasome, and epigenetic targets or using approaches derived from the immunotherapy. Despite the long list, only a limited number of substances are under investigation in T-ALL and none in T-LBL [135].

13.3.9 Conclusion

Despite the improved cure rates in the treatment of pediatric patients with lymphoblastic lymphoma, the most important challenge remains the increase of the survival and the reduction of relevant acute and long-term toxicity of today's treatment protocols. The implementations of new substances and in parallel the identification of valid prognostic parameters are essential prerequisites for the achievement of these aims.

13.4 Anaplastic Large Cell Lymphoma

13.4.1 Introduction

ALCL was first described in 1985 by Stein et al. when the expression of CD30, also known as Ki-1, was reported in a group of large cell neoplasms previously falsely diagnosed as malignant histiocytosis or metastases of undifferentiated non-hematopoietic neoplasms [136]. In 1988, ALCL was included in the revised Kiel classification as a separate entity, and subsequently, the Revised European American Lymphoma Classification incorporated ALCL in 1995 [137, 138]. Better understanding of the pathophysiology was obtained in 1994 when the gene product of the t(2;5)(p23;q35) translocation was cloned which led to the discovery of the anaplastic lymphoma kinase (ALK) [139]. More than 90% of childhood and adolescent ALCL are ALK positive. In the 2008 *WHO Classification of Tumours of Haematopoietic and Lymphoid Tissues*, ALK-positive ALCL is a distinct entity within the spectrum of mature T-cell lymphomas [140]. ALK-negative ALCL was recognized as a separate entity in 2016 [12]. Primary cutaneous ALCL accounts for 6–7% of pediatric ALCL and is associated with an excellent prognosis with local therapy [141]. Since these two entities do not commonly occur in childhood or adolescence, this chapter will concentrate on systemic ALK-positive ALCL. With improved understanding of the pathophysiology of ALCL, targeted therapies have been developed that are currently in clinical trials including the anti-CD30 antibody brentuximab and the tyrosine kinase inhibitor of ALK, crizotinib.

13.4.2 Epidemiology and Clinical Presentation

ALCL accounts for approximately 10–15% of childhood and adolescent lymphomas (SEERS data from 2010 to 2014) and is the only peripheral T-cell lymphoma frequently seen in childhood. The vast majority of ALK-positive ALCL occurs in the first three decades of life with the peak incidence in the 10–14 age groups. It is one of the most common lymphomas of the adolescent and young adult (AYA) population. There is a predominance of males with a M:F ratio of 1.5:1 [142]. In the United States, ALCL is more commonly seen in African Americans than in non-Hispanic Whites but is less common in Asians [143]. African Americans have an inferior prognosis compared to non-Hispanic Whites.

Approximately 60% of patients with ALCL present with disseminated disease often accompanied by systemic symptoms such as fever, weight loss, and night sweats (B-symptoms). While ALCL can present in any nodal area of the body, it commonly involves intraabdominal and mediastinal nodes with extensive disease that can lead to inflammatory reactions such as neoplastic or reactive pleural effusions and ascites. Extranodal dissemination to the skin, lungs, liver, and bone is frequently seen. Morphologic bone marrow involvement is found in less than 15% of cases, but minimal marrow disease can be detected in as much as 60% of cases using molecular techniques such as RT-PCR for NPM-ALK [144]. The small cell variant of ALK-positive ALCL can rarely present in a leukemic phase accounting for about 3% of cases [145–149]. Central nervous system disease is only found in 2% of patients at diagnosis but has been reported more commonly in cases with leukemic small cell variant ALCL [149].

13.4.3 Pathology

The morphology of ALCL has a wide spectrum, but the hallmark is a population of large cells that contain an eccentric, horseshoe- or kidney-shaped nucleus often with an eosinophilic region near the nucleus. Occasionally, cells appear to have nuclear inclusions which are not true inclusions but nuclear membrane invaginations.

There are five different morphologic patterns described in the 2008 WHO classification [140].

The "common pattern" accounting for about 60% of cases is characterized by tumor cells with abundant cytoplasm. Multiple nuclei can form a wreath-like pattern making the distinction from Reed-Sternberg cells difficult by morphology. In an only partially effaced lymph node, the tumor cells grow within the sinuses mimicking metastatic tumors.

The "lymphohistiocytic pattern" (10% of cases) contains a mixture of tumor cells and reactive histiocytes. Abundant reactive histiocytes can mask the tumors cells which tend to aggregate around vessels. Hemophagocytosis can be occasionally seen in this pattern.

The "small cell pattern" (5–10%) contains a predominant population of small- to medium-sized tumor cells with irregular nuclei that can have the appearance of "fried egg cells." In addition, signet ring-like cells can be seen, and on smear neoplastic cells in cases with peripheral blood involvement can appear as flower-like cells.

The "Hodgkin-like pattern" (3%) mimics the morphologic pattern of nodular-sclerosing Hodgkin disease.

About 15% of cases present with more than one pattern in single lymph nodes ("composite pattern"). Patterns can vary within the same lymph node, separate sites, or from diagnosis to relapse.

Neoplastic cells express CD30 on cell membranes and in the Golgi region with strongest expression in large cells. Small cell variants can be weakly positive to negative. In addition, ALK is expressed, usually in the cytoplasm and nucleus in large tumor cells but only in the nucleus in small cell variants. The majority of ALCL expresses one or more T-cell markers such as CD2, CD5, and CD4, but CD3 is negative in 70% cases. CD8 is also only rarely expressed; some cases have complete loss of expression of T-cell markers but show evidence of T-cell lineage at the genetic level. Since there are no other distinctions between cases with T-cell and null-cell phenotype, they are considered a single entity by the WHO [140]. In addition, most cases stain positive for proteins associated with cytotoxic T-cells such as TIA1, granzyme B, and perforin which has led to the assumption that peripheral cytotoxic T-cells are the cells of origin [140]. They are classified in the group of peripheral T-cell lymphomas (PTCL), but there is evidence on the molecular level that a more immature thymic precursor may be the cell of origin [150].

13.4.4 Genetic and Molecular Alterations

ALK-positive ALCL is characterized by ALK fusion genes. The most common translocation, t(2;5)(p23;q35), fuses the promoter and proximal part of nucleophosmin (NPM) gene on chromosome 5 to the ALK gene on chromosome 2 and is found in >80% of cases [140]. The second most common translocation t(1;2)(p25;P23) accounts for 10–15% of cases. There are several other fusion partners located on chromosomes 2, 3, 17, 19, 22, and X, each accounting for less than 1% of cases [151].

The expression of ALK is physiologically restricted to fetal neural cells and not found in normal postnatal tissue [152]. ALK encodes a tyrosine kinase belonging to the insulin receptor superfamily [139]. NPM is an ubiquitously expressed nonribosomal nucleolar phosphoprotein involved in trafficking between nucleus and cytoplasm [153]. NPM provides the active promoter that drives expression of NPM-ALK in tumor cells and the N-terminus with an oligomerization domain which leads to the formation of NPM-ALK homodimers mimicking ligand binding. ALK retains its intracellular portion with an intact tyrosine kinase domain that autophosphorylates through the dimerization. In the small variant, NPM-ALK dimerizes with wild-type NPM and co-localizes to the nucleus [154, 155].

NPM-ALK acts as a constitutionally active tyrosine kinase signaling through several pathways including the PI3 kinase, MAPK, mTOR, STAT3, and STAT5 pathways leading to increased survival and proliferation [156–161]. Marzec et al. showed that the gene expression profile induced by NPM-ALK significantly overlaps with genes induced by IL-2 signaling [162] Because IL-2 is critical for normal T-cell proliferation, this has led to the hypothesis that NPM-ALK mimics physiologic effects of IL-2 stimulation in ALCL albeit with constant activation giving it all the hallmarks of an oncogene [163]. Crescenzo et al. demonstrated that ALK- ALCL also depends on activation of the STAT3 pathway and activating mutations in Jak1 and STAT3 have been described in ALK- ALCL illuminating the crucial importance of the JAK/STAT pathway in the pathogenesis of both ALK+ and ALK- ALCL [164].

The activation of the STAT3 by NPM-ALK leads several oncogenic consequences including the suppression of antitumor responses and the methylation of tumor suppressor genes. ALCL tumor cells are able to create an immunosuppressive tumor microenvironment and evade the immune system by the STAT3-induced expression of transforming growth factor beta (TGF-beta), IL-10, and programmed death-ligand 1 (PD-L1) [157, 163, 165]. In addition, NPM-ALK-activated STAT3 activates several DNA methyltransferases and histone deacetylases that lead to epigenetic gene silencing of tumor suppressor genes including IL-2R-γ [166]. NPM-ALK makes the ALCL tumor cell IL-2 independent and downregulates in the expression of IL-2R-γ. Interestingly, re-expression of IL-2R-γ leads to loss of NPM-ALK and apoptosis [166].

ALCL is classified in the mature T and NK neoplasms by the WHO despite the loss of multiple or all T-cell antigens, but the cell of origin remains unknown [12, 140]. It has been proposed that ALCL is of activated T-cell origin because of the expression of cytotoxic proteins such as perforin and granzyme as well as T-cell receptor rearrangements [167, 168] or of T-regulatory origin because of expression of FoxP3 transcripts [169]. Because the t(2;5) translocation has been described in cord blood of healthy newborns, the hypothesis proposed that a more immature hematopoietic or T-cell precursor is the cell of origin [170]. This has been confirmed by gene expression profiling showing signatures more consistent with early thymic progenitors [150, 171].

13.4.5 Treatment of ALCL

The unique pathophysiology and molecular drivers of ALCL have led to three interesting observations in the treatment of ALCL, setting it apart from other childhood lymphomas. First, ALCL is extremely chemotherapy sensitive, and excellent response rates can be achieved with a variety of very different chemotherapy regimen of variable dose, interval intensity, and length of therapy. B-cell-directed therapy [172–175] led to similar outcome as leukemia-based therapy [176, 177]. Second, chemotherapy sensitivity is preserved at the time of relapse [178]. Second remissions can be achieved at higher rates than in other childhood lymphomas, and survival rates for relapsed ALCL approach 50–70% with stem cell transplantation [179–181]. Third, contrary to other childhood lymphomas, escalation of chemotherapy cumulative dosing and interval intensity has not increased cure rates [172, 182, 183]. Published EFS rates with frontline therapy remain between 65 and 75% which lacks behind the survival of most other childhood lymphomas [172, 183].

13.4.6 Frontline Therapy

The two most common frontline chemotherapy backbones are APO developed by the Pediatric Oncology Group and ALCL99 based on NHL-BFM90 protocol (Table 13.1) [172, 183]. Outcomes are similar with both treatment protocols. The Pediatric Oncology Group enrolled 86 patients with ALCL in a protocol for large cell lymphomas using the APO regimen and reported a 4-year EFS of 71.8% (SE, 6.1%) and OS of 88.1% (SE, 4.4%) in the ALCL group [182]. After a common APO induction, patients were randomized to 15 maintenance cycles every 21 days of either APO (doxorubicin, vincristine, prednisone, mercaptopurine ×5 cycles followed by methotrexate vincristine, prednisone, mercaptopurine ×10 cycles) or APO maintenance with every other cycle replaced by intermediate-dose methotrexate (1 g/m^2 over 24 h) followed by high-dose cytarabine (500 mg/m^2 bolus followed by a continuous infusion of 60 mg/m^2 over 48 h). Total treatment length was 52 weeks. Intensification with intermediate-dose methotrexate and high-dose cytarabine did not improve outcome. The follow-up study by the Children's Oncology Group ANHL0131 randomized between vincristine every 3 weeks and weekly vinblastine in the APO maintenance cycles 1–15 [183]. Overall outcome was similar with a 3-year EFS of 76% (95% CI of 67–83%) and OS of 85% (95% CI of 76–91%) in 129 patients. Vinblastine intensification did not improve outcome but was associated with increased toxicity, mainly myelosuppression leading to dose reductions, increased infections with neutropenia and febrile neutropenia, as well as sensory neuropathy. In summary, the American groups showed that the APO regimen leads to event-free survivals around 70–75% and intensification of this regimen with intermediate-dose methotrexate/high-dose cytarabine or vinblastine does not improve outcome.

ALCL99, the protocol of the European Intergroup Cooperation of Childhood and Adolescent NHL (EICNHL) showed 2-year EFS of 74.1% (95% CI of 69.2–78.4%) and 2-year OS of 92.5% (95% CI of 89.3–94.8%) [172]. Based on NHL-BFM-90, this protocol consisted of a 5-day prophase (dexamethasone, cyclophosphamide) followed by six induction courses every 21 days alternating between course A (dexamethasone, methotrexate, ifosfamide, cytarabine, etoposide, and vinblastine) and course B (dexamethasone, methotrexate, cyclophosphamide, doxorubicin, and vinblastine). Total treatment length was approximately 4 months. This trial included a methotrexate randomization between 3 g/m^2 intravenous methotrexate over 3 h without any intrathecal therapy and 1 g/m^2 intravenous methotrexate over 24 h with intrathecal triples (methotrexate, hydrocortisone/prednisolone, and cytarabine). Both methotrexate arms included leucovorin rescue. While there was no difference in outcome between both arms, the trial demonstrated that intrathecal chemotherapy could safely be eliminated with higher intravenous methotrexate dosing and that the shorter infusion rate of methotrexate at a higher dose without concomitant intrathecal methotrexate exposure reduced toxicities, namely, the incidence of grade 4 myelosuppression and grade 3/4 oral mucositis. In addition, ALCL99 included a randomization of high-risk patients with mediastinal, lung, liver, spleen, or skin involvement [184]. These patients were randomized between standard therapy and vinblastine intensification consisting in the addition of one dose of vinblastine 6 mg/m^2 to each course followed by weekly vinblastine for a total treatment length of 1 year. Interestingly, the rate of relapse was significantly reduced in the vinblastine arm during the first year of therapy (1-year EFS 91% vs. 74%), but this effect disappeared after completion of vinblastine, and the 2-year EFS was not significantly different (EFS 72.5% in the vinblastine arm vs. 70.1%). In summary, the European groups showed that ALCL99 also leads to cure rates of 70–75%, that intrathecal chemotherapy can be safely reduced to one initial dose by increasing methotrexate to 3 g/m^2 given over 3 h while also reducing toxicity, and that vinblastine intensification and maintenance therapy delay relapse but do not improve event-free survival. Most cooperative groups are currently using the ALCL99 backbone as their standard of care because of the shorter treatment length, the lower exposure to cumulative anthracyclines (150 mg/m^2 vs. 300 mg/m^2 in APO), and the reduction of intrathecal chemotherapy.

13.4.7 Prognostic Factors

Since approximately 30% of patients with ALCL fail therapy and 70% of patients can be cured with regimen of varying dose intensity, it is of great interest to identify prognostic factors for future clinical protocol development and risk stratification.

Most patients present with advanced stages making stage in itself not a useful predictor of outcome; however, a merged prognostic study of 225 pediatric patients enrolled on clinical protocols by the BFM, SFOP, and UKCCSG from 1987 to 1997 identified several clinical prognostic factors. In a multivariate analysis, three factors were significantly associated with inferior outcome [185]. Mediastinal involvement raised the relative risk of relapse by 2.1 (1.2–3.5), skin lesions by 1.9 (1.1–3.2), and spleen involvement by 1.9 (1.3–3.6). The 5-year PFS was 89% (82–96%) in patients without these risk factors, while involvement of the skin, spleen, or mediastinum reduced the PFS to 61% (53–69%).

In ALCL99, 32% of patients presented with small cell or lymphohistiocytic variant of ALCL, while 65% of patients have the common type [186]. Patients with small cell or lymphohistiocytic variant had a significantly higher risk for failure (HR, 2.0; 95% CI, 1.3–3.0; $P = 0.002$) controlling for clinical factors even though there was a higher incidence of skin and mediastinal involvement in this group of patients.

Circulating ALCL tumor cells can be detected in the peripheral blood at diagnosis in 50–60% of patients by using PCR of NPM-ALK and correlate with minimal disease in the bone marrow [187]. Several groups have shown an association of minimal disseminated disease (MDD) in either bone marrow or peripheral blood with prognosis [188, 189]. Progression-free survivals of 82–87% have been reported in MDD-negative patients compared to 38–54% in MDD-positive patients. In addition, anti-ALK antibodies can be found in the peripheral blood of more than 90% patients at diagnosis [190]. High titers were associated with lower stage, less minimal disseminated disease, and better outcome. Combining anti-ALK response with MDD, Mussolin et al. identified three biological risk groups: a high-risk group (20% of patients) that was MDD positive and had low anti-ALK titers with a PFS 28% and a low-risk group (31% of patients) with high anti-ALK titers and negative MDD with a PFS of 93% [189]. The remaining 48% of patients build an intermediate-risk group with PFS 68%. CD3 positivity was only associated with an inferior prognosis in univariant analysis [189]. In a multivariate analysis of stage, clinical prognostic factors, morphologic bone marrow involvement, pathological variant, and biological risk group, only pathological variant and biological risk group remained significantly associated with outcome.

13.4.8 Treatment Strategies at Relapse

Multiple different treatment strategies have been piloted at relapse, and there is no standard approach [178–180, 191]. Because ALCL retains chemosensitivity, a second remission can be achieved in more than half of all relapsed patients. Moreover, it is rare for patients to relapse on therapy [178]. Impressive results have been achieved with vinblastine monotherapy [178]. In a group of 36 patients with primary resistant disease ($n = 1$), first relapse ($n = 15$), second relapse ($n = 15$), and greater than two relapses ($n = 5$), 83% (25 of 30 evaluable patients) achieved a CR with weekly vinblastine at 6 mg/m^2. In 25 patients treated with vinblastine monotherapy, 9 (36%) achieved a lasting remission with a median follow-up of 7 years. Twelve of Nineteen patients with relapse received vinblastine as single agent again at the time of relapse, and 11 out of 12 received a second CR.

The experiences with autologous and allogeneic hematopoietic stem cell transplantation (HSCT) have been summarized by the French, German, and Japanese groups [179–181, 191, 192]. The French group used both autologous and allogeneic HSCT and concluded that autologous HSCT may not lead to better outcome than prolonged chemotherapy [180]. In 34 patients who underwent allogeneic HSCT, the EFS was 58% (SE = 8%) [181]. The BFM group reported 20 patients who underwent allogeneic HSCT for relapse during or shortly after therapy [192]. In this retrospective cohort, the EFS was 75%. Subsequently, they published their experience with autologous HSCT in 39 patients and reported EFS of 59% ± 8% [179]. Relapse during therapy and/or bone marrow or CNS involvement was associated with an inferior prognosis. The Japanese group reported superior outcome with allogeneic HSCT (relapse-free survival [RFS] 100%) compared to chemotherapy alone (RFS 53 ± 17%) or autologous stem cell transplantation (RFS 33% ± 18%) [191].

Because of the inconclusive results about the value of HSCT in relapsed or refractory ALCL and optimal relapse therapy, the EICNHL conducted a prospective ALCL relapse trial with risk-adapted therapy. Results of the trial were presented at the Fifth International Symposium on Childhood, Adolescent and Young Adult NHL in 2015 [193]. One hundred eighteen patients were stratified into four risk arms: progression during frontline therapy (risk arm 1), patients with CD3-positive relapse after initial therapy (risk arm 2), patients with CD3-negative relapse within 12 months of initial diagnosis (risk arm 3), and patients with CD3-negative relapse >12 months after initial diagnosis (risk arm 4). Patients with risk arms 1 and 2 were eligible for allogeneic HSCT (treatment arm A). Patients in risk arm 3 received consolidation with autologous HSCT (treatment arm B), and patients in risk arm 4 were treated with 24 months of weekly vinblastine (treatment arm C). The 3-year EFS of the entire cohort was 59 ± 5%, in treatment arm A 64 ± 7%, in treatment arm B 35± 9%, and in treatment arm C 85 ± 8%. The 3-year OS for the entire cohort was 78 ± 4%, in arm A 73 ± 7%, in arm B 77 ± 8%, and in arm C 90 ± 7%. While allogeneic HSCT offers a chance of cure in high-risk relapses, autologous HSCT with BEAM conditioning was not efficacious. Low-risk relapses can be treated with vinblastine monotherapy with excellent chance of cure. However, newer targeted therapies such as crizotinib and brentuximab may substitute or be incorporated with multi-agent chemotherapy, stem cell transplant, and vinblastine in the near future.

13.4.9 Novel and Targeted Therapies

There are two targeted therapies currently available for ALCL, crizotinib, a tyrosine kinase inhibitor (TKI) targeting ALK, and brentuximab vedotin, an anti-CD30 antibody conjugated to monomethyl auristatin E (MMAE), a microtubule inhibitor.

Crizotinib, an oral TKI, targeted ALK, and MET was developed for the treatment of ALK-driven non-small cell lung cancer [194]. There are several other ALK inhibitors currently in clinical trials [195]. Crizotinib as single agent has shown impressive results in ALCL. In a pediatric phase I trial, 7/8 relapsed ALCL patients achieved a CR [196]. There is emerging data, similar to vinblastine monotherapy in the relapsed setting, that relapse is rare on therapy, but it has not been established whether crizotinib will have to be administered continuously similar to other TKI like imatinib in chronic myeloid leukemia or whether cure can be achieved and crizotinib can be safely stopped [151]. Crizotinib was well tolerated in the pediatric age group without any development of resistance in the ALCL group [196]. In the relapse setting, it is being used as induction therapy to achieve CR prior to transplant. Crizotinib is also being evaluated as first-line therapy in combination with the ALCL99 backbone by the Children's Oncology Group, and the EICNHL is also planning a trial to evaluate it as first-line therapy in combination with chemotherapy.

Brentuximab vedotin, a conjugated anti-CD30 antibody, is approved in the United States and Europe for adults with relapsed ALCL after multi-agent chemotherapy based on high response rates in several phase II studies [151]. CD30, a transmembrane glycoprotein, is universally expressed in pediatric ALK+ ALCL [155]. Upon binding to CD30, brentuximab vedotin gets internalized and releases MMAE in the lysosome. MMAE, via its antitubulin activity, leads to M-phase arrest and induces apoptosis of the tumor cell [197]. MMAE shares the same tubulin binding site (vinca domain) as vinblastine [198]. In a phase II study of brentuximab vedotin as single agent in 58 patients with relapsed/refractory ALCL, 57% (33/58) achieved a CR [199]. The youngest patient enrolled on study was 14 years of age. The most common toxicities, grade III or greater, were neutropenia (21%), thrombocytopenia (14%), peripheral neuropathy (12%), and anemia (7%). Brentuximab vedotin has been evaluated in combination chemotherapy in adults with Hodgkin disease (HD) and ALCL. In a phase I study of adults with newly diagnosed HD, brentuximab vedotin led to excessive pulmonary toxicity when combined with bleomycin but was otherwise well tolerated [200]. Results of a phase II pediatric trial of brentuximab vedotin and gemcitabine in pediatric and young adults were presented at the American Society of Clinical Oncology Meeting in 2017 [201]. It showed that the combination of brentuximab and gemcitabine was well tolerated and highly active in children and young adults with refractory/relapsed HD. In addition, the St. Jude group published their experience of brentuximab in 16 patients with high-risk classical HD treated with brentuximab vedotin in combination with multi-agent chemotherapy showing that weekly administration of brentuximab vedotin was safe and tolerated in pediatric patients [202]. There are several case reports of brentuximab vedotin in pediatric patients with relapsed/refractory ALCL showing efficacy [203, 204]. A retrospective review identified five pediatric patients with refractory/relapsed HD and four pediatric patients with relapsed/refractory ALCL, age 12–17 years, enrolled on phase I and II studies with single-agent brentuximab vedotin [205]. Toxicity profile was similar to adult studies with three out of nine patients experiencing side effects, grade III or higher. All four patients with systemic ALCL achieved a CR.

The Children's Oncology Group is currently enrolling pediatric and adolescent patients with newly diagnosed CD30-positive ALK-positive ALCL on a phase II trial using the ALCL99 chemotherapy backbone with a randomization to either brentuximab or crizotinib.

In addition to the two targeted therapies currently in clinical trials, there are several other promising future treatment strategies in ALCL. Targeted therapies for downstream pathways of NPM-ALK such as inhibitors of JAK, mTOR, and PI3K are in clinical trials or development for other cancers and could be rationally tested in the treatment of ALCL [151]. PDGFR inhibition with imatinib markedly prolonged survival in NPM-ALK mice [206]. When combined with crizotinib, there was synergistic activity. Furthermore, a sustained remission was achieved with imatinib in a patient with refractory ALK+ ALCL [206]. Because STAT3 activation by NPM-ALK leads to epigenetic silencing of tumor suppressor genes, there may be a role of histone deacetylase inhibitors in ALK+ ALCL [166].

Lastly, immunological strategies are being studied for the treatment of ALCL. As previously discussed, ALK+ ALCL is a very immunogenic tumor with mechanisms to evade the immune system including expression of PD-L1 making checkpoint inhibition a potential therapeutic strategy. Furthermore, vinblastine did not improve outcome in the frontline therapy when combined with multi-agent chemotherapy but has shown impressive efficacy as single therapy in the relapsed setting [178, 183, 184]. This could suggest that vinblastine has immune modulatory effects in addition to cytotoxicity. Tanaka et al. demonstrated that vinblastine induces dendritic cell maturation and augments clonal expansion of tumor-specific cytotoxic T-cells when injected directly into the tumor in mouse models [207]. NPM-ALK-reactive CD8+ T-cell responses have been reported in children and adults with ALK+ ALCL [208, 209]. Because there is a correlation of anti-ALK antibody titer with outcome in ALK- ALCL, vaccination against ALK is another interesting strategy. In a mouse model, DNA vaccination with plasmids encoding several ALK fusion proteins protected mice from local and systemic lymphoma [210].

In summary, ALK+ ALCL accounts for 10–15% of childhood lymphomas. While the EFS lacks behind other childhood lymphomas, ALK+ ALCL retains its chemosensitivity, and about half of relapsed patients can be cured with further therapy. Because of its unique biology, targeted therapies are currently in clinical trials, and immunotherapies may further change the therapy of ALCL in the future in Table 13.5.

Table 13.5 Summary of clinical trials in pediatric patients with newly diagnosed ALCL

Protocol	Treatment	Patient number (*n*)	Stage	Median age in years (range)	EFS	OS	Reference
HM89 HM91	B-cell based: COP COPADMx2 Maintenance ×4 cycles No intrathecals	82	I–IV	10 (1.5–17)	83% (72–90%)	66% (54–76%)	Brugieres, 1998 [174]
NHL-BFM-90	Prephase K1 (stage I, II resected): 3 cycles K2 (II unresected, III): 6 alternating cycles K3 (IV or extensive bone involvement): 6 intensified cycles	89	I–IV	10.5 (0.8–17.3)	76 ± 5%		Seidemann, 2001 [175]
NHL 9001, 9002 and 9602	B-cell based: Stage I: 8 cycles with reduced doses Stage II–IV: COP COPADMx2 CYMx2 COPADMx1	72	I–IV	11.8 (1.1–16.4)	59% (47–70)	65% (53–76)	Williams, 2002 [173]
LNH-92	Leukemia based: Modified LSA2-L2	34	II–IV	11.6 (4.2–14.9)	85% (79–91)	65% (57–73)	Rosolen, 2005 [176]
POG-9315	APO	86	III–IV	13.7 (1.2–19.4)	71.8 ± 6.1%	88.1 ± 4.4%	Laver, 2005 [182]
ALCL99	Prephase Six alternating courses (A and B)	375	I–IV	11 (90.3–19.5)	74.1% (69.2–78.4)	92.5% (89.3–94.8)	Brugieres, 2009 [172]
ANHL1031	APO	125	III–IV	11.9	76% (67–93)	85% (76–91)	Alexander, 2014 [183]

13.5 Lymphoproliferation in Immunodeficiency

The link between immunodeficiency and increased risk of uncontrolled lymphoproliferation and lymphoma has long been recognized. In the 1950s, the concept of cellular immunity was emerging but poorly understood. At a New York Symposium in 1957, Lewis Thomas proposed the hypothesis that one purpose of cellular immunity consisted in early detection and elimination of neoplastic cells assuming that cancers are arising from small clones and exhibit something foreign on their surface; two hypotheses which have since been widely accepted [211]. Sir F. Macfarlane Burnet introduced the term immune surveillance in 1963 [212]. In addition, he postulated that if conditions associated with a suppressed immune system increase the likelihood of cancer, administration of immunosuppressive agents should facilitate the spontaneous appearance of cancer [212].

Children with primary and secondary immunodeficiency are at higher risk for a distinct set of malignancies that are often driven by viruses ("something foreign" [Thomas, 1957]). Data from the Australasian Society of Clinical Immunology and Allergy Primary Immunodeficiency Registry showed that children with primary immunodeficiency have an 8.82-fold excess relative risk of developing non-Hodgkin lymphoma [213]. The risk varies according to immune defect and appears highest in DNA repair defects such as ataxia telangiectasia and Nijmegen syndrome and lowest in antibody deficiencies (agammaglobulinemia, IgA deficiency, hyper IgM syndrome) [214]. Defects linked to immune dysregulation such as autoimmune lymphoproliferative disease (ALPS), X-linked lymphoproliferative disease (XLP), and MAGT1 deficiency predispose patients to autoimmune disease as well as lymphoproliferative disease [215]. The two most common acquired immunodeficiency states seen in childhood result from medically induced immunosuppression in transplant patients or infection with the human immunodeficiency virus (HIV). The incidence of the acquired immunodeficiency state (AIDS) has significantly decreased in childhood with maternal prenatal testing and perinatal prophylaxis and the use of highly active anti-retroviral therapy (HAART). With the rising prevalence of solid organ transplants (SOT) and allogeneic hematopoietic stem cell transplantation (HSCT), post-transplant lymphoproliferative disease (PTLD) has become the most common form of lymphoproliferation in childhood with estimated 150 pediatric cases per year, and more than 90% are Epstein-Barr virus (EBV) driven [216].

13.5.1 Epidemiology and Clinical Presentation of PTLD

The epidemiology and clinical presentation of PTLD is different in SOT versus HSCT recipients.

The incidence of PTLD ranges from 1 to 3% in allogeneic HSCT but can be as high as 11% depending on the degree of HLA mismatch between recipient and donor [217]. In a review of 272 umbilical cord blood transplants (UCBT) from two institutions, the incidence of PTLD was relatively low at 2%, but a subsequent study showed that nonmyleoablative preparatory regimen and the use of antithymocyte globulin increased the risk of PTLD [218, 219]. The most recent report of 175 UBCT recipients included only 4 patients with EBV-positive PTLD (2.3%) [220].

In data reported to the US Organ Procurement and Transplant Network and Scientific Registry of Transplant Recipients, the 5-year cumulative incidence of PTLD is 2.2% in kidney transplants, around 5% in liver and heart transplants, 15% in lung transplants, and up to 20% in small bowel and multiple organ transplants with large epithelial surfaces requiring higher immunosuppression and containing significant amounts of passenger lymphocytes [221].

PTLD in childhood tends to be an early event. In HSCT, almost all cases occur within the first 6–12 months posttransplant before immune reconstitution has occurred [217]. Data from the University of Minnesota showed patients with PTLD presented at a median of 0.3 years post-HSCT (range 0.1–7.3 years) [222]. Similarly, PTLD in pediatric SOT mostly occurs within the first 2 years of transplant during the time of most intense immunosuppression, but an increased risk persists lifelong because of ongoing immunosuppression [221].

The clinical presentation varies and can be non-specific. Fulminant PTLD is characterized by widespread disease with a rapidly progressive inflammatory process that can lead to multi-organ system failure and death without prompt intervention [223]. The incidence of fulminant PTLD without any well-defined tumor mass or lymphadenopathy is much higher in HSCT than in OLT. There is one report that a third of the cases of PTLD following BMT were found at autopsy with the antemortem cause of death originally felt to be severe graft-versus-host disease (GvHD) and/or infection because of widespread disease without any mass lesion but with a systemic inflammatory response that led to multi-organ failure [224].

Even in non-fulminant PTLD, constitutional symptoms are common and include fever, weight loss, fatigue, and pancytopenia. PTLD in SOT commonly affects the transplanted organ leading to clinical symptoms overlapping with rejection. Other tissues frequently involved include the lymph nodes, spleen, gastrointestinal (GI) tract, lung, and liver [225]. GI involvement can lead to intussusception, diarrhea, hypoalbuminemia, anemia from chronic blood loss, and even perforation from transmural involvement [225]. The spectrum of lung involvement goes from asymptomatic nodules to widespread interstitial disease with respiratory failure. Liver involvement can present as diffuse hepatitis and is difficult to distinguish from rejection in liver transplant recipients. Extranodular disease is much more common in PTLD than in immunocompetent children with lymphoma [225]. Nodal involvement is most common in the head and neck area, often with associated tonsillar and adenoid hypertrophy [221].

13.5.2 Risk Factors for PTLD

The highest risk factor for developing EBV-positive PTLD is the transplantation of an EBV-positive graft into an EBV-seronegative recipient. Attempts of matching donors and recipients by EBV status have proved difficult because 80–90% of the adult population is EBV positive, while only 30% of preschoolers are EBV positive.

The risk of PTLD in allogeneic HSCT is strongly associated with HLA disparity, T-cell depletion (TCD) of the stem cell graft, and use of antithymocyte globulin. Selective TCD, for example, sheep red blood cell resetting and the use of anti-T-cell monoclonal antibodies, confer a higher risk of PTLD compared with "pan-lymphocyte"-depleted stem cell grafts or CD34-positive selection of peripheral blood stem cell transplants. In the latter two methods, EBV-infected B-cells are also removed instead of just selectively removing T-cells.

The use of T-cell antibodies such as antithymocyte globulins also increases the risk of PTLD in SOT [225]. Recently, mTOR inhibition with sirolimus or everolimus has replaced calcineurin-based immunosuppression in renal and cardiac transplant recipients in some centers without any increase in the incidence of PTLD, and there is emerging evidence of benefit in PTLD because of preservation of T-regulatory cell function [226, 227]. Steroid intensification for rejection in pediatric SOT with PTLD was identified in a multivariate analysis [228].

The St. Jude staging and the recently introduced revised classification system, the International Paediatric Non-Hodgkin Lymphoma Staging System (IPNHLSS), are used for staging but have limited value in PTLD owing to the high predilection for extranodal involvement. Multiple (>2) sites of disease or CNS involvement are associated with poorer prognosis [225]. PTLD associated with primary EBV infection appears to have a superior prognosis [225].

13.5.3 The Epstein-Barr Virus

EBV is a double-stranded DNA virus containing 85 genes surrounded by a lipid envelope with immunogenic surface glycoproteins. Humans are the only known host of EBV and once infected harbor the virus lifelong. EBV infections usually originate in the oropharynx with the infection of mucosal cell by EBV-contaminated saliva, but

EBV infection can also be acquired from passenger lymphocytes in organ or HSCT transplants. EBV is released from infected mucosal cells or B-lymphocytes during the lytic phase and infects additional B-lymphocytes that disseminate throughout the body including the liver, spleen, bone marrow, and lymph nodes and persist lifelong.

At the time of primary EBV seroconversion, infected B-lymphocytes express viral antigens on their cell membranes which lead to a cytotoxic T-lymphocyte (CTL) response in the immunocompetent host [217]. After an initial expansion of $CD8^+$ CTL specific to viral lytic antigens, $CD8^+$ effector/memory T-lymphocytes against latent viral antigens develop and persist to provide lifelong immunosurveillance against EBV-induced B-lymphoproliferation. In the presence of EBV-specific CTL, the expression of viral antigens in infected B-cells is downregulated in a series of latent stages which are summarized. Viral antigens are expressed during periods of reactivation and replication, which in turn leads to expansion of EBV CTL that control the infection.

In immunosuppressed patients without the ability to mount a CTL response, there is no need to downregulate the expression of viral antigens, and EBV-transformed B-lymphocytes can proliferate uncontrollably leading to PTLD [229]. PTLD is characterized by the expression of the highly immunogenic antigens including EBNA1, 2, and 3 and LMP 1 and 2 associated with latency III [230].

13.5.4 Monitoring of EBV Viral Load

It is the standard of care to monitor EBV viral loads by quantitative polymerase chain reactions (PCR) in both HSCT and SOT recipients in the early posttransplant phase. Elevated EBV viral loads are a poor predictor of EBV-positive PTLD but highly sensitive in identifying patients at risk for PTLD [231]. Lack of EBV-specific cytotoxic T-lymphocytes in the presence of elevated EBV viral loads may add specificity, but testing is not routinely available [232]. There is no standardization of EBV PCR. Both plasma- or cell-based assays are being used, and the results between laboratories cannot be correlated. Plasma-based assays appear to be better in distinguishing untreated EBV+ PTLD from EBV+ PTLD in remission and EBV- lymphoma [233].

13.5.5 Pathology and Molecular Biology of Posttransplant Lymphoproliferative Disease

PTLD was first classified by a Society for Hematopathology workshop in 1997 which was included in a 2001 World Health Organization (WHO) classification of lymphomas and leukemias [142, 234]. PTLD is divided into four subtypes:

- **Early lesions** are also defined as mononucleosis like and are always EBV positive.
- **Polymorphic PTLD** is characterized by a mixture of B-lymphocytes with infiltrating T-lymphocytes without necrosis.
- The group of **monomorphic PTLD** includes all NHL histologies. The vast majority of monomorphic PTLD cases are diffuse large B-cell lymphomas (DLBCL). The second most common type is BL or Burkitt-like. T-cell neoplasms are also included in this category but are extremely rare in childhood without any standardized treatment approach. They are usually EBV negative and associated with a poor prognosis [235]. Other rare monomorphic subtypes of PTLD are multiple myeloma or plasmacytoma.
- EBV is found in greater than 90% of childhood monomorphic PTLD but only in about 70% of adult cases. Polymorphic and monomorphic PTLD has been described simultaneously in the same patient [236]. Thus, histology of a single biopsied site may not be representative of the entire disease process. Approximately two-thirds of DLBCL PTLD cases have diffuse expression of CD20, while the remaining cases expressed only focal CD20 expression. Typically, CD10 and bcl-6 expressions are

absent but Mum-1 is positive in the majority of cases, which suggests the post-GC-derived B-cell as the cell of origin [237].

- Classic Hodgkin lymphoma-like PTLD is rarely seen in childhood, has a late onset, but is generally EBV positive. It has also been described as a late-onset variant of polymorphic B-cell PTLD by some investigators [238].

Monoclonality, as defined by immunoglobulin gene rearrangements, occurs with a greater frequency in the monomorphic subtype of PTLD compared with the polymorphic subtype and shows that most cases of monomorphic PTLD have been differentiated past the germinal center stage [237]. There are no characteristic cytogenetic abnormalities in most subtypes of PTLD. In BL PTLD, 100% of cases have translocations involving the c-myc genes on 8q24 [239]. In DLBCL PTLD, rearrangements of the IgH locus have been reported [237].

Gene expression profiles of PTLD in small case series have found that PTLD clusters separately from DLBCL in nonimmunosuppressed patients and expression patterns can distinguish EBV-positive from EBV-negative disease [240]. In addition, gene expression profiling has been explored for predicting which EBV converters will progress to PTLD [241]. Further investigation is necessary to establish the value of gene profiling in the diagnosis and prognosis of this disease.

13.5.6 Treatment of PTLD

13.5.6.1 Reduction of Immunosuppression

First-line therapy in SOT recipients consists in reduction of immunosuppression to stimulate autologous EBV-specific cytotoxic T-cell activity [225]. In 20–80% of SOT recipients, reduction of immunosuppression leads to disease control, especially in localized PTLD and early lesions. Patients with polymorphic PTLD have a higher response rate than patients with monomorphic histology [225]. In HSCT recipients, reduction in immunosuppressive therapy may result in improvement of EBV viral load levels, but is usually not sufficient in treating PTLD after HSCT because it usually occurs before T-cell engraftment [242]. In addition, it increases the risk of graft-versus-host disease (GvHD).

13.5.6.2 Antiviral Therapy

Antiviral agents such as acyclovir or ganciclovir are being in the prophylaxis of viral infections or reactivation in the posttransplant period, but a prospective trial using ganciclovir prophylaxis failed to influence EBV load or the incidence of PTLD in SOT recipients [243]. Ganciclovir requires viral thymidine kinase, physiologically only expressed during the lytic phase, for conversion to its active metabolite. It is thus unlikely that ganciclovir has any efficacy in PTLD arising from latency stages unless expression of viral thymidine kinase can be induced. There is evidence that histone deacetylase inhibitors can stimulate expression of lytic-phase genes and sensitize cells to ganciclovir [244]. A phase I/II of the combination of arginine butyrate with ganciclovir enrolled 15 patients with EBV-associated malignancies that had failed prior therapy and showed four complete responses and six partial responses [245].

13.5.6.3 Anti-CD20 Antibody Therapy and Chemotherapy

PTLD has been treated with cytotoxic chemotherapy to achieve disease control while maintaining an immunosuppressive state to protect the allograft. In adult patients with PTLD, the use of conventionally dosed chemotherapy has been complicated by toxicity and infection, with regimen-related mortality as high as 50% [246]. This prompted a pilot study of a low-dose chemotherapy regimen with cyclophosphamide and prednisone (CP) for children with PTLD and resulted in a 77% CR rate. The 2-year failure-free survival, defined as alive, in continuous CR, and with original functioning allograft, was 67% (Table 13.6) [247].

Rituximab, a humanized chimeric monoclonal antibody against CD20 antibody, induces apoptosis in CD20-positive B-lymphocytes. In HSCT

Table 13.6 Summary of published treatment of PTLD in SOT with chemotherapy and rituximab

Treatment	Patient number (*n*)	Age	Pathology	EBV status	Outcome	Reference
Low-dose cyclophosphamide, prednisone	30	4.9 (0.8–17.2)	NA	Positive	2-year FFS: 69% 2-year OS: 73%	Gross, 2005 [247]
Rituximab	40	Pediatric	Polymorphic (27) DLBCL (9) BL (1) HD-like (1) Other high-grade B-cell lymphoma (1)	Positive (38/40)	CR 75%	Webber, 2005 [248]
Low-dose cyclophosphamide, prednisone, rituximab	55	4.9 (0.9–17.2)		Positive	2-year EFS 71% 2-year OS: 83%	Gross, 2012 [236]
Rituximab induction Good responders: rituximab Poor responders: mCOMP	49	9.8 (0.8–17.4)	Polymorphic (12) DLBCL (24 BL (7) Other high-grade B-cell lymphoma (6)	Positive (44/49)	2-year EFS: 67% 2-year OS: 86%	Maecker-Kohlhoff, 2014 [249]

recipients with rising EBV viral load, preemptive therapy with the anti-CD20 monoclonal antibody rituximab has been successful in reducing B-cell proliferation in up to 93% of patients [250, 251]. The efficacy of preemptive rituximab in response to rising EBV PCR's in SOT recipients has not been shown.

Rituximab is also used in the treatment of patients with established PTLD. The European Group for Blood and Bone Marrow Transplantation reported an event-free survival of 70% in children post-HSCT treated with rituximab as single agent [217]. In contrast, single-agent rituximab is only efficacious in about 50% of PTLD after SOT. Reported response rates range from 44.2 to 69% [221, 252]. Results from the German Ped-PTLD 2005 trial showed a good response rate of 64% to three doses of rituximab. In the group of good responders, 84% (53% of the entire study population) remained in remission after an additional three doses of rituximab [249]. Patients who had a poor response to three doses of rituximab received chemotherapy of moderate intensity with vincristine, prednisone, cyclophosphamide, and methotrexate (mCOMP), and only 66% (20% of the total study population) achieved a CR [249].

The COG phase II study ANHL0221 used the low-dose CP chemotherapy backbone in combination with rituximab with a 72% early response rate [236]. The 2-year event-free survival was 71%, and the 2-year overall survival was 83%. In summary, rituximab as single agent is efficacious in about 50% of patients. The addition of chemotherapy used either concurrently or sequentially leads to cure in an additional 20%. Since overall cure rates of PTLD in childhood are only around 70%, more efficacious strategies for treatment are needed.

13.5.6.4 Cellular Therapy

Donor lymphocyte infusions (DLI) were first piloted in the 1990s and showed durable completed remission in five HSCT patients [253]. However, DLI can be complicated by acute and chronic GvHD and only efficacious in 41% patients [251, 254, 255]. This led to the production of EBV-specific cytotoxic T-lymphocytes (CTL) [254]. B-lymphocytes isolated from peripheral blood mononuclear cells and infected with a laboratory strain of EBV are grown into EBV+ lymphoblastoid cell lines (LCL) over 4–6 weeks. Some laboratories additionally transfect LCLs with LMP-1 and LMP-2 to increase immunogenicity [254]. LCLs are then co-cultured with PBMC of the same donor to produce and expand a population of EBV-specific CTLs in the presence of interleukin-2 (IL-2) over a 4-week span. This leads to a 10-to-12-week delay in availability for a patient-specific product [254]. A rapid manufacturing practice using dendritic cells expressing immunogenic EBV genes (LMP1, LMP2) as antigen-expressing cells can reduce manufacturing time to 2–3 weeks [256].

Donor-derived EBV CTLs have been used prophylactically in HSCT recipients with EBV viremia or therapeutically in HSCT-related PTLD. They were effective in the prevention of PTLD in 101 patients with EBV viremia, and 24 out of 27 patients with established PTLD achieved a CR (Table 13.7) [254]. The treatment of PTLD in SOT is more complicated because PTLD usually arises from recipient cells and not donor lymphocytes, recipient and transplant organs are often not HLA matched, and donor-derived PBMCs are not available in cadaver transplants to produce EBV CTLs [221]. The production of autologous CTLs is complicated by the ongoing immunosuppression of the recipient as well as the delay in treatment caused by the production time of EBV CTLs. However, there are some successful reports [254].

Third-party EBV CTLs produced from healthy EBV-seropositive donors can be cryopreserved in banks that cover the most common HLA types [254, 256, 259, 262, 263]. Since HLA matching at 1–2 loci between CTL product and recipient is sufficient as long as the EBV activity is transmitted through shared alleles, a bank of approximately 30 donors with varied HLA types covers 80–90% of the population [259, 264, 265]. A multicenter phase II study of third-party EBV CTLs in 33 SOT and HSCT recipients including 11 children reported an overall response rate of 52% [257]. Other groups have shown overall responses from 67 to 80% [259, 262, 265].

The Children's Oncology Group is currently conducting a phase II trial using third-party EBV CTLs. Drawing from the German Ped-PTLD 2005 experience, patients receive induction with three doses of rituximab. Patients that do not achieve a complete response to induction are assigned to receive EBV CTLs. Depending on the response, patients are eligible to receive two to four doses of EBV CTLs. This is the first multicenter cooperative group trial using cellular therapy.

13.5.6.5 Other Emergent Treatments

Additional strategies to augment cellular therapy in EBV+ PTLD are being investigated. The bisphosphonate pamidronate leads to intracellular accumulation of isopentenyl pyrophosphate and activates natural killer cells able to induce apoptosis in EBV-infected B-cells [266]. In mice with EBV lymphoproliferative disease, intraperitoneal pamidronate induced tumor regression and prolonged survival [266].

Cellular therapy in PTLD is complicated by the need of immunosuppression for prevention of graft rejection or GvHD, which also affects virus-specific T-cells. Genetically engineered EBV CTLs resistant to calcineurin inhibitors can eradicate EBV+ B-cell lymphoma in mice with therapeutic tacrolimus levels [267]. The use of these modified cells could advance the treatment of PTLD without the need for reduction of immunosuppression, decreasing the risk of graft rejection or GvHD, but these modified cells have not been used in human trials thus decreasing the need for decreased immunosuppression.

Table 13.7 EBV-specific CTL in the treatment of PTLD

Donor source	Group	Number of patients	Type of transplant	Outcome	Reference
Third party	UK	2007	HSCT, SOT	CR: 52%	Haque, 2007 [257]
Donor	MSKCC	14	HSCT	CR: 64.3%	Doubrovina, 2012 [258]
Third party	MSKCC	5	HSCT	CR:80%	Doubrovina, 2012 [258]
Third party	Baylor	9	HSCT	CR: 67%	Leen, 2013 [259]
Third party	UK	11	SOT, HSCT	CR: 82%	Vickers, 2014 [260]
Donor	Baylor	13	HSCT	CR: 84.6	Bollard, 2016 [261]

13.6 Conclusion

PTLD, the most common form of childhood lymphoproliferation, is a heterogeneous disease ranging from polymorphic uncontrolled lymphoproliferation to monoclonal lymphomas. EBV and immunological defects are the main drivers of disease. Reduction of immunosuppression can lead to resolution by restoring T-cell function but is often not feasible due to risk of graft rejection. Rituximab is highly efficacious in preventing PTLD in HSCT and has response rates of 70–80% in HSCT and around 50% in SOT patients with established PTLD. EFS around 70% have been reported in combination low-dose chemotherapy with rituximab in SOT recipients. The combination of cellular therapy with rituximab may further improve the outcome of children with PTLD while avoiding the use of cytotoxic chemotherapy.

References

1. Reiter A. Diagnosis and treatment of childhood non-hodgkin lymphoma. Hematology Am Soc Hematol Educ Program. 2007;2007:285–96.
2. Burkhardt B, et al. The impact of age and gender on biology, clinical features and treatment outcome of non-Hodgkin lymphoma in childhood and adolescence. Br J Haematol. 2005;131(1):39–49.
3. Worch J, Rohde M, Burkhardt B. Mature B-cell lymphoma and leukemia in children and adolescents—review of standard chemotherapy regimen and perspectives. Pediatr Hematol Oncol. 2013;30(6):465–83.
4. Lange J, Burkhardt B. Treatment of adolescents with aggressive B-cell malignancies: the pediatric experience. Curr Hematol Malig Rep. 2013;8(3):226–35.
5. Sandlund JT, Downing JR, Crist WM. Non-Hodgkin's lymphoma in childhood. N Engl J Med. 1996;334(19):1238–48.
6. Burkhardt B, et al. Non-Hodgkin's lymphoma in adolescents: experiences in 378 adolescent NHL patients treated according to pediatric NHL-BFM protocols. Leukemia. 2011;25(1):153–60.
7. Salzburg J, et al. Prevalence, clinical pattern, and outcome of CNS involvement in childhood and adolescent non-Hodgkin's lymphoma differ by non-Hodgkin's lymphoma subtype: a Berlin-Frankfurt-Munster Group report. J Clin Oncol. 2007;25(25):3915–22.
8. Cairo MS, et al. Advanced stage, increased lactate dehydrogenase, and primary site, but not adolescent age (>/= 15 years), are associated with an increased risk of treatment failure in children and adolescents with mature B-cell non-Hodgkin's lymphoma: results of the FAB LMB 96 study. J Clin Oncol. 2012;30(4):387–93.
9. Abla O, et al. Primary CNS lymphoma in children and adolescents: a descriptive analysis from the International Primary CNS Lymphoma Collaborative Group (IPCG). Clin Cancer Res. 2011;17(2):346–52.
10. Thorer H, et al. Primary central nervous system lymphoma in children and adolescents: low relapse rate after treatment according to Non-Hodgkin-Lymphoma Berlin-Frankfurt-Munster protocols for systemic lymphoma. Haematologica. 2014;99(11):e238–41.
11. Swerdlow SH, et al., editors. WHO classification of tumours of haematopoietic and lymphoid tissue. World Health Organization classification of tumours. Lyon: IARC; 2008.
12. Swerdlow SH, et al. The 2016 revision of the World Health Organization classification of lymphoid neoplasms. Blood. 2016;127(20):2375–90.
13. A clinical evaluation of the International Lymphoma Study Group classification of non-Hodgkin's lymphoma. The Non-Hodgkin's Lymphoma Classification Project. Blood. 1997;89(11):3909–18.
14. Hummel M, et al. A biologic definition of Burkitt's lymphoma from transcriptional and genomic profiling. N Engl J Med. 2006;354(23):2419–30.
15. Dave SS, et al. Molecular diagnosis of Burkitt's lymphoma. N Engl J Med. 2006;354(23):2431–42.
16. Mbulaiteye SM, et al. Pediatric, elderly, and emerging adult-onset peaks in Burkitt's lymphoma incidence diagnosed in four continents, excluding Africa. Am J Hematol. 2012;87(6):573–8.
17. Boerma EG, et al. Gender and age-related differences in Burkitt lymphoma—epidemiological and clinical data from The Netherlands. Eur J Cancer. 2004;40(18):2781–7.
18. Molyneux EM, et al. Burkitt's lymphoma. Lancet. 2012;379(9822):1234–44.
19. Schmitz R, et al. Burkitt lymphoma pathogenesis and therapeutic targets from structural and functional genomics. Nature. 2012;490(7418):116–20.
20. Richter J, et al. Recurrent mutation of the ID3 gene in Burkitt lymphoma identified by integrated genome, exome and transcriptome sequencing. Nat Genet. 2012;44(12):1316–20.
21. Love C, et al. The genetic landscape of mutations in Burkitt lymphoma. Nat Genet. 2012;44(12):1321–5.
22. Campo E. New pathogenic mechanisms in Burkitt lymphoma. Nat Genet. 2012;44(12):1288–9.
23. Rohde M, et al. Relevance of ID3-TCF3-CCND3 pathway mutations in pediatric aggressive B-cell lymphoma treated according to the non-Hodgkin

Lymphoma Berlin-Frankfurt-Munster protocols. Haematologica. 2017;102(6):1091–8.
24. Rosenwald A, Staudt LM. Gene expression profiling of diffuse large B-cell lymphoma. Leuk Lymphoma. 2003;44(Suppl 3):S41–7.
25. Alizadeh AA, et al. Distinct types of diffuse large B-cell lymphoma identified by gene expression profiling. Nature. 2000;403(6769):503–11.
26. Rosenwald A, et al. The use of molecular profiling to predict survival after chemotherapy for diffuse large-B-cell lymphoma. N Engl J Med. 2002;346(25):1937–47.
27. Hans CP, et al. Confirmation of the molecular classification of diffuse large B-cell lymphoma by immunohistochemistry using a tissue microarray. Blood. 2004;103(1):275–82.
28. Choi WW, et al. A new immunostain algorithm classifies diffuse large B-cell lymphoma into molecular subtypes with high accuracy. Clin Cancer Res. 2009;15(17):5494–502.
29. Oschlies I, et al. Diffuse large B-cell lymphoma in pediatric patients belongs predominantly to the germinal-center type B-cell lymphomas: a clinicopathologic analysis of cases included in the German BFM (Berlin-Frankfurt-Munster) Multicenter Trial. Blood. 2006;107(10):4047–52.
30. Szczepanowski M, et al. Cell-of-origin classification by gene expression and MYC-rearrangements in diffuse large B-cell lymphoma of children and adolescents. Br J Haematol. 2017;179(1):116–9.
31. Salaverria I, et al. Translocations activating IRF4 identify a subtype of germinal center-derived B-cell lymphoma affecting predominantly children and young adults. Blood. 2011;118(1):139–47.
32. Miles RR, et al. Pediatric diffuse large B-cell lymphoma demonstrates a high proliferation index, frequent c-Myc protein expression, and a high incidence of germinal center subtype: report of the French-American-British (FAB) international study group. Pediatr Blood Cancer. 2008;51(3): 369–74.
33. Murphy SB. Classification, staging and end results of treatment of childhood non-Hodgkin's lymphomas: dissimilarities from lymphomas in adults. Semin Oncol. 1980;7(3):332–9.
34. Rosolen A, et al. Revised international pediatric non-Hodgkin lymphoma staging system. J Clin Oncol. 2015;33(18):2112–8.
35. Woessmann W, et al. The impact of the methotrexate administration schedule and dose in the treatment of children and adolescents with B-cell neoplasms: a report of the BFM Group Study NHL-BFM95. Blood. 2005;105(3):948–58.
36. Reiter A, et al. Improved treatment results in childhood B-cell neoplasms with tailored intensification of therapy: a report of the Berlin-Frankfurt-Munster Group Trial NHL-BFM 90. Blood. 1999;94(10):3294–306.
37. Fujita N, et al. Results of the Japan Association of Childhood Leukemia Study (JACLS) NHL-98 protocol for the treatment of B-cell non-Hodgkin lymphoma and mature B-cell acute lymphoblastic leukemia in childhood. Leuk Lymphoma. 2011;52(2):223–9.
38. Patte C, et al. The Societe Francaise d'Oncologie Pediatrique LMB89 protocol: highly effective multiagent chemotherapy tailored to the tumor burden and initial response in 561 unselected children with B-cell lymphomas and L3 leukemia. Blood. 2001;97(11):3370–9.
39. Patte C, et al. Results of the randomized international FAB/LMB96 trial for intermediate risk B-cell non-Hodgkin lymphoma in children and adolescents: it is possible to reduce treatment for the early responding patients. Blood. 2007;109(7):2773–80.
40. Cairo MS, et al. Results of a randomized international study of high-risk central nervous system B non-Hodgkin lymphoma and B acute lymphoblastic leukemia in children and adolescents. Blood. 2007;109(7):2736–43.
41. Pillon M, et al. Long-term results of the first Italian Association of Pediatric Hematology and Oncology protocol for the treatment of pediatric B-cell non-Hodgkin lymphoma (AIEOP LNH92). Cancer. 2004;101(2):385–94.
42. A predictive model for aggressive non-Hodgkin's lymphoma. The International Non-Hodgkin's Lymphoma Prognostic Factors Project. N Engl J Med. 1993;329(14):987–94.
43. Gerrard M, et al. Excellent survival following two courses of COPAD chemotherapy in children and adolescents with resected localized B-cell non-Hodgkin's lymphoma: results of the FAB/LMB 96 international study. Br J Haematol. 2008; 141(6):840–7.
44. Kikuchi A, et al. Outcome of childhood B-cell non-Hodgkin lymphoma and B-cell acute lymphoblastic leukemia treated with the Tokyo Children's Cancer Study Group NHL B9604 protocol. Leuk Lymphoma. 2008;49(4):757–62.
45. Jourdain A, et al. Outcome of and prognostic factors for relapse in children and adolescents with mature B-cell lymphoma and leukemia treated in three consecutive prospective "Lymphomes Malins B" protocols. A Societe Francaise des Cancers de l'Enfant study. Haematologica. 2015;100(6):810–7.
46. Anoop P, et al. Outcome of childhood relapsed or refractory mature B-cell non-Hodgkin lymphoma and acute lymphoblastic leukemia. Leuk Lymphoma. 2012;53(10):1882–8.
47. Gross TG, et al. Hematopoietic stem cell transplantation for refractory or recurrent non-Hodgkin lymphoma in children and adolescents. Biol Blood Marrow Transplant. 2010;16(2):223–30.
48. Fujita N, et al. The role of hematopoietic stem cell transplantation with relapsed or primary refractory childhood B-cell non-Hodgkin lymphoma and mature B-cell leukemia: a retrospective analysis of enrolled cases in Japan. Pediatr Blood Cancer. 2008;51(2):188–92.

49. Woessmann W, Reiter A. Re-induction approaches to relapsed/refractory childhood and adolescent non Hodgkin¢s lymphoma: BFM perspective. Br J Haematol. 2012;159(Suppl. 1):Abstract 71.
50. Griffin TC, et al. A study of rituximab and ifosfamide, carboplatin, and etoposide chemotherapy in children with recurrent/refractory B-cell (CD20+) non-Hodgkin lymphoma and mature B-cell acute lymphoblastic leukemia: a report from the Children's Oncology Group. Pediatr Blood Cancer. 2009;52(2):177–81.
51. Samochatova EV, et al. Therapy of advanced-stage mature B-cell lymphoma and leukemia in children and adolescents with rituximab and reduced intensity induction chemotherapy (B-NHL 2004M protocol): the results of a multicenter study. J Pediatr Hematol Oncol. 2014;36(5):395–401.
52. Meinhardt A, et al. Phase II window study on rituximab in newly diagnosed pediatric mature B-cell non-Hodgkin's lymphoma and Burkitt leukemia. J Clin Oncol. 2010;28(19):3115–21.
53. Lisfeld J, et al. Phase II window study on rituximab in newly diagnosed pediatric mature B-cell non-Hodgkin's lymphoma and Burkitt leukemia: dose-escalation does not increase the response rate. Br J Haematol. 2012;112(Suppl. 2012):Abstract 6.
54. Cairo M, et al. Safety, kinetics, and outcome following rituximab (R) in combination with FAB chemotherapy in children and adolescents (C+A) with stage III/IV (Group B) and BM+/CNS+ (Group C) mature B-NHL: a Children's Oncology Group report. JCO. 2010;28(15s):9536.
55. Frazer K, et al. Efficacy of rituximab plus FAB group C chemotherapy without CNS radiation in CNS-positive pediatric Burkitt lymphoma/leukemia: a report from the Children's Oncology Group. JCO. 2012;30(15_suppl):9501.
56. Goldman S, et al. Preliminary results of the addition of Rasburicase to the reduction cycle and rituximab to the induction and consolidation cycles of FAB Group C Chemotherapy in Children and Adolescents with Advanced Stage (Bone Marrow ±CNS) Mature B-Cell Non-Hodgkin Lymphoma (B-NHL): a Children's Oncology Group report. Blood. 2009;114:104.
57. Goldman S, et al. The efficacy of rasburicase and rituximab combined with FAB chemotherapy in children and adolescents with newly diagnosed stage III/IV, BM+ and CNS+ Mature B-NHL: a Children's Oncology Group Report. Blood. 2011;118:2702.
58. Goldman S, et al. Rituximab with chemotherapy in children and adolescents with central nervous system and/or bone marrow-positive Burkitt lymphoma/leukaemia: a Children's Oncology Group Report. Br J Haematol. 2014;167(3):394–401.
59. Goldman S, et al. Rituximab and FAB/LMB 96 chemotherapy in children with Stage III/IV B-cell non-Hodgkin lymphoma: a Children's Oncology Group report. Leukemia. 2013;27(5):1174–7.
60. Barth MJ, et al. Rituximab pharmacokinetics in children and adolescents with de novo intermediate and advanced mature B-cell lymphoma/leukaemia: a Children's Oncology Group report. Br J Haematol. 2013;162(5):678–83.
61. Worch J, Makarova O, Burkhardt B. Immunreconstitution and infectious complications after rituximab treatment in children and adolescents: what do we know and what can we learn from adults? Cancers (Basel). 2015;7(1):305–28.
62. Schmidt E, Burkhardt B. Lymphoblastic lymphoma in childhood and adolescence. Pediatr Hematol Oncol. 2013;30(6):484–508.
63. Oschlies I, et al. Clinical, pathological and genetic features of primary mediastinal large B-cell lymphomas and mediastinal gray zone lymphomas in children. Haematologica. 2011;96(2):262–8.
64. Ducassou S, et al. Clinical presentation, evolution, and prognosis of precursor B-cell lymphoblastic lymphoma in trials LMT96, EORTC 58881, and EORTC 58951. Br J Haematol. 2011;152(4):441–51.
65. Neth O, et al. Precursor B-cell lymphoblastic lymphoma in childhood and adolescence: clinical features, treatment, and results in trials NHL-BFM 86 and 90. Med Pediatr Oncol. 2000;35(1):20–7.
66. Bene MC, et al. Proposals for the immunological classification of acute leukemias. European Group for the Immunological Characterization of Leukemias (EGIL). Leukemia. 1995;9(10):1783–6.
67. Oschlies I, et al. Diagnosis and immunophenotype of 188 pediatric lymphoblastic lymphomas treated within a randomized prospective trial: experiences and preliminary recommendations from the European childhood lymphoma pathology panel. Am J Surg Pathol. 2011;35(6):836–44.
68. Patel JL, et al. The immunophenotype of T-lymphoblastic lymphoma in children and adolescents: a Children's Oncology Group report. Br J Haematol. 2012;159(4):454–61.
69. Smock KJ, et al. Characterization of childhood precursor T-lymphoblastic lymphoma by immunophenotyping and fluorescent in situ hybridization: a report from the Children's Oncology Group. Pediatr Blood Cancer. 2008;51(4):489–94.
70. Coustan-Smith E, et al. Early T-cell precursor leukaemia: a subtype of very high-risk acute lymphoblastic leukaemia. Lancet Oncol. 2009;10(2): 147–56.
71. You MJ, Medeiros LJ, Hsi ED. T-lymphoblastic leukemia/lymphoma. Am J Clin Pathol. 2015;144(3):411–22.
72. Haydu JE, Ferrando AA. Early T-cell precursor acute lymphoblastic leukaemia. Curr Opin Hematol. 2013;20(4):369–73.
73. Patrick K, et al. Outcome for children and young people with Early T-cell precursor acute lymphoblastic leukaemia treated on a contemporary protocol, UKALL 2003. Br J Haematol. 2014;166(3): 421–4.
74. Burkhardt B, et al. Current status and future directions of T-lymphoblastic lymphoma in children and adolescents. Br J Haematol. 2016;173(4):545–59.

75. Tubergen DG, et al. Comparison of treatment regimens for pediatric lymphoblastic non-Hodgkin's lymphoma: a Childrens Cancer Group study. J Clin Oncol. 1995;13(6):1368–76.
76. Abromowitch M, et al. High-dose methotrexate and early intensification of therapy do not improve 3 year EFS in children and adolescents with disseminated lymphoblastic lymphoma. Results of the randomized arms of COG A5971. Blood. 2008;112:3610.
77. Uyttebroeck A, et al. Treatment of childhood T-cell lymphoblastic lymphoma according to the strategy for acute lymphoblastic leukaemia, without radiotherapy: long term results of the EORTC CLG 58881 trial. Eur J Cancer. 2008;44(6):840–6.
78. Reiter A, et al. Results of the European intergroup trial EURO-LB02 on lymphoblastic lymphoma (LBL) in children/adolescents. Br J Haematol. 2012;159(Suppl. 1):38.
79. Burkhardt B. Paediatric lymphoblastic T-cell leukaemia and lymphoma: one or two diseases? Br J Haematol. 2010;149(5):653–68.
80. Basso K, et al. T-cell lymphoblastic lymphoma shows differences and similarities with T-cell acute lymphoblastic leukemia by genomic and gene expression analyses. Genes Chromosomes Cancer. 2011;50(12):1063–75.
81. Uyttebroeck A, et al. Is there a difference in childhood T-cell acute lymphoblastic leukaemia and T-cell lymphoblastic lymphoma? Leuk Lymphoma. 2007;48(9):1745–54.
82. Burkhardt B, et al. Loss of heterozygosity on chromosome 6q14-q24 is associated with poor outcome in children and adolescents with T-cell lymphoblastic lymphoma. Leukemia. 2006;20(8):1422–9.
83. Lones MA, et al. Chromosome abnormalities in advanced stage lymphoblastic lymphoma of children and adolescents: a report from CCG-E08. Cancer Genet Cytogenet. 2007;172(1):1–11.
84. Breit S, et al. Activating NOTCH1 mutations predict favorable early treatment response and long term outcome in child-hood precursor T-cell lymphoblastic leukemia. Blood. 2006;108(4):1151–7.
85. Kox C, et al. The favorable effect of activating NOTCH1 receptor mutations on long-term outcome in T-ALL patients treated on the ALL-BFM 2000 protocol can be separated from FBXW7 loss of function. Leukemia. 2010;24(12):2005–13.
86. Bonn BR, et al. Incidence and prognostic relevance of genetic variations in T-cell lymphoblastic lymphoma in childhood and adolescence. Blood. 2013;121(16):3153–60.
87. Callens C, et al. Clinical impact of NOTCH1 and/or FBXW7 mutations, FLASH deletion, and TCR status in pediatric T-cell lymphoblastic lymphoma. J Clin Oncol. 2012;30(16):1966–73.
88. Park MJ, et al. FBXW7 and NOTCH1 mutations in childhood T cell acute lymphoblastic leukaemia and T cell non-Hodgkin lymphoma. Br J Haematol. 2009;145(2):198–206.
89. Baleydier F, et al. T cell receptor genotyping and HOXA/TLX1 expression define three T lymphoblastic lymphoma subsets which might affect clinical outcome. Clin Cancer Res. 2008;14(3):692–700.
90. Burkhardt B, et al. Pediatric precursor T lymphoblastic leukemia and lymphoblastic lymphoma: differences in the common regions with loss of heterozygosity at chromosome 6q and their prognostic impact. Leuk Lymphoma. 2008;49(3):451–61.
91. Balbach ST, et al. Proposal of a genetic classifier for risk group stratification in pediatric T-cell lymphoblastic lymphoma reveals differences from adult T-cell lymphoblastic leukemia. Leukemia. 2016;30(4):970–3.
92. Song MS, Salmena L, Pandolfi PP. The functions and regulation of the PTEN tumour suppressor. Nat Rev Mol Cell Biol. 2012;13(5):283–96.
93. Hales EC, Taub JW, Matherly LH. New insights into Notch1 regulation of the PI3K-AKT-mTOR1 signaling axis: targeted therapy of gamma-secretase inhibitor resistant T-cell acute lymphoblastic leukemia. Cell Signal. 2014;26(1):149–61.
94. Bandapalli OR, et al. NOTCH1 activation clinically antagonizes the unfavorable effect of PTEN inactivation in BFM-treated children with precursor T-cell acute lymphoblastic leukemia. Haematologica. 2013;98(6):928–36.
95. Zuurbier L, et al. NOTCH1 and/or FBXW7 mutations predict for initial good prednisone response but not for improved outcome in pediatric T-cell acute lymphoblastic leukemia patients treated on DCOG or COALL protocols. Leukemia. 2010;24(12):2014–22.
96. Gutierrez A, et al. Absence of biallelic TCRgamma deletion predicts early treatment failure in pediatric T-cell acute lymphoblastic leukemia. J Clin Oncol. 2010;28(24):3816–23.
97. Yang YL, et al. Absence of biallelic TCRgamma deletion predicts induction failure and poorer outcomes in childhood T-cell acute lymphoblastic leukemia. Pediatr Blood Cancer. 2012;58(6):846–51.
98. Stark B, et al. Bone marrow minimal disseminated disease (MDD) and minimal residual disease (MRD) in childhood T-cell lymphoblastic lymphoma stage III, detected by flow cytometry (FC) and real-time quantitative polymerase chain reaction (RQ-PCR). Pediatr Blood Cancer. 2009;52(1):20–5.
99. Coustan-Smith E, et al. Minimal disseminated disease in childhood T-cell lymphoblastic lymphoma: a report from the Children's Oncology Group. J Clin Oncol. 2009;27(21):3533–9.
100. Mussolin L, et al. Detection and role of minimal disseminated disease in children with lymphoblastic lymphoma: the AIEOP experience. Pediatr Blood Cancer. 2015;62(11):1906–13.
101. Esteller M. CpG island hypermethylation and tumor suppressor genes: a booming present, a brighter future. Oncogene. 2002;21(35):5427–40.

102. Roman-Gomez J, et al. Poor prognosis in acute lymphoblastic leukemia may relate to promoter hypermethylation of cancer-related genes. Leuk Lymphoma. 2007;48(7):1269–82.
103. Bardi E, et al. Value of FDG-PET/CT examinations in different cancers of children, focusing on lymphomas. Pathol Oncol Res. 2014;20(1):139–43.
104. Nakatani K, et al. Roles and limitations of FDG PET in pediatric non-Hodgkin lymphoma. Clin Nucl Med. 2012;37(7):656–62.
105. Riad R, et al. Role of PET/CT in malignant pediatric lymphoma. Eur J Nucl Med Mol Imaging. 2010;37(2):319–29.
106. Riad R, et al. False-positive F-18 FDG uptake in PET/CT studies in pediatric patients with abdominal Burkitt's lymphoma. Nucl Med Commun. 2010;31(3):232–8.
107. Sioka C. The utility of FDG PET in diagnosis and follow-up of lymphoma in childhood. Eur J Pediatr. 2013;172(6):733–8.
108. Patte C, et al. Results of the LMT81 protocol, a modified LSA2L2 protocol with high dose methotrexate, on 84 children with non-B-cell (lymphoblastic) lymphoma. Med Pediatr Oncol. 1992;20(2):105–13.
109. Amylon MD, et al. Intensive high-dose asparaginase consolidation improves survival for pediatric patients with T cell acute lymphoblastic leukemia and advanced stage lymphoblastic lymphoma: a Pediatric Oncology Group study. Leukemia. 1999;13(3):335–42.
110. Reiter A, et al. Intensive ALL-type therapy without local radiotherapy provides a 90% event-free survival for children with T-cell lymphoblastic lymphoma: a BFM group report. Blood. 2000;95(2):416–21.
111. Burkhardt B, et al. Impact of cranial radiotherapy on central nervous system prophylaxis in children and adolescents with central nervous system-negative stage III or IV lymphoblastic lymphoma. J Clin Oncol. 2006;24(3):491–9.
112. Abromowitch M, et al. Shortened intensified multi-agent chemotherapy and non-cross resistant maintenance therapy for advanced lymphoblastic lymphoma in children and adolescents: report from the Children's Oncology Group. Br J Haematol. 2008;143(2):261–7.
113. Pillon M, et al. Long-term results of AIEOP LNH-92 protocol for the treatment of pediatric lymphoblastic lymphoma: a report of the Italian Association of pediatric hematology and oncology. Pediatr Blood Cancer. 2009;53(6):953–9.
114. Sandlund JT, et al. Effective treatment of advanced-stage childhood lymphoblastic lymphoma without prophylactic cranial irradiation: results of St Jude NHL13 study. Leukemia. 2009;23(6):1127–30.
115. Asselin BL, et al. Effectiveness of high-dose methotrexate in T-cell lymphoblastic leukemia and advanced-stage lymphoblastic lymphoma: a randomized study by the Children's Oncology Group (POG 9404). Blood. 2011;118(4):874–83.
116. Termuhlen AM, et al. Outcome of newly diagnosed children and adolescents with localized lymphoblastic lymphoma treated on Children's Oncology Group trial A5971: a report from the Children's Oncology Group. Pediatr Blood Cancer. 2012;59(7):1229–33.
117. Uyttebroeck A, et al. Dexamethasone (DEX) versus prednisone (PRED) in T-cell non Hodgkin lymphoma (T-NHL): results of the randomized phase III trial 58951 of the EORTC Children Leukemia Group. Br J Haematol. 2012;159(Suppl. 1):37.
118. Bergeron C, et al. Treatment of childhood T-cell lymphoblastic lymphoma-long-term results of the SFOP LMT96 trial. Pediatr Blood Cancer. 2015;62(12):2150–6.
119. Wollner N, et al. Non-Hodgkin's lymphoma in children. A comparative study of two modalities of therapy. Cancer. 1976;37(1):123–34.
120. Wollner N, Exelby PR, Lieberman PH. Non-Hodgkin's lymphoma in children: a progress report on the original patients treated with the LSA2-L2 protocol. Cancer. 1979;44(6):1990–9.
121. Reiter A, et al. Non-Hodgkin's lymphomas of childhood and adolescence: results of a treatment stratified for biologic subtypes and stage—a report of the Berlin-Frankfurt-Munster Group. J Clin Oncol. 1995;13(2):359–72.
122. Jin L, et al. Clinical features and prognosis of children with lymphoblastic lymphoma. Zhonghua Zhong Liu Za Zhi. 2012;34(2):138–42.
123. Kobayashi R, et al. Inferior outcomes of stage III T lymphoblastic lymphoma relative to stage IV lymphoma and T-acute lymphoblastic leukemia: long-term comparison of outcomes in the JACLS NHL T-98 and ALL T-97 protocols. Int J Hematol. 2014;99(6):743–9.
124. Sun XF, et al. Intensive chemotherapy improved treatment outcome for Chinese children and adolescents with lymphoblastic lymphoma. Int J Clin Oncol. 2008;13(5):436–41.
125. Gao YJ, et al. Clinical outcome of childhood lymphoblastic lymphoma in Shanghai China 2001-2010. Pediatr Blood Cancer. 2014;61(4):659–63.
126. Sunami S, et al. Prognostic impact of intensified maintenance therapy on children with advanced lymphoblastic lymphoma: a report from the Japanese Pediatric Leukemia/Lymphoma Study Group ALB-NHL03 study. Pediatr Blood Cancer. 2016;63(3):451–7.
127. Termuhlen AM, et al. Disseminated lymphoblastic lymphoma in children and adolescents: results of the COG A5971 trial: a report from the Children's Oncology Group. Br J Haematol. 2013;162(6):792–801.
128. Sterba J, et al. Capizzi methotrexate with BFM backbone without craniospinal irradiation is effective treatment for pediatric lymphoblastic lymphoma: results from 5 countries with I-BFM LL 09 protocol. Br J Haematol. 2015;171(Suppl.1):33.
129. Mitsui T, et al. Retrospective analysis of relapsed or primary refractory childhood lymphoblas-

tic lymphoma in Japan. Pediatr Blood Cancer. 2009;52(5):591–5.
130. Gross TG, et al. Hematopoietic stem cell transplantation for refractory or recurrent non-hodgkin lymphoma in children and adolescents. Biol Blood Marrow Transplant. 2009;16(2):223–30.
131. Burkhardt B, et al. Outcome of adolescents with Non-Hodgkin Lymphoma in the BFM studies: Relevance of gender and histological subtype. In: 3rd International Symposium on Childhood, adolescent and young adult Non-Hodgkin's Lymphoma. Frankfurt, Germany: Hematology meeting reports; 2009.
132. Cohen MH, et al. FDA drug approval summary: nelarabine (Arranon) for the treatment of T-cell lymphoblastic leukemia/lymphoma. Oncologist. 2008;13(6):709–14.
133. Dunsmore KP, et al. Pilot study of nelarabine in combination with intensive chemotherapy in high-risk T-cell acute lymphoblastic leukemia: a report from the Children's Oncology Group. J Clin Oncol. 2012;30(22):2753–9.
134. Winter SS, et al. Safe integration of nelarabine into intensive chemotherapy in newly diagnosed T-cell acute lymphoblastic leukemia: Children's Oncology Group Study AALL0434. Pediatr Blood Cancer. 2015;62(7):1176–83.
135. Raetz EA, Teachey DT. T-cell acute lymphoblastic leukemia. Hematology Am Soc Hematol Educ Program. 2016;2016(1):580–8.
136. Pileri SA, et al. Anaplastic large cell lymphoma: update of findings. Leuk Lymphoma. 1995;18(1–2):17–25.
137. Stansfeld AG, et al. Updated Kiel classification for lymphomas. Lancet. 1988;1(8580):292–3.
138. Harris NL, et al. A revised European-American classification of lymphoid neoplasms: a proposal from the International Lymphoma Study Group. Blood. 1994;84(5):1361–92.
139. Morris SW, et al. Fusion of a kinase gene, ALK, to a nucleolar protein gene, NPM, in non-Hodgkin's lymphoma. Science. 1994;263(5151):1281–4.
140. Delsol G, Jaffe ES, Falini B, Gascoyne RD, Muller-Hermelink HK, Stein H, Campo E, Kinney MC. Anaplastic Large Cell Lymphoma (ALCL), ALK-positive. In: Swerdlow S, Campo E, Harris NL, editors. WHO classification of tumors of the hematopoietic and lymphoid tissues. 4th ed. Lyon, France: IARC; 2008. p. 312–6.
141. Oschlies I, et al. ALK-positive anaplastic large cell lymphoma limited to the skin: clinical, histopathological and molecular analysis of 6 pediatric cases. A report from the ALCL99 study. Haematologica. 2013;98(1):50–6.
142. Swerdlow SH, Webber SA, Chadburn A. Post-Transplant lymphoproliferative disorders. In: Swerdlow SH, Campo E, Lee Harris N, editors. WHO classification of tumors of the hematopoietic and lymphoid tissues. Lyon, France: International Agency for Research on Cancer (IARC); 2008. p. 343–51.
143. Adams SV, Newcomb PA, Shustov AR. Racial patterns of peripheral T-cell lymphoma incidence and survival in the United States. J Clin Oncol. 2016;34(9):963–71.
144. Mussolin L, et al. Prevalence and clinical implications of bone marrow involvement in pediatric anaplastic large cell lymphoma. Leukemia. 2005;19(9):1643–7.
145. Grewal JS, et al. Highly aggressive ALK-positive anaplastic large cell lymphoma with a leukemic phase and multi-organ involvement: a report of three cases and a review of the literature. Ann Hematol. 2007;86(7):499–508.
146. Kinney MC, et al. A small-cell-predominant variant of primary Ki-1 (CD30)+ T-cell lymphoma. Am J Surg Pathol. 1993;17(9):859–68.
147. Bayle C, et al. Leukaemic presentation of small cell variant anaplastic large cell lymphoma: report of four cases. Br J Haematol. 1999;104(4):680–8.
148. Onciu M, et al. ALK-positive anaplastic large cell lymphoma with leukemic peripheral blood involvement is a clinicopathologic entity with an unfavorable prognosis. Report of three cases and review of the literature. Am J Clin Pathol. 2003;120(4):617–25.
149. Spiegel A, et al. Paediatric anaplastic large cell lymphoma with leukaemic presentation in children: a report of nine French cases. Br J Haematol. 2014;165(4):545–51.
150. Malcolm TI, et al. Anaplastic large cell lymphoma arises in thymocytes and requires transient TCR expression for thymic egress. Nat Commun. 2016;7:10087.
151. Turner SD, et al. Anaplastic large cell lymphoma in paediatric and young adult patients. Br J Haematol. 2016;173(4):560–72.
152. Iwahara T, et al. Molecular characterization of ALK, a receptor tyrosine kinase expressed specifically in the nervous system. Oncogene. 1997;14(4):439–49.
153. Borer RA, et al. Major nucleolar proteins shuttle between nucleus and cytoplasm. Cell. 1989;56(3):379–90.
154. Perkins SL, et al. Childhood anaplastic large cell lymphoma has a high incidence of ALK gene rearrangement as determined by immunohistochemical staining and fluorescent in situ hybridisation: a genetic and pathological correlation. Br J Haematol. 2005;131(5):624–7.
155. Stein H, et al. CD30(+) anaplastic large cell lymphoma: a review of its histopathologic, genetic, and clinical features. Blood. 2000;96(12):3681–95.
156. Zhang Q, et al. Multilevel dysregulation of STAT3 activation in anaplastic lymphoma kinase-positive T/null-cell lymphoma. J Immunol. 2002;168(1):466–74.
157. Kasprzycka M, et al. Nucleophosmin/anaplastic lymphoma kinase (NPM/ALK) oncoprotein induces the T regulatory cell phenotype by activating STAT3. Proc Natl Acad Sci U S A. 2006;103(26):9964–9.

158. Marzec M, et al. Oncogenic tyrosine kinase NPM/ALK induces activation of the rapamycin-sensitive mTOR signaling pathway. Oncogene. 2007;26(38):5606–14.
159. Marzec M, et al. Oncogenic tyrosine kinase NPM/ALK induces activation of the MEK/ERK signaling pathway independently of c-Raf. Oncogene. 2007;26(6):813–21.
160. Nieborowska-Skorska M, et al. Role of signal transducer and activator of transcription 5 in nucleophosmin/anaplastic lymphoma kinase-mediated malignant transformation of lymphoid cells. Cancer Res. 2001;61(17):6517–23.
161. Slupianek A, et al. Role of phosphatidylinositol 3-kinase-Akt pathway in nucleophosmin/anaplastic lymphoma kinase-mediated lymphomagenesis. Cancer Res. 2001;61(5):2194–9.
162. Marzec M, et al. Malignant transformation of CD4+ T lymphocytes mediated by oncogenic kinase NPM/ALK recapitulates IL-2-induced cell signaling and gene expression reprogramming. J Immunol. 2013;191(12):6200–7.
163. Werner MT, et al. Nucleophosmin-anaplastic lymphoma kinase: the ultimate oncogene and therapeutic target. Blood. 2017;129(7):823–31.
164. Crescenzo R, et al. Convergent mutations and kinase fusions lead to oncogenic STAT3 activation in anaplastic large cell lymphoma. Cancer Cell. 2015;27(4):516–32.
165. Marzec M, et al. Oncogenic kinase NPM/ALK induces through STAT3 expression of immunosuppressive protein CD274 (PD-L1, B7-H1). Proc Natl Acad Sci U S A. 2008;105(52):20852–7.
166. Zhang Q, et al. IL-2R common gamma-chain is epigenetically silenced by nucleophosphin-anaplastic lymphoma kinase (NPM-ALK) and acts as a tumor suppressor by targeting NPM-ALK. Proc Natl Acad Sci U S A. 2011;108(29):11977–82.
167. Krenacs L, et al. Cytotoxic cell antigen expression in anaplastic large cell lymphomas of T- and null-cell type and Hodgkin's disease: evidence for distinct cellular origin. Blood. 1997;89(3):980–9.
168. Foss HD, et al. Anaplastic large-cell lymphomas of T-cell and null-cell phenotype express cytotoxic molecules. Blood. 1996;88(10):4005–11.
169. Matsuyama H, et al. miR-135b mediates NPM-ALK-driven oncogenicity and renders IL-17-producing immunophenotype to anaplastic large cell lymphoma. Blood. 2011;118(26):6881–92.
170. Laurent C, et al. Circulating t(2;5)-positive cells can be detected in cord blood of healthy newborns. Leukemia. 2012;26(1):188–90.
171. Moti N, et al. Anaplastic large cell lymphoma-propagating cells are detectable by side population analysis and possess an expression profile reflective of a primitive origin. Oncogene. 2015;34(14):1843–52.
172. Brugieres L, et al. Impact of the methotrexate administration dose on the need for intrathecal treatment in children and adolescents with anaplastic large-cell lymphoma: results of a randomized trial of the EICNHL Group. J Clin Oncol. 2009;27(6):897–903.
173. Williams DM, et al. Anaplastic large cell lymphoma in childhood: analysis of 72 patients treated on The United Kingdom Children's Cancer Study Group chemotherapy regimens. Br J Haematol. 2002;117(4):812–20.
174. Brugieres L, et al. CD30(+) anaplastic large-cell lymphoma in children: analysis of 82 patients enrolled in two consecutive studies of the French Society of Pediatric Oncology. Blood. 1998;92(10):3591–8.
175. Seidemann K, et al. Short-pulse B-non-Hodgkin lymphoma-type chemotherapy is efficacious treatment for pediatric anaplastic large cell lymphoma: a report of the Berlin-Frankfurt-Munster Group Trial NHL-BFM 90. Blood. 2001;97(12):3699–706.
176. Rosolen A, et al. Anaplastic large cell lymphoma treated with a leukemia-like therapy: report of the Italian Association of Pediatric Hematology and Oncology (AIEOP) LNH-92 protocol. Cancer. 2005;104(10):2133–40.
177. Lowe EJ, et al. Intensive chemotherapy for systemic anaplastic large cell lymphoma in children and adolescents: final results of Children's Cancer Group Study 5941. Pediatr Blood Cancer. 2009;52(3):335–9.
178. Brugieres L, et al. Single-drug vinblastine as salvage treatment for refractory or relapsed anaplastic large-cell lymphoma: a report from the French Society of Pediatric Oncology. J Clin Oncol. 2009;27(30):5056–61.
179. Woessmann W, et al. Relapsed or refractory anaplastic large-cell lymphoma in children and adolescents after Berlin-Frankfurt-Muenster (BFM)-type first-line therapy: a BFM-group study. J Clin Oncol. 2011;29(22):3065–71.
180. Brugieres L, et al. Relapses of childhood anaplastic large-cell lymphoma: treatment results in a series of 41 children—a report from the French Society of Pediatric Oncology. Ann Oncol. 2000;11(1):53–8.
181. Strullu M, et al. Hematopoietic stem cell transplantation in relapsed ALK+ anaplastic large cell lymphoma in children and adolescents: a study on behalf of the SFCE and SFGM-TC. Bone Marrow Transplant. 2015;50(6):795–801.
182. Laver JH, et al. Advanced-stage large-cell lymphoma in children and adolescents: results of a randomized trial incorporating intermediate-dose methotrexate and high-dose cytarabine in the maintenance phase of the APO regimen: a Pediatric Oncology Group phase III trial. J Clin Oncol. 2005;23(3):541–7.
183. Alexander S, et al. Advanced stage anaplastic large cell lymphoma in children and adolescents: results of ANHL0131, a randomized phase III trial of APO versus a modified regimen with vinblastine: a report from the children's oncology group. Pediatr Blood Cancer. 2014;61(12):2236–42.
184. Le Deley MC, et al. Vinblastine in children and adolescents with high-risk anaplastic large-cell

lymphoma: results of the randomized ALCL99-vinblastine trial. J Clin Oncol. 2010;28(25):3987–93.
185. Le Deley MC, et al. Prognostic factors in childhood anaplastic large cell lymphoma: results of a large European intergroup study. Blood. 2008;111(3):1560–6.
186. Lamant L, et al. Prognostic impact of morphologic and phenotypic features of childhood ALK-positive anaplastic large-cell lymphoma: results of the ALCL99 study. J Clin Oncol. 2011;29(35):4669–76.
187. Damm-Welk C, et al. Prognostic significance of circulating tumor cells in bone marrow or peripheral blood as detected by qualitative and quantitative PCR in pediatric NPM-ALK-positive anaplastic large-cell lymphoma. Blood. 2007;110(2):670–7.
188. Damm-Welk C, et al. Flow cytometric detection of circulating tumour cells in nucleophosmin/anaplastic lymphoma kinase-positive anaplastic large cell lymphoma: comparison with quantitative polymerase chain reaction. Br J Haematol. 2007;138(4):459–66.
189. Mussolin L, et al. Use of minimal disseminated disease and immunity to NPM-ALK antigen to stratify ALK-positive ALCL patients with different prognosis. Leukemia. 2013;27(2):416–22.
190. Ait-Tahar K, et al. Correlation of the autoantibody response to the ALK oncoantigen in pediatric anaplastic lymphoma kinase-positive anaplastic large cell lymphoma with tumor dissemination and relapse risk. Blood. 2010;115(16):3314–9.
191. Mori T, et al. Recurrent childhood anaplastic large cell lymphoma: a retrospective analysis of registered cases in Japan. Br J Haematol. 2006;132(5):594–7.
192. Woessmann W, et al. Allogeneic haematopoietic stem cell transplantation in relapsed or refractory anaplastic large cell lymphoma of children and adolescents—a Berlin-Frankfurt-Munster group report. Br J Haematol. 2006;133(2):176–82.
193. Ruf S, et al. Risk-adapted therapy for patients with relapsed or refractory ALCL—Final Report of the Prospective ALCL-Relapse Trial of the EICNHL. In: Fifth International Symposium on Childhood Adolescent and Young Adult Non-Hodgkin Lymphoma. Varese, Italy: British Journal of Haematology; 2015. p. 45.
194. Shaw AT, et al. Crizotinib versus chemotherapy in advanced ALK-positive lung cancer. N Engl J Med. 2013;368(25):2385–94.
195. Li J, et al. Insight into drug resistance mechanisms and discovery of potential inhibitors against wild-type and L1196M mutant ALK from FDA-approved drugs. J Mol Model. 2016;22(9):231.
196. Mosse YP, et al. Safety and activity of crizotinib for paediatric patients with refractory solid tumours or anaplastic large-cell lymphoma: a Children's Oncology Group phase 1 consortium study. Lancet Oncol. 2013;14(6):472–80.
197. Thomas A, Teicher BA, Hassan R. Antibody-drug conjugates for cancer therapy. Lancet Oncol. 2016;17(6):e254–62.
198. Wang Y, et al. Structural insights into the pharmacophore of vinca domain inhibitors of microtubules. Mol Pharmacol. 2016;89(2):233–42.
199. Pro B, et al. Brentuximab vedotin (SGN-35) in patients with relapsed or refractory systemic anaplastic large-cell lymphoma: results of a phase II study. J Clin Oncol. 2012;30(18):2190–6.
200. Younes A, et al. Brentuximab vedotin combined with ABVD or AVD for patients with newly diagnosed Hodgkin's lymphoma: a phase 1, open-label, dose-escalation study. Lancet Oncol. 2013;14(13):1348–56.
201. Cole PD, et al. Phase 2 trial of brentuximab vedotin and gemcitabine for pediatric and young adult patients with relapsed or refractory Hodgkin Lymphoma (HL): a Children's Oncology Group (COG) report. J Clin Oncol. 2017;35:7527.
202. Flerlage JE, et al. Pharmacokinetics, immunogenicity, and safety of weekly dosing of brentuximab vedotin in pediatric patients with Hodgkin lymphoma. Cancer Chemother Pharmacol. 2016;78(6):1217–23.
203. Mikles B, et al. Brentuximab vedotin (SGN-35) in a 3-year-old child with relapsed systemic anaplastic large cell lymphoma. J Pediatr Hematol Oncol. 2014;36(2):e85–7.
204. Koh KN, et al. Successful use of brentuximab vedotin for refractory anaplastic large cell lymphoma as a bridging therapy to haploidentical stem cell transplantation and maintenance therapy post-transplantation. Pediatr Blood Cancer. 2015;62(6):1063–5.
205. Fanale M, et al. Complete Remissions Observed in a Subset of Pediatric Patients with CD30-expressing Malignant Lymphomas Treated in Clinical Studies of Brentuximab Vedotin (SGN-35). In: European Multidisciplinary Cancer Congress; 2011; Stockholm, Sweden. p. S640.
206. Laimer D, et al. PDGFR blockade is a rational and effective therapy for NPM-ALK-driven lymphomas. Nat Med. 2012;18(11):1699–704.
207. Tanaka H, et al. Dual therapeutic efficacy of vinblastine as a unique chemotherapeutic agent capable of inducing dendritic cell maturation. Cancer Res. 2009;69(17):6987–94.
208. Singh VK, et al. Analysis of nucleophosmin-anaplastic lymphoma kinase (NPM-ALK)-reactive CD8(+) T cell responses in children with NPM-ALK(+) anaplastic large cell lymphoma. Clin Exp Immunol. 2016;186(1):96–105.
209. Ait-Tahar K, et al. B and CTL responses to the ALK protein in patients with ALK-positive ALCL. Int J Cancer. 2006;118(3):688–95.
210. Chiarle R, et al. The anaplastic lymphoma kinase is an effective oncoantigen for lymphoma vaccination. Nat Med. 2008;14(6):676–80.
211. Thomas L. On immunosurveillance in human cancer. Yale J Biol Med. 1982;55(3–4):329–33.
212. Burnet FM. Immunological surveillance in neoplasia. Transplant Rev. 1971;7:3–25.

213. Vajdic CM, et al. Are antibody deficiency disorders associated with a narrower range of cancers than other forms of immunodeficiency? Blood. 2010;116(8):1228–34.
214. Shapiro RS. Malignancies in the setting of primary immunodeficiency: implications for hematologists/oncologists. Am J Hematol. 2011;86(1):48–55.
215. Hayashi RJ, Wistinghausen B, Shiramazu B. Lymphoproliferative disorders and malignancies related to immunodeficiencies. In: Pizzo PA, Poplack DG, editors. Principles and practice of pediatric oncology. Philadelphia: Wolters Kluwers; 2016. p. 604–16.
216. Gross TG, Termuhlen AM. Pediatric non-Hodgkin lymphoma. Curr Hematol Malig Rep. 2008;3(3):167–73.
217. Styczynski J, et al. Response to rituximab-based therapy and risk factor analysis in Epstein Barr Virus-related lymphoproliferative disorder after hematopoietic stem cell transplant in children and adults: a study from the Infectious Diseases Working Party of the European Group for Blood and Marrow Transplantation. Clin Infect Dis. 2013;57(6):794–802.
218. Barker JN, et al. Low incidence of Epstein-Barr virus-associated posttransplantation lymphoproliferative disorders in 272 unrelated-donor umbilical cord blood transplant recipients. Biol Blood Marrow Transplant. 2001;7(7):395–9.
219. Brunstein CG, et al. Umbilical cord blood transplantation after nonmyeloablative conditioning: impact on transplantation outcomes in 110 adults with hematologic disease. Blood. 2007;110(8):3064–70.
220. Dumas PY, et al. Incidence and risk factors of EBV reactivation after unrelated cord blood transplantation: a Eurocord and Societe Francaise de Greffe de Moelle-Therapie Cellulaire collaborative study. Bone Marrow Transplant. 2013;48(2):253–6.
221. Wistinghausen B, Gross TG, Bollard C. Post-transplant lymphoproliferative disease in pediatric solid organ transplant recipients. Pediatr Hematol Oncol. 2013;30(6):520–31.
222. Baker KS, et al. New malignancies after blood or marrow stem-cell transplantation in children and adults: incidence and risk factors. J Clin Oncol. 2003;21(7):1352–8.
223. Sanz J, Andreu R. Epstein-Barr virus-associated posttransplant lymphoproliferative disorder after allogeneic stem cell transplantation. Curr Opin Oncol. 2014;26(6):677–83.
224. Collins MH, et al. Autopsy pathology of pediatric posttransplant lymphoproliferative disorder. Pediatrics. 2001;107(6):E89.
225. Gross TG, Savoldo B, Punnett A. Posttransplant lymphoproliferative diseases. Pediatr Clin N Am. 2010;57(2):481–503, table of contents.
226. Matthews K, et al. Indications, tolerance and complications of a sirolimus and calcineurin inhibitor immunosuppression regimen: intermediate experience in pediatric heart transplantation recipients. Pediatr Transplant. 2010;14(3):402–8.
227. Gibelli NE, et al. Sirolimus in pediatric liver transplantation: a single-center experience. Transplant Proc. 2009;41(3):901–3.
228. Weintraub L, et al. Identifying predictive factors for posttransplant lymphoproliferative disease in pediatric solid organ transplant recipients with Epstein-Barr virus viremia. J Pediatr Hematol Oncol. 2014;36(8):e481–6.
229. Allen UD. The ABC of Epstein-Barr virus infections. Adv Exp Med Biol. 2005;568:25–39.
230. San-Juan R, et al. Epstein-Barr virus-related post-transplant lymphoproliferative disorder in solid organ transplant recipients. Clin Microbiol Infect. 2014;20(Suppl 7):109–18.
231. Stevens SJ, Pronk I, Middeldorp JM. Toward standardization of Epstein-Barr virus DNA load monitoring: unfractionated whole blood as preferred clinical specimen. J Clin Microbiol. 2001;39(4):1211–6.
232. Savoldo B, et al. Cellular immunity to Epstein-Barr virus in liver transplant recipients treated with rituximab for post-transplant lymphoproliferative disease. Am J Transplant. 2005;5(3):566–72.
233. Kanakry JA, et al. The clinical significance of EBV DNA in the plasma and peripheral blood mononuclear cells of patients with or without EBV diseases. Blood. 2016;127(16):2007–17.
234. Harris NL, Ferry JA, Swerdlow SH. Posttransplant lymphoproliferative disorders: summary of Society for Hematopathology Workshop. Semin Diagn Pathol. 1997;14(1):8–14.
235. Miloh T, et al. T-cell PTLD presenting as acalculous cholecystitis. Pediatr Transplant. 2008;12(6):717–20.
236. Gross TG, et al. Low-dose chemotherapy and rituximab for posttransplant lymphoproliferative disease (PTLD): a Children's Oncology Group Report. Am J Transplant. 2012;12(11):3069–75.
237. Gulley ML, et al. Tumor origin and CD20 expression in posttransplant lymphoproliferative disorder occurring in solid organ transplant recipients: implications for immune-based therapy. Transplantation. 2003;76(6):959–64.
238. Ranganathan S, Jaffe R. Is there a difference between Hodgkin's disease and a Hodgkin's-like posttransplant lymphoproliferative disorder, and why should that be of any interest? Pediatr Transplant. 2004;8(1):6–8.
239. Capello D, Gaidano G. Post-transplant lymphoproliferative disorders: role of viral infection, genetic lesions and antigen stimulation in the pathogenesis of the disease. Mediterr J Hematol Infect Dis. 2009;1(2):e2009018.
240. Morscio J, et al. Gene expression profiling reveals clear differences between EBV-positive and EBV-negative posttransplant lymphoproliferative disorders. Am J Transplant. 2013;13(5):1305–16.
241. Allen U, et al. Gene expression using microarrays in transplant recipients at risk of EBV lymphoproliferation after organ transplantation:

preliminary proof-of-concept. Pediatr Transplant. 2009;13(8):990–8.
242. Styczynski J, et al. Management of HSV, VZV and EBV infections in patients with hematological malignancies and after SCT: guidelines from the Second European Conference on Infections in Leukemia. Bone Marrow Transplant. 2009;43(10):757–70.
243. Humar A, et al. A randomized trial of ganciclovir versus ganciclovir plus immune globulin for prophylaxis against Epstein-Barr virus related posttransplant lymphoproliferative disorder. Transplantation. 2006;81(6):856–61.
244. Ghosh SK, et al. Histone deacetylase inhibitors are potent inducers of gene expression in latent EBV and sensitize lymphoma cells to nucleoside antiviral agents. Blood. 2012;119(4):1008–17.
245. Perrine SP, et al. A phase 1/2 trial of arginine butyrate and ganciclovir in patients with Epstein-Barr virus-associated lymphoid malignancies. Blood. 2007;109(6):2571–8.
246. Hayashi RJ, et al. Posttransplant lymphoproliferative disease in children: correlation of histology to clinical behavior. J Pediatr Hematol Oncol. 2001;23(1):14–8.
247. Gross TG, et al. Low-dose chemotherapy for Epstein-Barr virus-positive post-transplantation lymphoproliferative disease in children after solid organ transplantation. J Clin Oncol. 2005;23(27):6481–8.
248. Webber SA, Harmon W, Faro A, Green M, Sarwal M, Hayashi R, Canter C, Thomas D, Jaffe R, Fine R. Anti-CD20 Monoclonal Antibody (rituximab) for Refractory PTLD after Pediatric Solid Organ Transplantation: Multicenter Experience from a Registry and from a Prospective Clinical Trial. In: American Society of Hematology Annual Meeting; 2004. p. Abstract 746.
249. Maecker-Kohlhoff B, Beier R, Zimmermann M, Schlegelberger B, Baumann U, Mueller CM, Pape L, Reiter A, Rossig C, Schubert S, Toenshoff B, Wingen A, Meissner B, Kebelmann-Betzing C, Henze G, Kreipe HH, Klein C. Response-adapted sequential immuno-chemotherapy of post-transplant lymphoproliferative disorders in pediatric solid organ transplant recipients: results from the prospective ped-PTLD 2005 trial. In: Loewenberg B, editor. American Society of Hematology. San Francisco, CA: The American Society of Hematology; 2014. p. 4468.
250. van Esser JW, et al. Prevention of Epstein-Barr virus-lymphoproliferative disease by molecular monitoring and preemptive rituximab in high-risk patients after allogeneic stem cell transplantation. Blood. 2002;99(12):4364–9.
251. Styczynski J, et al. Outcome of treatment of Epstein-Barr virus-related post-transplant lymphoproliferative disorder in hematopoietic stem cell recipients: a comprehensive review of reported cases. Transpl Infect Dis. 2009;11(5):383–92.
252. Choquet S, et al. Efficacy and safety of rituximab in B-cell post-transplantation lymphoproliferative disorders: results of a prospective multicenter phase 2 study. Blood. 2006;107(8):3053–7.
253. Papadopoulos EB, et al. Infusions of donor leukocytes to treat Epstein-Barr virus-associated lymphoproliferative disorders after allogeneic bone marrow transplantation. N Engl J Med. 1994;330(17):1185–91.
254. Bollard CM, Rooney CM, Heslop HE. T-cell therapy in the treatment of post-transplant lymphoproliferative disease. Nat Rev Clin Oncol. 2012;9(9): 510–9.
255. O'Reilly RJ, et al. Biology and adoptive cell therapy of Epstein-Barr virus-associated lymphoproliferative disorders in recipients of marrow allografts. Immunol Rev. 1997;157:195–216.
256. Bollard CM, et al. Good manufacturing practice-grade cytotoxic T lymphocytes specific for latent membrane proteins (LMP)-1 and LMP2 for patients with Epstein-Barr virus-associated lymphoma. Cytotherapy. 2011;13(5):518–22.
257. Haque T, et al. Allogeneic cytotoxic T-cell therapy for EBV-positive posttransplantation lymphoproliferative disease: results of a phase 2 multicenter clinical trial. Blood. 2007;110(4):1123–31.
258. Doubrovina E, et al. Adoptive immunotherapy with unselected or EBV-specific T cells for biopsy-proven EBV+ lymphomas after allogeneic hematopoietic cell transplantation. Blood. 2012;119(11):2644–56.
259. Leen AM, et al. Multicenter study of banked third-party virus-specific T cells to treat severe viral infections after hematopoietic stem cell transplantation. Blood. 2013;121(26):5113–23.
260. Anurathapan U, et al. Kinetics of tumor destruction by chimeric antigen receptor-modified T cells. Mol Ther. 2014;22(3):623–33.
261. Bollard CM, Heslop HE. T cells for viral infections after allogeneic hematopoietic stem cell transplant. Blood. 2016;127(26):3331–40.
262. Vickers MA, et al. Establishment and operation of a Good Manufacturing Practice-compliant allogeneic Epstein-Barr virus (EBV)-specific cytotoxic cell bank for the treatment of EBV-associated lymphoproliferative disease. Br J Haematol. 2014;167(3):402–10.
263. Heslop HE, et al. Long-term outcome of EBV-specific T-cell infusions to prevent or treat EBV-related lymphoproliferative disease in transplant recipients. Blood. 2010;115(5):925–35.
264. Naik S, et al. Adoptive immunotherapy for primary immunodeficiency disorders with virus-specific T lymphocytes. J Allergy Clin Immunol. 2016;137(5):1498–1505 e1.
265. O'Reilly RJ, et al. Virus-specific T-cell banks for 'off the shelf' adoptive therapy of refractory infections. Bone Marrow Transplant. 2016;51(9):1163–72.
266. Dharnidharka VR, Mohanakumar T. New approaches to treating B-cell cancers induced by Epstein-Barr virus. N Engl J Med. 2015;372(6):569–71.
267. Ricciardelli I, et al. Towards gene therapy for EBV-associated posttransplant lymphoma with genetically modified EBV-specific cytotoxic T cells. Blood. 2014;124(16):2514–22.

Part III

Future Directions in Aggressive Lymphomas

Role of Modern Imaging with FDG-PET/CT in Aggressive Lymphoma

14

Judith Trotman and Michel Meignan

14.1 Staging of Aggressive Lymphoma

When the Ann Arbor staging system for lymphoma was drafted in 1971, the authors acknowledged two aims of staging: to facilitate communication and exchange information and to guide prognosis and assist in therapeutic decisions. The former could only be done at the expense of a loss of some information, as it is necessary to condense in one number a considerable amount of data, while the latter aim was best achieved if the greatest amount of information was given for each patient. These two aims highlighted a tension that has existed in lymphoma staging ever since: between being succinct and comprehensive; a lumper vs. a splitter; providing a simple standardised staging paradigm vs. a more complicated individualised approach. Furthermore, it was acknowledged that intercomparison demands that all the staging procedures performed should be as similar as possible in each centre to avoid bias in staging and interpretation of the therapeutic results.

A diagnosis of aggressive lymphoma is most commonly made after a standard CT scan has been performed and mapped the presence of lymphadenopathy, including the node/lesion most suitable for core or ideally excision biopsy. CT-based anatomic extent of lymphoma has traditionally defined stage, but, with aggressive lymphomas being invariably glucose- avid, in 2007 the IHP defined PET-CT as the principal imaging modality for staging aggressive lymphoma [1, 2]. Therefore once a diagnosis is made, whole body PET-CT is performed. PET-CT is the most sensitive imaging modality, particularly in identifying extranodal disease [3–5]. Indeed, the more recent, international staging criteria noted significant (~20%) stage migration, particularly upstaging with the more sensitive PET-CT scanning [6, 7]. It has been shown recently that the detection of extranodal involvement by PET has improved the prognostic value of IPI, R-IPI and NCCN-IPI [3]. While still separating lymphomas into localised or advanced stage, it was recognised that distinguishing nodal vs. extranodal status and unidimensional measurement of bulk was of limited use in an era of widespread use of systemic and multimodality approaches.

As a full-dose contrast-enhanced CT has commonly already been performed when diagnosing aggressive lymphoma, the most common PET-CT performed for staging purposes utilises 18F-FDG

J. Trotman (✉)
Department of Haematology, Concord Repatriation General Hospital, University of Sydney, Concord, NSW, Australia
e-mail: judith.trotman@health.nsw.gov.au

M. Meignan
LYSA Imaging, Hôpitaux Universitaires Henri Mondor, Créteil, France
e-mail: michel.meignan@aphp.fr

G. Lenz, G. Salles (eds.), *Aggressive Lymphomas*, Hematologic Malignancies,
https://doi.org/10.1007/978-3-030-00362-3_14

(administered 60 +/− 5′ after resting) and low-dose CT to minimise the impact of contrast on attenuation correction: the correction made for the loss of detection of photons because of spatially dependent absorption. When precise anatomical definition of disease is required, say for consideration of radiotherapy, a full contrast-enhanced CT scan is also required, either with, or more commonly separate to the PET scan.

Staging PET scans are to be reported using visual assessment [8], noting the location of increased focal uptake in nodal and extranodal sites, which is distinguished from physiological uptake and other patterns of disease that may have increased FDG uptake including infection and inflammation [9, 10], according to the distribution and/or CT characteristics. PET scans should be reported using a fixed display and a grey or colour table which can be scaled to the standardised uptake value (SUV) [11]. The SUV is the measured radioactivity corrected for patient weight and administered activity.

Focal FDG uptake within the bone/bone marrow, liver and spleen is highly sensitive for involvement in aggressive NHL [12–15], and the presence of focal lesions in the bone marrow may obviate the need for bone marrow biopsy [4, 16, 17]. Indeed PET detects BM involvement more often than BMB, and patients with a positive BMB generally have other factors consistent with advanced stage or poor prognosis. Where the PET scan shows no focal marrow uptake, the clinical value of performing a bone marrow biopsy outside of clinical trials to exclude concurrent low-grade disease is debatable as it generally would not change the prognosis and management. High physiological FDG uptake occurs in the brain, and although intracerebral lymphoma is often highly FDG-avid [18], diffuse and low-volume leptomeningeal disease may be missed. MRI is preferred to assess suspected CNS involvement.

Prior to our capacity to measure both anatomic and metabolic extent of lymphoma, various surrogates of tumour burden, including CT and BM biopsy-based stage, presence of extranodal disease and the lactate dehydrogenase level (a surrogate of both bulk and proliferation) have been included in the prognostic indices of all aggressive lymphoma subtypes (the IPI [19] and revised IPI [20] and NCCN-IPI [21] in DLBCL and the PIT in PTCL [22].

More recently, PET studies across a range of lymphomas including DLBCL and peripheral T-cell lymphoma suggest that quantifying the baseline total metabolic tumour volume (TMTV), the sum of the three-dimensional measurements of lesions with FDG uptake: a measure of the viable fraction of tumours and microenvironment may more accurately quantify tumour burden for determining prognosis. In two retrospective DLBCL series, the median TMTV was reported around 320 cm^3 using the 41% thresholding method [23]. Patients with a large baseline metabolic volume (>300 cm^3) had a significantly worse outcome than those with a volume ≤300 cm^3 [24, 25]. The populations could be stratified according to TMTV, with risk increasing with each TMTV distribution quartile [25]. Combining these two PET series resulted in a cohort of 187 patients (44% >60 years old, 81% Ann Arbor Stage III/IV, 66% with aaIPI 2–3, 75% treated by R-CHOP) confirming that TMTV with a 300 cm^3 cut-off was predictive of both 5-year PFS and OS [24], Fig. 14.1. In 167 young patients with an aaIPI score of 2–3 enrolled in a prospective study and treated with either R/CHOP14 or R/ACVBP, the median TMTV was 380 cm^3. A 6.6% increase in risk of events for each 100 cm^3 increase of TMTV was observed, and a TMTV >660 cm^3 was the strongest predictor of inferior PFS and OS [26]. In primary mediastinal B-cell lymphoma, TMTV was shown to be predictive of outcome in 103 patients included in the series of the International Extranodal Lymphoma Study Group (IELSG26 trial) [27]. In a retrospective study including 108 patients with nodal PTCL (PTCL NOS, AITL, ALCL), the median TMTV at staging was 220 cm^3. It was shown that TMTV with a threshold >230 cm^3 was strongly prognostic independent of either IPI or PIT [24].

Not only can TMTV "per se" be used to stratify patient prognosis, but it has been shown in several studies to be independent to risk assignment using the current clinical prognostic indi-

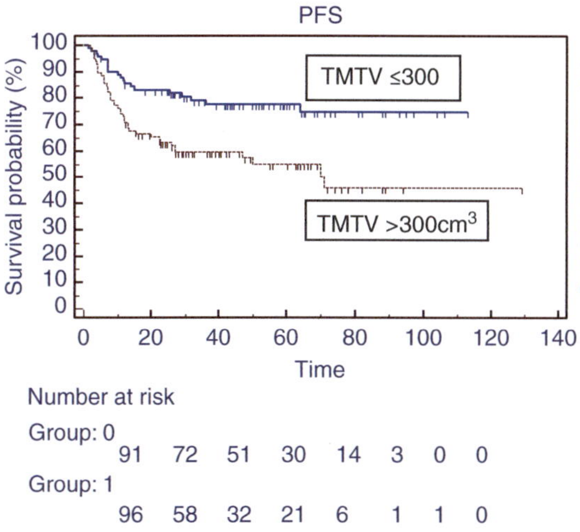

Fig. 14.1 TMTV impacts PFS and OS in 187 patients with DLBCL. Kaplan-Meier curves show that patients with TMTV>300 cm³, Group 1, have lower 5-year PFS and OS than patients with TMTV≤300 cm³, Group 0 (54.7% vs. 77%, HR = 2.32, $p = 0.013$ and 55% vs. 85%, HR = 3.03, $p = 0.0002$, respectively). Note that when the best cut-off of 205 cm³ determined for PFS by ROC and X-tile analysis is taken, the 5-year PFS is 55% when >205 cm³ and 82% when ≤205 cm³, HR = 2.96, $p = 0.0002$

ces. In DLBCL, TMTV stratified patients with high NCCN-IPI into two risk groups, a group with high TMTV, with a very poor outcome (5-year PFS 35%, 5-year OS 42%), and a group with low TMTV, with a much better outcome (5-year PFS 64%, 5-year OS 69%, $P = 0.001$ and $P = 0.01$, respectively) [24]. Patients with low NCCN-IPI had an excellent outcome irrespective of their TMTV (5-year PFS 80%, 5-year OS 77%). Moreover, TMTV has potential to refine cell of origin risk assignment in DLBCL. Both patients with GCB genotype and a high volume and patients with ABC disease with a small TMTV had a 5-year PFS of around 50% [24]. Similarly, in patients with PTCL, TMTV0 combined with PIT discriminated outcome better than TMTV0 alone, identifying patients with an adverse outcome (TMTV0 > 230 cm³ and PIT >1, $n = 33$) from those with good prognosis (TMTV0 ≤ 230 cm³ and PIT ≤1, $n = 40$): 19% vs. 73% 2-year PFS ($p < 0.0001$) and 43% vs. 81% 2-year OS ($p = 0.0002$), respectively.

An alternative interest in TMTV measurement is around measurement of drug delivery. It has recently been shown in 108 patients with DLBCL that the TMTV influenced rituximab pharmacokinetics. Exposure to rituximab decreased as TMTV increased with a decrease of the area under concentration-time curve (AUC). Small volume and high AUC were associated with a better response and a longer PFS. These results suggested that TMTV measurement could be helpful for optimising rituximab dose individualisation in DLBCL [28].

With standardisation of PET acquisition and software packages to assist with measurement of TMTV, we may be getting closer to providing a single staging parameter (Fig. 14.2). However, we must remain committed to systematically addressing the challenges of volume calculation and the appropriate choice of TMTV software algorithms to provide reproducible measurements of TMTV across prospective multisite studies. No method is always the most accurate: performance varies as a function of the activity distribution, noise, spatial resolution and contrast. The cut-off volume separating high vs. lower tumour volume across patients depends upon the method. With evolving scanner performance, relative methods relying on internal standards such as fixed percentage thresholding or adaptive methods are the most reproducible, but it has been shown that even if the cut-off varies with a

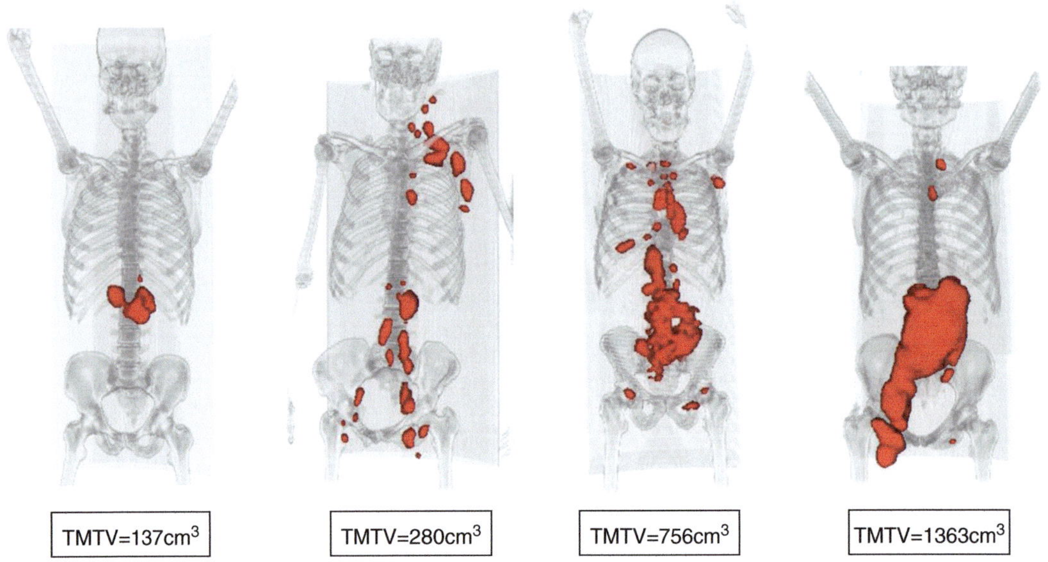

Fig. 14.2 Different total metabolic tumour volume observed in patients with DLBCL (from Cottereau et al. Clin Cancer Res, 2016)

given method, the predictive value remains quite similar once a method is chosen.

With widespread use of multi-agent systemic therapies, the Ann Arbor staging is no longer fit for purpose. TMTV has the potential to provide the single most efficient and relevant means of informing clinicians and patients of their disease burden. With reliable software and consensus, TMTV may in time replace the Ann Arbor system and become the new standard to convey prognosis and rationale for tailored therapy to our patients.

14.2 PET to Assess Therapeutic Response

One of the advantages of metabolic imaging is the capacity to accurately chart early metabolic response to therapy. The high FDG avidity of the aggressive lymphoma cells results from increased cellular turnover and internal trapping of glucose by tumour and stromal cells. Decreased glucose metabolism during treatment may be a surrogate of treatment efficiency. Chemotherapy-induced reduction of lymphoma metabolism is a nonlinear process influenced by chemotherapy regimen, the schedule and number of cycles and the effect of the chemotherapy on the surrounding microenvironment. End-of-induction PET-CT is necessary for response assessment in aggressive lymphoma, and the poorer prognosis of patients who remain PET-positive after completion of therapy has driven study of interim PET assessment seeking to identify such patients earlier where it is hoped that a change, often intensification of therapy, will improve outcomes.

14.2.1 Interim PET

In both clinical trials and in practice, the decision of when to perform interim PET (iPET) is driven by the clinical tension between the very good negative predictive value (NPV) of the test in identifying patients with a good prognosis and obtaining a sufficiently high positive predictive value (PPV) at an early enough time point so that PET-positive patients can be salvaged with a change in therapeutic approach. Therefore in most studies, iPET is performed after 2 and/or 4 cycles of chemotherapy. Resolution of FDG uptake at sites of initial disease indicates a complete metabolic response with a very good negative predictive value with a 2-year PFS rate of 73–85% [6].

The limitations of iPET are twofold. Firstly, the positive predictive value of iPET is too low as cited to range from 18 to 74% [6]. Secondly, no prospective randomised study has clearly demonstrated that either intensification of chemotherapy or change in therapeutic agent can improve the poorer prognosis of patients who remain PET-positive.

One study highlights the low PPV of iPET, particularly when applying the now outdated IHP criteria (using background FDG uptake as reference) [29]. All patients who remained PET-positive after 4 cycles of R-CHOP-14 underwent systematic biopsy. The 23% with biopsy-confirmed disease had an inferior outcome. However, the PFS in PET-positive biopsy-negative patients was comparable to that of PET-negative patients. The observation of a high false PET-positive rate in this series did not deny a clinically relevant prognostic value to early PET. It rather highlighted the key challenge for early PET reporting: to establish reproducible interpretation criteria able to discriminate FDG uptake associated with active disease from that related to non-specific post-therapy inflammatory changes. Indeed, visual interpretation can significantly change depending on the reference background used. Clearly for the same residual FDG uptake, increasing the reference for measuring background uptake can change a PET-positive scan to a negative one and the cut-off must be chosen carefully. In DLBCL the signal decreases continuously during induction treatment in parallel with tumour destruction, and the residual uptake decreases with each cycle. The degree of uptake that is indicative of response [8] is dependent on the timing of the scan during treatment [30, 31] and on the clinical context, including prognosis, lymphoma subtype [32–34] and treatment regimen [35, 36]. It is also dependent on the presence of inflammatory cells induced by rituximab and on microenvironmental cells. In addition there are difficulties in a qualitative visual comparison between residual uptake and background since visual reporting is highly observer dependent.

The 5-PS was developed as a simple, reproducible scoring method for response assessment (Table 14.1). It provides flexibility to change the threshold between good/poor response according to the clinical context and treatment strategy [37]. For example, a lower level of FDG uptake might be preferred to define a "negative result" in a clinical trial exploring de-escalation to avoid undertreatment. A higher level of uptake might be preferred to define a "positive result" in a trial exploring escalation to avoid overtreatment. The 5-PS has been validated for use at interim and at the end of treatment and in the last decade has been adopted as the preferred reporting method for response assessment [8].

Table 14.1 The 5-PS (also called Deauville criteria) scores the most intense uptake in a site of initial disease, if present as follows

1.	No uptake
2.	Uptake ≤ mediastinum
3.	Uptake > mediastinum but ≤ liver
4.	Uptake moderately higher than the liver
5.	Uptake markedly higher than liver and/or new lesions

Good interobserver agreement has been reported in DLBCL [38]. Scores 1, 2 and for the most part 3 are defined as CMR. When a score 1 or 2 is achieved at interim, an end of treatment scan is not required [39]. Score 3 also likely represents CMR at interim [40] and a good prognosis at completion of standard treatment ([41] (suppl 1; abst 15); [42]). One issue to be resolved with the 5PS is the lack of definition of the terms "moderately "and "markedly" which are not yet defined in quantitative terms. However, the 2014 Lugano guidelines recommend that a score of 4 should apply to uptake greater than the max SUV of the liver and a score of 5 to uptake 2–3 times greater than the SUVmax liver. In these guidelines a score of 4–5 with uptake reduced from baseline represents a partial metabolic response, while a score of 5 with no decreased uptake or with new FDG-avid foci consistent with lymphoma represents treatment failure and/or progression.

The problem of interobserver variability for reporting according to the 5PS has been pointed out recently. Concordance was excellent with the liver threshold but decreased for all the other thresholds. In this regard a quantitative approach measuring delta (Δ)SUVmax between baseline and interim PET would add value, and such quantitative reporting is being encouraged both clinically and in trials. It decreases the interobserver variability seen with visual reporting and integrates kinetic information by comparing baseline PET with interim PET [38]. The maximum SUV is measured in the hottest lesion before treatment and after 2 or 4 cycles of treatment. The change in SUV is expressed as a percentage of the initial uptake: referred to as the ΔSUVmax (Itti et al. 0.2009). When calculating the ΔSUVmax, it is important to appreciate that the lesion containing the SUVmax on iPET may not be the same as the lesion with the SUVmax at baseline. One challenge is the difficulty applying the ΔSUVmax method in patients with low baseline SUV which cannot reach the cut-off ΔSUVmax (between 66 and 72%) to determine a good response. The use of this metric has been adopted in two large clinical prospective trials (PETAL and GAINED), but there has been no prospective within-study comparison of the performance of the 5PS and ΔSUVmax. Another interesting quantitative approach has been recently proposed by a group from Beijing. They showed in DLBCL that using a ratio of 1.6 between the residual uptake and the liver, they could better discriminate patient outcomes than using 5PS or ΔSUVmax approach [43].

Although there is no prospective comparison between these methods, several exploratory investigations compare qualitative visual and nonvisual quantitative PET assessment [38]. Even while these studies have limitations, they all conclude in favour of quantitative methods.

The more significant limitation of iPET relates not to the scans themselves per se but the failure observed in some iPET-directed escalation studies to improve outcomes for patients who remain PET-positive. The most notable study in this respect was the PETAL (positron emission tomography-guided therapy of aggressive non-Hodgkin lymphomas) trial, where patients who failed to have a ΔSUVmax of 66% after 4 cycles of R-CHOP were escalated to a Burkitt-like regimen. iPET remained positive in 13% of patients and was highly predictive of inferior outcome with a 2-year TTF of 79% vs. 47% ($p < 0.001$), but a benefit from escalation could not be demonstrated (Duhrsen et al. 2014). To the contrary, in the Australasian Leukaemia and Lymphoma Group phase II escalation study, patients with DLBCL remaining PET-positive after 4 cycles of R-CHOP 14 and changed to R-ICE followed by ASCT had similar survival as PET-negative patients who completed six cycles of R-CHOP, (Hertzberg et al. 2017). However in this trial, iPET were reported using the now outdated IHP criteria. A reanalysis of PET-positive patients with the 5PS showed that the subset with score 5 had a poor prognosis and were refractory to the intensification approach.

In contrast to the challenges of interpreting an iPET-positive result, the very good negative predictive value of interim PET in DLBCL allows us to consider studies of de-escalation strategies in PET-negative patients. Furthermore, the reassurance to the patient in achieving iPET-negativity and a favourable prognosis cannot be underestimated. The results of the French LNH073B trial studying patients <60 years, with age adjusted IPI > 1, showed that 79% of patients became PET-negative using a ΔSUVmax approach. The results suggested that the quantitative approach could better characterise the majority of patients eligible for continued standard immunochemotherapy and select the presumably small subset of patients likely to benefit from upfront ASCT consolidation and those refractory ones early needing alternative strategies [44].

In peripheral T-cell lymphoma (PTCL), retrospective studies have reported conflicting results on the value of iPET. However, the largest retrospective multicentre French and Danish series applying the 5PS in 140 patients for interim PET performed either after two or after 3/4 cycles have shown that interim PET was predictive of outcome [45]. PFS and OS for iPET3/4 positive and iPET3/4 negative patients were 16% and 32% vs. 75% and 85%, respectively. Moreover baseline TMTV helped stratify the early PET responders into different risk categories.

The complexity of interpreting iPET demands that it be assessed in a multidisciplinary setting aware of the clinical context of such interpretation before influencing the ongoing therapeutic approach for patients with aggressive lymphoma.

14.2.2 Postinduction PET

End-of-induction (EOI) PET is the standard imaging modality for end-of-induction response assessment of aggressive lymphoma with demonstrated greater accuracy than CT scanning. PET should be performed at least 3 weeks after last cycle of chemotherapy or 8–12 weeks after radiotherapy, given the propensity for inflammatory reactions after this modality of therapy.

The current recommendation for end-of-induction PET is to apply the 5PS, where a score of 4 or 5 represents residual metabolic disease and treatment failure [7]. There is insufficient evidence to specify a target ΔSUVmax at end-of-induction PET that predicts a high probability of cure in DLBCL, and so the 5PS remains the recommended guide to subsequent prognosis and clinical approach. The NPV of end-of-induction PET is reported to be 80–100%, but again PET assessment is plagued with a low PPV ranging from 50 to 100% [6]. Therefore, if further treatment, beyond consolidation radiotherapy to a single residual FDG-avid lesion, is being considered, a biopsy or follow-up imaging is advised. One DLBCL subtype with excellent long-term response rates despite frequent persistence of FDG uptake is primary mediastinal B-cell lymphoma with data suggesting that a score of 4 on the 5PS is not associated with as poor a prognosis as score 5 [46]. In this lymphoma where consolidation radiotherapy is commonly used, a prospective randomised IELSG is assessing whether it is safe to omit radiotherapy in patients who become PET-negative.

There is data to suggest that the anatomic CT response may also play a complementary role with a greater reduction in mass associated with improved outcome both in patients who remain PET-positive and who achieve PET-negative status. The recently published response evaluation criteria in lymphoma (RECIL), recommended for use patients in basket clinical trials with novel agents, outlines the predictive power of a reduction by ≥30% in the sum of the longest diameters of three target lesions [47]. This supports an ongoing value to anatomic reduction of masses, although how these criteria can be applied outside of clinical trials is unclear and for now the Lugano criteria remain central to response assessment for aggressive lymphomas in clinical practice.

14.3 Assessment Before High-Dose Therapy (HDT) and Autologous Stem Cell Transplant (ASCT)

Several studies have reported that PET is prognostic in patients with relapsed or refractory DLBCL after salvage chemotherapy for whom high-dose chemotherapy and autologous stem cell transplantation are considered. In the context of this population of patients having a poorer prognosis, overall PET separates out a 3-year PFS/EFS of 30–40% in patients who remain PET-positive, vs. 75–82% for those who become PET-negative after salvage. The PET results, particularly in the context of a comparison with PET prior to salvage therapy, and the context of patient age, fitness and alternative clinical trial options serve to assist the clinician in deciding the merits of transplantation +/− consolidation radiotherapy.

14.4 Peripheral T cell Lymphoma

In 130 patients with relapsed or refractory PTCL treated by romidepsin, end of treatment PET reported with outdated criteria appeared superior to conventional CT assessment to determine prognosis [48]. In a recent retrospective study including 140 PTCL patients, the prognostic value of end of treatment PET reported with Lugano criteria has been confirmed, Cottereau et al. 2017). In extranodal NK/T-cell lymphoma, it has been shown that posttreatment 5PS and

Epstein-Barr virus DNA positivity were independently associated with progression-free and overall survival in a multivariable analysis (for posttreatment 5PS of 3–4, PFS hazard ratio [HR] 3.607, 95% CI 1.772–7.341, univariable $p < 0.0001$; for posttreatment Epstein-Barr virus DNA positivity, progression-free survival HR 3.595, 95% CI 1.598–8.089, univariable $p < 0.0001$) [49].

14.5 Remission Surveillance

There is no evidence-based role for either PET or CT in the routine surveillance of remission in aggressive lymphoma. Educating the patient about signs and symptoms of relapse and clinical follow-up at initially three and then six monthly intervals is more appropriate. In the absence of prospective data demonstrating its benefit, surveillance imaging with either PET or standard contrast-enhanced CT for aggressive lymphoma generates unnecessary cost, anxiety and radiation exposure as most relapses are detected clinically. The 2014 Lugano guidelines cite a false positive rate of 20% which results in unnecessary biopsies for such patients. There was an estimated 91–255 scans performed for every relapse detected and no clear demonstrated improvement in patient outcome in the small proportion of patients whose relapse is detected initially with imaging [50, 51].

14.6 The Future for Imaging in Response Assessment of Aggressive Lymphoma

Despite considerable enthusiasm for identifying blood biomarkers for prognosis and response prediction, PET imaging remains the central biomarker at both baseline and end of immunochemotherapy in aggressive lymphoma. It is hoped that future combinations of baseline TMTV, the biologic profile of the lymphoma (particularly DLBCL), iPET and EOI PET assessment may be sufficiently prognostic to provide a platform for PET-adapted approaches in aggressive lymphomas in future clinical trials. For such approaches to be successful however, the results from the PETAL study suggest that simply intensification of chemotherapy may not be sufficient, and rationally biologic targeted therapies need to be developed.

References

1. Cheson BD, Pfistner B, Juweid ME, Gascoyne RD, Specht L, Horning SJ, Coiffier B, Fisher RI, Hagenbeek A, Zucca E, Rosen ST, Stroobants S, Lister TA, Hoppe RT, Dreyling M, Tobinai K, Vose JM, Connors JM, Federico M, Diehl V. Revised response criteria for malignant lymphoma. J Clin Oncol. 2007;25(5):579–86. https://doi.org/10.1200/jco.2006.09.2403.
2. Juweid ME, Stroobants S, Hoekstra OS, Mottaghy FM, Dietlein M, Guermazi A, Wiseman GA, Kostakoglu L, Scheidhauer K, Buck A, Naumann R, Spaepen K, Hicks RJ, Weber WA, Reske SN, Schwaiger M, Schwartz LH, Zijlstra JM, Siegel BA, Cheson BD. Use of positron emission tomography for response assessment of lymphoma: consensus of the imaging Subcommittee of International Harmonization Project in lymphoma. J Clin Oncol. 2007;25(5):571–8. https://doi.org/10.1200/jco.2006.08.2305.
3. El-Galaly TC, Villa D, Alzahrani M, Hansen JW, Sehn LH, Wilson D, de Nully Brown P, Loft A, Iyer V, Johnsen HE. Outcome prediction by extranodal involvement, IPI, R-IPI, and NCCN-IPI in the PET/CT and rituximab era: a Danish–Canadian study of 443 patients with diffuse-large B-cell lymphoma. Am J Hematol. 2015;90(11):1041–6.
4. Khan AB, Barrington SF, Mikhaeel NG, Hunt AA, Cameron L, Morris T, Carr R. PET-CT staging of DLBCL accurately identifies and provides new insight into the clinical significance of bone marrow involvement. Blood. 2013;122(1):61–7.
5. Raanani P, Shasha Y, Perry C, Metser U, Naparstek E, Apter S, Nagler A, Polliack A, Ben-Bassat I, Even-Sapir E. Is CT scan still necessary for staging in Hodgkin and non-Hodgkin lymphoma patients in the PET/CT era? Ann Oncol. 2006;17(1):117–22. https://doi.org/10.1093/annonc/mdj024.
6. Barrington SF, Mikhaeel NG, Kostakoglu L, Meignan M, Hutchings M, Müeller SP, Schwartz LH, Zucca E, Fisher RI, Trotman J. Role of imaging in the staging and response assessment of lymphoma: consensus of the International Conference on Malignant Lymphomas Imaging Working Group. J Clin Oncol. 2014;32(27):3048–58.
7. Cheson BD, Fisher RI, Barrington SF, Cavalli F, Schwartz LH, Zucca E, Lister TA. Recommendations for initial evaluation, staging, and response assessment

of Hodgkin and non-Hodgkin lymphoma: the Lugano classification. J Clin Oncol. 2014;32(27):3059–67.
8. Meignan M, Gallamini A, Haioun C. Report on the First International Workshop on interim-PET-scan in lymphoma. Leuk Lymphoma. 2009;50(8):1257–60. https://doi.org/10.1080/10428190903040048.
9. Barrington SF, O'Doherty MJ. Limitations of PET for imaging lymphoma. Eur J Nucl Med Mol Imaging. 2003;30:S117–27. https://doi.org/10.1007/s00259-003-1169-2.
10. Cook GJ, Wegner EA, Fogelman I. Pitfalls and artifacts in 18FDG PET and PET/CT oncologic imaging. Semin Nucl Med. 2004;34(2):122–33.
11. Barrington SF, Mikhaeel NG. When should FDG-PET be used in the modern management of lymphoma? Br J Haematol. 2013;164(3):315–28.
12. Berthet L, Cochet A, Kanoun S, Berriolo-Riedinger A, Humbert O, Toubeau M, Dygai-Cochet I, Legouge C, Casasnovas O, Brunotte F. In newly diagnosed diffuse large B-cell lymphoma, determination of bone marrow involvement with 18F-FDG PET/CT provides better diagnostic performance and prognostic stratification than does biopsy. J Nucl Med. 2013;54(8):1244–50.
13. Mittal BR, Manohar K, Malhotra P, Das R, Kashyap R, Bhattacharya A, Varma N, Varma S. Can fluorodeoxyglucose positron emission tomography/computed tomography avoid negative iliac crest biopsies in evaluation of marrow involvement by lymphoma at time of initial staging? Leuk Lymphoma. 2011;52(11):2111–6. https://doi.org/10.3109/10428194.2011.593273.
14. Ngeow JY, Quek RH, Ng DC, Hee SW, Tao M, Lim LC, Tan YH, Lim ST. High SUV uptake on FDG-PET/CT predicts for an aggressive B-cell lymphoma in a prospective study of primary FDG-PET/CT staging in lymphoma. Ann Oncol. 2009;20(9):1543–7. https://doi.org/10.1093/annonc/mdp030.
15. Pelosi E, Penna D, Douroukas A, Bello M, Amati A, Arena V, Passera R, Bisi G. Bone marrow disease detection with FDG-PET/CT and bone marrow biopsy during the staging of malignant lymphoma: results from a large multicentre study. Q J Nucl Med Mol Imaging. 2011;55(4):469–75.
16. Cheson BD. Hodgkin lymphoma: protecting the victims of our success. J Clin Oncol. 2012;30(36):4456–7.
17. El-Galaly TC, d'Amore F, Mylam KJ, de Nully Brown P, Bogsted M, Bukh A, Specht L, Loft A, Iyer V, Hjorthaug K, Nielsen AL, Christiansen I, Madsen C, Johnsen HE, Hutchings M. Routine bone marrow biopsy has little or no therapeutic consequence for positron emission tomography/computed tomography-staged treatment-naive patients with Hodgkin lymphoma. J Clin Oncol. 2012;30(36):4508–14.
18. O'Doherty MJ, Barrington SF, Campbell M, Lowe J, Bradbeer CS. PET scanning and the human immunodeficiency virus-positive patient. J Nucl Med. 1997;38(10):1575–83.
19. Solal-Céligny P, Roy P, Colombat P, White J, Armitage JO, Arranz-Saez R, Au WY, Bellei M, Brice P, Caballero D. Follicular lymphoma international prognostic index. Blood. 2004;104:1258.
20. Sehn LH, Berry B, Chhanabhai M, Fitzgerald C, Gill K, Hoskins P, Klasa R, Savage KJ, Shenkier T, Sutherland J. The revised International Prognostic Index (R-IPI) is a better predictor of outcome than the standard IPI for patients with diffuse large B-cell lymphoma treated with R-CHOP. Blood. 2007;109(5):1857–61.
21. Zhou Z, Sehn LH, Rademaker AW, Gordon LI, LaCasce AS, Crosby-Thompson A, Vanderplas A, Zelenetz AD, Abel GA, Rodriguez MA. An enhanced International Prognostic Index (NCCN-IPI) for patients with diffuse large B-cell lymphoma treated in the rituximab era. Blood. 2014;123(6):837–42.
22. Gallamini A, Stelitano C, Calvi R, Bellei M, Mattei D, Vitolo U, Morabito F, Martelli M, Brusamolino E, Iannitto E. Peripheral T-cell lymphoma unspecified (PTCL-U): a new prognostic model from a retrospective multicentric clinical study. Blood. 2004;103(7):2474–9.
23. Meignan M, Sasanelli M, Casasnovas RO, Luminari S, Fioroni F, Coriani C, Masset H, Itti E, Gobbi PG, Merli F, Versari A. Eur J Nucl Med Mol Imaging. 2014;41(6):1113–22. https://doi.org/10.1007/s00259-014-2705-y. Epub 2014 Feb 26.
24. Cottereau A-S, Lanic H, Mareschal S, Meignan M, Vera P, Tilly H, Jardin F, Becker S. Molecular profile and FDG-PET/CT total metabolic tumor volume improve risk classification at diagnosis for patients with diffuse large B-cell lymphoma. Clin Cancer Res. 2016a;22(15):3801–9.
25. Sasanelli M, Meignan M, Haioun C, Berriolo-Riedinger A, Casasnovas R-O, Biggi A, Gallamini A, Siegel BA, Cashen AF, Véra P. Pretherapy metabolic tumour volume is an independent predictor of outcome in patients with diffuse large B-cell lymphoma. Eur J Nucl Med Mol Imaging. 2014;41(11):2017–22.
26. Casasnovas O, Cottereau ASKS, Oberic L, Thieblemont C, Haioun C, et al. Baseline total metabolic volume (TMTV0) predicts the outcome of patients with diffuse large B cell lymphoma (DLBCL) enrolled in the LNH07-3B LYSA trial. Hematol Oncol. 2015;33:100–80.
27. Ceriani L, Martelli M, Zinzani PL, Ferreri AJM, Botto B, Stelitano C, Gotti M, Cabras MG, Rigacci L, Gargantini L, Merli F, Pinotti G, Mannina D, Luminari S, Stathis A, Russo E, Cavalli F, Giovanella L, Johnson PWM, Zucca E. Blood. 2015. https://doi.org/10.1182/blood-2014-12-616474.
28. Tout M, Casasnovas O, Meignan M, Lamy T, Morschhauser F, Salles G, Gyan E, Haioun C, Mercier M, Feugier P, Boussetta S, Paintaud G, Ternant D, Cartron G. Blood. 2017. https://doi.org/10.1182/blood-2016-10-744292.
29. Moskowitz CH, Schöder H, Teruya-Feldstein J, Sima C, Iasonos A, Portlock CS, Straus D, Noy A, Palomba ML, O'Connor OA, Horwitz S, Weaver SA, Meikle JL, Filippa DA, Caravelli JF, Hamlin PA, Zelenetz AD. Risk-adapted dose-dense Immunochemotherapy

determined by interim FDG-PET in advanced-stage diffuse large B-cell lymphoma. J Clin Oncol. 2010;28(11):1896–903. https://doi.org/10.1200/jco.2009.26.5942.
30. Itti E, Lin C, Dupuis J, Paone G, Capacchione D, Rahmouni A, Haioun C, Meignan M. Prognostic value of interim 18F-FDG PET in patients with diffuse large B-cell lymphoma: SUV-based assessment at 4 cycles of chemotherapy. J Nucl Med. 2009;50(4):527–33. https://doi.org/10.2967/jnumed.108.057703.
31. Lin C, Itti E, Haioun C, Petegnief Y, Luciani A, Dupuis J, Paone G, Talbot JN, Rahmouni A, Meignan M. Early 18F-FDG PET for prediction of prognosis in patients with diffuse large B-cell lymphoma: SUV-based assessment versus visual analysis. J Nucl Med. 2007;48(10):1626–32. https://doi.org/10.2967/jnumed.107.042093.
32. Barnes JA, LaCasce AS, Zukotynski K, Israel D, Feng Y, Neuberg D, Toomey CE, Hochberg EP, Canellos GP, Abramson JS. End-of-treatment but not interim PET scan predicts outcome in nonbulky limited-stage Hodgkin's lymphoma. Ann Oncol. 2011;22(4):910–5. https://doi.org/10.1093/annonc/mdq549.
33. Gallamini A, Rigacci L, Merli F, Nassi L, Bosi A, Capodanno I, Luminari S, Vitolo U, Sancetta R, Iannitto E, Trentin L, Stelitano C, Tavera S, Biggi A, Castagnoli A, Versari A, Gregianin M, Pelosi E, Torchio P, Levis A. The predictive value of positron emission tomography scanning performed after two courses of standard therapy on treatment outcome in advanced stage Hodgkin's disease. Haematologica. 2006;91(4):475–81.
34. Pregno P, Chiappella A, Bello M, Botto B, Ferrero S, Franceschetti S, Giunta F, Ladetto M, Limerutti G, Menga M, Nicolosi M, Priolo G, Puccini B, Rigacci L, Salvi F, Vaggelli L, Passera R, Bisi G, Vitolo U. Interim 18-FDG-PET/CT failed to predict the outcome in diffuse large B-cell lymphoma patients treated at the diagnosis with rituximab-CHOP. Blood. 2012;119(9):2066–73.
35. Gallamini A, Hutchings M, Rigacci L, Specht L, Merli F, Hansen M, Patti C, Loft A, Di Raimondo F, D'Amore F, Biggi A, Vitolo U, Stelitano C, Sancetta R, Trentin L, Luminari S, Iannitto E, Viviani S, Pierri I, Levis A. Early interim 2- F-18 Fluoro-2-deoxy-D-glucose positron emission tomography is prognostically superior to international prognostic score in advanced-stage Hodgkin's lymphoma: a report from a joint Italian-Danish study. J Clin Oncol. 2007;25(24):3746–52. https://doi.org/10.1200/jco.2007.11.6525.
36. Markova J, Kobe C, Skopalova M, Klaskova K, Dedeckova K, Plutschow A, Eich HT, Dietlein M, Engert A, Kozak T. FDG-PET for assessment of early treatment response after four cycles of chemotherapy in patients with advanced-stage Hodgkin's lymphoma has a high negative predictive value. Ann Oncol. 2009;20(7):1270–4. https://doi.org/10.1093/annonc/mdn768.
37. Barrington SF, Qian W, Somer EJ, Franceschetto A, Bagni B, Brun E, Almquist H, Loft A, Hojgaard L, Federico M, Gallamini A, Smith P, Johnson P, Radford J, O'Doherty MJ. Concordance between four European centres of PET reporting criteria designed for use in multicentre trials in Hodgkin lymphoma. Eur J Nucl Med Mol Imaging. 2010;37(10):1824–33. https://doi.org/10.1007/s00259-010-1490-5.
38. Itti E, Meignan M, Berriolo-Riedinger A, Biggi A, Cashen AF, Vera P, Tilly H, Siegel BA, Gallamini A, Casasnovas RO, Haioun C. An international confirmatory study of the prognostic value of early PET/CT in diffuse large B-cell lymphoma: comparison between Deauville criteria and DeltaSUVmax. Eur J Nucl Med Mol Imaging. 2013;40(9):1312–20.
39. Strobel K, Schaefer NG, Renner C, Veit-Haibach P, Husarik D, Koma AY, Hany TF. Cost-effective therapy remission assessment in lymphoma patients using 2-[fluorine-18]fluoro-2-deoxy-D-glucose-positron emission tomography/computed tomography: is an end of treatment exam necessary in all patients? Ann Oncol. 2007;18(4):658–64.
40. Biggi A, Gallamini A, Chauvie S, Hutchings M, Kostakoglu L, Gregianin M, Meignan M, Malkowski B, Hofman MS, Barrington SF. International validation study for interim PET in ABVD-treated, advanced-stage Hodgkin lymphoma: interpretation criteria and concordance rate among reviewers. J Nucl Med. 2013;54(5):683–90.
41. Mamot C, Klingbiel D, Renner C, Pabst T, Hitz F, Mey U, Pless M, Bargetzi M, Krasniqi F, Gigli F, Hany T, Samarin A, Rusterholz C, Biaggi C, Zucca E, Martinelli G. (Suppl 1; abst 15) final results of a prospective evaluation of the predictive value of interim PET in patients with DLBCL under R-CHOP-14 (SAKK 38/07). Hematol Oncol. 2013;31:100–1.
42. Dupuis J, Berriolo-Riedinger A, Julian A, Brice P, Tychyj-Pinel C, Tilly H, Mounier N, Gallamini A, Feugier P, Soubeyran P, Colombat P, Laurent G, Berenger N, Casasnovas RO, Vera P, Paone G, Xerri L, Salles G, Haioun C, Meignan M, Ghesquieres H, Cartron G, Seymour JF, Delfau-Larue MH, Offner F, Soubeyran P, Perrot A, Brice P, Bouabdallah R, Sonet A, Dupuis J, Catalano JV, Delmer A, Jardin F, Verney A, Dartigues P, Salles G, Le Gouill S, De Guibert S, Planche L, Brice P, Dupuis J, Cartron G, Van Hoof A, Gyan E, Tilly H, Fruchart C, Deconinck E, Fitoussi O, Gastaud L, Delwail V, Gabarre J, Gressin R, Blanc M, Foussard C, Salles G. Impact of [18F]Fluorodeoxyglucose positron emission tomography response evaluation in patients with high-tumor burden follicular lymphoma treated with Immunochemotherapy: a prospective study from the Groupe d'Etudes des Lymphomes de l'Adulte and GOELAMS. J Clin Oncol. 2012;30(35):4317–22.
43. Fan Y, Zhang Y, Yang Z, Ying Z, Zhou N, Liu C, Song Y, Zhu J, Wang X. Evaluating early interim fluorine-18 fluorodeoxyglucose positron emission tomography/computed tomography with the SUVmax-liver-

based interpretation for predicting the outcome in diffuse large B-cell lymphoma. Leuk Lymphoma. 2017;58:1–9.
44. Casasnovas RO, Ysebaert L, Thieblemont C, Bachy E, Feugier P, Delmer A, Tricot S, Gabarre J, Andre M, Fruchart C, Mounier N, Delarue R, Meignan M, Berriolo-Riedinger A, Bardet S, Emile JF, Jais JP, Haioun C, Tilly H, Morschhauser F. Blood. 2017;130(11):1315–26. https://doi.org/10.1182/blood-2017-02-766691. Epub 2017 Jul 12.
45. Cottereau A, Becker S, Broussais F, Casasnovas O, Kanoun S, Roques M, Charrier N, Bertrand S, Delarue R, Bonnet C. Prognostic value of baseline total metabolic tumor volume (TMTV0) measured on FDG-PET/CT in patients with peripheral T-cell lymphoma (PTCL). Ann Oncol. 2016b;27(4):719–24.
46. Martelli M, Ceriani L, Zucca E, Zinzani PL, Ferreri AJ, Vitolo U, Stelitano C, Brusamolino E, Cabras MG, Rigacci L. [18F] fluorodeoxyglucose positron emission tomography predicts survival after chemoimmunotherapy for primary mediastinal large B-cell lymphoma: results of the International Extranodal Lymphoma Study Group IELSG-26 Study. J Clin Oncol. 2014;32(17):1769–75.
47. Younes A, Hilden P, Coiffier B, Hagenbeek A, Salles G, Wilson W, Seymour J, Kelly K, Gribben J, Pfreunschuh M. International Working Group consensus response evaluation criteria in lymphoma (RECIL 2017). Ann Oncol. 2017;28(7):1436–47.
48. Horwitz S, Coiffier B, Foss F, Prince H, Sokol L, Greenwood M, Caballero D, Morschhauser F, Pinter-Brown L, Iyer SP. Utility of 18fluoro-deoxyglucose positron emission tomography for prognosis and response assessments in a phase 2 study of romidepsin in patients with relapsed or refractory peripheral T-cell lymphoma. Ann Oncol. 2015;26(4):774–9.
49. Kim SJ, Choi JY, Hyun SH, Ki C-S, Oh D, Ahn YC, Ko YH, Choi S, Jung S-H, Khong P-L. Risk stratification on the basis of Deauville score on PET-CT and the presence of Epstein-Barr virus DNA after completion of primary treatment for extranodal natural killer/T-cell lymphoma, nasal type: a multicentre, retrospective analysis. Lancet Haematol. 2015;2(2):e66–74.
50. El-Galaly TC, Mylam KJ, Bøgsted M, Brown P, Rossing M, Gang AO, Haglund A, Arboe B, Clausen MR, Jensen P, Pedersen M, Bukh A, Jensen BA, Poulsen CB, d'Amore F, Hutchings M. Role of routine imaging in detecting recurrent lymphoma: a review of 258 patients with relapsed aggressive non-Hodgkin and Hodgkin lymphoma. Am J Hematol. 2014;89(6):575–80. https://doi.org/10.1002/ajh.23688.
51. Truong Q, Shah N, Knestrick M, Curley B, Hu Y, Craig M, Hamadani M. Limited utility of surveillance imaging for detecting disease relapse in patients with non-Hodgkin lymphoma in first complete remission. Clin Lymphoma Myeloma Leuk. 2014;14(1):50–5.

15 Kinase Inhibitors in Large Cell Lymphoma

Franck Morschhauser, Salomon Manier, and Nathan Fowler

15.1 Introduction

Regulation of a broad array of cellular functions in both normal cells and cancer is controlled through the phosphorylation of unique proteins within multistep signaling pathways. Phosphorylation is directed through hundreds of specific kinases which can be activated through a variety of mechanisms. Not surprisingly, these tightly regulated networks are critical to nearly all cellular functions and can be abnormally activated or suppressed in cancer through both genetic and epigenetic mechanisms [1]. Often, these alterations in kinase activity result in tumorigenic changes leading to increased survival and resistance, as well as tumor growth and spread (Fig. 15.1). It has also become evident that aberrant kinase activity plays a central role in a tumor's ability to evade immune surveillance. As a result, kinase inhibition has emerged as a field of intense study across multiple cancer subtypes, and currently over 25 oncology drugs that target kinases are approved in the United States [1].

F. Morschhauser · S. Manier
Department of Hematology, Lille University Hospital, Lille, France
e-mail: f-morschhauser@chru-lille.fr

N. Fowler (✉)
Department of Lymphoma/Myeloma, MD Anderson Cancer Center, Houston, TX, USA
e-mail: nfowler@mdanderson.org

Recently, insights into important kinase-controlled pathways in aggressive B-cell malignancies have led to the development of several inhibitors with potential in lymphoma. Unfortunately, due to the overlapping and redundant nature of most signaling cascades, single agent activity has been low, resistance is common, and most patients still relapse following initial response. Toxicity has also been difficult to predict, likely due to the ubiquitous nature of several targets and their multifunction role across cell types. Despite these setbacks, promising kinase-based combinations are emerging, and research on predictive biomarkers is underway.

This chapter will review some of the current classes of tyrosine kinase inhibitors being studied in aggressive B-cell lymphomas, along with recent clinical outcomes seen with the leading novel agents in each class.

15.2 The B-Cell Receptor Pathway

The B-cell receptor (BCR) pathway is essential for the development of both normal B cells and their malignant brethren. The B-cell receptor consists of a highly variable extracellular antigen-binding domain and an intracellular cytoplasmic tail consisting of immunoreceptor tyrosine-based activation motifs (ITAMs) which further generate intracellular signals [2]. The initiation/activation and maintenance of BCR signaling appear to

G. Lenz, G. Salles (eds.), *Aggressive Lymphomas*, Hematologic Malignancies,
https://doi.org/10.1007/978-3-030-00362-3_15

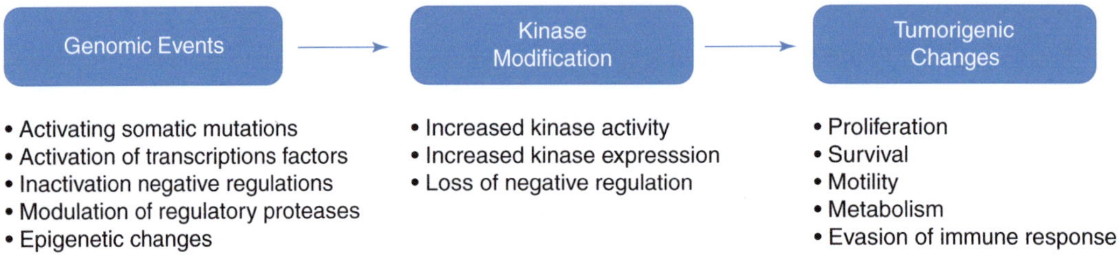

Fig. 15.1 Kinase alterations in aggressive lymphoma

differ in subtypes of aggressive B-cell malignancies, and interruption of this pathway through inhibition of critical kinases represents a viable strategy for targeting aggressive B-cell lymphomas [3]. Although the exact mechanisms of pathway activation are still being elucidated, activated B-cell (ABC) DLBCL likely depends on "chronic active" BCR signaling mediated through receptor clustering, while germinal center B-cell (GCB) DLBCLs may be stimulated in an antigen-independent manner through receptor cross-linking leading or "tonic" signaling [4, 5]. Furthermore, gain-of-function mutations in the BCR subunit CD79 occur more frequently in ABC subtype compared to GCB.

15.2.1 BTK Inhibitors

Bruton's tyrosine kinase (BTK), a member of the TEC family kinases, lies proximal in the BCR and is required for pathway signaling. BTK is activated by Src family kinases Blk and Lyn and phosphorylates phospholipase Cγ (PLC gamma). Signaling through BTK eventually leads to downstream activation of both NF-kB and MAP kinase pathways [6]. Inhibition of BTK as a therapeutic strategy has been extremely successful in chronic lymphocytic leukemia (CLL) and mantle cell lymphoma and has modest but consistent activity in aggressive large cell lymphomas.

15.2.1.1 Ibrutinib

Ibrutinib is an oral, covalent irreversible inhibitor of BTK. Initial phase I studies of ibrutinib reported responses in two of seven DLBCL patients [7]. A subsequent phase I/II study by Wilson and colleagues enrolled patients with both relapsed ABC and GCB diffuse large B-cell lymphoma. The study enrolled 80 patients, including 54% of patients who were refractory to prior therapy and 23% who had failed a prior stem cell transplant. All patients received standard dosing with 560 mg once daily. The overall response rate across subtypes of DLBCL was 22% including 9% of patients who achieved a complete remission. Progression-free survival was 5 months. As part of the initial study design, all patients underwent analysis of their primary tumor by gene expression profiling to determine the cell of origin. Interestingly, although patient characteristics were common between groups, inhibition of BTK was dramatically different between subtypes of DLBCL. Patients with ABC DLBCL achieved an overall response rate of 37%, including 16% who achieved complete remission. The response rate in GCB DLBCL was only 5%. Furthermore, ABC lymphomas with mutations in the BCR were especially sensitive to ibrutinib therapy with an overall response rate of 56%. Common toxicities associated with ibrutinib include fatigue, atrial fibrillation, bruising, and hypertension [8]. A subsequent phase Ib study combined ibrutinib with R-CHOP in patients with untreated DLBCL. Younes and colleagues reported a 94% overall response rate with the combination without an evident increase in toxicity [9]. Phase III studies of R-CHOP with or without ibrutinib in DLBCL are underway.

15.2.1.2 Tirabrutinib

Tirabrutinib (ONO-4059) is a selective and reversible inhibitor of BTK with a 50% inhibitory concentration (IC50) of 2 nmol/L and an

IC50 of greater than 300-fold selectivity for other kinases. Of the 35 patients with DLBCL recruited in the phase I trial, 31 were classified as ABC DLBCL using the Hans immunohistochemical algorithm. Median number of prior treatments was three (range two to ten), and 30/35 patients were refractory to their last line of chemotherapy. 11/31 (35%) of ABC subtype responded with two confirmed complete responses and one CRu. Median time on treatment was 12 weeks. Tirabrutinib was generally very well tolerated. The most common (75%) were grade 1 or 2 in severity. Grade 3 or 4 toxicities were mainly hematological, occurred early during therapy, and recovered spontaneously. There were no grade 3 or 4 episodes of hemorrhage. Diarrhea and arthralgia were classified as grade 2 toxicity in their most severe forms (Walter et al. Blood. 2016;127(4):411–9. https://doi.org/10.1182/blood-2015-08-664,086. Epub 2015 Nov 5).

15.2.1.3 Acalabrutinib and BGB-3111

Several other inhibitors of BTK are also in development. Acalabrutinib is a covalent inhibitor of BTK with a more selective profile than ibrutinib. A phase I study of acalabrutinib in relapsed chronic lymphocytic leukemia (CLL) demonstrated a response rate of 95% when the drug was given twice daily. The most common side effects reported included headache and diarrhea [10]. Studies are ongoing with acalabrutinib as a single agent and in combination with chemotherapy in patients with untreated and relapsed DLBCL. BGB-3111 is another specific, irreversible inhibitor of BTK. Preclinical studies suggest greater selectivity for BTK versus other TEC- and EGFR-family kinases compared to ibrutinib [11]. Phase Ib studies of BGB-3111 in 46 patients with aggressive lymphomas, including mantle cell lymphoma, demonstrated an overall response rate of 61% to the drug as a single agent. Frequent side effects included bruising, changes in bowel habits, fatigue, and upper respiratory tract infections [12]. How the activity of next-generation BTK inhibitors compare to ibrutinib in aggressive lymphoma will require further study.

15.2.2 SYK Inhibitors

The cytoplasmic non-receptor tyrosine kinase, SYK, is constitutively activated in B-cell lymphomas and plays a critical role in BCR signaling. SYK amplification of the BCR signal promotes subsequent downstream signaling through BTK and PI3K, and the kinase has been shown to act as an oncogene in certain hematologic malignancies [13]. Several SYK inhibitors are currently in clinical trials for hematologic malignancies including fostamatinib, entospletinib, cerdulatinib, and TAK-659.

15.2.2.1 Fostamatinib

Fostamatinib was one of the first oral SYK inhibitors to enter into clinical studies for lymphoma. In a pilot phase I/II study of 22 patients with refractory DLBCL, the overall response rate was 22% with a median progression-free survival of 2.7 months. Side effects of the drug included diarrhea, neutropenia, and thrombocytopenia [14]. Unfortunately, larger phase II studies at various doses demonstrated minimal activity in aggressive lymphoma (overall response rate of 3%) with similar adverse events [15]. Responses also did not appear to differ regardless of cell of origin.

15.2.2.2 Entospletinib

Entospletinib (GS-9973) is another orally available selective inhibitor of SYK. The agent has shown promising activity in relapsed and refractory CLL with up to 61% of patients demonstrating response [16]. In pretreated indolent lymphoma, approximately 13% of patients responded to the drug. Common adverse events associated with the drug included dyspnea, pneumonia, neutropenia, transaminitis, and fever [16]. Although clinical data is lacking in DLBCL, preclinical models in aggressive hematologic malignancies including a DLBCL cell lines suggest SYK inhibition can lead to cell cycle arrest and apoptosis by preventing SYK-dependent activation of PLCγ2 and AKT [17]. Combination studies with the PI3K inhibitor idelalisib and entospletinib in relapsed NHL and CLL were halted due to unexpected and often severe immune toxicities [18].

15.2.2.3 Cerdulatinib

Cerdulatinib (PRT062070) is a dual JAK/SYK total inhibitor which has shown promising activity in CLL and in preclinical models of large cell lymphoma. In ABC and GCB cell lines, cerdulatinib induced cell death associated with caspase-3 cleavage [19]. Phase I studies with cerdulatinib in relapsed CLL, indolent lymphoma, and DLBCL are underway with interim results demonstrating tolerable safety profiles [20].

15.3 PI3K/mTOR/AKT Pathway

The phosphoinositide 3-kinases (PI3Ks) play a pivotal role in multiple cellular processes, including cell differentiation, proliferation, cell cycle, cellular metabolism, angiogenesis, survival, apoptosis, and motility [21]. PI3Ks are intracellular lipid kinases that transmit extracellular signals from transmembrane receptors such as G-protein-coupled receptors (GPCRs) and receptor tyrosine kinases (RTKs) to the cytoplasm and thereby regulate key cellular processes [22]. Downstream effectors of PI3K signaling include the AKT/mTOR pathway, which governs oncogenic processes such as metabolism, chemoresistance, cell cycle regulation, growth, and proliferation [23, 24]. The PI3K/AKT/mTOR pathway is deregulated in a subset of cases in a variety of lymphoma subtypes including Hodgkin, diffuse large B-cell, mantle cell, and follicular lymphoma [25–28].

15.3.1 PI3K Inhibitors

Class I PI3Ks are heterodimers consisting of regulatory (p85) and catalytic (p110) subunits. The p110 subunit exists as four isoforms (α, β, γ, δ) with nonoverlapping functions and different expression profiles. The α and β isoforms are expressed ubiquitously, while the γ and δ isoforms are expressed primarily in the hematopoietic tissues. Knockout studies in mice have shown that lack of p110c and p110d is associated with an impaired immune response and B-cell development [29]. Due to its prominent role in lymphoma, there is great interest in the development of PI3K inhibitors in clinical trials.

15.3.1.1 Idelalisib

Idelalisib is a PI3K delta inhibitor and has been extensively studied in indolent lymphoma [30, 31] but not significantly in DLBCL. In mantel cell lymphoma, a phase I trial investigated idelalisib as a single agent in 40 patients with a median of four prior therapies [32]. The ORR was 40% including two patients who attained complete remission (CR). Despite promising response rates, single agent therapy rarely resulted in durable remissions, prompting subsequent combination studies. A separate phase I study combines idelalisib with everolimus or bortezomib or rituximab and bendamustine, with a response rate of 46% [33]. Other combination studies with idelalisib and BTK inhibitors are currently under investigation in patients with B-cell malignancies including non-GC DLBCL. Regarding toxicity, elevation of liver transaminase is frequently observed as well as the class-specific side effect diarrhea (reported in approximately 25% of patients). Neutropenia has also been reported and occurs in a dose-independent manner. Pneumonitis was seen in 3% of patients treated on single agent studies and generally occurred after several months of treatment [33].

15.3.1.2 Duvelisib

Duvelisib is an oral, dual inhibitor of the PI3K delta and gamma isoforms which is also being investigated in lymphoid diseases. In a phase I trial, including relapsed/refractory NHL patients, duvelisib has demonstrated clinical activity and a safety profile similar to idelalisib [34, 35]. Although the maximum tolerated dose was 75 mg BID, concurrent pharmacokinetic (PK) studies suggested full target inhibition at lower doses, and 25 mg BID was selected for further testing. The 26 patients with aggressive B-cell NHL who enrolled in the phase I study achieved an ORR of 19% (8% CR). The overall response rate was 50% in MCL (5/10 including 1 CR), 50% in peripheral T-cell lymphoma—including 3 CR out of 16 patients—and 32% in cutaneous T-cell lymphoma. Severe adverse events (≥ 3) occurred in 84% of patients, mainly neutropenia, thrombocytopenia, and transamanitis [35].

15.3.1.3 Copanlisib

Copanlisib is a novel dual inhibitor of PI3K delta and gamma isoforms. In preclinical models, copanlisib was predominantly active in ABC DLBCL [36]. A phase II study by Lenz and colleagues evaluated copanlisib in 67 patients with relapsed or refractory DLBCL and three or more prior therapies. The overall response rate was 25% with a median of PFS of 8.1 months in responders. The main adverse events included hypertension and hyperglycemia. Twenty-five percent of patients with ABC DLBCL achieved a complete remission [37]. Another phase II trial evaluated copanlisib in 33 patients with indolent lymphoma and 51 with aggressive lymphoma, mostly T-cell lymphoma. The overall response rate was 27% in the aggressive cohort with a PFS of 70 days. Similar adverse events were observed. Interestingly, a predominant activity was observed in tumors with up-regulation of PI3K pathway [38].

15.3.1.4 Umbralisib

Umbralisib (TGR-1202) is a potent and selective inhibitor of p110δ, with a unique molecular structure. Umbralisib has been shown to induce cytotoxicity, and inhibit AKT phosphorylation at submicromolar concentrations in cell lines regardless of 17p deletion, and was equipotent to idelalisib [39]. TGR-1202 has shown promising activity in patients, with a 94% nodal response rate observed in CLL patients treated with umbralisib monotherapy. Preliminary results suggest that hepatotoxicity, colitis, and opportunistic infections, such as pneumonia and pneumonitis, were less common, possibly due to conservation of Th2 cytokine expression and GATA-3 mRNA compared to other PI3Kδ inhibitors as well as a differential effect on regulatory T cells [40]. To date, little data has been reported with umbralisib as a single agent in DLBCL. O'Connor and colleagues reported responses in 3 out of 12 patients from a single agent monotherapy study [41]. A subsequent combination trial with anti-CD20 therapy reported partial remissions in 4 out of 12 patients with DLBCL [42]. Larger studies are underway in DLBCL, stratifying patients according to cell of origin (GCB/ABC).

15.3.2 mTOR Inhibitors

The mechanistic target of rapamycin (mTOR) is a core component of mTOR complex 1 and mTOR complex 2, which regulates different cellular processes such as cell growth, cell proliferation, cell motility, cell survival, protein synthesis, autophagy, and transcription. The most established mTOR inhibitors are called rapalogs (rapamycin and its analogs).

15.3.2.1 Temsirolimus

Temsirolimus has significant activity in relapsed mantle cell lymphoma. Single agent studies have shown response rates of 38% or combined with rituximab (ORR of 59%) [43]. Based on these trials, temsirolimus has received orphan drug approval for relapsed mantle cell lymphoma in Europe. Early studies also suggest temsirolimus has efficacy in other NHL subtypes, including DLBCL [44].

15.3.2.2 Everolimus

Everolimus is an oral mTORC1 inhibitor that is approved by the Food and Drug Administration for relapsed renal cell, brain, neuroendocrine, and hormone receptor-positive breast cancers. A phase II trial of everolimus in relapsed aggressive lymphoma demonstrated an ORR of 30% [45]. Everolimus was also evaluated in combination with the histone deacetylase inhibitor panobinostat in relapsed or refractory lymphomas. Toxicities were mild, and the ORR was 33% with complete response rate of 15% in heavily pretreated lymphoma. The limiting dose toxicity was thrombocytopenia [46]. Unfortunately, in a subsequent a phase III trial, adjuvant everolimus in patients with poor-risk DLBCL demonstrated no improvement in disease-free survival [47]. A newer generation of mTOR inhibitors, which are now entering clinical trials, is able to block mTORC1 and mTORC2 and might allow greater efficacy and avoidance of the compensatory phosphorylation of AKT.

15.3.3 AKT Inhibitors

Perifosine is a first-generation AKT inhibitor that functions via inhibition of AKT translocation to the cell membrane. Combined in a phase II trial, sorafenib and perifosine had an ORR of 22% in relapsed or refractory lymphoproliferative diseases [48]. Due to limited efficacy and moderate toxicities, there are currently no ongoing clinical trials evaluating perifosine in patients with lymphoma.

A second-generation AKT inhibitor, MK-2206, was tested in a phase II trial including 59 patients with relapsed or refractory lymphoma. The ORR was 14% including two CR and six PR, with a median duration of response of 5.8 months [49].

15.4 Anaplastic Lymphoma Kinase Inhibitors

15.4.1 Role in T-cell and B-cell lymphomas

Chromosomal translocation t(2;5) is associated with approximately 60% of anaplastic large cell lymphomas (ALCLs). The translocation creates a fusion gene consisting of the anaplastic lymphoma kinase (ALK) gene and the nucleophosmin (NPM) gene. The product of the NPM-ALK fusion gene is oncogenic. In other cases, ALK is fused to TPM3 or more rarely to other partners, such as TFG, ATIC, CLTC1, TPM4, MSN, ALO17, and MYH9 [50]. ALK-positive DLBCL is a rare variant of DLBCL. In a retrospective cohort of 38 cases of ALK-positive DLBCL, most patients had an aggressive clinical course with advanced stage at diagnosis and poor outcome. Overall survival was 20.3 months in this CHOP and CHOP-like regimen-treated cohort [51].

15.4.2 Overview of Active Studies

Limited data exists utilizing ALK inhibitors in lymphoma. In a retrospective cohort of 11 patients with relapsed ALK-positive ALCLs treated with the ALK inhibitor, ceritinib, the overall response rate was 90%, with seven patients in durable CR. OS and PFS at 2 years were 72.7% and 63.7%, respectively [52]. Safety and tolerability of ceritinib were evaluated in a phase I trial enrolling 304 patients with ALK-positive tumors, among which three had relapsed ALK-positive ALCL. Two of them achieved a durable CR and one a PR [53]. Given the high remission rate, long duration of remission, and acceptable tolerability of treatment, ALK inhibitors may have promise in the treatment of patients with ALK-positive ALCL. Phase II studies are ongoing to evaluate the activity of ceritinib as single agent in patients affected by resistant or refractory ALK-positive lymphoma.

15.5 Aurora Kinase Inhibitors

The aurora family of kinases regulate key cell cycle events including mitotic processes such as chromosome alignment and segregation. Overexpression of aurora kinases has been observed in several malignancies including aggressive lymphomas, and efforts have been made recently to develop agents targeting members of the kinase family. Preclinical studies suggest that inhibition of aurora kinases can result in mitotic arrest, chromosome misalignment, and apoptosis [54].

15.5.1 Alisertib

Alisertib (MLN8237) is an orally available selective aurora A kinase inhibitor with antiproliferative activity across several human tumor cell lines [54]. The agent has also been shown to inhibit tumor growth in mouse xenograft models with DLBCL [55]. Initial phase I studies in relapsed myeloma, non-Hodgkin's lymphoma, and CLL were recently reported. Responses were observed and 13% of patients with 2 out of 17 patients with DLBCL attaining partial remission. The drug was associated with revisable neutropenia, thrombocytopenia, and leukopenia [56].

Friedberg and colleagues reported a subsequent phase II study of alisertib in aggressive B- and T-cell non-Hodgkin's lymphomas. Forty-eight patients were enrolled, including 21 patients with relapsed DLBCL. Although the drug was well tolerated, only 3 out of 21 patients (14%) with DLBCL responded [57]. Single agent and combination studies of alisertib in aggressive B-cell and T-cell lymphoma are ongoing.

15.6 Conclusion

With improved understanding of key cellular pathways and their respective kinase drivers, more therapeutic targets in DLBCL are emerging. Unfortunately, most studies targeting single kinases in aggressive lymphoma have been met with low response rates and short remissions. Toxicity modeling has also been challenging due to several inhibitors' lack of specificity and the ubiquitous nature of many kinase targets. Next-generation agents and studies will focus on gaining a deeper understanding of not only the effect of target inhibition on both malignant and normal cells but developing predictive biomarkers for efficacy and toxicity.

References

1. Gross S, Rahal R, Stransky N, et al. Targeting cancer with kinase inhibitors. J Clin Invest. 2015;125:1780–9.
2. Liu W, Meckel T, Tolar P, Sohn HW, Pierce SK. Antigen affinity discrimination is an intrinsic function of the B cell receptor. J Exp Med. 2010;207:1095–111.
3. Neimann C, Weistner A. B-cell receptor signaling as a driver of lymphoma development and evolution. Semin Cancer Biol. 2015;23:410–21.
4. Davis E, Ngo V, Lenz G, et al. Chronic active B-cell receptor signaling in diffuse large B-cell lymphoma. Nature. 2010;463:88–92.
5. Havranek O, Xu J, Davis E, et al. Molecular aspects of tonic B-cell receptor signaling in diffuse large B-cell lymphoma provide biomarkers and targets for specific inhibition. Blood. 2016;128:779.
6. Honigberg L, Smith A, Sirisawad M, et al. The Bruton tyrosine kinase inhibitor PCI-32765 blocks B-cell activation and is efficacious in models of autoimmune disease and B-cell malignancy. PNAS. 2010;107:13075–80.
7. Advani R, Buggy J, Sharman J, et al. Bruton tyrosine kinase inhibitor Ibrutinib (PCI-32765) has significant activity in patients with relapsed/refractory B-cell malignancies. J Clin Oncol. 2013;31(1):88–94.
8. Wilson W, Young R, Schmitz R, et al. Targeting B cell receptor signaling with ibrutinib in diffuse large B cell lymphoma. Nat Med. 2015;21(8):922–6.
9. Younes A, Theiblemont C, Morchhauser F, et al. Combination of ibrutinib with rituximab, cyclophosphamide, doxorubicin, vincristine, and prednisone (R-CHOP) for treatment-naive patients with CD20-positive B-cell non-Hodgkin lymphoma: a non-randomised, phase 1b study. Lancet Oncol. 2015;15(9):1019–26.
10. Byrd J, Harrington B, O'Brien S, et al. Acalabrutinib in relapsed chronic lymphocytic leukemia. N Eng J Med. 2016;374:323–32.
11. Li C, Yang L, Bell T, et al. Novel Bruton's tyrosine kinase inhibitor Bgb-3111 demonstrates potent activity in mantle cell lymphoma. Blood. 2016;128:5374.
12. Tam C, Simpson D, Opat S, et al. Safety and activity of the highly specific BTK inhibitor BGB-3111 in patients with indolent and aggressive non Hodgkin's lymphoma. Blood. 2017;130:152.
13. Mocsai A, Ruland J, Tybulewiicz V, et al. The SYK tyrosine kinase: a crucial player in diverse biological functions. Nat Rev Immunol. 2010;10(6):387–402.
14. Friedberg J, Sharman J, Sweetenham J, et al. Inhibition of Syk with fostamatinib disodium has significant clinical activity in non-Hodgkin lymphoma and chronic lymphocytic leukemia. Blood. 2010;115:2578–85.
15. Flinn I, Bartlett N, Blum K, et al. A phase II trial to evaluate the efficacy of fostamatinib in patients with relapsed or refractory diffuse large B-cell lymphoma (DLBCL). Eur J Cancer. 2016;54:11–7.
16. Sharman J, Klein L, Boxer M, et al. Phase 2 trial of Entospletinib (GS-9973), a selective Syk inhibitor, in indolent non-Hodgkin's lymphoma (iNHL). Blood. 2015;126:1545.
17. Cheng S, Coffey G, Zhang XH, et al. SYK inhibition and response prediction in diffuse large B-cell lymphoma. Blood. 2011;118:6342–52.
18. Barr P, Saylors G, et al. Phase 2 study of idelalisib and entospletinib: pneumonitis limits combination therapy in relapsed refractory CLL and NHL. Blood. 2016;127(20):2411–5.
19. Ma J, Xing W, Coffey G, et al. Cerdulatinib, a novel dual SYK/JAK kinase inhibitor, has broad anti-tumor

activity in both ABC and GCB types of diffuse large B cell lymphoma. Oncotarget. 2015;22:43881–96.
20. Hamlin P, Farber C, Fenske T, et al. The dual SYK/JAK inhibitor cerdulatinib demonstrates rapid tumor responses in a Phase 2 Study in patients with relapsed B-cell malignancies. Hematol Oncol. 2017;35:74.
21. Cantley LC. The phosphoinositide 3-kinase pathway. Science. 2002;296(5573):1655–7.
22. Liu P, Cheng H, Roberts TM, Zhao JJ. Targeting the phosphoinositide 3-kinase pathway in cancer. Nat Rev Drug Discov. 2009;8(8):627–44.
23. Engelman JA. Targeting PI3K signalling in cancer: opportunities, challenges and limitations. Nat Rev Cancer. 2009;9(8):550–62.
24. Hennessy BT, Smith DL, Ram PT, Lu Y, Mills GB. Exploiting the PI3K/AKT pathway for cancer drug discovery. Nat Rev Drug Discov. 2005;4(12):988–1004.
25. Meadows SA, Vega F, Kashishian A, Johnson D, Diehl V, Miller LL, et al. PI3Kdelta inhibitor, GS-1101 (CAL-101), attenuates pathway signaling, induces apoptosis, and overcomes signals from the microenvironment in cellular models of Hodgkin lymphoma. Blood. 2012;119(8):1897–900.
26. Go H, Jang JY, Kim PJ, Kim YG, Nam SJ, Paik JH, et al. MicroRNA-21 plays an oncogenic role by targeting FOXO1 and activating the PI3K/AKT pathway in diffuse large B-cell lymphoma. Oncotarget. 2015;6(17):15035–49.
27. Psyrri A, Papageorgiou S, Liakata E, Scorilas A, Rontogianni D, Kontos CK, et al. Phosphatidylinositol 3′-kinase catalytic subunit alpha gene amplification contributes to the pathogenesis of mantle cell lymphoma. Clin Cancer Res. 2009;15(18):5724–32.
28. Yahiaoui OI, Nunes JA, Castanier C, Devillier R, Broussais F, Fabre AJ, et al. Constitutive AKT activation in follicular lymphoma. BMC Cancer. 2014;14:565.
29. Rommel C, Camps M, Ji H. PI3K delta and PI3K gamma: partners in crime in inflammation in rheumatoid arthritis and beyond? Nat Rev Immunol. 2007;7(3):191–201.
30. Flinn IW, Kahl BS, Leonard JP, Furman RR, Brown JR, Byrd JC, et al. Idelalisib, a selective inhibitor of phosphatidylinositol 3-kinase-delta, as therapy for previously treated indolent non-Hodgkin lymphoma. Blood. 2014;123(22):3406–13.
31. Gopal AK, Kahl BS, de Vos S, Wagner-Johnston ND, Schuster SJ, Jurczak WJ, et al. PI3Kdelta inhibition by idelalisib in patients with relapsed indolent lymphoma. N Engl J Med. 2014;370(11):1008–18.
32. Kahl BS, Spurgeon SE, Furman RR, Flinn IW, Coutre SE, Brown JR, et al. A phase 1 study of the PI3Kdelta inhibitor idelalisib in patients with relapsed/refractory mantle cell lymphoma (MCL). Blood. 2014;123(22):3398–405.
33. Wagner-Johnston ND, De Vos S, Leonard J, Sharman JP, Schreeder MT, Fowler NH. Preliminary results of PI3Kδ inhibitor idelalisib (GS-1101) treatment in combination with everolimus, bortezomib, or bendamustine/rituximab in patients with previously treated mantle cell lymphoma (MCL). ASCO Meeting Abstr. 2013;31:8501.
34. Flinn I, Patel MR, Maris MB, Matous J, Cherry M, Berdeja JG. An open-label, phase Ib study of Duvelisib (IPI-145) in combination with Bendamustine, Rituximab or Bendamustine/Rituximab in select subjects with lymphoma or chronic lymphocytic leukemia. Blood. 2014;124:4422.
35. Horwitz SM, Porcu P, Flinn I, Kahl BS, Sweeney J, Stern HM, Douglas M, Allen K, Kelly P, Foss FM. Duvelisib (IPI-145), a Phosphoinositide-3-Kinase-δ,γ inhibitor, shows activity in patients with relapsed/refractory T-cell lymphoma. Blood. 2014;124:803.
36. Erdmann T, Klener P, Lynch JT, Grau M, Vockova P, Molinsky J, et al. Sensitivity to PI3K and AKT inhibitors is mediated by divergent molecular mechanisms in subtypes of DLBCL. Blood. 2017;130(3):310–22.
37. Lenz G, Hawkes E, Verhoef G, et al. Clinical outcomes and molecular characterization from a phase II study of copanlisib in patients with relapsed or refractory diffuse large B-cell lymphoma. Hematol Oncol. 2017;35:68–9.
38. Dreyling M, Morschhauser F, Bouabdallah K, Bron D, Cunningham D, Assouline SE, et al. Phase II study of copanlisib, a PI3K inhibitor, in relapsed or refractory, indolent or aggressive lymphoma. Ann Oncol. 2017;28(9):2169–78.
39. Freidman D, Lanasa M, Brander D, et al. Comparison of the PI3K-δ inhibitors TGR1202 and GS-1101 in inducing cytotoxicity and inhibiting phosphorylation of Akt in CLL cells in vitro. Blood. 2012;120:3914.
40. Maharaj KK, Powers J, Fonseca R, et al. Abstract 545: differential regulation of human T-cells by TGR-1202, a novel PI3Kδ inhibitor. Cancer Res. 2016;76(14 Supplement):545.
41. O'Connor OO, Flinn IW, Patel MR, et al. TGR-1202, a novel once daily PI3K-delta inhibitor, demonstrates clinical activity with a favorable safety profile in patients with CLL and B-cell lymphoma [abstract]. Blood. 2015;126(23).
42. Lunning MA, Vose J, Fowler N, et al. Ublituximab + TGR-1202 demonstrates activity and a favorable safety profile in relapsed/refractory B-cell NHL and high-risk CLL: phase I results [abstract]. Blood. 2015;126(23). Abstract 1538.
43. Witzig TE, Geyer SM, Ghobrial I, Inwards DJ, Fonseca R, Kurtin P, et al. Phase II trial of single-agent temsirolimus (CCI-779) for relapsed mantle cell lymphoma. J Clin Oncol. 2005;23(23):5347–56.
44. Smith SM, van Besien K, Karrison T, Dancey J, McLaughlin P, Younes A, et al. Temsirolimus has activity in non-mantle cell non-Hodgkin's lymphoma subtypes: the University of Chicago phase II consortium. J Clin Oncol. 2010;28(31):4740–6.
45. Witzig TE, Reeder CB, LaPlant BR, Gupta M, Johnston PB, Micallef IN, et al. A phase II trial of the oral mTOR inhibitor everolimus in relapsed aggressive lymphoma. Leukemia. 2011;25(2):341–7.

46. Oki Y, Buglio D, Fanale M, Fayad L, Copeland A, Romaguera J, et al. Phase I study of panobinostat plus everolimus in patients with relapsed or refractory lymphoma. Clin Cancer Res. 2013;19(24):6882–90.
47. Witzig TE, Tobinai K, Rigacci L, Lin T, Ikeda T, Vanazzi A. PILLAR-2: a randomized, double-blind, placebo-controlled, phase III study of adjuvant everolimus (EVE) in patients (pts) with poor-risk diffuse large B-cell lymphoma (DLBCL). J Clin Oncol. 2016;34:7506.
48. Guidetti A, Viviani S, Marchiano A, et al. Dual targeted therapy with the AKT inhibitor perifosine and the multikinase inhibitor sorafenib in patients with relapsed/refractory lymphomas: final results of a phase II trial. Blood. 2012;120:3679.
49. Oki Y, Fanale M, Romaguera J, Fayad L, Fowler N, Copeland A, et al. Phase II study of an AKT inhibitor MK2206 in patients with relapsed or refractory lymphoma. Br J Haematol. 2015;171(4):463–70.
50. Hapgood G, Savage KJ. The biology and management of systemic anaplastic large cell lymphoma. Blood. 2015;126(1):17–25.
51. Laurent C, Do C, Gascoyne RD, Lamant L, Ysebaert L, Laurent G, et al. Anaplastic lymphoma kinase-positive diffuse large B-cell lymphoma: a rare clinicopathologic entity with poor prognosis. J Clin Oncol. 2009;27(25):4211–6.
52. Shaw AT, Kim DW, Mehra R, Tan DS, Felip E, Chow LQ, et al. Ceritinib in ALK-rearranged non-small-cell lung cancer. N Engl J Med. 2014;370(13): 1189–97.
53. Richly H, Kim TM, Schuler M, Kim DW, Harrison SJ, Shaw AT, et al. Ceritinib in patients with advanced anaplastic lymphoma kinase-rearranged anaplastic large-cell lymphoma. Blood. 2015;126(10):1257–8.
54. Bavetsias V, Linardopoulos S. Aurora kinase inhibitors: current status and outlook. Front Oncol. 2015;5:278.
55. Manfredi MG, Ecsedy JA, Chakravarty A, et al. Characterization of Alisertib (MLN8237), an investigational small-molecule inhibitor of aurora A kinase using novel in vivo pharmacodynamic assays. Clin Cancer Res. 2011;17:7614–24.
56. Kelly KR, Shea TC, Goy A, Berdeja JG, Reeder CB, McDonagh KT, et al. Phase I study of MLN8237—investigational aurora A kinase inhibitor—in relapsed/refractory multiple myeloma, non-Hodgkin lymphoma and chronic lymphocytic leukemia. Investig New Drugs. 2014;32:489–99.
57. Friedberg JW, Mahadevan D, Cebula E, Persky D, Lossos I, Agarwal AB, et al. Phase II study of alisertib, a selective aurora A kinase inhibitor, in relapsed and refractory aggressive B- and T-cell non-Hodgkin lymphomas. J Clin Oncol. 2014;32:44–50.

16 Immunological Approaches

Guillaume Cartron, F. Frontzek, and N. Schmitz

16.1 Introduction

Diffuse large B-cell lymphoma (DLBCL) is currently treated with immunochemotherapy based on the R-CHOP regimen (see Chap. 5). Depending on the clinical risk factors summarized by the International Prognostic Index (IPI) and some molecular characteristics of the tumor, about two thirds of patients are cured with standard first-line therapy, whereas one third is primarily refractory or relapse in the further course of disease [1]. Thus, the addition of rituximab to CHOP chemotherapy has dramatically improved survival of patients with DLBCL and largely contributed to the development of monoclonal antibodies (mAbs) in DLBCL and more generally in cancer [2]. This first clinical success of immunotherapy led different companies to develop new mAbs targeting new surface molecules or being modified to elicit increased immune activity or to bring chemotherapy or a radioactive isotope closer to the tumor cells. Patients who relapse after R-containing first-line therapy [3] showed their dismal prognosis; the recently published SCHOLAR-1 study described an objective response rate of only 26% (complete response rate 7%) and a median overall survival of 6.3 months for patients with refractory DLBCL [4]. Taken together, the enormous difficulties in successfully managing patients suffering from refractory or relapsed DLBCL demonstrate that novel therapeutic approaches are urgently required. In contrast to other novel approaches discussed below, chimeric antigen receptor T cells (CAR-T) showed remarkable response rates and ongoing remissions in early clinical trials, even in heavily pretreated patients who had failed multiple salvage regimens. Thus, CAR T cells seem to become an important pillar in the therapeutic management of lymphoma even when immunochemotherapy, radiotherapy, and the use of small molecules fail.

16.2 Monoclonal Antibody Therapy

Monoclonal antibodies (mAbs) are undoubtedly one of the therapeutic revolutions of the last 10 years in oncology. Because of the absolute specificity of the antibody for its target, they perfectly illustrate the concept of targeted therapy highlighted at the end of the nineteenth century. Their success can be explained by the progress of

G. Cartron (✉)
Department of Hematology, CHU Montpellier; CNRS UMR 5235, University of Montpellier, Montpellier, France
e-mail: g-cartron@chu-montpellier.fr

F. Frontzek · N. Schmitz
Department of Medicine A, Hematology, Oncology, Hemostaseology and Pneumonology, University Hospital Münster, Münster, Germany

G. Lenz, G. Salles (eds.), *Aggressive Lymphomas*, Hematologic Malignancies,
https://doi.org/10.1007/978-3-030-00362-3_16

biotechnologies made in the 1980s, allowing their humanization. Rituximab (MabThera®, Rituxan®) was the first "humanized" mAb marketed worldwide. The results obtained in non-Hodgkin's lymphomas, especially in DLBCL, and the rapidity of its clinical development largely explain the enthusiasm for this class of drugs. The progress made in understanding the mechanisms of action of this antibody and its ability to interact with the immune system have consequences applicable to all monoclonal antibodies and have allowed the development of new format of mAbs and gave us way to better use these compounds. These successes explain why this antibody is a hope for patients and a model for doctors, scientists, and drug manufacturers.

Given the success of rituximab, various companies first developed monoclonal antibodies that recognize the different proteins expressed on the surface of the B lymphocyte. To date, no other monoclonal antibody targeting a protein expressed by DLBCL cells has been approved. Other strategies were then developed. All of them aim to improve the cellular cytotoxicity of the antibody either by modifying the Fc portion of the antibody itself, enabling it to better recruit the immune effector cells, or by directing one of the two Fab against a protein expressed by immune cells. In the first case, it is essentially the natural killer (NK) cells and the macrophages which are recruited by the optimized Fc portion allowing an improvement of the antibody-dependent cellular cytotoxicity (ADCC); in the other case, the bispecific antibody will recruit the T lymphocytes via CD3 allowing a T-cell killing.

More recently, the demonstration of the mechanisms controlling the immune response during tumorigenesis has made possible identification of key proteins (immune checkpoint) that can be targeted by monoclonal antibodies. It is still too early to say how this strategy will modify the management of DLBCL, but these antibodies could at least in combination contribute to improve long-term control of this disease.

16.2.1 Anti-CD20 Monoclonal Antibodies

In 1984, the second workshop of human leukocyte differentiation antigens identified 11 new clusters of differentiation (CD16 to CD26), including CD20, expressed by all B lymphocytes and B-cell lymphoma. Among the antibodies of this CD20 cluster, clone 1F5 (mouse IgG2a) was selected by Oncogen in Seattle and tested in four patients with lymphomas at the University of Washington [5]. The patient receiving the highest dose experienced a 90% reduction in tumor mass, but the remission lasted only 6 weeks. At that time, IDEC Pharmaceuticals developed a chimeric monoclonal antibody from the murine monoclonal anti-CD20 2B8 antibody (mu-2B8). This antibody was chimerized with the constant domains κ and γ1 (human IgG1 version or ch-C2B8) or κ and γ4 (human IgG4 version) [6]. Only the human IgG1 version was able to activate the complement and recruit the effectors of the immunity, proved to be lymphopenic in the macaque and was developed under the name of rituximab.

Rituximab, combined with chemotherapy, is now the gold standard for treatment of DLBCL [2, 3]. A better knowledge of its mechanisms of action allowed to understand the development of novel anti-CD20 antibodies and, in a broader sense, part of recent development in DLBCL immunotherapy.

16.2.1.1 Rituximab: Mechanisms of Action

Rituximab is a "bifunctional" molecule combining functions related to the recognition of the antigen (and, therefore, specific for the epitope) and functions related to the Fc portion (crystallizable fragment) common to all IgG1. The properties related to the Fc portion make it possible to distinguish the IgG1 monoclonal antibodies from the different isotype monoclonal antibodies (Table 16.1). Thus, IgG1 and IgG3 are the classes of IgG with the greatest capacity to recruit the immune system (effector cells and complement). In mice, however, IgG2a and, to a lesser extent,

Table 16.1 Ability to recruit cellular effectors (A) and complement (B) by immunoglobulins according to their isotype

A

Human		Mouse	
IgG1	++	IgG1	+
IgG2	–	IgG2a	+++
IgG3	++	IgG2b	++
IgG4	–	IgG3	+
IgM	–	IgGM	–

B

	IgG1	IgG2	IgG3	IgM
Classical pathway	+++	+	+++	–
Alternate pathway	–	+	–	–

IgG2b have this property. This difference underlines the difficulties to interpret experiments using humanized monoclonal antibodies in the murine model. The Fc portion of the IgGs is also capable to bind to a receptor named FcRn (or Brambell factor) expressed by endothelial cells, epithelial cells, and syncytiotrophoblast cells. Interaction with this receptor ensures their transplacental or transepithelial passage and allows IgGs to escape the lysosomal degradation that accounts for the longer half-life of IgG compared to other immunoglobulins.

Mechanisms Related to Target Recognition

CD20 is the target antigen of rituximab, and the advent of this therapeutic antibody has led to important advances in the knowledge of this protein and its functions. CD20 is a transmembrane protein (Fig. 16.1) that has characteristics that make it a therapeutic target of choice [7]. Thus, CD20 is expressed by most B lymphocytes but is absent or poorly expressed by B-progenitors or plasma cells, thus maintaining immunoglobulin levels and peripheral lymphoid reconstitution after treatment. After binding to the antibody, CD20 is neither regulated nor released from the plasma surface. This is the extracellular domain, which carries the epitopes recognized by anti-CD20 antibodies. The homology with murine CD20 is 73% and is located essentially in the transmembrane regions. The extracellular domain of murine CD20 differs from that of human CD20 for 16 of the 43 amino acids explaining [8] the lack of rituximab binding to murine CD20.

The function of CD20 has remained unknown for a long time, and its role as a calcium channel has been now demonstrated [9]. However, knockout mice for the gene coding for CD20 do not show phenotypic abnormalities [10], which could testify either to the minor role of CD20 in the physiology of the B lymphocyte or to a certain biological redundancy with other proteins. The use of antibodies directed against CD20 has long been the only method of understanding its function. Two types of properties reported initially to the recognition of two different epitopes could be identified: the first, found with rituximab, but also with other types of anti-CD20 (2H7, B1), leads to inhibitory signals inducing apoptosis and/or antiproliferative activity, whereas the 1F5 antibody activates cell proliferation. In reality, there is a wide variety of epitopes within the extracellular domains, although some residues are critical for antiproliferative activity (Fig. 16.1) [8]. The binding of the antibody to its target induces, under certain conditions, the migration of the antigen within lipid rafts present on the surface of the plasma membrane [11]. This movement is dependent on an amino acid sequence (219–225) located within the intracytoplasmic portion and not present in the mouse. This property allowed the identification of antibodies inducing (type I antibodies: rituximab, 2H7, etc.) or not (type II antibodies: B1, Ly1, etc.) this migration. The translocation of CD20 within these structures allows its colocalization with proteins ensuring the signal transduction. Only the antibodies inducing this migration are able to complement activation (see below) [12]. In vitro and in some cell models, rituximab induces apoptotic cell death. Several pathways for apoptosis activation have been described, in particular by the mitogen-activated protein kinase (MAPK), NFκB, protein kinase C (PKC), or ceramides or BCL-2. The activation of such pathways would explain the synergies observed with certain chemotherapeutic agents (fludarabine, cisplatin, anthracyclines).

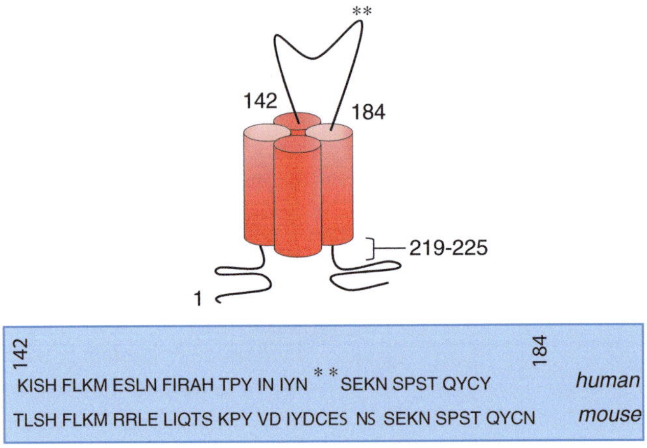

Fig. 16.1 Structure of human CD20. CD20 is a non-glycosylated protein with four transmembrane domains (Tetraspan). The extracellular domain carries the epitopes recognized by the various anti-CD20 antibodies. Alanine and proline located at positions 170 and 172 are important residues in the determination of the rituximab epitope. The sequence between residues 219 and 225 plays an important role in the migration of CD20 into lipid rafts

Mechanisms Related to the Fc Portion

The ability of the Fc portion of IgG1 to interact with cellular immune effectors or complement confers on the set of monoclonal antibodies belonging to this class of common cytolytic properties which largely explain the therapeutic activity of these molecules.

Complement-Dependent Cell Lysis

Complement is an important actor in the eradication of malignant cells. The activation of the classical complement pathway by immunoglobulins (IgG1, IgG3, and IgM) requires the binding of the antibody to its target allowing the binding of the C1q protein to the Fc portion of the antibody. This binding will trigger a proteolytic cascade leading to the formation of a large amount of C3b allowing the formation of the membrane attack complex (MAC) and the destruction of the cell (complement-dependent cell lysis or CDC). It also allows the migration of cells from inflammation (via C3a and C5a) to the activation site and the opsonization of C3b on the target cell allowing its interaction with complement receptors (CR3 and CR4) expressed by immune cells (NK cells, monocytes, neutrophils). Thus, the complement constitutes a system allowing both the direct lysis of the target cell and the establishment of a cytolytic cellular response.

Many in vitro studies have shown that rituximab induces CDC on fresh lymphoma cells. The activation of complement by rituximab was perfectly shown in a syngeneic model of murine lymphoma expressing human CD20 (EL4-huCD20) [13]. In this model, the therapeutic activity of rituximab was not found with mice deficient for C1Q. In humans, administration of rituximab is accompanied by increased concentrations of complement degradation products (C3b/c, C4b/c) [14]. It has been observed in vitro that the complement activation may be different depending on the histological type of lymphoma. The role of the expression level of CD20 or proteins that negatively regulate complement (CD46, CD55, and CD59) on this activity has long been discussed. Recent results have clearly demonstrated that CDC is correlated with the expression level of CD20 by the target cell [15]. The ability of an anti-CD20 antibody to activate complement is also related to the recognized epitope and its ability to relocate CD20 within the lipid rafts. Thus, rituximab or 2H7 that induce effective redistribution (type I) results in CDC, while murine B1 or Ly1 antibodies do not induce CDC due to their inability to migrate CD20 within lipid rafts (type II).

Receptor-Dependent Cellular Lysis at the Fc Portion of the Antibody

The Fc portion of rituximab is capable to interact with receptors at the Fc portion of IgG or FcγRs (Fig. 16.2). By the recruitment of cells expressing these receptors (Table 16.2), immunoglobulins participate in the implementation of immune effector mechanisms such as antibody-dependent cell phagocytosis (ADCP) and ADCC.

The ability of rituximab to induce an ADDC or to mediate ADPC has been demonstrated in vitro on human lymphomatous lines, and the involvement of FcγRs has been shown in a mouse model [16]. The involvement of these receptors and particularly FcγRIIIa has been shown in humans. In fact, this receptor exhibits a nucleotide polymorphism leading to the substitution of the amino acid located at position 158. Thus, two variants of the receptor are possible, one with a valine at position 158 (FcγRIIIa-158 V) and the other with a phenylalanine (FcγRIIIa-158F). This substitution is accompanied by a modification of the affinity between the FcγRIIIa receptor and the Fc portion of the IgG1 [17]. The influence of this amino acid is not surprising since it is located in the site of interaction between these two proteins. A study including patients with follicular lymphoma showed that patients homozygous for the high-affinity receptor for the Fc fragment (FcγRIIIa-158 V) had a better clinical response to

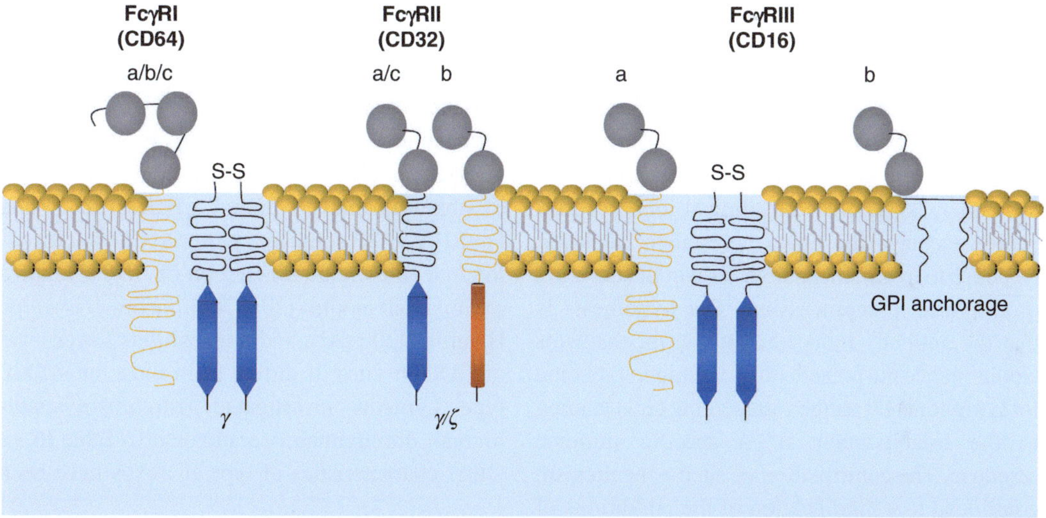

Fig. 16.2 Structure of the different receptors for the Fc portion of IgG immunoglobulins (FcγRs). FcγRIIb is the only inhibitory receptor due to the presence of an ITIM motif (immunoreceptor tyrosine-based inhibition motif) in its intracytoplasmic portion. The presence of an ITAM motif (immunoreceptor tyrosine-based activation motif) in the intracytoplasmic domain or within an associated accessory chain gives to the other FcγRs activating properties

Table 16.2 Cell expression of different receptors for the IgG1 (FcγRs)

	FcγRI	FcγRIIa	FcγRIIb	FcγRIIc	FcγRIIIa	FcγRIIIb
Monocyte/macrophage	+	+	+		+	
NK cells				+	+	
Neutrophil	+/−	+				+
B lymphocyte			+			
Dendritic cell	+	+	+		+	
Mastocyte	+/−	+	+			
Platelet		+				

NK natural killer

rituximab [18]. Since this receptor is expressed by monocytes and NK cells, essential actors of ADCC, this cytolytic mechanism is considered today as an important mode of action of rituximab. Above all, this work emphasized the importance of the interaction between FcγRs and the Fc portion of the antibody. The influence of FcγRIIIa-158 V/F polymorphism on rituximab response was however inconstantly found in DLBCL clinical trials. This could be related either to the lack of importance of ADCC in this histology or by the chemotherapy associated with rituximab which could reduce rituximab-mediated ADCC.

Anti-Lymphoma-Specific Immunity

There are a number of arguments for the initiation of specific anti-lymphoma immunity during treatment with rituximab that murine models seem to confirm [19]. Indeed, most antigen-presenting cells (dendritic cells, macrophages) express FcγRs whose role in the therapeutic activity of the mAbs has been demonstrated. Moreover, a number of clinical observations could account for this mechanism: delayed response to treatment and increase in the duration of response to reprocessing. The hypothesis is that the antibody-induced cytolytic mechanisms would induce the presentation of antigens specific for lymphoma by antigen-presenting cells leading to the establishment of a specific immune response. The confirmation of such a mechanism could lead to a modification of the conditions of rituximab use and would open up new ways to optimize its therapeutic activity.

16.2.1.2 Other Anti-CD20 Monoclonal Antibodies

Glyco-Modified Anti-CD20 Monoclonal Antibodies

The principle of these mAbs is to modify the Fc portion in order to obtain a better affinity for FcγRIIIa. These can be obtained either by modifying the oligosaccharide located between the two Fc arms of the antibody (obinutuzumab, ublituximab) or by mutating the region of the Fc portion involved in the interaction with FcγRIIIa (ocaratuzumab, PRO131921). To date, only obinutuzumab has been tested in clinical trials in DLBCL, and ocaratuzumab and PRO131921 development are stopped.

Obinutuzumab

Obinutuzumab is the first humanized glycoengineered IgG1 anti-CD20 mAb to be tested in clinical trials. Obinutuzumab has been humanized by grafting the complementarity-determining region sequences from the murine antibody B-ly1 into human VH and VL acceptor frameworks [20]. Obinutuzumab was expressed from Chinese hamster ovary (CHO) K1 cell lines engineered to constitutively overexpress the heavy and light chains of obinutuzumab. Those cell lines also express recombinant wild-type β-1,4-*N*-acetyl-glucosaminyltransferase III and wild-type Golgi α-mannosidase II leading to accumulation of antibody glycoforms containing bisected, non-fucosylated oligosaccharides attached to asparagine 297 in the Fc region.

Such modifications induce increased affinity of obinutuzumab to both FcγRIIIa-158 V and FcγRIIIa-158F compared with rituximab translating into an increased induction of ADCC relative to rituximab in vitro [20]. Obinutuzumab is a type II anti-CD20 mAbs and thus exhibits lower level of CDC in vitro. It differs from most anti-CD20 type I mAbs investigated (rituximab, ofatumumab, ublituximab, ocaratuzumab) (Table 16.3). Other characteristics of type II mAbs have been

Table 16.3 In vitro properties of recombinant anti-CD20 monoclonal antibodies

Type I mAbs (rituximab, ofatumumab, veltuzumab, ublituximab, ocaratuzumab, ocrelizumab, PRO131921)	Type II mAbs (obinutuzumab)
Translocate CD20 into lipid rafts → CDC	Do not translocate CD20 into lipid rafts → no CDC
No homotypic adhesion	Homotypic adhesion
Caspase-dependent cell death	Lysosome-dependent cell death
CD20 modulation	No CD20 modulation
ADCC	
ADCP	

ADCC antibody-dependent cellular cytotoxicity; *ADCP* antibody-dependent cell phagocytosis; *CDC* complement-dependent cell lysis

described differentiating these mAbs from type I antibodies: homotypic adhesion resulting in non-caspase-dependent direct cell death, half-maximal CD20 binding at saturating conditions, and less or no CD20 modulation. Except lack of CD20 modulation, all these in vitro properties have been described for obinutuzumab [21] and thus enhance direct cell death compared to rituximab [22]. Preclinical development of obinutuzumab elucidated such differences, leading to the proposal of a model of mechanism of action [20, 23]. Obinutuzumab conformational structure is different to that of rituximab. Firstly, obinutuzumab binds CD20 in a different overlapping epitope than rituximab and in a different orientation [24, 25]. In comparison with rituximab, obinutuzumab is rotated 90° around the Fab middle axis and tilts 70° toward the carboxy-terminus of the CD20 epitope. Moreover, the elbow angle between VH and CH1 is 30° wider. This characteristic could be related to amino acid substitution at position 11 substituting a leucine for a valine [20]. This results in a new spatial arrangement between CD20 and the antibody, and, unlike rituximab, obinutuzumab can bind its two Fab arms on the same CD20 tetramer. This difference in binding CD20 antigen (i.e., intra-CD20 tetramer for type II vs. inter-CD20 tetramer for type I) led authors to propose a dynamic model of interaction [24] explaining the majority of in vitro observations.

An obinutuzumab phase I/II study [26], including previously rituximab-treated DLBCL patients, demonstrated an overall response rate of 30%, which was not different from that obtained with rituximab [27]. Untreated DLBCL patients were randomized to receive eight cycles of either rituximab-$CHOP_{21}$ or obinutuzumab-$CHOP_{21}$ in the GOYA study [28]. No difference was found in terms of overall response rate or progression-free survival (PFS). Such results indicate that the improvement of FcγRIIIA-mediated mechanisms and/or enhancement of direct cytotoxicity does not translate into higher clinical activity in DLBCL, possibly due to low-level CDC observed with obinutuzumab. Final results of randomized phase III GAINED study including younger DLBCL patients receiving more intensive chemotherapy with obinutuzumab or rituximab are awaited soon.

Ublituximab

Ublituximab is a chimeric IgG1k produced by rat hybridoma YB2/0 cells [29] resulting in low percentage of fucosylated glycoforms. In vitro data demonstrated higher ADCC than rituximab but similar direct toxic effect or CDC. No trial testing of ublituximab in DLBCL is ongoing (Table 16.4).

16.2.1.3 Anti-CD20 Monoclonal Antibodies with Increased Affinity for CD20

Ofatumumab is the only representative of this anti-CD20 class. It was selected because its affinity for CD20 appeared to be greater than that observed with rituximab [30]. In fact, it is also a type I antibody, but its off-rate is decreased contributing to a greater aggregation of ofatumumab-CD20 complexes within the lipid rafts, a condition favorable to the recruitment of C1Q, leading to CDC activation. Thus, ofatumumab is characterized by a better CDC than rituximab, especially when antibody concentrations or CD20 expression is low [31, 32]. This property appears to be related to the recognition of a different CD20 epitope [31], ofatumumab, recognizing two epitope

Table 16.4 Anti-CD20 monoclonal antibodies in development

Name	Company	Type (all IgG1κ)	Status
Rituximab	Roche/Genentech	Chimeric	Approved
Ofatumumab	Novartis	Fully human	Approved
Obinutuzumab	Roche/Genentech	Humanized, glycoengineered	Approved
Ublituximab	TG Therapeutics	Chimeric, glycoengineered	Phase III
Veltuzumab	Immunomedics	Humanized	Phase II
Ocaratuzumab	Mentrik Biotech	Humanized, Fc-mutant	Apparently stopped
Ocrelizumab	Roche/Genentech	Humanized	Stopped in hematology
PRO131921	Roche/Genentech	Humanized, Fc-mutant	Stopped

sites with which it interacts via strong bonds [33]. Unfortunately, ofatumumab failed to demonstrate any clinical advantage in relapse/refractory DLBCL compared to rituximab when associated with chemotherapy (Table 16.4) [34].

16.2.2 Bispecific Monoclonal Antibodies

Bispecific mAbs are able to bind two different targets simultaneously and might potentially induce more powerful antitumor response. Different formats of bispecific antibodies are developing. Blinatumomab is a single-chain protein comprising the antigen-binding domains of two different antibodies joined by a non-immunogenic linker that allows for the rotational flexibility to bind two different antigen epitopes on separate cells in close proximity. Blinatumomab contains binding regions for the B-cell lineage-specific antigen, CD19, as well as the invariant CD3ε subunit of the T-cell receptor (TCR) present on all T lymphocytes. Compared to full IgG antibodies (150 KDa), bispecific antibodies exhibit improved tissue distribution and better tumor penetration. Their bivalent nature confers them probably a prolonged target retention. All these characteristics may result in synergistic effect on tumor destruction. A phase II evaluated blinatumomab in 25 DLBCL patients [35]. Among 21 evaluable patients, the overall response after one cycle was 43%, including complete response in 19%, and three patients experienced late complete response in follow-up. Patients experienced grade 3 neurologic events with encephalopathy and aphasia (each 9%) and tremor, speech disorder, dizziness, somnolence, and disorientation (each 4%). Those neurological adverse events are presumably caused by release cytokines. Importantly, continuous infusion is required to ensure sustained effective serum concentration due to a very short half-time of less than 2 h related to the absence of Fc portion and renal excretion. Larger trials evaluating blinatumomab in relapse/refractory DLBCL are ongoing.

The progress of biotechnologies allows today to design new generation of bispecific monoclonal antibodies. Indeed, it is now possible to construct bispecific antibodies while preserving the properties of interest of the Fc portion. For example, the bispecific can retain the format of an IgG1, thus preserving a favorable pharmacokinetic profile of this isotype (in relation to its binding to FcRn) and mutating the CH2 region involved in the interaction with FcγR and C1Q, allowing to repeal any ADCC or CDC. Of course, the absence of such modifications of this region will make it possible to obtain a trifunctional antibody (e.g., CD16xCD3xCD20).

16.2.3 Monoclonal Antibodies Targeting Immune Cells

The emergence of treatments targeting immune checkpoints owes much to the advances in biotechnologies and the ability to produce mAbs directly targeting proteins involved in controlling the immune response. At the same time, considerable progress has been made since the 1970s to better understand the role of the immune response in the development of tumorigenesis. Today, and following the success of targeting immune checkpoints, monoclonal antibodies against proteins involved in immune control are an emerging treatment of DLBCL.

16.2.3.1 Monoclonal Antibodies Targeting Inhibitory Checkpoints

The concept of immune checkpoint emerged when we understood the role of immunological surveillance made by the immune system during tumor development. Thus, the tumor is able to regulate negatively the immune system allowing it to escape to its control. Immune evasion by cancers is accomplished through a variety of mechanisms, including upregulation of negative costimulatory molecules, such as PD1 and CTLA-4.

Three inhibitory checkpoints are currently targeted in DLBCL (Table 16.5).

Antigen-Presenting Cell (APC)/T-Cell Interactions: CTLA-4 Pathway

TCR stimulation by an antigenic peptide in the context of a major histocompatibility complex (MHC) molecule leads to CTLA-4 upregulation on the plasma membrane of the activated T cell

Table 16.5 Anti-immune checkpoint monoclonal antibodies in development

Target	Name	Isotype	Clinical phase	Company
PD1	AMP-224	PD-L2 Ig2a fusion protein	Not available	Amplimmune/GSK
	AMP-514 (MEDI0680)	PD-L2 fusion protein	Phase I	MedImmune/Astra Zeneca
	Nivolumab (Opdivo, BMS-936558, MDX1106)	Human IgG4	Approved	BMS
	Pidilizumab (CT-011)	Humanized IgG1k	Phase I/II	Cure Tech
	Pembrolizumab (MK-3475, lambrolizumab)	Humanized IgG4	Approved	Merck
PD-L1	BMS-936559 (MDX1105)	Human IgG4	Phase I	BMS
	MEDI-4736/Durvalumab	Fc-modified human IgG1k	Phase I–III	MedImmune/ AstraZeneca
	MPDL32801/Atezolizumab	Fc-modified human IgG1k	Phase I–III	Roche
	MSB0010718C/Avelumab	Human IgG1	Approved	Merck/Serono

where it outcompetes CD28 for B7 ligand binding, resulting in costimulation and downregulation of effector T-cell functions. CTLA-4 expression is mainly expressed by T cells in the lymph nodes where initial tumor antigen presentation is thought to occur. Anti-CTLA4 antibody ipilimumab has been tested in phase I trial [36]. Objective response rate was low (11%), but durable complete response suggested that ipilimumab may have additive and durable effect as combination therapy.

Tumor Cell/Activating T-Cell Interactions: PD1 Pathway

PD1 is expressed by activated T cells located in peripheral tissues, including those residing within the tumor. PD1 interacts with PD-L1, which is broadly expressed, and with PD-L2 expressed mainly on hematopoietic cells. The upregulation of PD-1, which occurs after tumor antigen recognition and its binding to PD-L1 or PD-L2 ligands, inhibits intracellular signaling pathways and blocks further T-cell activation. PD-L1 expression is usually induced by inflammatory signals, such as IFNγ produced by activated T cells attempting to execute an active antitumor response (adaptive resistance). In some tumor, PD-L1 expression could be induced through activation of the AKT pathway or gene amplifications, outside inflammatory signals (innate resistance). Primary mediastinal lymphomas exhibit gene fusions between MHC class II transactivator (CIITA) and *PD-L1* or *PD-L2* placing those genes under the transcriptional control of the CIITA promoter leading to expression of PD-L1 in around 40% of cases [37]. A subset of Epstein-Barr virus (EBV)-associated lymphomas also display gene amplification leading to PD-L1 and PD-L2 overexpression. Outside specific mechanisms leading to PD-L1 (over)expression, PD-L1 is expressed in around 30% of DLBCL [37]. In a phase II study including 66 DLBCL patients [38], three doses of pidilizumab were infused after autologous stem cell transplantation. The 16-month PFS was 70%, and among the 35 patients with measurable disease after autologous stem cell transplantation, the overall response rate after pidilizumab treatment was 51%.

Tumor Cell/Macrophage Interactions: CD47 Pathway

CD47 is now recognized as a "marker of self" and broadly expressed by tumor cells. Its ligand, signal regulatory protein alpha (SIRPα), is expressed by macrophage and, when it is engaged by CD47, decreases phagocytosis and cytotoxicity. CD47/SIRPα inhibits therefore the activation of macrophages and other myeloid cells against tumors and thereby acts as a myeloid-specific immune checkpoint. CD47 expression is increased in DLBCL, correlates with cells of origin, and confers worse clinical prognosis [39]. Blocking antibodies against CD47 enable phagocytosis of lymphoma cells by macrophages and synergize with rituximab in vitro. Combination therapy with anti-CD47 antibody and rituximab eliminates lymphoma in xenograft mouse model [39]. Phase I testing CD47/SIRPα-targeting therapeutics is ongoing.

In the future, characterization of multiple immune checkpoints will drive the further clinical development of other checkpoint inhibitors, such as TIM3, LAG-3, KIR, and VISTA.

16.2.3.2 Monoclonal Antibodies Targeting Costimulatory Receptors

Another attractive alternative is to use agonistic antibodies that target stimulatory molecules expressed by T cells; CD137 and CD40 are the most prominent of these molecules. Activation of T cells by antibodies may lead to critical adverse events warranting particular attention during clinical development.

CD137 (4-1BB) is a surface glycoprotein belonging to the tumor necrosis factor receptor family. CD137 is an inducible costimulatory molecule expressed on a variety of immune cells, including activated $CD4^+$ and $CD8^+$, T cells, NK cells, monocytes, and dendritic cells. Agonistic mAbs against this receptor have been shown to induce tumor-specific T-cell responses able to eradicate tumor cells in murine models [40]. In a syngeneic murine lymphoma model and in a xenotransplanted human lymphoma model, sequential administration of rituximab followed by anti-CD137 mAb has potent anti-lymphoma activity in vivo [41]. These results suggested that stimulation of CD137 could enhance NK cell killing by ADCC and thereby augment rituximab efficacy. A phase I trial evaluating utomilumab in combination with rituximab in patients with relapsed or refractory CD20-positive lymphomas demonstrated a significant antitumor efficacy and no dose-limiting toxicities. In addition, no patients discontinued treatment due to treatment-related adverse events [42].

CD40 is also a tumor necrosis factor receptor family member expressed on APC, B cells, and monocytes. In murine models, CD40 agonistic antibodies have shown exceptional therapeutic activity in the treatment of CD40-positive B-cell lymphomas with 80–100% of mice cured [43].

Despite some success achieved by mAbs targeting immune cells in DLBCL patients, there are still a number of patients who do not benefit from single-agent therapy. To enhance efficacy, synergistic combinations are now proposed including co-targeting of inhibitory checkpoint (anti-CTLA-4 and anti-PD1/PD-L1) or co-targeting of inhibitory checkpoint and costimulatory receptors (anti-PD1/PDL1 and anti-CD137).

16.3 CAR T-Cell Therapy

16.3.1 Design and Differences

CAR T cells are T cells expressing a chimeric antigen receptor (CAR) introduced in vitro by varying vector systems. The CAR consists of three major structural elements: an extracellular domain with an antibody-derived single-chain variable fragment (scFv), a spacer and linker domain, and finally an intracellular signaling domain like CD3ζ connected to important costimulatory domains like CD28 (KTE-C19) or CD137 (4-1BB) (CTL019, JCAR017) (Fig. 16.3) [44]. Most CAR T-cells are autologous, but allogeneic CAR T cells are also being developed. To overcome critical HLA barriers and to allow evading to host-mediated immunity and deliver anti-lymphoma effects without graft versus host disease (GVHD), a smart method is used to target the constant region of the T-cell receptor alpha chain (TRAC), thereby disrupting cell surface expression of TCRαβ [45]. Such allogenic CAR T cells are also named universal CAR T cells (UCAR-T) reflecting their ability to be effective in all patients without restriction to distinct HLA molecules.

For treatment of B-cell malignancies, the scFv has been directed against the B-cell surface antigen CD19 representing an ideal therapeutic target since apart from virtually all B-cell lymphomas only normal B cells and follicular dendritic cells express CD19 [46]. CAR T cells directed against CD19 specifically bind to B cells, get activated by downstream signaling, and initiate a cytotoxic response and cytokine release. In contrast to normal T cells, which for different reasons are not completely understood (e.g., checkpoint inhibition, immunosuppressive tumor environment, downregulation of MHC-presented tumor antigens) and fail to induce effective tumor lysis, CAR T cells induce rigorous killing of

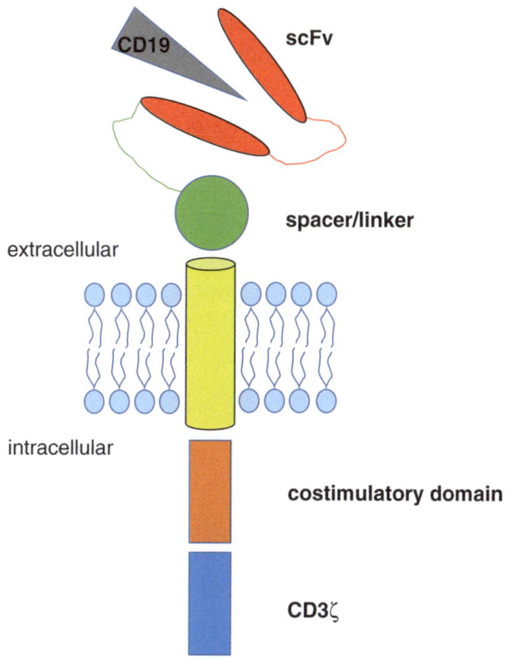

Fig. 16.3 Structure of chimeric antigen receptor. A chimeric antigen receptor (CAR) consists of an antibody-derived single-chain variable fragment (scFv) binding to the tumor antigen (e.g., CD19), a spacer and linker region, and an intracellular signaling domain activating the T cell

lymphoma cells. The binding affinity as well as the exact epitope location the scFv binds to will finally determine the efficacy of the CAR system.

The off-tumor toxicity of CD19-binding CAR T cells is limited with the resulting B-cell aplasia being clinically well manageable. The lack of an in many respects ideal target like CD19 explains the difficulty to design appropriate CAR T cells for other hematological malignancies and especially for solid tumors although important progress is being made [47].

The so-called first-generation CAR T cells consisted of the scFv and the CD3ζ domain; clinical responses to these constructs were still limited [48]. By the adding costimulatory domains like CD28 or 4-1BB (second-generation CARs), a significantly higher antitumor activity as well as an increased persistence of CAR T cells could be achieved [49]. Interestingly, costimulation via CD28 was associated with strong activation, increased cytokine release, and enhanced tumor lysis, whereas costimulation using the 4-1BB domain is said to induce longer persistence of CAR T cells and more durable tumor control [48]. Further benefit of CARs with several costimulatory domains (third generation) was reported in preclinical settings although clinical experience with such molecules is limited. Overstimulation may not only decrease the tumor response but also induce severe side effects.

The transmembrane and extracellular spacer and linker domain is a pivotal structural element for the stability and functionality of the CAR optimizing the T cell to target cell engagement. The phenotype of the transduced T cells represents a further key point. More immature T cells with a phenotype of memory T cells show a significant better tumor control and a longer survival compared to more differentiated effector and effector memory T cells. In most clinical trials, investigators used unselected transduced T cells. Therefore, the importance of specifically selected T cells for the success of CAR T-cell therapy is not yet clear, and further investigation is highly warranted.

16.3.2 Practical Aspects

Autologous CAR T-cell manufacturing starts with leukapheresis from the patient's blood. The apheresis product is transported to a central manufacturing facility where T cells are isolated from the collected blood cells. It is possible to enrich T-cell subsets such as CD4+, CD8+, CD25+, or CD62L+ T cells. The isolated T cells are expanded by T-cell activation via different systems using, e.g., beads coated with anti-CD3 and anti-CD28 antibodies. The expanded and activated T cells are finally transduced with the CAR system, most often using lentiviral or γ-retroviral vector systems. The final product is cryopreserved and shipped back to the study site. The time from leukapheresis to delivery of the ready-to-use CAR T-cell product may take between 14 and 40 days. This time period is relatively long and may necessitate administration of further chemo-immunotherapy to the patient in order to prevent massive tumor growth and further worsening of the patient's performance status.

T-cell-depleting chemotherapy prior to CAR T-cell infusion is associated with an impairment of regulatory T cells, an increase of T-cell-activating cytokines like IL-15, and an activation of antigen-presenting cells [50, 51] and may contribute to the success of CAR T-cell therapy.

The limitation of autologous CAR T cells is that they need to be customized, whereas allogenic CAR T cells (UCART) could be produced independently of the patient and the tumor and can be taken off the shelf when needed.

16.3.3 CAR T Cells for Treatment of Relapsed and Refractory B-Cell Lymphoma

Clinically, three CD19 CAR T-cell constructs have been used for treatment of refractory B-cell lymphoma: CTL019 (tisagenlecleucel, Novartis Pharmaceuticals, Basel, Switzerland), KTE-C19 (axicabtagene ciloleucel (axi-cel), Kite Pharma, Santa Monica, USA) and JCAR017 (lisocabtagene maraleucel (liso-cel), Juno Therapeutics, Seattle, USA; Celgene, New Jersey, USA) (Table 16.6).

CTL019 uses the CD137 costimulatory domain and a lentiviral vector transduction. Since August 2017, CTL019 is approved by the FDA to treat children and young adult patients up to 25 years with refractory disease or in relapse of B-cell precursor acute lymphoblastic leukemia. KTE-C19 uses CD28 as costimulatory domain and was originally constructed at the National Cancer Institute [52]. In October 2017, the FDA approved KTE-C19 for adult patients with refractory or relapsed DLBCL after at least two different therapy lines. JCAR017 was developed by Juno Therapeutics and Celgene Corporation and is under investigation for treatment of relapsed and/or refractory DLBCL. In January 2018, Celgene announced the acquisition of Juno Therapeutics. Regulatory approval for JCAR017 in the USA is expected in 2019.

16.3.3.1 Clinical Experience with CAR T Cells

Based on the promising initial results at the NCI, the phase II multicenter study ZUMA-1 (NCT02348216) enrolled 111 patients with refractory DLBCL, primary mediastinal B-cell

Table 16.6 Three different CAR T-cell constructs have been used for the treatment of refractory/relapsed B-cell lymphoma

	CTL019	KTE-C19	JCAR017
Name	Tisagenlecleucel (tisa-cel)	Axicabtagene ciloleucel (axi-cel)	Lisocabtagene maraleucel (liso-cel)
Pharma	Novartis	Kite/Gilead	Juno/Celgene
Target	CD19	CD19	CD19
Costimulatory domain	CD137 (4-1BB)	CD28	CD137 (4-1BB)
FDA approval	Children and young adult patients (≤25 years) with refractory disease or relapse of B-cell precursor acute lymphoblastic leukemia	Refractory/relapsed DLBCL after at least 2 therapy lines	Expected in 2019
Trial	JULIET (NCT02445248)	ZUMA-1 (NCT02348216)	TRANSCEND (NCT02631044)
Patients enrolled	147	111	68 (DLBCL cohort)
Responses	CRR 40% After 3 months: 30% CR After 6 months: 30% CR	CRR 54% After median FU of 15 months: 40%	CRR 56% After 3 months: 40% CR After 6 months: 40% CR
Product delivery in days	39	17	Unknown
Non-hematological adverse effects (≥grade 3)	23% CRS 12% NE	13% CRS ~30% NE	1% CRS (grade 4) 14% NE

This table shows the main characteristics of CTL09, KTE-C19, and JCAR017
CR complete response; *CRR* complete response rate; *CRS* cytokine release syndrome; *NE* neurologic events

lymphoma, or transformed follicular lymphoma to be treated with KTE-C19 CAR T cells [53]. Refractory disease was defined as progressive or stable disease after the most recent therapy or relapse within 12 months after autologous transplantation. The patients received a conditioning regimen of fludarabine (30 mg/m^2) and cyclophosphamide (500 mg/m^2) on days −5 to −3 before administration of a target dose of two million of CAR T cells per kilogram body weight on day 0. The conditioning regimen as well as the minimum number of CAR T cells necessary to elicit reliable tumor responses had been examined in previous studies.

Among patients who received KTE-C19, the objective response rate was 82%, with complete responses in 54% of cases. With a median follow-up of 15.4 months, remissions were ongoing in 42% (including 40% complete response (CR) remissions). The overall survival rate at 18 months was 52%. Three patients died during treatment. The time from leukapheresis to final delivery of the CAR T-cell product took a median of only 17 days.

The major side effects developing after infusion of CAR T cells were myelosuppression, occurrence of the cytokine release syndrome (CRS), and neurologic side effects. 93% of patients suffered from CRS with 13% of patients experiencing CRS of grade 3 or higher. The symptoms resolved within a median of 8 days except for two patients who died due to hemophagocytic lymphohistiocytosis and cardiac arrest.

Severe neurologic events (grade 3 or higher) comprising encephalopathy, confusion, aphasia, or somnolence occurred in about one third of cases. Except for four events occurring in patients who eventually died, all neurologic symptoms resolved over a median time of 17 days after infusion. Altogether, 43% of patients needed tocilizumab (a humanized monoclonal antibody against the interleukin-6 receptor) and 27% received glucocorticoids to handle CRS and/or neurologic events. Interestingly, high numbers of CAR T cells in peripheral blood were correlated with clinical response and the occurrence of neurologic events but not with the severity of CRS.

The second CAR T-cell system CTL-019 was studied in the JULIET trial [54]. JULIET enrolled 147 patients with chemorefractory DLBCL after at least two different therapies. Patients had to be ineligible for or had to have failed to autologous transplantation. JULIET was an international study with participation of 27 centers in 10 different countries. The time from apheresis to delivery to the treating physician was 39 days. Ninety-nine patients received a single infusion of CTL019 CAR T cells at a median dose of 3.1×10^8 cells. In 16 of 48 cases, CAR T cells could not be infused because the patient had died prior to delivery. Like in the ZUMA trial, most patients received conditioning with fludarabine (25 mg/m^2) and cyclophosphamide (250 mg/m^2) for 3 days or bendamustine (90 mg/m^2) for 2 days. Of the 81 patients infused, 40% achieved a CR which was maintained in 30% of cases after 3 and 6 months, respectively. The response rates were consistent across disease subgroups. Three patients died due to disease progression; no death was reported due to CTL09 infusion.

Looking at adverse events, CRS occurred in about two thirds of patients, and 15% of patients experienced grade 3 and 8% grade 4 toxicity. 15% of patients received tocilizumab in order to control CRS. Neurological events (of grade 3 or 4) occurred in 12% of cases. Infections of higher grade were described in about one of five patients.

In the TRANSCEND trial patients with refractory DLBCL, but also PMBL, follicular lymphoma of grade 3B and mantle cell lymphoma were enrolled and treated with JCAR017 [55]. All patients received fludarabine (30 mg/m^2) and cyclophosphamide (300 mg/m^2) for 3 days prior to CAR T-cell infusion. In contrast to the previously described trials, patients in TRANSCEND received transduced CD4-positive and CD8-positive CAR T cells in a predefined 1:1 ratio at different dose levels.

In the DLBCL cohort, 68 patients could be evaluated: 56% of patients achieved a CR, and almost 40% maintained CR at 3 and 6 months follow-up. Remarkably, the rate of CRS was rather low (30%) with only 1% of grade 4 toxicity. Severe neurotoxicity (grades 3–4) occurred in 14% of cases.

To summarize, clinical experience with second-generation CAR T cells used in order to treat refractory DLBCL and other aggressive

B-cell malignancies appears very promising. The patients treated with CAR T cells were true poor-risk patients with dismal prognosis whatever salvage treatment would have been administered. The SCHOLAR-1 study attributed a median overall survival of 6 months to such patients [4]. In this poor prognostic setting, treatment with CAR T cells resulted in a CR rate of approximately 50%. Most of the complete remissions were durable although follow-up times are still limited. As an important caveat, it must be taken into account that only those patients surviving rather long periods of time without or with mild chemotherapy were put on CAR T-cell trials. The typical patient suffering from refractory or multiple relapsed aggressive B-cell lymphoma, however, will need immediate and aggressive therapy. It is difficult to understand that many patients on CAR T-cell trials treated with mild and atypical chemotherapy survived time periods up to 145 days before CAR T cells were infused.

The major acute toxicities of CAR T-cell infusion represent the cytokine release syndrome and neurologic events. CRS and neurologic events can be severe to life-threatening and need immediate therapy. Over time, management of CRS and neurologic side effects substantially improved. With the use of tocilizumab and glucocorticoids, both CRS and neurologic complications are mostly reversible, and severe adverse events seem to be observed less frequently.

16.3.4 Perspectives

CAR T cells hold great promise in clinical settings with very poor prognosis. To further optimize the potential of CAR T cells, the aim must be to investigate what kind of CAR T-cell system is most powerful for which malignancy and how to further boost its therapeutic power. Target selection is one crucial issue. CAR T cells for B-cell neoplasia so far address the antigen CD19. One new approach in order to avoid tumor cell escape is the development of bispecific CAR T cells directed against two antigens, like CD19 and CD20 (Fig. 16.4a) [56]. The infusion of a mixture of different CAR T cells and the creation of T cells with different CARs are possible approaches to prevent tumor escape.

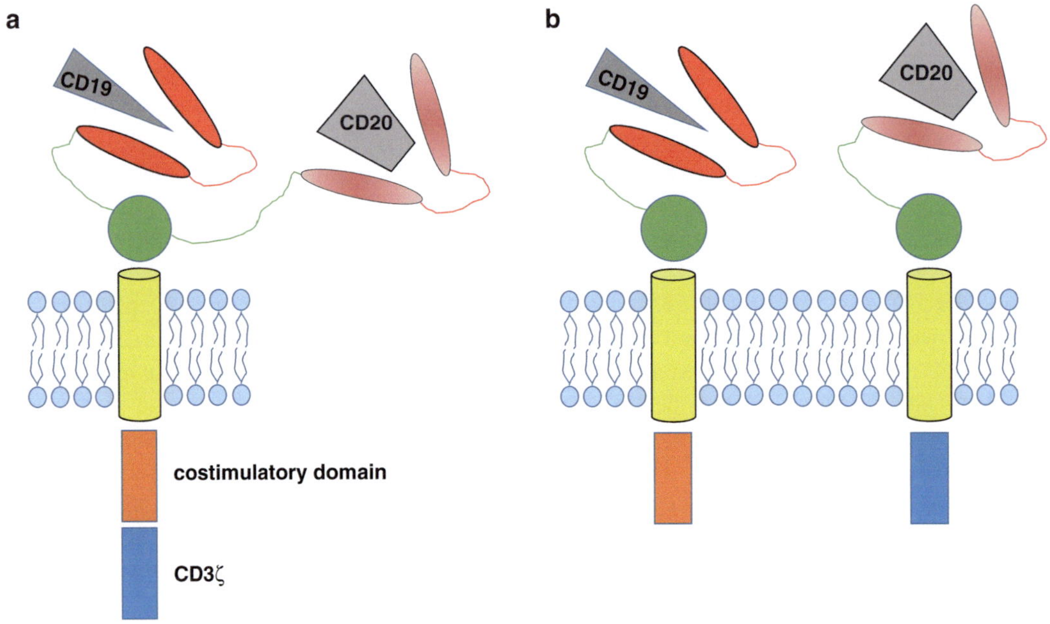

Fig. 16.4 Activation of bispecific CAR T cells. (**a**) Bispecific CAR T cells can be activated by two different antigens (e.g., CD19 and CD20) and minimize the risk of tumor escape by downregulation of surface proteins. (**b**) These CAR T cells express two different CARs: one connected to CD3ζ and the other to the costimulatory domain. Only when both CARs bind to their target (e.g., CD19 and CD20), the full T-cell activation is triggered

To further enhance tumor binding, CAR T cells expressing two different CARs directed against different antigens have been constructed. One CAR is linked to CD3ζ, and the other CAR is linked to the costimulatory domain: only when both antigens are bound the full CAR T-cell reaction is triggered (Fig. 16.4b) [57]. With an alternative approach, both antigens must be present on the target cell: a NOTCH receptor binds to the first antigen, gets cleaved within the cell membrane, and translocates into the nucleus to induce expression of the "effector CAR." Only if the effector CAR binds to the second target, a cytotoxic response occurs [58, 59].

Even if CAR T cells succeed in recognizing the malignant cells, there are multiple inhibitory effects that may hinder efficient tumor lysis. One important player is PD1. Theoretically, the combination of CAR T cells with checkpoint inhibitors (PD1-inhibitors) may enhance antitumor effects. In mouse models, the CAR T-cell efficacy could indeed be boosted by the simultaneous use of PD1 inhibitors [59].

The combination of CAR T cells with small molecules also holds great potential. Pretreatment with ibrutinib may improve expansion of CAR T cells in vitro and in vivo. In mouse models of CLL, the combination of ibrutinib and CAR T cells led to enhanced tumor clearance and survival [60].

The most serious side effects of CAR T cells are the cytokine release syndrome and neurologic events. To better control potentially life-threatening side effects, researchers develop CAR T-cell systems which are transient or can be destroyed on demand. Introduction of suicide genes or transient transduction of CAR T cells via RNA electroporation represents examples on how to create CAR T cells that can be irreversibly destroyed if clinically necessary [61]. Of course, the irreversible depletion of CAR T cells will increase the risk of relapse. Therefore, the next logical step was the development of ON-OFF switch CAR T-cell systems. One established system is a chimeric CAR that dimerizes only in presence of a small molecule. Only the dimerized CAR transduces downstream signaling and hence activation of the T cells (Fig. 16.5) [62]. A further advancement is the development of switchable

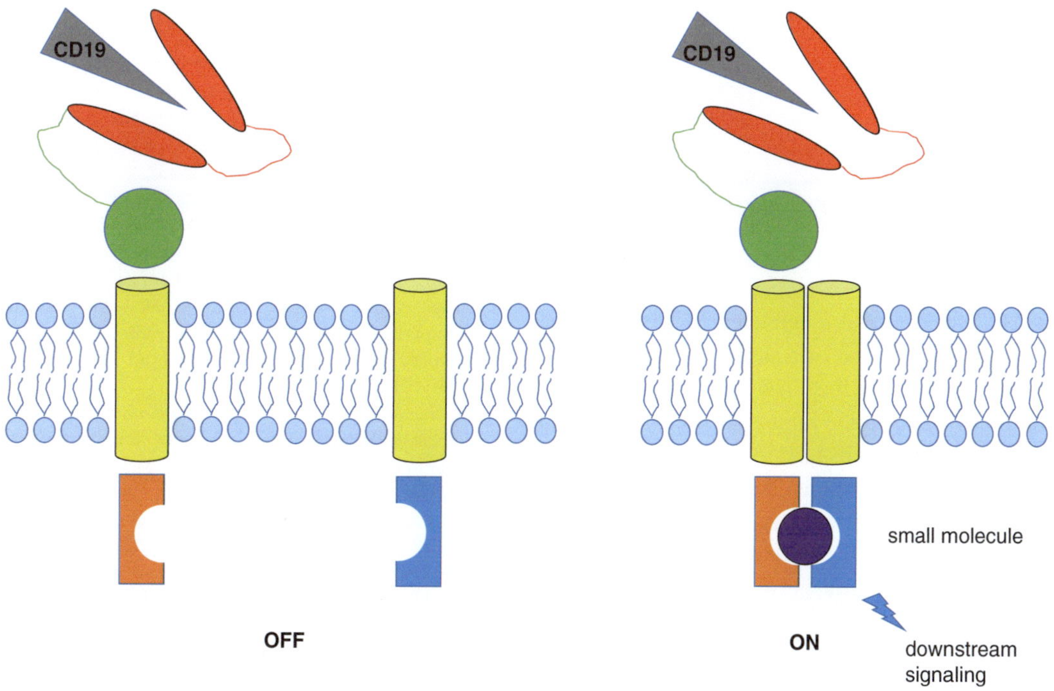

Fig. 16.5 ON-OFF switch CARs dimerize in the presence of a small molecule (ON). Only the dimerized CAR transduces the downstream signaling and hence activation of the T cell

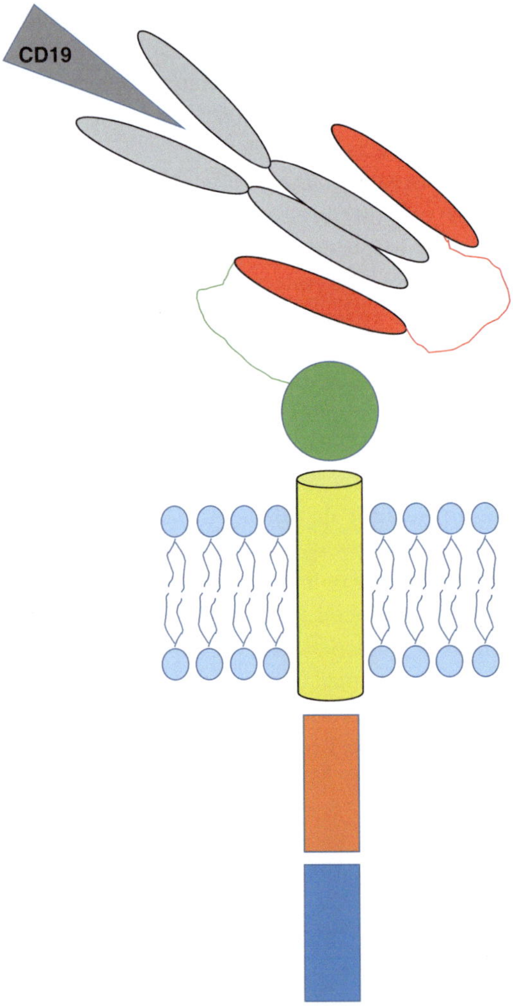

Fig. 16.6 A tumor antigen-specific Fab molecule binds to the tumor target (e.g., CD19), and the CAR is directed vs. the Fab molecule

CAR T cells that are activated by binding to a peptide neo-epitope of a tumor antigen-specific Fab molecule. Not the CAR itself but the infused antibody binds to the tumor surface. In a second step, the CAR T cells bind to the antibody and get activated. This technique leads to a tunable control of CAR T-cell activity. Moreover, different tumor antigens can be addressed with the same CAR T cells by infusing a mixture of different antibodies (Fig. 16.6) [63]. Clinical trials will show to what extent these technologies can further improve the long-term response rates of CAR T cells.

References

1. Friedberg JW. Relapsed/refractory diffuse large B-cell lymphoma. Hematol Am Soc Hematol Educ Program. 2011;2011:498–505.
2. Coiffier B, Lepage E, Briere J, et al. CHOP chemotherapy plus rituximab compared with CHOP alone in elderly patients with diffuse large-B-cell lymphoma. N Engl J Med. 2002;346(4):235–42.
3. Gisselbrecht C, Glass B, Mounier N, et al. Salvage regimens with autologous transplantation for relapsed large B-cell lymphoma in the rituximab era. J Clin Oncol. 2010;28(27):4184–90.
4. Crump M, Neelapu SS, Farooq U, et al. Outcomes in refractory diffuse large B-cell lymphoma: results from the international SCHOLAR-1 study. Blood. 2017;130(16):1800–8.
5. Press OW, Appelbaum F, Ledbetter JA, et al. Monoclonal antibody 1F5 (anti-CD20) serotherapy of human B cell lymphomas. Blood. 1987;69(2):584–91.
6. Reff ME, Carner K, Chambers KS, et al. Depletion of B cells in vivo by a chimeric mouse human monoclonal antibody to CD20. Blood. 1994;83(2):435–45.
7. Cartron G, Watier H, Golay J, Solal-Celigny P. From the bench to the bedside: ways to improve rituximab efficacy. Blood. 2004;104(9):2635–42.
8. Polyak MJ, Deans JP. Alanine-170 and proline-172 are critical determinants for extracellular CD20 epitopes; heterogeneity in the fine specificity of CD20 monoclonal antibodies is defined by additional requirements imposed by both amino acid sequence and quaternary structure. Blood. 2002;99(9):3256–62.
9. Li H, Ayer LM, Lytton J, Deans JP. Store-operated cation entry mediated by CD20 in membrane rafts. J Biol Chem. 2003;278(43):42427–34.
10. O'Keefe TL, Williams GT, Davies SL, Neuberger MS. Mice carrying a CD20 gene disruption. Immunogenetics. 1998;48(2):125–32.
11. Polyak MJ, Tailor SH, Deans JP. Identification of a cytoplasmic region of CD20 required for its redistribution to a detergent-insoluble membrane compartment. J Immunol. 1998;161(7):3242–8.
12. Cragg MS, Morgan SM, Chan HT, et al. Complement-mediated lysis by anti-CD20 mAb correlates with segregation into lipid rafts. Blood. 2003;101(3):1045–52.
13. Di Gaetano N, Cittera E, Nota R, et al. Complement activation determines the therapeutic activity of rituximab in vivo. J Immunol. 2003;171(3):1581–7.
14. van der Kolk LE, Grillo-Lopez AJ, Baars JW, Hack CE, van Oers MH. Complement activation plays a key role in the side-effects of rituximab treatment. Br J Haematol. 2001;115(4):807–11.
15. van Meerten T, van Rijn RS, Hol S, Hagenbeek A, Ebeling SB. Complement-induced cell death by rituximab depends on CD20 expression level and acts complementary to antibody-dependent cellular cytotoxicity. Clin Cancer Res. 2006;12(13):4027–35.

16. Clynes RA, Towers TL, Presta LG, Ravetch JV. Inhibitory Fc receptors modulate in vivo cytotoxicity against tumor targets. Nat Med. 2000;6(4):443–6.
17. Dall'Ozzo S, Tartas S, Paintaud G, et al. Rituximab-dependent cytotoxicity by natural killer cells: influence of FCGR3A polymorphism on the concentration-effect relationship. Cancer Res. 2004;64(13):4664–9.
18. Cartron G, Dacheux L, Salles G, et al. Therapeutic activity of humanized anti-CD20 monoclonal antibody and polymorphism in IgG Fc receptor FcgammaRIIIa gene. Blood. 2002;99(3):754–8.
19. Abes R, Gelize E, Fridman WH, Teillaud JL. Long-lasting antitumor protection by anti-CD20 antibody through cellular immune response. Blood. 2010;116(6):926–34.
20. Mossner E, Brunker P, Moser S, et al. Increasing the efficacy of CD20 antibody therapy through the engineering of a new type II anti-CD20 antibody with enhanced direct and immune effector cell-mediated B-cell cytotoxicity. Blood. 2010;115(22): 4393–402.
21. Alduaij W, Ivanov A, Honeychurch J, et al. Novel type II anti-CD20 monoclonal antibody (GA101) evokes homotypic adhesion and actin-dependent, lysosome-mediated cell death in B-cell malignancies. Blood. 2011;117(17):4519–29.
22. Bologna L, Gotti E, Manganini M, et al. Mechanism of action of type II, glycoengineered, anti-CD20 monoclonal antibody GA101 in B-chronic lymphocytic leukemia whole blood assays in comparison with rituximab and alemtuzumab. J Immunol. 2011;186(6):3762–9.
23. Dalle S, Reslan L, Besseyre de Horts T, et al. Preclinical studies on the mechanism of action and the anti-lymphoma activity of the novel anti-CD20 antibody GA101. Mol Cancer Ther. 2011;10(1):178–85.
24. Klein C, Lammens A, Schafer W, et al. Epitope interactions of monoclonal antibodies targeting CD20 and their relationship to functional properties. MAbs. 2013;5(1):22–33.
25. Niederfellner G, Lammens A, Mundigl O, et al. Epitope characterization and crystal structure of GA101 provide insights into the molecular basis for type I/II distinction of CD20 antibodies. Blood. 2011;118(2):358–67.
26. Morschhauser FA, Cartron G, Thieblemont C, et al. Obinutuzumab (GA101) monotherapy in relapsed/refractory diffuse large b-cell lymphoma or mantle-cell lymphoma: results from the phase II GAUGUIN study. J Clin Oncol. 2013;31(23):2912–9.
27. Coiffier B, Haioun C, Ketterer N, et al. Rituximab (anti-CD20 monoclonal antibody) for the treatment of patients with relapsing or refractory aggressive lymphoma: a multicenter phase II study. Blood. 1998;92(6):1927–32.
28. Vitolo U, Trneny M, Belada D, et al. Obinutuzumab or rituximab plus cyclophosphamide, doxorubicin, vincristine, and prednisone in previously untreated diffuse large B-cell lymphoma. J Clin Oncol. 2017;35(31):3529–37.
29. de Romeuf C, Dutertre CA, Le Garff-Tavernier M, et al. Chronic lymphocytic leukaemia cells are efficiently killed by an anti-CD20 monoclonal antibody selected for improved engagement of FcgammaRIIIA/CD16. Br J Haematol. 2008;140(6):635–43.
30. Teeling JL, French RR, Cragg MS, et al. Characterization of new human CD20 monoclonal antibodies with potent cytolytic activity against non-Hodgkin lymphomas. Blood. 2004;104(6):1793–800.
31. Teeling JL, Mackus WJ, Wiegman LJ, et al. The biological activity of human CD20 monoclonal antibodies is linked to unique epitopes on CD20. J Immunol. 2006;177(1):362–71.
32. Bleeker WK, Munk ME, Mackus WJ, et al. Estimation of dose requirements for sustained in vivo activity of a therapeutic human anti-CD20 antibody. Br J Haematol. 2008;140(3):303–12.
33. Du J, Yang H, Guo Y, Ding J. Structure of the Fab fragment of therapeutic antibody Ofatumumab provides insights into the recognition mechanism with CD20. Mol Immunol. 2009;46(11–12):2419–23.
34. van Imhoff GW, McMillan A, Matasar MJ, et al. Ofatumumab versus rituximab salvage chemoimmunotherapy in relapsed or refractory diffuse large B-cell lymphoma: the ORCHARRD study. J Clin Oncol. 2017;35(5):544–51.
35. Viardot A, Goebeler ME, Hess G, et al. Phase 2 study of the bispecific T-cell engager (BiTE) antibody blinatumomab in relapsed/refractory diffuse large B-cell lymphoma. Blood. 2016;127(11):1410–6.
36. Ansell SM, Hurvitz SA, Koenig PA, et al. Phase I study of ipilimumab, an anti-CTLA-4 monoclonal antibody, in patients with relapsed and refractory B-cell non-Hodgkin lymphoma. Clin Cancer Res. 2009;15(20):6446–53.
37. Menter T, Bodmer-Haecki A, Dirnhofer S, Tzankov A. Evaluation of the diagnostic and prognostic value of PDL1 expression in Hodgkin and B-cell lymphomas. Hum Pathol. 2016;54:17–24.
38. Armand P, Nagler A, Weller EA, et al. Disabling immune tolerance by programmed death-1 blockade with pidilizumab after autologous hematopoietic stem-cell transplantation for diffuse large B-cell lymphoma: results of an international phase II trial. J Clin Oncol. 2013;31(33):4199–206.
39. Chao MP, Alizadeh AA, Tang C, et al. Anti-CD47 antibody synergizes with rituximab to promote phagocytosis and eradicate non-Hodgkin lymphoma. Cell. 2010;142(5):699–713.
40. Takeda K, Kojima Y, Uno T, et al. Combination therapy of established tumors by antibodies targeting immune activating and suppressing molecules. J Immunol. 2010;184(10):5493–501.
41. Kohrt HE, Houot R, Goldstein MJ, et al. CD137 stimulation enhances the antilymphoma activity of anti-CD20 antibodies. Blood. 2011;117(8):2423–32.
42. Gopal AK, Bartlett NL, Levy R, et al. A phase I study of PF-05082566 (anti-4-1BB) + rituximab in patients with CD20+ NHL. J Clin Oncol. 2015;33(15_suppl):3004.

43. Tutt AL, O'Brien L, Hussain A, Crowther GR, French RR, Glennie MJ. T cell immunity to lymphoma following treatment with anti-CD40 monoclonal antibody. J Immunol. 2002;168(6):2720–8.
44. Priceman SJ, Forman SJ, Brown CE. Smart CARs engineered for cancer immunotherapy. Curr Opin Oncol. 2015;27(6):466–74.
45. Poirot L, Philip B, Schiffer-Mannioui C, et al. Multiplex genome-edited T-cell manufacturing platform for "off-the-shelf" adoptive T-cell immunotherapies. Cancer Res. 2015;75(18):3853–64.
46. Wang K, Wei G, Liu D. CD19: a biomarker for B cell development, lymphoma diagnosis and therapy. Exp Hematol Oncol. 2012;1(1):36.
47. Till BG, Jensen MC, Wang J, et al. Adoptive immunotherapy for indolent non-Hodgkin lymphoma and mantle cell lymphoma using genetically modified autologous CD20-specific T cells. Blood. 2008;112(6):2261–71.
48. van der Stegen SJ, Hamieh M, Sadelain M. The pharmacology of second-generation chimeric antigen receptors. Nat Rev Drug Discov. 2015;14(7): 499–509.
49. Carpenito C, Milone MC, Hassan R, et al. Control of large, established tumor xenografts with genetically retargeted human T cells containing CD28 and CD137 domains. Proc Natl Acad Sci U S A. 2009;106(9):3360–5.
50. Klebanoff CA, Khong HT, Antony PA, Palmer DC, Restifo NP. Sinks, suppressors and antigen presenters: how lymphodepletion enhances T cell-mediated tumor immunotherapy. Trends Immunol. 2005;26(2):111–7.
51. Kochenderfer JN, Somerville RPT, Lu T, et al. Lymphoma remissions caused by anti-CD19 chimeric antigen receptor T cells are associated with high serum Interleukin-15 levels. J Clin Oncol. 2017;35(16):1803–13.
52. Kochenderfer JN, Dudley ME, Feldman SA, et al. B-cell depletion and remissions of malignancy along with cytokine-associated toxicity in a clinical trial of anti-CD19 chimeric-antigen-receptor-transduced T cells. Blood. 2012;119(12):2709–20.
53. Neelapu SS, Locke FL, Bartlett NL, et al. Axicabtagene Ciloleucel CAR T-cell therapy in refractory large B-cell lymphoma. N Engl J Med. 2017;377(26):2531–44.
54. Schuster SJ, Svoboda J, Chong EA, et al. Chimeric antigen receptor T cells in refractory B-cell lymphomas. N Engl J Med. 2017;377(26):2545–54.
55. Abramson JS, Lia Palomba P, Gordon LI, et al. High durable CR rates in relapsed/refractory (R/R) aggressive B-NHL treated with the CD19-directed CAR T cell product JCAR017 (TRANSCEND NHL 001): defined composition allows for dose-finding and definition of pivotal cohort 59th annual meeting & exposition of the American Society of Hematology. Atlanta. 2017.
56. Zah E, Lin MY, Silva-Benedict A, Jensen MC, Chen YY. T cells expressing CD19/CD20 bispecific chimeric antigen receptors prevent antigen escape by malignant B cells. Cancer Immunol Res. 2016;4(6):498–508.
57. Kloss CC, Condomines M, Cartellieri M, Bachmann M, Sadelain M. Combinatorial antigen recognition with balanced signaling promotes selective tumor eradication by engineered T cells. Nat Biotechnol. 2013;31(1):71–5.
58. Morsut L, Roybal KT, Xiong X, et al. Engineering customized cell sensing and response behaviors using synthetic Notch receptors. Cell. 2016;164(4):780–91.
59. John LB, Kershaw MH, Darcy PK. Blockade of PD-1 immunosuppression boosts CAR T-cell therapy. Oncoimmunology. 2013;2(10):e26286.
60. Fraietta JA, Beckwith KA, Patel PR, et al. Ibrutinib enhances chimeric antigen receptor T-cell engraftment and efficacy in leukemia. Blood. 2016;127(9):1117–27.
61. Di Stasi A, Tey SK, Dotti G, et al. Inducible apoptosis as a safety switch for adoptive cell therapy. N Engl J Med. 2011;365(18):1673–83.
62. Wu CY, Roybal KT, Puchner EM, Onuffer J, Lim WA. Remote control of therapeutic T cells through a small molecule-gated chimeric receptor. Science. 2015;350(6258):aab4077.
63. Rodgers DT, Mazagova M, Hampton EN, et al. Switch-mediated activation and retargeting of CAR-T cells for B-cell malignancies. Proc Natl Acad Sci U S A. 2016;113(4):E459–68.

Therapeutic Modulators of Apoptosis and Epigenetics in Aggressive Lymphoma

17

Michael J. Dickinson and John F. Seymour

17.1 Introduction

Elsewhere throughout this text, other authors have discussed the role of targeted immunotherapies, small molecules targeting the B-cell receptor complex and tyrosine kinases that regulate cellular function. In this chapter we address other small molecules that target cellular signalling pathways involved in malignant cell survival, not otherwise addressed in this book.

Inhibition of BCL-2 promises to change the treatment approach for chronic lymphocytic leukaemia following the emergence of striking single-agent activity of navitoclax and its subsequent derivative venetoclax and the approval of the latter for CLL with deletion of 17p. We discuss emerging clinical data for this agent in aggressive lymphomas which show activity but without the same dramatic single-agent effect. We explore rational combinations for future research of other inhibitors of cell survival that are emerging in early phase trials.

Over the last decade, we have seen that it is possible to selectively target the cancer epigenome to induce a clinical anticancer response. Inhibition of histone deacetylases and methyltransferases has led to clinical responses in lymphoid malignancies and myeloid malignancies, respectively. Several histone deacetylase inhibitors have been approved for the treatment of T-cell lymphoma, and we review that data here. With the knowledge that mutations within epigenetic machinery can be drivers of lymphoid malignancy, we have seen the development of novel agents that target mutated EZH2 or BET bromodomain-containing proteins. We present recent data regarding agents which show the most promise in the management of diffuse large B-cell lymphoma.

M. J. Dickinson · J. F. Seymour (✉)
Department of Haematology, Peter MacCallum Cancer Centre and Royal Melbourne Hospital, Melbourne, VIC, Australia

Sir Peter MacCallum Department of Oncology, University of Melbourne, Parkville, VIC, Australia
e-mail: Michael.Dickinson@petermac.org; John.Seymour@petermac.org

17.2 BH3-Mimetic Agents in B-Cell Lymphoma: Venetoclax

17.2.1 Role of BCL-2 in Apoptosis

The BCL-2 family of intracellular proteins regulate the intrinsic pathway of apoptosis through the balance of effects of its pro-apoptotic and anti-apoptotic members. All members of the group have in common the presence of one of four BH (BCL-2 homology) domains. The BCL-2 family of proteins comprises three functionally distinct subgroups: pro-apoptotic BH3-only proteins, pro-survival proteins like BCL-2

G. Lenz, G. Salles (eds.), *Aggressive Lymphomas*, Hematologic Malignancies,
https://doi.org/10.1007/978-3-030-00362-3_17

and the apoptotic effector proteins. Members of these three subgroups interact specifically with each other in a complex, highly regulated interplay to regulate the propensity of a cell to undergo apoptotic cell death. It is the overall balance between the pro-survival and pro-apoptotic members of the BCL-2 family that ultimately determines cellular fate. Expression of the pro-apoptotic BH3-only proteins is increased in response to physiologic or pharmacologic stress signals such as cytokine or nutrient deprivation, oxidative stress, DNA damage or proliferative stress. These proteins include BIM, BID, PUMA and NOXA, and they work in two ways: through selective binding to, and inhibition of, the pro-survival BCL-2 proteins and in some contexts they can also interact directly with the pro-apoptotic effectors to initiate cell death. The pro-survival subgroup of BCL-2 family proteins include BCL-2 itself, $BCLx_L$, BCLw, MCL1 and A1. These proteins have a complex but defined repertoire of binding capacity with specific BH3-only family members. The pro-survival proteins function to prevent cell death by binding to and inhibiting the third subgroup of proteins: the pro-apoptotic effectors. These are BAK and BAX that are activated by their homo- or hetero-dimerisation, which is normally physiologically inhibited through binding to members of the pro-survival proteins. Once activated, BAK and BAX initiate apoptosis through mitochondrial outer membrane permeabilisation, leading to cytochrome C release and consequential caspase activation [1, 2].

In multiple malignancies, resistance to apoptosis is mediated by a relative increase in activity of BCL-2 and associated pro-survival proteins, although through a variety of underlying mechanisms. In follicular lymphoma, t(14;18) leads to BCL-2 overexpression through juxtaposition of the BCL-2 gene to the immunoglobulin heavy chain enhancer locus. This same mechanism is present in a subset of BCL-2 rearranged diffuse large B-cell lymphoma. However gene amplification and other mechanisms are more often responsible for BCL-2 overexpression in this disease.

The presence of BCL-2 protein expression and gene rearrangements is of prognostic importance in diffuse large B-cell lymphoma. Increased protein expression, as assessed by immunohistochemistry, occurs in 20–40% of DLBCL and is associated with more advanced disease stage that is relatively less sensitive to standard induction chemotherapies and in general portends a poorer prognosis [3–5]. The prognostic impact of BCL-2 protein expression is less clear in the era of chemoimmunotherapy, and the presence or absence of the t(14;18) translocation also does not appear to independently portend poor prognosis [3–5]. In the presence of other known oncogenic drivers, especially protein overexpression or rearrangements of c-MYC, BCL-2 overexpression provides a collaborating oncogenic "hit" that portends chemo-refractoriness, a high risk of relapse and a poor overall prognosis [6–10]. Inhibiting BCL-2 is therefore an attractive therapeutic target in B-cell lymphoma.

The BH3-mimetic class of drugs inhibits BCL-2 through molecular mimicry of BH3-only proteins. Apoptosis is induced through binding to the activation groove in BCL-2, preventing its binding to and competitive release of bound BH3-only proteins such as bim/bid. The first clinical agents with demonstrated efficacy in B-cell malignancy to achieve this are the orally bioavailable small molecules navitoclax (ABT-263) and venetoclax (ABT-199).

Navitoclax, which is selective for BCL-2 and BCLxl and BCLw, provided the first proof that targeting BCL-2 induces clinically striking responses in B-cell malignancies. A phase 1 study included 55 patients with a range of lymphoma subtypes treated at doses ranging from 10 to 425 mg daily. None of the four patients with DLCBL responded to treatment. A single patient with NK/T-cell lymphoma had a complete remission [11]. A phase 1 study of patients with highly refractory chronic lymphocytic leukaemia produced a 35% partial response rate in the 26 patients evaluable at or above the active dose of 110 mg/day [12]. A further trial demonstrated that response rates in follicular lymphoma could be augmented with the addition of rituximab [13]. However, navitoclax induces a dose-dependent, reproducible on-target thrombocytopenia owing to its inhibitory effect on BCLxl which is required to maintain normal platelet lifespan [11, 12, 14, 15]. Venetoclax is a more selective and specific inhibitor of BCL-2 and has therefore become the focus of clinical development in most B-cell malignancies.

17.2.2 Venetoclax Has Excellent Activity in Chronic Lymphocytic Leukaemia

A phase 1 study of venetoclax in a highly refractory population of patients with CLL, of whom 90% had poor risk features, produced a 79% response rate in 116 patients. Three patients developed clinical tumour lysis syndrome and there was one death [16]. A gradual ramp-up dosing strategy introduced during the trial lessened the risk of tumour lysis. The final go-forward dose in CLL was 400 mg/day after a ramp-up over 5 weeks. Apoptosis occurred through a p53-independent mechanism [17] and was equally active in the typically chemotherapy treatment-refractory population of patients with del(17p). An analysis of the features of the clinical features of 67 patients treated across three early trials of this agent showed a 25% rate of progression with Richter's transformation [18]. The drug continues development for CLL. In phase 1b study of the combination of venetoclax with rituximab, the complete remission (CR) and marrow MRD negativity rate was 51%(21/49) and 57% (28/49), higher than the 20% CR rate achieved in the monotherapy study. This was achieved without a significant safety signal. Venetoclax monotherapy has recently been approved in many regions for the treatment of CLL with deletions of 17p.

17.2.3 Venetoclax Monotherapy in Aggressive Lymphoma

A second arm of the phase 1 study of venetoclax assessed its activity in patients with non-Hodgkin lymphoma [19]. A total of 106 patients with relapsed or refractory non-Hodgkin lymphoma received doses of venetoclax once a day ranging from 200 to 1200 mg. Treatment was commenced with a 3-week ramp-up approach. A range of histological subtypes were recruited, including aggressive and indolent forms of lymphoma. A total of 34 patients had diffuse large B-cell lymphoma, and 28 had mantle cell lymphoma. A further seven patients had Richter's transformation from chronic lymphocytic leukaemia. Patients in these aggressive lymphoma cohorts had received a median of three prior therapies (range one to eight), but only 13 patients had had prior autologous stem cell transplantation. In the diffuse large B-cell lymphoma cohort, 59% of patients had an LDH higher than the upper limit of normal, and this was the case in 25% of patients with mantle cell lymphoma.

No maximal tolerated dose was identified. Despite the inclusion of nine patients with bulky lymphadenopathy greater than 10 cm diameter within these two disease subtypes, only three developed criteria for laboratory tumour lysis syndrome within 24 h of initial dosing, and there were no episodes of clinical tumour lysis syndrome. The two dose-limiting toxicities observed were grade 4 neutropenia in one patient with prior Richter's transformation and one episode of grade 3 febrile neutropenia. Importantly, 9 of the 51 patients across the entire study who received 1200 mg required dose reductions for nausea or diarrhoea. Treatment was interrupted on eight occasions across the cohort due to neutropenia. This is generally considered a well-tolerated drug, but in this trial about half of patients reported diarrhoea or nausea, usually of low-grade, approximately 40% reported fatigue and a fifth of patients reported decreased appetite.

The overall response rate in diffuse large B-cell lymphoma was 18%; 12% of patients achieved a complete remission. No complete remissions were observed in patients with Richter's transformation. In striking contrast, mantle cell lymphoma appeared to be exquisitely sensitive to ABT-199 with an overall response rate of 75% and a complete remission rate of 21%. Only 1 of the 28 patients with mantle cell lymphoma did not experience some degree of measurable tumour shrinkage. Complete remissions were only observed in the diffuse large B-cell lymphoma group at doses greater than or equal to 600 mg a day, whereas in the mantle cell lymphoma group, two complete remissions were observed at a dose of 400 mg a day. It should be noted, however, that the potential requirement for higher doses in the diffuse large B-cell lymphoma group did not translate into a consistent dose effect as of the 26 patients treated at 1200 mg; 16 had progression as their best response and were completely refractory to treatment.

There was an apparent difference in durability of response between lymphoma subtypes. Mantle cell lymphoma had a median progression-free survival of 14 months, whereas diffuse large B-cell lymphoma had a median progression-free survival of only 1 month (follicular lymphoma had a PFS of 11 months). Only one patient with DLBCL had not progressed when censored at 12 months. The numbers of patients with diffuse large B-cell lymphoma who were recruited were too small to assess the role of BCL-2 expression or cell of origin. However, it is noteworthy that BCL-2 and MYC double-expressing lymphoma was observed in four of six available tumours and two patients with double-expressing disease achieved an objective response. The authors concluded that for non-Hodgkin lymphoma subtypes, other than mantle cell lymphoma, the recommended dose was 1200 mg daily, using a ramp-up strategy starting at 400 mg daily for a week. In mantle cell lymphoma, the target dose recommended was 800 mg daily, ramping up from 100 mg daily for the first week (to 200 mg, 400 mg and 800 mg), with continued vigilance regarding tumour lysis prophylaxis and monitoring still required.

17.2.4 Venetoclax Combinations

The observation that combinations of venetoclax with anti-CD20 antibody are significantly more efficacious than monotherapy in CLL suggests that anti-CD20 antibodies are attractive partners for inclusion in combination approaches. A recent randomised, open label, phase 3 study confirmed that the combination of venetoclax and rituximab significantly improved progression-free survival compared to bendamustine and rituximab in patients with relapsed CLL. This may well lead to broad registration of the venetoclax in this setting [20]. Safety of the combination of the BTK inhibitor ibrutinib with venetoclax is well tolerated in mantle cell lymphoma and in chronic lymphocytic leukaemia and may also be employed in combinations for diffuse large B-cell lymphoma [21].

Combinations are clearly required given the low response rate of 18% to venetoclax monotherapy in diffuse large B-cell lymphoma. A randomised phase 2 study of bendamustine/rituximab versus venetoclax/rituximab/bendamustine (CONTRALTO: NCT02187861) is currently underway in patients with follicular lymphoma with overall response rates of 77% and 75%, respectively, in a preliminary analysis (Zinzani ASH 2016; abstract 617). We await the final results of combinations with rituximab-CHOP or G-CHOP (NCT02055820). Preliminary results showed a significant increase of neutropenia complicating a combination of venetoclax with CHOP mandating reduction from an initial planned administration of daily venetoclax to administration on days 1 to 10 [22, 23]. Efficacy appears promising with ORR of 100% (88% CR) in frontline FL with R-CHOP and 89% (78% CR) with G-CHOP. In the DLBCL cohort, ORR was 87% (all CR). Venetoclax is also being assessed in combination with R-EPOCH in patients with chronic lymphocytic leukaemia and Richter's transformation and in a second study in patients with double-hit lymphoma (NCT03036904). Venetoclax has also been studied in the setting of relapsed lymphoma in combination with ICE chemotherapy and is a partner in many novel-novel drug combination trials currently recruiting patients (see Table 17.1).

Table 17.1 Venetoclax, selected combination studies 1

Combination/mechanism	Venetoclax combination partner (s)	Disease indication	Design	Expected accrual (n)	Location	NCT
BTK inhibition	Ibrutinib	Mantle cell lymphoma	Phase 3	287	Global	NCT03112174
BTK inhibition	Ibrutinib, obinutuzumab	B-cell lymphoma	1/2	38	USA	NCT03223610
BTK inhibition	Ibrutinib, rituximab	DLBCL	1	30	Global	NCT03136497
Chemotherapy and BTK inhibition	Bendamustine, rituximab, ibrutinib	Mantle cell lymphoma	Phase 1	18	New York	NCT03295240
MDM inhibition	Obinutuzumab, idasanutlin	DLBCL	Phase 1/2	140	Global	NCT03135262
PDL1 inhibition	Atezolizumab, obinutuzumab	R/R lymphoma	Phase 2	138	Global	NCT03276468
Antibody/drug conjugate	Obinutuzumab, polatuzumab vedotin	FL and DLBCL	Phase 2	134	Global	NCT02611323
BET inhibition	RO6870810 (Ten-010) +/− Rituximab	DLBCL	Phase 1/2	94	Global	NCT03255096
Immunomodulatory	Lenalidomide	Mantle cell lymphoma	Phase 1/2	77	Global	NCT03505944
Chemotherapy	Bendamustine, rituximab	R/R lymphoma	2	60	Global	NCT01594229
Chemotherapy	ICE chemotherapy	DLCBL	1/2	18	USA	NCT03064867
Chemotherapy	DA-EPOCH-R	DLBCL	1	18	USA	NCT03036904
SYK inhibition	TAK-659	R/R NHL	1/2	53	Global	NCT03357627
BCL-2-family inhibition	Navitoclax	Acute lymphoblastic lymphoma/leukaemia	Phase 1	42	Global	NCT03181126

BTK Bruton tyrosine kinase; *ICE* ifosfamide, etoposide, carboplatin; *DLBCL* diffuse large B-cell lymphoma; *DA-EPOCH-R* dose-adjusted etoposide, prednisolone, vincristine, cyclophosphamide, etoposide, rituximab; *PDL-1* programmed death ligand-1; *BET* bromodomain and extra-terminal repeats; *MDM-2* mouse double-minute homolog-2

17.3 Epigenetic Agents

The term epigenetics has been defined in several ways, but it is most commonly taken to refer to heritable or even dynamic cellular processes affecting the phenotype of cells without alterations in the genetic sequence of the underlying DNA [24, 25]. Because epigenetic alterations in cells may be dynamic, they are potentially druggable. The best described and understood epigenetic changes in cancer medicine are chemical modifications of histones that result in altered chromatin structure and gene expression profiles and methylation of CpG-rich gene promoter regions which also alter expression of target genes. An expanding drug armamentarium seeks to target these and other epigenetic mechanisms, following the proof of principle provided by histone deacetylase inhibitors and the DNA methyltransferase-inhibiting agents. Histone deacetylase inhibitors have been approved in the treatment of T-cell lymphoma, while DNA hypomethylating agents are approved in MDS and AML but also appear active in T-cell lymphoma but remain under investigation. Drugs that target mutated EZH2 and the BET inhibitors can also be considered as epigenetics agents, are emerging as active agents in lymphoid malignancies and are addressed in this section.

17.3.1 Histone Deacetylase Inhibitors for T-Cell Lymphoma

Histone deacetylases modify the acetylation status of lysine chains on histones. This leads to conformational change of chromatin and the co-location of transcriptional factors to target genes. Histone deacetylase inhibitors selectively inhibit specific histone deacetylases (HDAC); however the aggregate effect on the cell is multifaceted with multiple cellular pathways being influenced by the activity of these drugs [26]. A full review of the activity of histone deacetylase inhibitors is beyond the scope of this chapter; however it should be broadly understood that these agents are classified as either pan histone deacetylase inhibitors (targeting the class I, II and IV HDACs) or selective histone deacetylase inhibitors. The differential effects on cellular pathways are affected by histone selectivity; however in the clinic clear differences in activity according to HDACs targeted are yet to be observed. Histone deacetylase inhibitors induce selective cancer cell death probably through induction of intrinsic and extrinsic apoptotic pathways, disruption of the misfolded protein response, cell cycle arrest, modulation of the JAK/STAT survival pathways and potentially multiple immune mechanisms [27, 28].

Histone deacetylase inhibitors have shown their greatest efficacy in T-cell lymphoma. The original observations were made in cutaneous T-cell lymphoma, but activity has also been demonstrated in peripheral T-cell lymphoma. Romidepsin and belinostat have been approved in the USA for the treatment of relapsed peripheral T-cell lymphoma. Romidepsin has approval for cutaneous T-cell lymphoma as does vorinostat. We will not discuss the management of cutaneous T-cell lymphoma in this section and will focus predominantly on the evidence of these agents in systemic T-cell lymphoma. The activity of approved HDACi in T-cell lymphoma is summarised in Table 17.2.

17.3.1.1 Romidepsin

Two pivotal phase 2 studies have confirmed the activity of romidepsin in peripheral T-cell lymphoma and ultimately led to its approval in the USA and in several other jurisdictions. The treatment schedule was identical across both studies, 14 mg/m^2 intravenously, days 1, 8 and 15 of a 28-day cycle [29, 30]. Romidepsin has only a moderate overall response rate, 23% across these studies, in which 175 patients were treated. Interestingly, however, the response duration is clinically meaningful: medians of 9 and 17 months overall for CR and PR, respectively, for the aggregated patient groups across these two trials. Stable disease lasted a median of only 4 months. Responses were seen as early as the first response assessment at week 8, and in our clinical experience, responses typically

Table 17.2 Patient characteristics and responses to HDAC inhibitors in T-cell lymphoma

Drug	Romidepsin		Belinostat
First author and reference	Piekarz [30]	Coiffier [29]	O'Connor [34]
Total patient number	47	130	129
Median age (range)	59 (27–84)	61 (20–83)	64 (29–81)
Stage III/IV (%)	45 (96%)	70 (53%)	90 (91%)
Marrow involvement (%)	14 (28%)		35 (29%)
PTCL NOS	27 (57%)	27 (21%)	77 (64%)
Angioimmunoblastic	7 (15%)	27 (21%)	22 (18.3%)
ALCL ALK positive	2 (4%)	1 (0.7%)	2 (1.7%)
ALCL ALK negative	2 (4%)	21 (16%)	13 (10.8%)
Cutaneous ALCL	2 (4%)	–	0
Other	4 (8%)	12 (9.2%)	
DLBCL	1 (2%)		0
Overall response	16 (38%)	38 (39%)	31 (25.8%)
Complete response	8 (18%)	18 (14%)	11 (9.2%)
Median response duration, months (range)	8.9 (2–74)	3 (<1–28+)	12 (4.7–19.8)
Median time to response, months	1.8	2	1.5
Response duration in complete responders, months (range)	29.4 (3–74)	14 (1.2–26.7+)	NR (>29 m)
Median duration of treatment, months (range)	3 (1–57)		1.75 (0.75–34)

occur between the first and second cycles of therapy. Very extended responses were seen in patients with angioimmunoblastic T-cell lymphoma with some patients reported to be in an ongoing complete remission after as long as 34 months. Long-term follow-up showed that 10 of 19 patients in a complete remission sustained that remission for more than 12 months, some patients recording a remission of more than 48 months [31]. Responsiveness does not appear to depend upon the number of prior therapies, with no difference seen between patients who have had one, two or greater than two prior therapies within the pivotal studies [32]. At our centre we have several patients who have been on romidepsin for a variety of subtypes of T-cell lymphoma in excess of 5 years. Romidepsin has been approved in the USA for patients who have relapsed after one prior therapy and represents an important treatment option in patients who are refractory to conventional chemotherapeutic agents. An intergroup collaborative trial of romidepsin in combination with CHOP as frontline therapy for peripheral T-cell lymphoma is currently underway. Coordinated by LYSA, the study randomises patients to receive either CHOP or romidepsin with CHOP (Ro-CHOP) [33]. Results are eagerly awaited in the study and represent a major undertaking in a relatively rare cancer. A recent phase 1 study of romidepsin and pralatrexate in relapsed NHL showed that these drugs could be feasibly combined at a recommended phase 2 dose of romidepsin 12 mg/m^2 and pralatrexate 25 mg/m^2 every other week. Eighteen of 29 patients had T-cell lymphoma. At the dose ranges assessed within the trial, the overall response rate was 57 and 71% of PTCL (10/14). The response rate for T-cell lymphoma likely warrants further exploration in a phase 2 trial. There is no evidence that romidepsin is active in other subtypes of aggressive lymphoma. It has not been systematically assessed in B-cell lymphoma.

17.3.1.2 Belinostat

Belinostat is a hydroxamic acid derivative and is considered a pan histone deacetylase inhibitor. Like romidepsin, its best evidence of activity is in peripheral T-cell lymphoma. It was assessed in a single pivotal phase 2 trial of 120 evaluable patients who had received a median of two prior therapies [34]. Belinostat is given intravenously at a dose of 1 g/m^2 days 1 to 5 of a 21-day cycle. The study reported overall and complete remission rates of 26 and 11%, respectively, with a median time to response of 5.6 weeks. The median duration of response is 14 months but was shown to be more than 29 months in those achieving a complete remission. These findings led to the approval of this drug for treatment of patients with relapsed peripheral T-cell lymphoma in the USA.

17.3.1.3 Other HDACi

Beyond the T-cell lymphomas, the HDACi have most thoroughly been studied as monotherapy in Hodgkin lymphoma. Both panobinostat and mocetinostat have been the subject of large phase 2 studies in this disease which have not demonstrated sufficient activity or durability of response to result in registration [35, 36]. In non-Hodgkin lymphoma, efficacy has been less promising. However a recent study of panobinostat with or without rituximab in relapsed DLBCL demonstrated a 28% response rate (11/40) and a median duration of response of 14.5 months [37]. Multiple combinations of HDACi with chemotherapy and other novel agents and chemotherapy have been tested over the last decade of development, with none that we are aware of demonstrating a sufficient efficacy to warrant further development.

17.3.1.4 Toxicities of HDACi

The histone deacetylase inhibitors demonstrate a class effect with respect to common toxicities. The most common treatment-limiting side effect is thrombocytopenia. In the romidepsin trial grade, 3/4 thrombocytopenia was reported in about 1/3 of patients, and severe neutropenia was reported on about fifth. Interestingly, belinostat is reported to cause grade 3–4 thrombocytopenia in only 7% of patients. This is unexpected because other HDACi (panobinostat, mocetinostat) cause thrombocytopenia in rates similar to romidepsin. In our experience the cytopenia related to histone deacetylase inhibitors responds well to dose adjustment. Thrombocytopenia may be an on-target effect arising from an impact on megakaryocytic budding of platelets during therapy [38]. Prolongation of the QT interval was previously a concern following the phase 1 study of romidepsin; however detailed analysis from the phase 2 studies suggests ECG changes following treatment with this class of agents are unlikely to be clinically significant [39]. Care needs to be taken not to combine these drugs with agents that prolong the QT interval. Belinostat was not associated with prolongation of the QT interval [40].

17.3.1.5 HDACi: Future Directions

Whether the histone deacetylase inhibitors have a future beyond their current indication remains to be seen. Approvals for romidepsin are now almost a decade old, and there is no evidence that the indication will be expanded to other subtypes of lymphoma. Integration into frontline treatment of T-cell lymphoma is still under investigation. Molecular subtyping of T-cell lymphoma and the apparent specific sensitivity of angioimmunoblastic lymphomas to these epigenetic therapies raise the possibility of improving response rates and clinical applicability through more careful patient selection. While panobinostat has been shown to have some activity in B-cell lymphoma, and molecular markers for sensitivity to this agent have been described, further development in this space is considered by these authors to be unlikely [37].

17.3.1.6 DNA Demethylation

Inhibition of DNA methyltransferases (DNMT) is a proven mechanism of anticancer therapy in the myelodysplastic syndromes and acute myeloid leukaemia where azacitidine and decitabine are approved therapies. Recurrent mutations in genes coding for the epigenetic cellular machinery (such as TET2) may predict responsiveness to azacitidine in these diseases

[41, 42]. Mutational analyses of T-cell lymphomas reveal an overlap of the mutational profile with myeloid disease, with TET2 and RHOA mutations amongst the more frequently mutated genes [43–47]. This provides one of several rationales for the assessment of azacitidine in T-cell lymphoma. We and others have successfully treated several cases of angioimmunoblastic T-cell lymphoma successfully with standard doses of azacitidine [48, 49]. Azacitidine upregulates genes associated with cancer immunogenicity and so for multiple cancers has been used in combinations with other conventional therapies in an attempt to augment cancer-associated immune responses [50–54]. Authors have also observed that prolonged inhibition of DNMT resensitises cells to doxorubicin [55]. Together, these observations have driven over 40 combinations of azacitidine or its oral analogue CC486 alone or in combination for T- and B-cell lymphomas. Combination partners include PD1/L1 inhibitors (NCT02951156, NCT03161223, NCT03240211), cytotoxic T-lymphocytes, pralatrexate, HDAC inhibitors and more recently R-CHOP for patients with high-risk diffuse large B-cell lymphoma [56–60].

17.4 EZH2 Inhibition: Tazemetostat

Tazemetostat (EPZ-6438, Epizyme) is a selective, orally available inhibitor of enhancer of zeste homolog 2 (EZH2). EZH2 is a histone methyltransferase, a catalytic subunit of the polycomb repressor complex 2 (PRC2), and is responsible for methylating lysine 27 in histone H3 (H3K27). This leads to a closed chromatin structure and transcriptional silencing of regulated genes [25, 61]. Alterations in EZH2 function can arise due to both gain or loss of function mutations and altered protein expression. Gain of function mutations occur in approximately a fifth of germinal centre B-cell diffuse large B-cell lymphoma and in 10–15% of follicular lymphomas and are thought to be drivers of lymphoma proliferation and survival through maintenance of the germinal centre phenotype [62–67]. Several inhibitors have been developed, and one, tazemetostat, is most advanced in clinical development. Tazemetostat binds to both mutated and wild-type EZH2 to inhibit its enzymatic function. The other EZH2 molecules in development (e.g. GSK126) can be differentiated from each other by their relative selectivity for mutated EZH2 over wild-type EZH2 and for EZH2 over other methyltransferases [61, 68–70].

The phase 1 study of tazemetostat explored doses ranging from 100 mg twice daily to 1600 mg twice daily, with a classical 3 + 3 dose-escalation study. Twenty-one patients with relapsed non-Hodgkin lymphoma and 43 with relapsed solid tumours were assessed [71]. The drug was well tolerated, and the single DLT was thrombocytopenia at a dose of 1600 mg bd. The recommended phase 2 dose was 800 mg bd [71]. Tazemetostat has received fast-track approval in the USA for treatment of relapsed follicular lymphoma and DLBCL bearing mutations of EZH2 on the basis of early data from the currently accruing phase 2 study (NCT01897571) [72].

Preliminary results from the phase 2 study were presented at the ICML meeting in 2017 [73]. The trial allowed recruitment of patients into one of five cohorts. All received a dose of tazemetostat 800 mg twice a day continuously. Prior to study entry, patients underwent screening for the presence of one of three mutations (Y646X, A682G, A692V) in formalin-fixed, paraffin-embedded tissue. Patients were streamed into one of five cohorts on the basis of the presence or absence of EZH2 mutation in either follicular lymphoma or diffuse large B-cell lymphoma (cohorts one to four) or into a fifth cohort with activated B-cell type diffuse large B-cell lymphoma. A further cohort was subsequently added during the conduct of the study which allowed patients with wild-type EZH2 to be recruited to a prednisone combination arm. Molecular results were required prior to allocation to treatment arm.

As expected, EZH2 wild-type arms rapidly recruited, while the relative rarity of the patient population bearing the mutant EZH2 leads to slow recruitment of those arms. Two hundred and three patients were evaluable for response, and

210 patients were evaluable for safety. Only 13 patients with EZH2-mutated follicular lymphoma and 17 patients with EZH2-mutated diffuse large B-cell lymphoma were available for response evaluation. Patients with follicular lymphoma had a median of four prior lines of treatment, and patients with diffuse large B-cell lymphoma had a median of three prior treatments. The objective response rate in EZH2-mutated follicular lymphoma was 92% (12 of 13 patients); in mutated diffuse light B-cell lymphoma, 29% (5 of 17 patients); in wild-type follicular lymphoma, 26% (4 of 14 patients); and in wild-type diffuse large B-cell lymphoma, 15% (18 of 119 patients). In follicular lymphoma, even allowing for the small number of cases presented, there was a clear difference in the EZH2-mutated subset both in terms of response rate and durability of responses. No patients with EZH2 mutant FL came off study due to disease progression. The finding that responses occurred later than with conventional therapies was consistent with the epigenetic mechanism of action.

The most common side effect was thrombocytopenia attributed to drug in 13% of patients and of grade III/IV severity in just 6%. Neutropenia occurred in 9% and was grade III/IV in 6%. Adverse events related to treatment led to dose reduction in 3% of patients studied and withdrawal in 2% of patients. Overall, tazemetostat is very well tolerated.

Positive predictors of response, as expected, were the presence of the EZH2 mutation and interestingly the presence of activating mutations in MYD88, while mutations of MYC, TP53 and HIST1H1E were associated with lower response rates.

The phase 2 study continues and a combination study with CHOP in the frontline setting is planned.

A clear message from the clinical trial is the difficulty in screening patients for relatively rare mutations in the context of haematological malignancy and in the context of follicular lymphoma and diffuse large B-cell lymphoma specifically. Although this paradigm has penetrated solid tumour oncology and the treatment of acute myeloid leukaemia, it is the first such study to seek relatively rare mutations in lymphoma during screening. The low response rates, the unmutated arms and apparently short responses in mutated diffuse large B-cell lymphoma suggest that tazemetostat requires a combination partner for enhanced efficacy. However, the initial signal albeit from very low patient numbers in EZH2-mutated follicular lymphoma is promising.

17.5 BET Inhibitors

Bromodomain and end-terminal repeat proteins (BET) are part of the transcriptional apparatus and recruit transcription factors to chromatin. By preferentially locating to histones with acetyl modification, BET proteins have considered epigenetic "readers" of the "histone code" [25]. Several inhibitors of BET proteins have been developed, and clinical trials in haematological and non-haematological malignancies have been underway for some years. Inhibition of BRD4 leads to downregulation of MYC-associated pathways; hence inhibition may be considered an attractive approach to drugging diseases driven by active mutations or amplifications of MYC [74].

17.5.1 OTX015

OTX015 (MK-8628) binds to bromodomain BRD4, BRD3 and BRD2 in BET proteins. OTX015 was assessed preclinically in cell line models of B-cell lymphoma. Consistent with observations with another BET inhibitor, JQ1, it was shown to downregulate signalling pathways associated with MYC, E2F1 and NFKB [75]. Interestingly this drug was shown to be predominantly cytostatic in the cell lines, and only 14% of cell lines (3 of 22) demonstrated dose- and time-dependent apoptosis. Those three cell lines were derived from ABC lymphoma and had mutated MYD88, wild-type p53 and mutations in CD79b or CARD 11. The gene expression profile signature generated from exposure to OTX015 was similar to that seen in prior publications of expression profile changes following treatment with JQ1 in different tumour models.

A clinical trial investigating this agent was sponsored by OncoEthix, a wholly owned subsidiary of Merck Corporation [76]. The study was conducted across seven sites in Europe, and patients were treated with daily oral dosing ranging between 10 mg and 100 mg daily. The study had a conventional 3 + 3 dose escalation design with the primary endpoint being dose-limiting toxicity in the first treatment cycle of 21 days. The study recruited patients with refractory lymphoma or multiple myeloma and required a baseline platelet count of more than 50 × 10^9/L and a neutrophil count of >1.0 × 10^9/L and creatinine clearance of 30 mL/min or more. Thirty-three patients with lymphoma and 12 patients with myeloma were recruited to the trial. The median age was 63 years with a preponderance of males to females (2:1). In the lymphoma cohort, patients had received a median of three prior lines of therapy, and 7 of 33 patients (21%) had prior autologous stem cell transplantation. All patients entered the study with a normal platelet count. A total of 22 of 33 patients (67%) had a diagnosis of diffuse large B-cell lymphoma, of whom five were shown to have expression by immunohistochemistry of both Bcl-2 and c-Myc. Eleven cases had insufficient material for this assessment. Ten cases had transformed B-cell lymphoma. The remainder of patients had a range of lymphoma subtypes, including peripheral T-cell lymphoma (n = 2), Hodgkin lymphoma (2) and mantle cell lymphoma (2), as well as several other indolent lymphoma subtypes. One patient had Burkitt lymphoma [76].

Three patients were evaluable for dose-limiting toxicity in each of the first three cohorts (10 mg, 20 mg, 40 mg daily), and no dose-limiting toxicity was observed. However, when the study switched to 40 mg twice a day, five of six patients reported grade 4 thrombocytopenia lasting more than 3 days. The study returned to once-daily dosing and the dose escalated to 120 mg a day, and again, a dose-limiting toxicity of grade 4 thrombocytopenia (four of six patients) was observed, with one patient experiencing grade 4 neutropenia. A go-forward dose of 80 mg once a day on a continuous 21-day cycle was chosen. This dose is currently being explored in diffuse large B-cell lymphoma expansion cohort.

As with other BET inhibitors, thrombocytopenia appears to be dose-limiting [77]. The nadir platelet count occurred after 18 days of treatment and was reversible, usually observed after 7–15 days of treatment interruption. No observation of cumulative toxicity was made. Apart from thrombocytopenia, the other main related adverse events were haematological toxicities which included anaemia in 41 patients (91%) and neutropenia in 23 (51%).The most common non-haematological adverse events were diarrhoea in 47% of patients and nausea in 24% of patients, as well as fatigue in 27% of patients. These appeared to be dose-related effects. Intriguingly, a reduction in coagulation factor VII of 20% to 30% was observed in three patients receiving a dose of 80 mg and 120 mg once a day without clinically significant bleeding or alteration in the international normalised ratio. This may be an on-target effect, as it has been observed in other BET inhibitor trials [77].

Only three patients (14%) with diffuse large B-cell lymphoma reported objective responses. One had time to progression of 6 months, two had complete responses with time to progression of 4.5 and 13.7 months and two patients had tumour shrinkage not meeting objective response criteria with a time to progression of 3.6 months. Although the numbers are small, the authors looked at the response rate according to cell of origin and showed that 40% (4 of 10) of patients with non-germinal centre phenotype had evidence of clinical activity versus 2 of 12 (17%) of those with germinal centre-like diffuse large B-cell lymphoma. Only one of five patients with c-Myc-positive diffuse large B-cell lymphoma responded to treatment. As an aside, no patients with myeloma responded.

17.5.2 Other BET Inhibitors in Development

Several other BET inhibitors are currently in development with clinical studies investigating them alone or in combinations in the setting of aggressive lymphoma. GSK 525762 is an orally available inhibitor of BRD4, BRD2 and BRD3 and is being investigated in a phase 1 trial exploring its role in acute myeloid leukaemia, lymphoma and myeloma [77, 78]. Results of this study are expected in 2018.

RO6870810 (Roche; formerly Ten-010, Tensure) is a subcutaneously administered BET inhibitor chemically similar to JQ1, which was widely used in preclinical mechanistic studies. It has been assessed in a phase 1 study that included 53 patients and which was completed in October 2017 (NCT01987362). At least 20 patients with diffuse large B-cell lymphoma were recruited. Preliminary or final results are not available; however the drug is being taken forward in combination with venetoclax for relapsed lymphoma (NCT03255096), testing the preclinical observation that the combination may regulate expression of BCL-2 proteins epigenetically, providing synergistic inhibition of BCL-2 with venetoclax [79]. If the preclinical observations with respect to downregulation of the MYC pathway bear fruit, the combination may be attractive as a treatment for DLBCL expressing both MYC and BCL-2 [79, 80].

17.6 Inhibitors of MDM-2

Loss or dysfunction of the tumour suppressor gene *p53* is amongst the most frequent drivers of cancer. The protein it encodes is a transcription factor that leads to cell cycle arrest and apoptosis. It is regulated through several negative feedback loops including via MDM-2 (murine double minute) and MDM4 [81]. MDM-2 directly suppresses the transcriptional activity of p53 as well as mediating its ubiquitination and degradation. Loss of p53 is a driver of disease in many subtypes of lymphoma, and mutation of p53 is a common pathway of transformation from low- to high-grade disease and acquisition of chemotherapy resistance across a range of lymphoma subtypes [82–86]. Overexpression of p53 without biallelic mutation is frequently observed in B- and T-cell lymphomas, as is independent overexpression of MDM2. MDM2 expression is not associated with altered prognosis in DLBCL [87]. Inhibition of MDM2 is therefore an attractive target in several B- and T-cell aggressive lymphoma subtypes and is theoretically most appealing in disease with residual wild-type p53 function [82, 83, 87].

Idasanutlin (RG7388, Roche) is an orally available inhibitor of the interaction between MDM2 and p53, belonging to a class of agents termed "nutlins". Preclinically, inhibition of MDM2 by nutlins inhibits lymphomagenesis in a range of B- and T-cell lymphoma subtypes (88–90). Mouse models of B-cell lymphoma suggest that BCL-2 overexpression can be overcome as a driver of disease and that combination with anti-CD20 antibody or venetoclax potentiates its action [88–90]. Idasanutlin was first tested in humans in the context of AML, where haematological toxicity, particularly thrombocytopenia, was dose-limiting [91, 92]. At lower doses, it is currently the subject of a global phase 1/2 study of the triplet of an obinutuzumab and venetoclax in DLBCL (see Table 17.1). Other MDM2 inhibitors are also under evaluation, with Aileron Therapeutics currently investigating its stapled-peptide MDM2 inhibitor in T-cell lymphomas amongst other diseases.

17.7 Future Directions

Over the last year, several pivotal studies have reported and summarised the genomic complexity of DLBCL [93–96]. These papers provide further evidence that in the future DLBCL will be classified according to the presence of mutations as well as copy number alterations and structural rearrangements that cluster together into broad definable entities large enough to be addressed through clinical trials of targeted approaches [93–96]. Frequently altered pathways include disruption of epigenetically active genes (e.g. KMT2D, CREBBP/EP300); dysregulation of the germinal centre programme via BCL6; immune surveillance avoidance via loss of MHC class I and II; gains and rearrangements of PD-L1 and PD-L2; mutations in CD79b NOTCH1, NOTCH2, SPEP, ARID1A and EZH2; and MYC and BCL-2 rearrangements and dysregulation [93, 97].

As we have seen from the development approach in venetoclax (Table 17.1), the agents in this chapter are likely to have their strongest future in combinations with immunotherapies, chemotherapy and targeted pathway/tyrosine kinase inhibitors. The rationales provided for these combinations in lymphoma are strong enough that there are a large number of potential combinations that merit exploration and will require structured prioritisation based on preclinical criteria [98]. The lesson from the tazemetostat experience is that development of even simple mutation-driven treatments in lymphoma is logistically and commercially challenging. The genomics data and the experience from the clinic tell us that the future of lymphoma treatment is likely to demand combinations that harness the immune system and target the epigenome and cell cycle regulation, MYC and its associated pathways and apoptosis pathways and (in the case of B-cell lymphoma) the B-cell receptor and its post-receptor signalling cascade. Hopefully these recent papers on the genomic landscape in DLBCL indicate that we will identify disease groups large enough in prevalence to allow rapid trials of these targeted agents and their rational combination partners.

References

1. Cory S, Roberts AW, Colman PM, Adams JM. Targeting BCL-2-like proteins to kill cancer cells. Trends Cancer. 2016;2(8):443–60.
2. Roberts AW, Huang D. Targeting BCL2 with BH3 mimetics: basic science and clinical application of Venetoclax in chronic lymphocytic leukemia and related malignancies. Clin Pharmacol Ther. 2017;101(1):89–98.
3. Hermine O, Haioun C, Lepage E, d'Agay MF, Briere J, Lavignac C, et al. Prognostic significance of bcl-2 protein expression in aggressive non-Hodgkin's lymphoma. Groupe d'Etude des Lymphomes de l'Adulte (GELA). Blood. 1996;87(1):265–72.
4. Gascoyne RD, Adomat SA, Krajewski S, Krajewska M, Horsman DE, Tolcher AW, et al. Prognostic significance of Bcl-2 protein expression and Bcl-2 gene rearrangement in diffuse aggressive non-Hodgkin's lymphoma. Blood. 1997;90(1):244–51.
5. Winter JN, Andersen J, Reed JC, Krajewski S, Variakojis D, Bauer KD, et al. BCL-2 expression correlates with lower proliferative activity in the intermediate- and high-grade non-Hodgkin's lymphomas: an Eastern Cooperative Oncology Group and Southwest Oncology Group Cooperative Laboratory Study. Blood. 1998;91(4):1391–8.
6. Friedberg JW. Double-hit diffuse large B-cell lymphoma. J Clin Oncol. 2012;30(28):3439–43.
7. Green TM, Young KH, Visco C, Xu-Monette ZY, Orazi A, Go RS, et al. Immunohistochemical double-hit score is a strong predictor of outcome in patients with diffuse large B-cell lymphoma treated with rituximab plus cyclophosphamide, doxorubicin, vincristine, and prednisone. J Clin Oncol. 2012;30(28):3460–7.
8. Pedersen MO, Gang AO, Poulsen TS, Knudsen H, Lauritzen AF, Nielsen SL, et al. Double-hit BCL2/MYC translocations in a consecutive cohort of patients with large B-cell lymphoma—a single centre's experience. Eur J Haematol. 2012;89(1):63–71.
9. Landsburg DJ, Nasta SD, Svoboda J, Morrissette JJ, Schuster SJ. 'Double-Hit' cytogenetic status may not be predicted by baseline clinicopathological characteristics and is highly associated with overall survival in B cell lymphoma patients. Br J Haematol. 2014;166(3):369–74.
10. Landsburg DJ, Petrich AM, Abramson JS, Sohani AR, Press O, Cassaday R, et al. Impact of oncogene rearrangement patterns on outcomes in patients with double-hit non-Hodgkin lymphoma. Cancer. 2016;122(4):559–64.
11. Wilson WH, O'Connor OA, Czuczman MS, LaCasce AS, Gerecitano JF, Leonard JP, et al. Navitoclax, a targeted high-affinity inhibitor of BCL-2, in lymphoid malignancies: a phase 1 dose-escalation study of safety, pharmacokinetics, pharmacodynamics, and antitumour activity. Lancet Oncol. 2010;11(12):1149–59.
12. Roberts AW, Seymour JF, Brown JR, Wierda WG, Kipps TJ, Khaw SL, et al. Substantial susceptibility of chronic lymphocytic leukemia to BCL2 inhibition: results of a phase I study of navitoclax in patients with relapsed or refractory disease. J Clin Oncol. 2012;30(5):488–96.
13. Kipps TJ, Eradat H, Grosicki S, Catalano J, Cosolo W, Dyagil IS, et al. A phase 2 study of the BH3 mimetic BCL2 inhibitor navitoclax (ABT-263) with or without rituximab, in previously untreated B-cell chronic lymphocytic leukemia. Leuk Lymphoma. 2015;56(10):2826–33.
14. Mason KD, Carpinelli MR, Fletcher JI, Collinge JE, Hilton AA, Ellis S, et al. Programmed anuclear cell death delimits platelet life span. Cell. 2007;128(6):1173–86.
15. Souers AJ, Leverson JD, Boghaert ER, Ackler SL, Catron ND, Chen J, et al. ABT-199, a potent and selective BCL-2 inhibitor, achieves antitumor activity while sparing platelets. Nat Med. 2013;19(2):202–8.
16. Roberts AW, Stilgenbauer S, Seymour JF, Huang DCS. Venetoclax in patients with previously treated chronic lymphocytic leukemia. Clin Cancer Res. 2017;23(16):4527–33.

17. Anderson MA, Deng J, Seymour JF, Tam C, Kim SY, Fein J, et al. The BCL2 selective inhibitor venetoclax induces rapid onset apoptosis of CLL cells in patients via a TP53-independent mechanism. Blood. 2016;127(25):3215–24.
18. Anderson MA, Tam C, Lew TE, Juneja S, Juneja M, Westerman D, et al. Clinicopathological features and outcomes of progression of CLL on the BCL2 inhibitor venetoclax. Blood. 2017;129(25): 3362–70.
19. Davids MS, Roberts AW, Seymour JF, Pagel JM, Kahl BS, Wierda WG, et al. Phase I first-in-human study of Venetoclax in patients with relapsed or refractory non-Hodgkin lymphoma. J Clin Oncol. 2017;35(8):826–33.
20. Seymour JF, Kipps TJ, Eichhorst B, Hillmen P, D'Rozario J, Assouline S, et al. Venetoclax-Rituximab in relapsed or refractory chronic lymphocytic leukemia. N Engl J Med. 2018;378(12):1107–20.
21. Tam CS, Anderson MA, Pott C, Agarwal R, Handunnetti S, Hicks RJ, et al. Ibrutinib plus Venetoclax for the treatment of mantle-cell lymphoma. N Engl J Med. 2018;378(13):1211–23.
22. Zelenetz AD, Salles GA, Mason KD, Casulo C, Gouill SL, Sehn LH, et al. Phase 1b study of venetoclax plus R- or G-CHOP in patients with B-cell non-Hodgkin lymphoma. J Clin Oncol. 2016;34.(15_suppl:7566.
23. Zelenetz AD, Salles GA, Mason KD, Casulo C, Le Gouill S, Sehn LH, et al. Results of a Phase Ib study of Venetoclax Plus R- or G-CHOP in patients with B-cell non-Hodgkin lymphoma. Blood. 2016;128:3032.
24. Berger SL, Kouzarides T, Shiekhattar R, Shilatifard A. An operational definition of epigenetics. Genes Dev. 2009;23(7):781–3.
25. Dawson MA, Kouzarides T, Huntly BJ. Targeting epigenetic readers in cancer. N Engl J Med. 2012;367(7):647–57.
26. Bertrand P. Inside HDAC with HDAC inhibitors. Eur J Med Chem. 2010;45(6):2095–116.
27. Dickinson M, Johnstone RW, Prince HM. Histone deacetylase inhibitors: potential targets responsible for their anti-cancer effect. Invest New Drugs. 2010;28(Suppl 1):S3–20.
28. Bolden JE, Peart MJ, Johnstone RW. Anticancer activities of histone deacetylase inhibitors. Nat Rev Drug Discov. 2006;5(9):769–84.
29. Coiffier B, Pro B, Prince HM, Foss F, Sokol L, Greenwood M, et al. Results from a pivotal, open-label, phase II study of romidepsin in relapsed or refractory peripheral T-cell lymphoma after prior systemic therapy. J Clin Oncol. 2012;30(6):631–6.
30. Piekarz RL, Frye R, Prince HM, Kirschbaum MH, Zain J, Allen SL, et al. Phase 2 trial of romidepsin in patients with peripheral T-cell lymphoma. Blood. 2011;117(22):5827–34.
31. Coiffier B, Pro B, Prince HM, Foss F, Sokol L, Greenwood M, et al. Romidepsin for the treatment of relapsed/refractory peripheral T-cell lymphoma: pivotal study update demonstrates durable responses. J Hematol Oncol. 2014;7:11.
32. Foss F, Pro B, Miles Prince H, Sokol L, Caballero D, Horwitz S, et al. Responses to romidepsin by line of therapy in patients with relapsed or refractory peripheral T-cell lymphoma. Cancer Med. 2017;6(1):36–44.
33. Dupuis J, Morschhauser F, Ghesquieres H, Tilly H, Casasnovas O, Thieblemont C, et al. Combination of romidepsin with cyclophosphamide, doxorubicin, vincristine, and prednisone in previously untreated patients with peripheral T-cell lymphoma: a non-randomised, phase 1b/2 study. Lancet Haematol. 2015;2(4):e160–5.
34. O'Connor OA, Horwitz S, Masszi T, Van Hoof A, Brown P, Doorduijn J, et al. Belinostat in patients with relapsed or refractory peripheral T-cell lymphoma: results of the pivotal phase II BELIEF (CLN-19) study. J Clin Oncol. 2015;33(23):2492–9.
35. Younes A, Sureda A, Ben-Yehuda D, Zinzani PL, Ong TC, Prince HM, et al. Panobinostat in patients with relapsed/refractory Hodgkin's lymphoma after autologous stem-cell transplantation: results of a phase II study. J Clin Oncol. 2012;30(18):2197–203.
36. Younes A, Oki Y, Bociek RG, Kuruvilla J, Fanale M, Neelapu S, et al. Mocetinostat for relapsed classical Hodgkin's lymphoma: an open-label, single-arm, phase 2 trial. Lancet Oncol. 2011;12(13):1222–8.
37. Assouline SE, Nielsen TH, Yu S, Alcaide M, Chong L, MacDonald D, et al. Phase 2 study of panobinostat with or without rituximab in relapsed diffuse large B-cell lymphoma. Blood. 2016;128(2):185–94.
38. Bishton MJ, Harrison SJ, Martin BP, McLaughlin N, James C, Josefsson EC, et al. Deciphering the molecular and biologic processes that mediate histone deacetylase inhibitor-induced thrombocytopenia. Blood. 2011;117(13):3658–68.
39. Cabell C, Bates S, Piekarz R, Whittaker S, Kim Y, Godfrey C, et al. Systematic assessment of potential cardiac effects of the novel histone deacetylase (HDAC) inhibitor romidepsin. ASCO Meeting Abstr. 2009;27(15S):e19533 EP.
40. Pohlman B, Advani R, Duvic M, Hymes K, Intragumtornchai T, Lekhakula A, et al. Final results of a phase II trial of Belinostat (PXD101) in patients with recurrent or refractory peripheral or cutaneous T-cell lymphoma. ASH Annual Meeting Abstr. 2009;114(22):920 EP.
41. Solary E, Bernard OA, Tefferi A, Fuks F, Vainchenker W. The Ten-Eleven Translocation-2 (TET2) gene in hematopoiesis and hematopoietic diseases. Leukemia. 2014;28(3):485–96.
42. Itzykson R, Kosmider O, Cluzeau T, Mansat-De Mas V, Dreyfus F, Beyne-Rauzy O, et al. Impact of TET2 mutations on response rate to azacitidine in myelodysplastic syndromes and low blast count acute myeloid leukemias. Leukemia. 2011;25(7):1147–52.
43. Couronne L, Bastard C, Bernard OA. TET2 and DNMT3A mutations in human T-cell lymphoma. N Engl J Med. 2012;366(1):95–6.
44. Lemonnier F, Couronne L, Parrens M, Jais JP, Travert M, Lamant L, et al. Recurrent TET2 mutations in peripheral T-cell lymphomas correlate with

TFH-like features and adverse clinical parameters. Blood. 2012;120(7):1466–9.
45. Van Arnam JS, Lim MS, Elenitoba-Johnson KSJ. Novel insights into the pathogenesis of T-cell lymphomas. Blood. 2018.
46. Fujisawa M, Sakata-Yanagimoto M, Nishizawa S, Komori D, Gershon P, Kiryu M, et al. Activation of RHOA-VAV1 signaling in angioimmunoblastic T-cell lymphoma. Leukemia. 2018;32(3):694–702.
47. Muto H, Sakata-Yanagimoto M, Nagae G, Shiozawa Y, Miyake Y, Yoshida K, et al. Reduced TET2 function leads to T-cell lymphoma with follicular helper T-cell-like features in mice. Blood Cancer J. 2014;4:e264.
48. Saillard C, Guermouche H, Derrieux C, Bruneau J, Frenzel L, Couronne L, et al. Response to 5-azacytidine in a patient with TET2-mutated angioimmunoblastic T-cell lymphoma and chronic myelomonocytic leukaemia preceded by an EBV-positive large B-cell lymphoma. Hematol Oncol. 2017;35(4): 864–8.
49. Cheminant M, Bruneau J, Kosmider O, Lefrere F, Delarue R, Gaulard P, et al. Efficacy of 5-azacytidine in a TET2 mutated angioimmunoblastic T cell lymphoma. Br J Haematol. 2015;168(6):913–6.
50. Moreno A, Szmania S, Shi J, Barlogie B, Prentice G, van Rhee F. Induction of the cancer-testis antigen MAGE-A3 in myeloma cell lines by 5'azacitidine and MGCD0103. ASCO Meeting Abstr. 2008;26(15_suppl):14008.
51. Goodyear O, Agathanggelou A, Ryan G, Novitsky-Basso I, Stankovic T, Moss P, et al. The epigenetic therapies Azacitidine and Sodium Valproate augment immune responses to the MAGE cancer testis antigen in acute myeloid leukemia and myeloma. ASH Annual Meeting Abstr. 2009;114(22):2086 EP.
52. Goodyear O, Agathanggelou A, Novitzky-Basso I, Siddique S, McSkeane T, Ryan G, et al. Induction of a CD8+ T-cell response to the MAGE cancer testis antigen by combined treatment with azacitidine and sodium valproate in patients with acute myeloid leukemia and myelodysplasia. Blood. 2010;116(11):1908–18.
53. Li H, Chiappinelli KB, Guzzetta AA, Easwaran H, Yen RW, Vatapalli R, et al. Immune regulation by low doses of the DNA methyltransferase inhibitor 5-azacitidine in common human epithelial cancers. Oncotarget. 2014;5(3):587–98.
54. Toor AA, Payne KK, Chung HM, Sabo RT, Hazlett AF, Kmieciak M, et al. Epigenetic induction of adaptive immune response in multiple myeloma: sequential azacitidine and lenalidomide generate cancer testis antigen-specific cellular immunity. Br J Haematol. 2012;158(6):700–11.
55. Clozel T, Yang S, Elstrom RL, Tam W, Martin P, Kormaksson M, et al. Mechanism-based epigenetic chemosensitization therapy of diffuse large B-cell lymphoma. Cancer Discov. 2013;3(9):1002–19.
56. Moss JJ, Howard D, Van Meter E, Hayslip J. A phase I study of the combination of Azacitidine, Cyclophosphamide, Vincristine, and Rituximab in relapsed and refractory lymphoma. Blood. 2011;118:1624.
57. Martin P, Bartlett NL, Rivera IIR, Revuelta M, Chavez JC, Reagan JL, et al. A phase I, open label, multicenter trial of oral Azacitidine (CC-486) Plus R-CHOP in patients with high-risk, previously untreated diffuse large B-cell lymphoma, Grade 3B follicular lymphoma, or transformed lymphoma. Blood. 2017;130:192.
58. Laille E, Shi T, Garcia-Manero G, Cogle CR, Gore SD, Hetzer J, et al. Pharmacokinetics and pharmacodynamics with extended dosing of CC-486 in patients with hematologic malignancies. PLoS One. 2015;10(8):e0135520.
59. Wang W, Wang J, Li M, Ying J, Jing H. 5-Azacitidine induces demethylation of PTPL1 and inhibits growth in non-Hodgkin lymphoma. Int J Mol Med. 2015;36(3):698–704.
60. Hiraga J, Tomita A, Suzuki N, Takagi Y, Narita M, Kagami Y. Partial restoration of CD20 protein expression and rituximab sensitivity after treatment with azacitidine in CD20-negative transformed diffuse large B cell lymphoma after using rituximab. Ann Hematol. 2018.
61. Kim KH, Roberts CW. Targeting EZH2 in cancer. Nat Med. 2016;22(2):128–34.
62. Yap DB, Chu J, Berg T, Schapira M, Cheng SW, Moradian A, et al. Somatic mutations at EZH2 Y641 act dominantly through a mechanism of selectively altered PRC2 catalytic activity, to increase H3K27 trimethylation. Blood. 2011;117(8): 2451–9.
63. Ryan RJ, Nitta M, Borger D, Zukerberg LR, Ferry JA, Harris NL, et al. EZH2 codon 641 mutations are common in BCL2-rearranged germinal center B cell lymphomas. PLoS One. 2011;6(12):e28585.
64. Bodor C, O'Riain C, Wrench D, Matthews J, Iyengar S, Tayyib H, et al. EZH2 Y641 mutations in follicular lymphoma. Leukemia. 2011;25(4):726–9.
65. Velichutina I, Shaknovich R, Geng H, Johnson NA, Gascoyne RD, Melnick AM, et al. EZH2-mediated epigenetic silencing in germinal center B cells contributes to proliferation and lymphomagenesis. Blood. 2010;116(24):5247–55.
66. Nikoloski G, Langemeijer SM, Kuiper RP, Knops R, Massop M, Tonnissen ER, et al. Somatic mutations of the histone methyltransferase gene EZH2 in myelodysplastic syndromes. Nat Genet. 2010;42(8):665–7.
67. Morin RD, Johnson NA, Severson TM, Mungall AJ, An J, Goya R, et al. Somatic mutations altering EZH2 (Tyr641) in follicular and diffuse large B-cell lymphomas of germinal-center origin. Nat Genet. 2010;42(2):181–5.
68. Qi W, Chan H, Teng L, Li L, Chuai S, Zhang R, et al. Selective inhibition of Ezh2 by a small molecule inhibitor blocks tumor cells proliferation. Proc Natl Acad Sci U S A. 2012;109(52):21360–5.
69. McCabe MT, Ott HM, Ganji G, Korenchuk S, Thompson C, Van Aller GS, et al. EZH2 inhibition

as a therapeutic strategy for lymphoma with EZH2-activating mutations. Nature. 2012;492(7427):108–12.
70. Knutson SK, Wigle TJ, Warholic NM, Sneeringer CJ, Allain CJ, Klaus CR, et al. A selective inhibitor of EZH2 blocks H3K27 methylation and kills mutant lymphoma cells. Nat Chem Biol. 2012;8(11):890–6.
71. Italiano A, Soria JC, Toulmonde M, Michot JM, Lucchesi C, Varga A, et al. B-cell non-Hodgkin lymphoma and advanced solid tumours: a first-in-human, open-label, phase 1 study. Lancet Oncol. 2018;19(5):649–59.
72. Wire GN. Epizyme announces Tazemetostat fast track designation for follicular lymphoma and plenary session on Phase 2 NHL data at ICML 2017. https://globenewswire.com/news-release/2017/04/25/970819/0/en/Epizyme-Announces-Tazemetostat-Fast-Track-Designation-for-Follicular-Lymphoma-and-Plenary-Session-on-Phase-2-NHL-Data-at-ICML.html. Accessed 10 Jan 2018.
73. Morschhauser F, Salles G, McKay P, Tilly H, Schmitt A, Gerecitano J, et al. Interim report from phase 2 multicentre study of tazemetostat, an EZH2 inhibitor, in patients with relapsed or refractory B cell non-Hodgkin lymphomas. 2017. http://www.epizyme.com/wp-content/uploads/2017/06/ICML-Tazemetostat-F-Morschhauser-FINAL-2.pdf.
74. Delmore JE, Issa GC, Lemieux ME, Rahl PB, Shi J, Jacobs HM, et al. BET bromodomain inhibition as a therapeutic strategy to target c-Myc. Cell. 2011;146(6):904–17.
75. Boi M, Gaudio E, Bonetti P, Kwee I, Bernasconi E, Tarantelli C, et al. The BET bromodomain inhibitor OTX015 affects pathogenetic pathways in preclinical B-cell tumor models and synergizes with targeted drugs. Clin Cancer Res. 2015;21(7):1628–38.
76. Amorim S, Stathis A, Gleeson M, Iyengar S, Magarotto V, Leleu X, et al. Bromodomain inhibitor OTX015 in patients with lymphoma or multiple myeloma: a dose-escalation, open-label, pharmacokinetic, phase 1 study. Lancet Haematol. 2016;3(4):e196–204.
77. Dawson M, Stein EM, Huntly BJP, Karadimitris A, Kamdar M, Fernandez de Larrea C, et al. A phase I study of GSK525762, a selective bromodomain (BRD) and extra terminal protein (BET) inhibitor: results from part 1 of phase I/II open label single agent study in patients with acute myeloid leukemia (AML). Blood. 2017;130:1377.
78. Borthakur G, Dawson MA, Stein EM, Karadimitris A, Huntly BJP, Dickinson MJ, et al. A phase I/II open-label, dose escalation study to investigate the safety, pharmacokinetics, pharmacodynamics and clinical activity of GSK525762 in subjects with relapsed, refractory hematologic malignancies. Blood. 2016;128:5223.
79. Hogg SJ, Newbold A, Vervoort SJ, Cluse LA, Martin BP, Gregory GP, et al. BET inhibition induces apoptosis in aggressive B-cell lymphoma via epigenetic regulation of BCL-2 family members. Mol Cancer Ther. 2016;15(9):2030–41.
80. Johnson-Farley N, Veliz J, Bhagavathi S, Bertino JR. ABT-199, a BH3 mimetic that specifically targets Bcl-2, enhances the antitumor activity of chemotherapy, bortezomib and JQ1 in "double hit" lymphoma cells. Leuk Lymphoma. 2015;56(7):2146–52.
81. Li Q, Lozano G. Molecular pathways: targeting Mdm2 and Mdm4 in cancer therapy. Clin Cancer Res. 2013;19(1):34–41.
82. Moller MB, Ino Y, Gerdes AM, Skjodt K, Louis DN, Pedersen NT. Aberrations of the p53 pathway components p53, MDM2 and CDKN2A appear independent in diffuse large B cell lymphoma. Leukemia. 1999;13(3):453–9.
83. Vasmatzis G, Johnson SH, Knudson RA, Ketterling RP, Braggio E, Fonseca R, et al. Genome-wide analysis reveals recurrent structural abnormalities of TP63 and other p53-related genes in peripheral T-cell lymphomas. Blood. 2012;120(11):2280–9.
84. Solenthaler M, Matutes E, Brito-Babapulle V, Morilla R, Catovsky D. p53 and mdm2 in mantle cell lymphoma in leukemic phase. Haematologica. 2002;87(11):1141–50.
85. Lo Coco F, Gaidano G, Louie DC, Offit K, Chaganti RS, Dalla-Favera R. p53 mutations are associated with histologic transformation of follicular lymphoma. Blood. 1993;82(8):2289–95.
86. Tzardi M, Kouvidou C, Panayiotides I, Stefanaki K, Rontogianni D, Zois E, et al. p53 protein expression in non-Hodgkin's lymphoma. Comparative study with the wild type p53 induced proteins mdm2 and p21/waf1. Clin Mol Pathol. 1996;49(5):M278–82.
87. Xu-Monette ZY, Moller MB, Tzankov A, Montes-Moreno S, Hu W, Manyam GC, et al. MDM2 phenotypic and genotypic profiling, respective to TP53 genetic status, in diffuse large B-cell lymphoma patients treated with rituximab-CHOP immunochemotherapy: a report from the International DLBCL Rituximab-CHOP Consortium Program. Blood. 2013;122(15):2630–40.
88. Drakos E, Singh RR, Rassidakis GZ, Schlette E, Li J, Claret FX, et al. Activation of the p53 pathway by the MDM2 inhibitor nutlin-3a overcomes BCL2 overexpression in a preclinical model of diffuse large B-cell lymphoma associated with t(14;18)(q32;q21). Leukemia. 2011;25(5):856–67.
89. Herting F, Herter S, Friess T, Muth G, Bacac M, Sulcova J, et al. Antitumour activity of the glycoengineered type II anti-CD20 antibody obinutuzumab (GA101) in combination with the MDM2-selective antagonist idasanutlin (RG7388). Eur J Haematol. 2016;97(5):461–70.
90. Herting F, Friess T, Umana P, Middleton S, Klein C. Chemotherapy-free, triple combination of obinutuzumab, venetoclax and idasanutlin: antitumor activity in xenograft models of non-Hodgkin lymphoma. Leuk Lymphoma. 2018;59(6):1482–5.
91. Yee K, Martinelli G, Vey N, Dickinson MJ, Seiter K, Assouline S, et al. Phase 1/1b study of RG7388, a potent MDM2 antagonist, in acute myelogenous leukemia (AML) patients (Pts). Blood. 2014;124(21):116.
92. Reis B, Jukofsky L, Chen G, Martinelli G, Zhong H, So WV, et al. Acute myeloid leukemia patients' clinical

response to idasanutlin (RG7388) is associated with pre-treatment MDM2 protein expression in leukemic blasts. Haematologica. 2016;101(5):e185–8.
93. Schmitz R, Wright GW, Huang DW, Johnson CA, Phelan JD, Wang JQ, et al. Genetics and pathogenesis of diffuse large B-cell lymphoma. N Engl J Med. 2018;378(15):1396–407.
94. Karube K, Enjuanes A, Dlouhy I, Jares P, Martin-Garcia D, Nadeu F, et al. Integrating genomic alterations in diffuse large B-cell lymphoma identifies new relevant pathways and potential therapeutic targets. Leukemia. 2018;32(3):675–84.
95. Chapuy B, Stewart C, Dunford AJ, Kim J, Kamburov A, Redd RA, et al. Molecular subtypes of diffuse large B cell lymphoma are associated with distinct pathogenic mechanisms and outcomes. Nat Med. 2018;24(5):679–90.
96. Reddy A, Zhang J, Davis NS, Moffitt AB, Love CL, Waldrop A, et al. Genetic and functional drivers of diffuse large B cell lymphoma. Cell. 2017;171(2):481–94 e15.
97. Pasqualucci L, Dalla-Favera R. Genetics of diffuse large B cell lymphoma. Blood. 2018;131(21):2307–19.
98. Stathis A, Iasonos A, Seymour JF, Thieblemont C, Ribrag V, Zucca E, et al. Report of the 14th International Conference on Malignant Lymphoma (ICML) closed workshop on future design of clinical trials in lymphomas. Clin Cancer Res. 2018;24(13):2993–8.

18 Targeted Therapeutics for Lymphoma: Using Biology to Inform Treatment

T. E. C. Cummin, M. S. Cragg, J. W. Friedberg, and P. W. M. Johnson

18.1 Introduction

Aggressive lymphomas are among the most highly proliferating cancers and are fatal without treatment. The vast majority of lymphoma-related mortality is attributable to aggressive subtypes of B- and T-cell non-Hodgkin lymphoma (NHL), which result in 20,400 deaths annually in the United States [1]. Approximately 40% of patients with diffuse large B-cell lymphoma (DLBCL) are not cured by first-line therapy, and 50% of those with peripheral T-cell lymphomas do not survive in 5 years [2, 3]. Our knowledge of the normal biology of lymphocytes and the events associated with malignant transformation is extensive, suggesting that this may be a means to improve the outcomes of treatment, translating molecular insights into more specific forms of therapy. To date the clinical data supporting this approach is limited, but a number of possible opportunities are under investigation.

The move towards targeted therapy is in part driven by the recognition that adjustment of conventional cytotoxic treatment may have reached the limits of usefulness in these illnesses. Increasing the intensity of first-line therapy has not improved overall survival (OS) for the majority of cases and, in any case, is constrained by the patient demographics, with more than half now presenting over the age of 65. The dose-dense infusional anthracycline-containing regimen DA-EPOCH-R (dose-adjusted etoposide + prednisone + vincristine + cyclophosphamide + doxorubicin + rituximab) did not apparently improve disease control or survival in DLBCL when directly compared with standard R-CHOP (rituximab + cyclophosphamide + doxorubicin + vincristine + prednisolone) [4], despite promising results from single-arm studies. High-dose therapy with autologous progenitor cell rescue (HDT + PSCT) does not appear to improve outcomes when used in first remission as part of front-line therapy for DLBCL [4]. For aggressive T-cell lymphomas, the role of high-dose consolidation in first remission is debated, lacking randomised controlled trial results to support its use, but cohort data suggests outcomes may be improved [5]. A large proportion of patients with aggressive T-cell lymphoma are unsuitable for HDT + PSCT in the

T. E. C. Cummin · P. W. M. Johnson
Cancer Research UK Centre, University of Southampton, Southampton, UK
e-mail: johnsonp@soton.ac.uk

M. S. Cragg
Antibody and Vaccine Group, Cancer Sciences Unit, Faculty of Medicine, University of Southampton, Southampton, UK

J. W. Friedberg (✉)
Department of Medicine, Wilmot Cancer Institute, University of Rochester Medical Center, Rochester, NY, USA
e-mail: jonathan_friedberg@urmc.rochester.edu

G. Lenz, G. Salles (eds.), *Aggressive Lymphomas*, Hematologic Malignancies,
https://doi.org/10.1007/978-3-030-00362-3_18

Table 18.1 Phase III clinical trials comparing investigational regimens with R-CHOP21 with results for overall survival

Regimen compared with R-CHOP21 [references]	Study	Population	Overall survival (OS) time point	Hazard ratio (HR)	*P*-value	Year
R-CHOP14 [8]	R-CHOP-14v21 UK NCRI	Stage IA–IV	2 years	0.90	0.38	2013
DA R-EPOCH [4]	CALG B50303	>Stage II	5 years	1.19	0.40	2016
R-ACVBP [9]	LNH-032B	Low/Int risk IPI	3 years	0.44	0.007	2011
R-CHOP + rituximab maintenance [10]	NHL13	CR/CRu	3 years	0.81	0.41	2015
R-CHOP + enzastaurin maintenance [11]	PRELUDE	IPI ≥3 and CR/CRu	48 months	1.04	0.81	2013
R-CHOP + everolimus maintenance [12]	PILLAR-2	Stage III/IV CR by PET/CT	50.4 months	0.75	Not significant	2016
Obinutuzumab + CHOP [13]	GOYA	IPI ≥2, or 0–1 with >7.5 cm bulk	3 years	0.99	0.99	2016
R-CHOP + lenalidomide maintenance [14]	REMARC	Elderly CR or PR	40 months	1.22	0.26	2016
R-CHOP + bortezomib [15]	REMoDL-B	Stage IAX, IB–IV	30 months	0.91	0.55	2017

CR complete response; *CRu* unconfirmed complete response; *IPI* international prognostic index

first remission, attributable to lack of response to induction chemotherapy or ineligibility with poor premorbid status [6]. There is some evidence that patients with high-risk DLBCL may benefit from more intensive regimens such as R-CODOX-M/IVAC (rituximab + cytarabine + vincristine + doxorubicin + methotrexate/ifosfamide + etoposide + cytarabine + methotrexate) (overall response rates (ORR) 92%), dose-adjusted R-EPOCH or R-hyper-CVAD (rituximab + cyclophosphamide + doxorubicin + vincristine + dexamethasone + methotrexate + cytarabine) (3-year progression-free survival (PFS) 75.7%). However, where DLBCL and PTCL have respective median ages of approximately 70, more tolerable novel approaches are clearly needed.

The first targeted agent to significantly improve outcomes was the anti-CD20 monoclonal antibody (mAb), rituximab, showing an overall survival benefit across subgroups in combination with CHOP chemotherapy for DLBCL [7]. However since then, progress has slowed: a number of large clinical trials in DLBCL have investigated novel agents in addition to R-CHOP standard of care, but none has significantly improved overall survival, including enzastaurin, lenalidomide, everolimus and bortezomib (Table 18.1) [12, 14, 15]. Early phase trials investigating novel agents as monotherapy in aggressive lymphomas rarely produce ORR greater than 30%, although occasional exceptional responders are identified (Table 18.2). To date, the evidence for directing therapy based upon molecular characterisation is limited. Where biology is complex and subtypes are rare, understanding mechanisms in the context of heterogeneity is important. Targeting actionable mutations or oncogenic addictions is a rational approach to using biology to guide therapy, but this requires the incorporation of a thorough preclinical mechanistic work alongside clinical trials where extensive characterisation is included.

Table 18.2 Response rates to novel agents in aggressive lymphomas

Pathway	Target	Agent	Disease overall response rate (reference)	
			DLBCL	PTCL
B-cell receptor (BCR)	Syk	Fostamatinib	3% [16]	–
	Btk	Ibrutinib	26% [17]	–
Apoptosis	BCL-2	Venetoclax	18% [18]	–
Immune checkpoint	PD-1	Nivolumab	36% [19]	66% [19]
PI3K/AKT/mTOR	PI3K-δ,γ	Duvelisib	0% [20]	42% [21]
	AKT	MK2206	0% [20]	0% [20]
	mTOR	Everolimus	30% [22]	63% [23]
Epigenetic	BET BRD	RG6146	17% [24]	–
	EZH2	Tazemetostat	29% (MT) 15% (WT) [25]	–
	Histone deacetylase	Romidepsin	–	15% [26]

18.2 Molecular Diagnostic Techniques for Aggressive Lymphomas

The 2016 update to the WHO classification of lymphomas increased the incorporation of molecular features within lymphoma diagnostics. Gene rearrangements (*MYC*, *BCL2*, *BCL6* and *ALK*) and gene expression signatures of germinal-centre B-cell (GCB) and activated B-cell (ABC) DLBCL were included [27]. Modern techniques for molecular characterisation include next-generation sequencing (NGS) and gene expression profiling (GEP). In addition to genomic and transcriptomic changes, epigenetic dysregulation is an increasingly recognised feature of lymphomas, albeit less well understood [28].

Whole genome sequencing (WGS) and whole exome sequencing (WES) have been applied to aggressive lymphomas. Within DLBCL more than 200 recurrent somatic mutations have been identified although very few have a prevalence of greater than 5% [29, 30]. WGS analyses the entire genome, comprising roughly three billion base pairs, whilst WES assesses only transcribed sequences, of which there are around 30 million base pairs [31]. These techniques are relatively expensive and time-consuming and also bring their own technical and logistical challenges, such as determining the consequence and pathogenicity of multiple variants. Next-generation sequencing (NGS) technology, also known as massive parallel sequencing, allows millions of DNA fragments to be sequenced simultaneously without prior sequence knowledge. Technical advances leading to improved reliability and reduced costs have made NGS feasible in clinical practice for somatic mutation and copy number analysis and characterisation using a "liquid biopsy" [31]. Given sufficiently large cohorts, NGS allows the characterisation of specific somatic mutations in the context of clinical outcomes to produce prognostic scores. The French Lymphoma Study Association (LYSA) group and UK Precision Medicine for Aggressive Lymphoma (PMAL) have developed and reported on lymphoma-specific NGS mutation panels for DLBCL within clinical trials, identifying patterns of mutation that correlated well with those expected for cell of origin subtypes [32, 33].

Gene expression profiling (GEP) is a technique which utilises microarrays or RNA sequencing to provide data on patterns of gene expression. Advances in GEP technologies have facilitated its application to formalin-fixed paraffin-embedded (FFPE) tissue allowing systems-level measures of cellular function in large cohorts [34]. This technique has identified subgroups with differing biology. The "cell of origin" (COO) classification for DLBCL distinguishes lymphoma based on the point in B-cell ontogeny at which transformation to malignancy apparently occurred. Subtypes include germinal-centre B-cell (GCB), activated B-cell (ABC), primary mediastinal B-cell (PMBL) and an unclassified group [35]. An alternative system, the consensus clustering classification (CCC), delineates subtypes by shared functional features: B-cell receptor (BCR) signalling, oxidative phosphorylation (OxPhos) and host response (HR) [36]. The subtypes have differing molecular features, which present opportunities for therapeutic intervention and can be targeted in preclinical models, to provide a rational methodology for treatment stratification within trials. It is likely that further endotypes based on expression patterns lie among these defined subgroups, providing potential opportunities for further stratification.

High-throughput molecular biology techniques such as these can also be used to inform diagnostic classification. Just as DLBCL has been further characterised by gene expression profiling, so the diagnostic criteria for aggressive T-cell lymphoma have been informed. For example, peripheral T-cell lymphoma not otherwise specified (PTCL-NOS) constitutes around a third of cases of peripheral T-cell lymphoma (PTCL), where further characterisation by standard immunostaining techniques has not been possible [37]. GEP and NGS have allowed further categorisation of this previously ill-defined disease entity, so that GEP applied to cases of aggressive T and NK NHL produced robust gene expression classifiers [38, 39]. One study was able to redefine 37% of previously diagnosed PTCL-NOS as more definitive lymphoma subtypes, such as angioimmunoblastic T-cell lymphoma (AITL), based on their gene signature. Analysis also isolates prognostic groups and identifies important oncogenic pathways [38, 39]. High mRNA expression of *GATA3* or *TBX21* defines distinct subgroups within PTCL-NOS. GATA3-high lymphoma signifies worse OS, potentially due to its association with high MYC protein expression and oncogenic PI3K pathway activation [38, 40]. Such characterisation provides opportunities for therapeutic targeting within clinical trials.

18.3 Lymphoma Subtypes to Guide Therapy

Characterisation of lymphomas identifies those with distinct biological features, including high-risk subtypes and those displaying differential responses to standard therapy. Dysregulated MYC and BCL-2 have consistently been implicated in conferring poor outcomes on patients with DLBCL [41]. *MYC* and *BCL-2* gene rearrangements are present in 5–14% and 10–40% of cases, respectively [42, 43]. Cases with concomitant *MYC* and *BCL-2* gene rearrangements are referred to as double-hit lymphomas (DHL) and arise almost exclusively within GCB-DLBCL [44]. A number of studies have demonstrated that these lymphomas have increased rates of early progression and lower 2-year survival of 35–60% [4, 45, 46]. A single-arm phase II trial of DHL treated with DA-R-EPOCH reported an encouraging 87% progression-free survival (PFS) at a median follow-up time of 14 months, suggesting a potential alternative therapy to R-CHOP [45]. In contrast, a retrospective analysis of two trials concluded that among 13 cases of DLBCL with MYC rearrangement treated with DA-EPOCH-R, the OS was 63.5% [47]. Recent analyses of prospective clinical trials, involving patients receiving R-CHOP (the NCRI R-CHOP14v21 and GOYA trials), appear to show DHLs having similar outcomes to those seen in the DA-EPOCH-R studies [46, 48], highlighting the need for careful randomised comparison following on from the phase II series.

Retrospective analyses have shown that the ABC-DLBCL subtype is associated with worse outcomes than GCB-DLBCL, although within subsequent large prospective studies, the prognostic power is less clear [49, 50]. One important consideration is that the proportion of DLBCL with this subtype increases with age, where full-intensity R-CHOP may be impractical, and novel approaches capable of targeting this entity become increasingly important [51]. In contrast, biomarker analysis of the LNH 03-2b trial found non-GCB cases identified by the Hans immunohistochemical (IHC) algorithm (of which ABC are the majority), to derive benefit from the more intensive R-ACVBP regimen, which increased PFS and OS compared with R-CHOP (HR, 6.09; 95% CI, 1.37 to 27.03). This was an unplanned secondary analysis with COO status only available for comparison between 61 cases in one arm and 67 in the other. The regime increased rates of febrile neutropenia (9% vs. 38%) and non-GCB cases included PMBL that did poorly with R-CHOP [9, 52].

Within retrospective analyses of trial participants, GCB-DLBCL has been associated with different responses to standard immunochemotherapy regimens. A retrospective analysis looking for biological correlates within 249 patients from the CORAL trial comparing R-ICE (rituximab + ifosfamide + carboplatin + etoposide) and R-DHAP (rituximab + cytarabine + cisplatin) salvage chemotherapy found survival differences based on COO. Three-year PFS for GCB-DLBCL was significantly higher within the R-DHAP arm than for R-ICE (100% vs. 27%, $p = 0.01$). Other prognostic features such as *MYC* and *BCL-2* rearrangements were not incorporated in this particular analysis, and validation within a prospective study would be needed to confirm the relationship. It was hypothesised that cytarabine may modulate BCL-6 expression to directly repress TP53, where BCL-6 activation is a hallmark of the subtype [53]. An analysis of 245 patients from a Danish lymphoma cohort examined biological correlates including COO (determined by IHC) with survival in patients treated with R-CHOP or R-CHOEP. It was reported that PFS (HR, 2.9; 95% CI, 1.5–5.9) and OS (HR, 3.4; 95% CI, 1.5–7.8) were significantly superior in the GCB group treated with R-CHOEP than R-CHOP [54]. Despite confirming that the treatment benefit was independent of IPI, age and gender using multivariate analysis, high-risk DHLs were not characterised and may have been disproportionately represented in the R-CHOP group. It is also important to remember that retrospective analysis may be unreliable where no randomisation has occurred, and clinician choice for treatment based on patient-specific factors may also affect survival.

The small molecule inhibitors, ibrutinib and lenalidomide, appear to have preferential single-agent activity within the ABC-DLBCL subtype [55]. In relapsed and refractory DLBCL, ibrutinib induced responses in 37% (14/38) of ABC-DLBCL but only 5% (1/20) of GCB-DLBCL, resulting in significantly higher median OS [56]. This observation may reflect the relative importance of Btk- and BCR-signalling to cell survival in the two subtypes [17]. Within ABC-DLBCL, the presence of concomitant *MYD88* and *CD79B* mutations was associated with higher sensitivity to ibrutinib. However, a majority of patients who responded lacked any BCR-related mutations, supporting the role of BCR activation per se, in the sensitisation of ABC-DLBCL to treatment with ibrutinib. Preclinical ABC-DLBCL models suggest that binding of self-antigen may be critical for cell survival and could explain chronic BCR-signalling in cases that lack BCR-related mutations [53]. Whilst, genetic screens in *MYD88* mutant cell lines demonstrated the assembly of a "super-pathway" of signalling adapters, including MYD88 and the CBM complex facilitated by TLR9 and IgM, which is thought to drive powerful activation of NF-κB and termed the "My-T-BCR" supercomplex [57, 58]. It is argued that this hyper-addiction could explain the sensitivity of patients with *MYD88* and *CD79B* mutations to treatment with Btk inhibitors. Studying biopsy material from patients in a trial of ibrutinib in DLBCL using proximity ligation assay, cases that responded to the inhibitor were significantly enriched for presence of the My-T-BCR. Also, patient samples of lymphoplasmocytic lymphoma, ABC-DLBCL and primary central nervous system lymphoma had increased evidence of activity of the My-T-BCR, are all lymphomas known to have encouraging responses to Btk inhibition. The functional relationship of the components of the supercomplex also suggests rational combinations: the addition of a dual mTORC1/2 inhibitor (AZD2014) in addition to ibrutinib further reduced formation of the My-T-BCR and downstream NF-κB activity [58].

An alternative class of therapeutic is the immunomodulating drugs (imids) such as lenalidomide and pomalidomide. Lenalidomide has demonstrated preferential activity as single-agent therapy in non-GCB-DLBCL where ORR was 52.9% vs. 8.7% in GCB-DLBCL [59]. Although median PFS was only 6.2 months in ABC-DLBCL, when lenalidomide was combined with R-CHOP in a phase II trial, it appeared to overcome the worse outcomes previously seen in ABC-DLBCL with R-CHOP treatment alone [59]. However, within prospective trials, where selection bias may contribute to excluding elderly patients or those that require prompt treatment, the ABC subtype appears to do better [60]. One important lesson from these studies is that small trials or those lacking a control arm are difficult to interpret convincingly, particularly where known prognostic features are not accounted for. Investigating lenalidomide as maintenance following R-CHOP in a randomised phase III clinical trial, there was significant improvement in PFS but not OS [61]. Unexpectedly, PFS was only significantly improved in the GCB cases, identified using Hans criteria (HR, 0.49; $P = 0.04$), but not the non-GCB cases (HR, 1.08; $p = 0.75$) [62]. A prospective analysis of lenalidomide in combination with R-CHOP in ABC-DLBCL, defined by GEP, is ongoing, and it remains to be seen if the ABC subtype derives significant benefit with the combination (ROBUST study, NCT02285062).

Germinal-centre DLBCL show features consistent with their derivation from germinal-centre B-cells. The malignancy is characterised by PI3K pathway activation, BCL-6 transcription factor activity and characteristic patterns of somatic mutations, suggesting a prominent role for epigenetic dysregulation. GCB-DLBCL is enriched for mutations in genes encoding histone-modifying proteins: *EZH2*, *CREBBP*, *EP300*, *MLL2* (*KMT2D*) and *MEF2B* [29, 63, 64]. Constitutive, tonic BCR-signalling is found in a high number of GCB-DLBCL, where ITAM phosphorylation results in recruitment and activation of Syk [63]. In preclinical models, tonic BCR-signalling has been associated with response to Syk inhibition [65], and aberrant PI3K-related signalling may be a similarly useful target in the subtype. However, BCR-signalling and PI3K/AKT/mTOR inhibitors have demonstrated variable efficacy within trials [16, 20, 66]. Everolimus used as maintenance in first-line DLBCL failed to significantly improve disease-free survival [67]. The PI3K pathway contains several upstream and downstream regulators complicated by a high-level of crosstalk between multiple other signalling pathways involving several transcription factors [68]. In a heterogeneous disease, predicting responsive biology and appropriate patient selection is a challenge. However, loss of PTEN protein expression, a tumour suppressor, can lead to hyperactive PI3K signalling and may provide a predictor of PI3K-related dependence. PTEN loss is identified in 55% of GCB-DLBCLs and indicates targetable addiction to the PI3K/Akt/mTOR pathway which may in part be mediated through MYC [69].

An alternative predictive biomarker was identified in a phase II trial of copanlisib, a pan-class 1 PI3K inhibitor with greater activity against the α and δ isoforms. PI3K pathway gene expression was more associated with cases that responded across multiple lymphoma subtypes [70]. Interestingly, two studies have described the sensitivity of ABC-DLBCL rather than GCB-DLBCL to the combined inhibition of two class I PI3K isoforms (α and δ) [71, 72]. This has led to the incorporation of the PI3K dual α/δ inhibitor in combination with ibrutinib in MasterLymph, a stratified clinical trial in DLBCL. Identification of driver mutations, oncogene addictions and potential predictive biomarkers is starting to emerge in DLBCL through preclinical research. It appears that by inhibiting crucial cell signalling pathways or where actionable mutations are present, new methods to treat DLBCL may be identified. However, crosstalk between pathways in addition to multiple concurrent genomic aberrations contributes to the difficulty in selecting appropriate therapy for sensitive subgroups with our present state of knowledge.

Two recent studies have proposed new classifications of DLBCL based upon genomic aberrations and related them to COO subtypes. These have highlighted the prognostic and pathogenic importance of somatic number variants (SNVs) and structural variants in addition to somatic mutations and how they may cluster in DLBCL. They also suggest putative targets for therapy. Encouragingly, two studies have identified similar clusters independently using different techniques. The group at NCRI used an algorithm to best fit to predetermined seeds and cases were enriched for ABC and unclassified cases, reporting on three new groups. The Harvard group used unbiased clustering and identified five distinct clusters [73, 74]. An example of their similarities are the MCD and C5 groups that have striking similarities, specifically *MYD88*^{L265P} and *CD79B* mutations/amplification. Such cases were enriched for extranodal involvement, had BCL-2 perturbation and were associated with inferior survival. It was not reported whether they encompass a large number of the double-expressor lymphoma cases that are enriched in ABC-DLBCL and have worse prognosis. However, when cases with the MCD seed feature (*MYD88*^{L265P} and *CD79B* mutations) were identified within a phase III trial population they were not associated with worse survival [75]. It will be important to validate these new groups and refine them but also design clinical trials so that they do not exclude the worst cases exhibiting these likely high-risk subtypes. ABC cases tend to be older, if the higher risk cases tend to be MCD/C5 trials may miss patients of highest clinical need. The biology of the class suggest actionable targets for investigation and may be amenable to ibrutinib, mTOR pathways inhibitors and BCL-2 BH3 mimetics.

C3 and EZB also shared similar features: frequent *BCL-2* rearrangements and epigenetic modifier mutations (*CREBBP, KMT2D, EP300*). It is presumed that they share pathogenic processes with follicular lymphomas; EZB were the strongest confidence GCB classification cases in the NCRI study. It appeared that these cases may also have significantly worse survival. GCB cases are thought to have a better outcome overall in DLBCL. Most of the concomitant *MYC* and *BCL-2* rearranged cases, DHLs, are GCB subtype and have poor clinical outcomes. This was not explained in the studies and it may be that outcomes can be bisected based on the presence of *MYC*- and *BCL-2* rearrangement. It will be interesting to understand how DEL and DHL fit within the proposed taxonomy and whether they retain prognostic importance (Fig. 18.1).

These subgroups provide a framework to divide DLBCL and better understand the complexity of this disease. Preclinical models reflecting these subtypes, pre-classified xenografts and genetically engineered mouse models, may be used to support targeting biology for stratified studies. Refining the classifications and developing NGS platforms may also be required to deliver prospective stratification within studies or retrospective understanding of these subgroups' outcomes following novel approaches. Entities that ultimately display different responses to treatment and determine patient management are those that will persist.

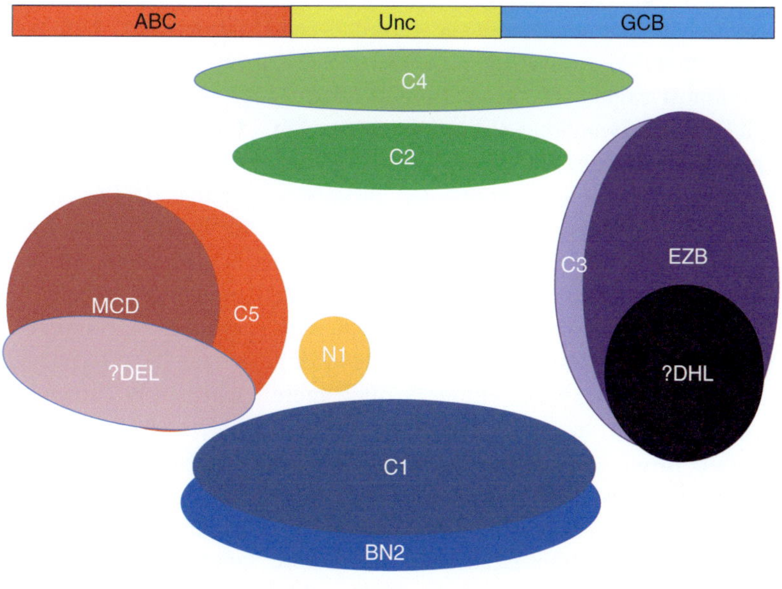

Fig. 18.1 Pictorial representation of the new genetic taxonomy of DLBCL

18.4 Actionable Somatic Lymphoma Aberrations

Actionable mutations have been used to select successful targeted agents in solid tumours. For example, the anaplastic lymphoma kinase *(*ALK) inhibitor crizotinib is employed in the treatment of non-small-cell lung cancer (NSCLC) carrying ALK mutations [76]. Recently evidence is emerging for similar promise in lymphoma. The t(2;5)(q23;q35) translocation which results in *NPM1/ALK* fusions was the first recurrent genetic abnormality identified in PTCL [77] and is involved in ~ 50% of anaplastic large-cell lymphomas, where it confers a favourable prognosis. Alternative translocations with ALK are present in a further 15–25% of cases [78]. Precision therapy for this subset has been attempted with crizotinib, and a small case series of relapsed/refractory patients showed a 91% ORR with a 2-year PFS of 63.7% [79]. A more potent ALK inhibitor alectinib has improved outcomes in non-small-cell lung cancer (NSCLC) in direct comparison with crizotinib as part of a phase III study and may warrant investigation in lymphoma [80].

The catalytic subunit of polycomb repressive complex 2, EZH2, is involved in trimethylation of histone 3 on lysine 27 (H3K27), required for maintenance of the germinal-centre reaction [81]. Activating mutations in EZH2 are almost exclusively seen in GCB-DLBCL and follicular lymphoma (FL), being present in approximately 20% of these types [81, 82]. Clinical trials have demonstrated promising responses in patients treated with EZH2 inhibitors such as the orally available tazemetostat [83]. There was a significantly higher response to tazemetostat in cases of DLBCL with activating mutations of EZH2 (29% vs 15%), although there were numerically more responses seen in wild-type (WT) DLBCL overall, owing to the low prevalence of the mutation. Whilst the testing of EZH2 inhibitors may be most appropriate in *EZH2* mutant cases, the premature stratification to these cases alone would have missed activity in WT cases. Further biomarkers may be found to explain responses related to the activity of EZH2 in epigenetic regulation. A phase II clinical trial investigating panobinostat, a histone deacetylase inhibitor, in combination with rituximab for relapsed and refractory DLBCL found that mutations in *MEF2B* were significantly associated with clinical response with a subset of extreme responders remaining in remission beyond 3 years [84].

Further specific actionable aberrations have been identified within aggressive lymphomas which may benefit from further investigation. Seventy percent of Burkitt lymphomas (BL) have mutations in *ID3* or *TCF-3*, the gene products of which act as partners regulating TCF-3 transcriptional activation [85]. Resulting increases in TCF-3 activity upregulate cyclin-dependent kinase 3 (CCND3), proliferation and cell cycle progression and contribute to the expression of genes that define BL in classifier gene sets [86]. Additionally, *CCND3* mutations occur in 38% of sporadic BL [86]. These mutant isoforms of cyclin D3 are found to accumulate to levels tenfold greater than wild-type cyclin D3, suggesting the aberrations increase protein stability. TCF3 activation appears to play a role in PI3K pathway signalling similar to that seen in tonic-BCR-signalling [86]. There is evidence of activity with CDK inhibitors and PI3K in BL models, and these are just entering clinical testing [87, 88].

Angioimmunoblastic T-cell lymphoma (AITL) and PTCL-NOS contain frequent mutations in genes involved in regulating DNA methylation: *TET2*, *IDH2* and *DNMT3A* [89]. Global DNA and histone hypermethylation are the product of these inactivating or gain-of-function mutations, evoking widespread gene expression changes in comparison to the proposed cell of origin [89]. Hypomethylating agents have been extensively studied in myelodysplastic syndrome where *TET2* mutations are associated with higher response rates to 5-azacytidine than wild-type cases [90]. In a small case series, 5-azacytidine treatment resulted in an ORR of 75% for AITL with 42% attaining CR. For other PTCL entities where *TET2* mutations are less frequent, a disappointing 15% ORR was observed [91].

18.5 BCL-2 Proteins and BH3 Mimetics

Two recent studies used CRISP-R (Clustered Regularly Interspaced Short Palindromic Repeats) screens in DLBCL cell lines to identify critical functional dependencies. They both identified BCL-2 family members, *BCL-2* and *MCL-1*, as driver genes, suggesting them as promising targets in the disease [58, 92]. Anti-apoptotic BCL-2 proteins serve to prevent mitochondrial or intrinsic apoptosis and are consistently associated with chemotherapy resistance in cancer [7, 93, 94]. These proteins serve as a bridge between pro-apoptotic family members such as BAX and BAK and the initiator BH3-only proteins, which are typically induced following apoptotic stimuli [95]. High BCL-2 expression through gene amplification or rearrangement is associated with poor outcomes in DLBCL [41]. Venetoclax is a second-generation BH3 mimetic that selectively binds and inhibits BCL-2 and has been approved by the FDA for treatment of CLL following rapid and impressive responses in clinical trials, increasing interest in the drug's applicability to other lymphoproliferative disorders [96]. Unfortunately, single agent used in DLBCL induces only low response rates (18%) which do not appear to correlate with BCL-2 expression, in the small numbers of patients studied [18]. However, there is a significant appeal to combine BCL-2 inhibitors with cytotoxic chemotherapy. The US National Clinical Trials Network is planning a randomised trial in patients with high-grade lymphoma with *MYC* and *BCL-2* translocations of DA-EPOCH-R with or without venetoclax. There is evidence that upregulation of alternative pro-survival BCL-2 proteins can drive resistance to BH3 mimetics in preclinical models [97]. Dependence on specific pro-survival BCL-2 proteins appears to predict the response to these therapeutic molecules in other cancer models and may act in part by reducing the threshold for apoptosis with other agents by "priming" cells for death [97, 98]. A number of newer agents are emerging that target alternative BCL-2 family proteins, including CDK9 inhibitors such as dinaciclib, which reduces MCL-1 expression and may be beneficial in "MCL-1-dependent" lymphomas [99].

18.6 Targeting the Immune Microenvironment in Lymphoma

Advances in immunotherapy for solid tumours using checkpoint blockade therapy (CBT) have transformed the clinical course of some malignancies, leading to exponential growth in the field [100]. Programmed death 1 (PD-1) is expressed by activated T-cells and serves to limit T-cell expansion during acute immune responses. However, during chronic activation, PD-1 can mark exhausted T-cells and serves as a key immune checkpoint receptor that mediates potent immune suppression when engaged by its ligands PDL-1 or PDL-2. Among lymphomas and solid tumours, classical Hodgkin lymphoma (cHL) has demonstrated the most striking ORRs to CBT with the anti-PD-1 mAbs pembrolizumab, achieving 65% ORR [90], and nivolumab, 87% [101, 102], in the relapsed/refractory setting. cHL is morphologically characterised by a dense immune cell infiltrate surrounding the malignant cell, including "exhausted" effector T-cells which tolerate the malignant clone. The Reed-Sternberg cell exhibits amplification of 9p24.1 in 85% of cHL, which drives PD-L1 and PD-L2 overexpression, providing the clear rationale for targeting this interaction with anti-PD-1. This success demonstrates the potential for linkage between a molecular aberration and translation into therapeutic benefit [103]. In most other lymphoma types, the response to CBT in lymphoma has been less impressive, although there is evidence of activity in PMBL [19]. The COO for malignant transformation in PMBL is believed to be related to that of cHL, the thymic B-cell; 70% of cases demonstrate a 9p24.1 amplification with associated PD-L1/PD-L2 expression [104]. PD-1 ligand expression is also common in primary CNS lymphoma (PCNSL) and primary testicular lymphoma (PTL), where copy number alterations of 9p24.1 are frequently identified [105]. A small case series of five patients with PCNSL and

PTL all responded to PD-1 mAb treatment, with three patients remaining progression-free beyond 13 months [106].

Nivolumab has a reported ORR of 37% among 11 cases of relapsed/refractory DLBCL [107]. A subpopulation of cases appears to respond to checkpoint inhibitors, and reliable predictors of response are needed. The consensus clustering classification (CCC) by GEP identifies DLBCL with a prominent immune cell infiltrate, referred to as the "host response" (HR) subtype, and this may prove relevant. Other malignancies exhibiting an "immune-inflamed" phenotype with immune cell infiltrate on histological examination are associated with responses to CBT [108]. Only around 24% of cases of DLBCL express PD-L1, whilst PD-L2 expression is even rarer, and immune cell infiltrates are not a universal feature of DLBCL in the manner seen in cHL [104, 109]. Interestingly, high levels of soluble PD-L1 at diagnosis have been independently associated with a poorer prognosis in DLBCL [110]. Conversely, PD-L1 copy number is associated with clinical response to nivolumab in cHL, where amplification was associated with greater responses than copy number gains [111]. These genomic changes also correlated to relative protein PD-L1 expression.

Clearly, immune-modulation coupled to small molecule targeting is also attractive. However, one potential factor that may complicate translational development in this area is the fact that small molecules also have activity against tumour immune cell infiltrates, such as Btk and PI3K inhibitors [112, 113]. In some contexts, this may be harnessed. Inhibition of PI3Kδ has been implicated in downregulation of regulatory T-cells that dampen T-cell responses to tumour-antigen [114]. Clinical trials in solid tumour patients have been instigated to utilise this mechanism of action. Alternatively, inhibition of Btk in macrophages has been used to upregulate CD8+ T-cells in solid tumour models associated with reduced tumour growth supporting incorporation into clinical trials [115]. Furthermore, immunomodulatory antibodies may be used in a similar manner. Targeting CD27, a co-stimulatory receptor on T and NK cells, in lymphoma models resulted in myeloid cell infiltration to allow greater phagocytosis of tumour cells opsonised by rituximab [116]. This combination is now being investigated in a phase Ib clinical trial of lymphomas. A precision medicine approach may be appropriate in this context also, targeting the specific immune cells that make up patient's tumour microenvironment. However, the effects upon anticancer immunity are unpredictable. Novel assays will be needed to accurately represent lymphoma and immune biology and allow the development of these treatments for potential combination.

18.7 Circulating Tumour DNA to Guide Therapy

Applying precision therapy requires accurate and reliable characterisation of a malignancy and is limited by acquisition of tumour material both spatially and temporally. Advances in detecting and analysing circulating tumour DNA (ctDNA) from plasma for somatic mutations and copy number alterations are being extensively investigated in the management of many cancers.

An early study used NGS to detect a tumour-specific clonotype, based on VDJ gene segments of the rearranged immunoglobulin receptor genes, in pretreatment specimens for DLBCL patients [117]. A clonotype was identified successfully in the tumour for 126 of 198 patients, so that serum ctDNA encoding the VDJ rearrangements could then be quantified. CtDNA quantity correlated significantly with lymphoma tumour burden and international prognostic index (IPI). Sequential monitoring demonstrated that 98% of the cases that remained progression-free from lymphoma had undetectable ctDNA. Patterns of sequential measurable ctDNA levels were more variable for cases that exhibited progressive disease; for some cases ctDNA quantity increased around the time of progression whilst others never cleared detectable ctDNA or had no rise associated with progression. Overall, ctDNA levels taken at cycle 3 day 1 provided a positive predictive value of 63% and negative predictive value of 80% for disease progression. Failure to identify a disease-specific marker for a third of cases and relatively poor reliability to predict all relapses reduce the applicability of the technique for risk-adapted therapy without incorporating other techniques, although it may allow earlier identification of refractory patients.

A larger study used 217 DLBCL patients split between a discovery and two validation sets to investigate the dynamics of ctDNA by targeted sequencing using cancer personalised profiling by deep sequencing (CAPP-Seq). 2-log reduction in ctDNA, early molecular response (EMR), or 2.5 log decrease, major molecular response (MMR) were significantly associated with superior event-free survival in the first-line or salvage settings [118]. Molecular response (EMR or MMR where available) was associated with worse OS independent of IPI or interim PET result. Incorporating molecular response with IPI or interim PET results further discriminated outcome by EFS and OS. The value of using the prognostic implications of dynamic ctDNA response would be as a risk-adapted approach intensifying therapy or incorporating novel agents for high-risk patients or potentially de-escalating molecular responders. A small number failed to achieve molecular response and had a positive interim PET and exhibited extremely poor OS. They progressed rapidly and it is likely this would be apparent clinically prior to requiring molecular results. It is possible that these cases had known high-risk features such as being double-hit lymphomas, which was not reported in the study. If this is the case, it would be rational to select these patients for investigation of novel approaches based on baseline features rather than commencing standard of care to later adapt therapy. The differences in survival between cases with negative interim PET but with or without molecular response were not large limiting the prognostic utility. It may be that incorporating molecular subtyping such as COO, or the newer genomic subtypes, with other prognostic features such as total metabolic tumour volume or interim PET response may allow better stratification for prospective risk-adapted clinical studies.

A phase II study of panobinostat and rituximab in relapsed and refractory (R/R) DLBCL examined ctDNA for recurrent somatic mutations using a combination of hybridisation capture sequencing of lymphoma-related genes (modelled after Capp-Seq) followed by deep sequencing and droplet digital polymerase chain reaction (ddPCR) in 92 cases [84]. Similar to the ctDNA study above, at treatment day 15, those patients with a reduction in ctDNA level all had clinical responses to the experimental therapy, whilst none with an elevated level at this time point subsequently responded. CtDNA as an early biomarker of response requires further investigation, and optimal time points are certain to be treatment-specific. The particular utility of this approach is that it provides information on driver mutations, without the need for tumour sampling.

Further studies have utilised a similar approach using NGS for ctDNA with encouraging results. A study of 92 patients with DLBCL used CAPP-Seq to profile somatic alterations [119]. In 8 of 11 patients who subsequently relapsed, ctDNA was detectable prior to clinical relapse. The median time between first detectable ctDNA result and radiographic disease recurrence was 188 days, highlighting possible early opportunities for prediction of progression using ctDNA for minimal residual disease monitoring. Genotyping using ctDNA of three patients who progressed whilst receiving ibrutinib identified *BTK* emergent mutations thought to represent clonal evolution. A further study employing CAPP-Seq to sequentially study ctDNA in 50 DLBCL patients found the technique had >90% sensitivity and ~100% specificity for somatic gene mutations represented in >20% of alleles, compared with tumour DNA [120]. Among patients who relapsed or were primary refractory to immunochemotherapy, new mutations appeared in the ctDNA at the time of progression conceivably reflecting the emergence of treatment-resistant clones not detected at diagnosis. It appears that there is an excellent concordance between ctDNA and the tumour-derived mutational landscape which may allow monitoring of mutation-directed therapy [121]. Patterns of somatic mutations found in the plasma of DLBCL patients also associate closely with COO status for DLBCL cases and may be used as a surrogate where IHC and GEP cannot be performed [122]. Subclonal populations may be identifiable with DNA shed from locations apart from tumour biopsy sites. Clonal evolution and emergence of new mutations may also be monitored due to the ease of plasma sampling over tumour, possibly revealing mechanisms of resistance.

The group from Stanford University Medical Center applied Capp-Seq to identify somatic copy number alterations (SCNAs) in clinically relevant genes in plasma samples from DLBCL patients. When 23 of these cases were compared with corresponding tumour biopsy results, there was good concordance; sensitivity and specificity were 77% and 97%, respectively [123]. Interestingly, PD-L1 amplification was significantly enriched in relapsed cases (43.5% vs. 19.2%). The relative ease of plasma sampling can provide information on treatment resistance, less available using standard approaches.

18.8 Challenges Incorporating Biology into Future Studies

Disease heterogeneity determines that understanding responses to new and existing therapies is difficult, particularly without large datasets. Where patient selection within clinical trials is agnostic, researchers may overlook understanding of which subgroups may actually benefit from a novel therapy. Thorough molecular characterisation is necessary to understand novel approaches applied to aggressive lymphomas and should be incorporated within clinical studies. However, unplanned retrospective analyses to seek understanding of responders are likely to be underpowered and may risk false positives from multiple analyses. Conversely, premature selection may misunderstand mechanisms of action of the investigational drug, such as indicated in the

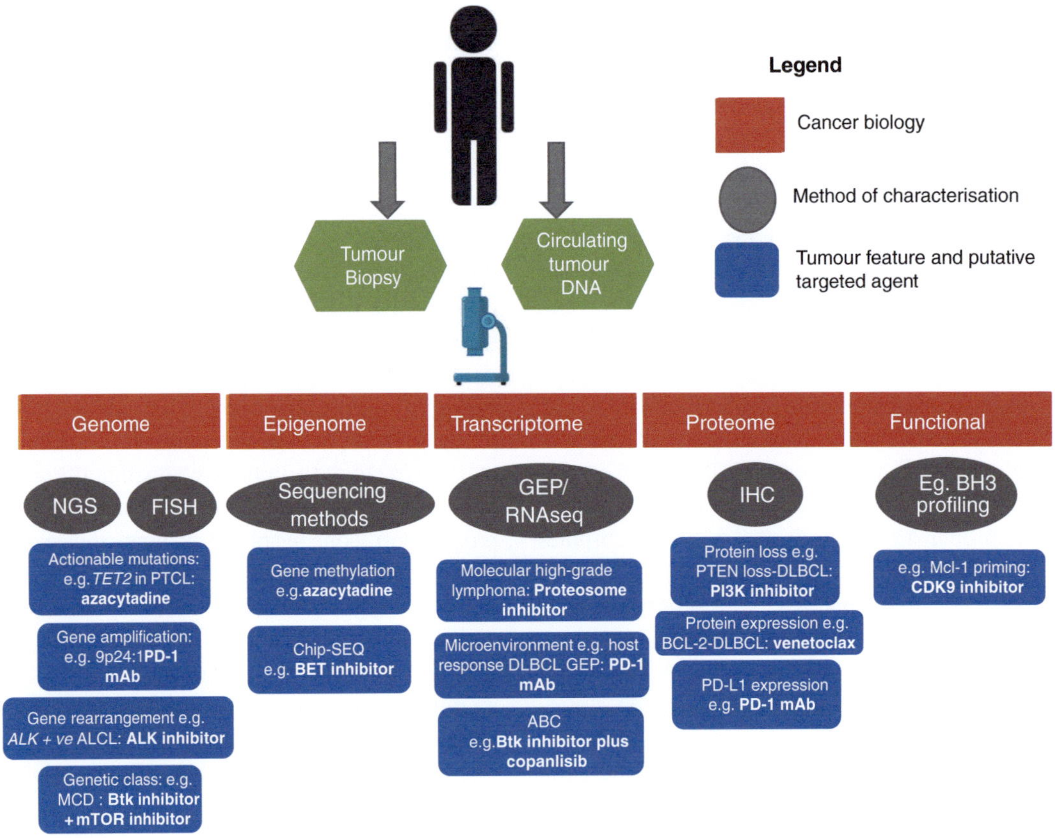

Fig. 18.2 Aggressive lymphoma characterisation and putative targets for therapy

case of EZH2 inhibitors which have demonstrable activity in *EZH2* WT cases as well as mutants.

Basic science can be used to understand mechanisms of effect in the context of lymphoma biology; however models that reflect diverse lymphomas are limited, elucidating mechanisms that are time-consuming where clinical need is ongoing. Predictive biomarkers must be explored within early phase clinical trials to guide future directions with agent-specific measures in addition to diverse and thorough characterisation. Several large precision medicine trials across a variety of malignancies have failed to improve outcomes for the majority of patients, suggesting the approach is not straightforward [124, 125]. A number of studies with targeted agents have failed to improve outcomes for aggressive lymphomas. The reasons for these failures are almost certainly multifactorial. In addition to pleotropic effects of presumed "targeted" agents, rigorous inclusion criteria and cumbersome central pathology review may inadvertently exclude high-risk patients from enrolling on precision medicine studies. Ensuring homogeneity to the patient population without excluding high-risk patients represents a major challenge in clinical trial design. Disease heterogeneity is a further challenge. Within DLBCL the majority of recurrent somatic mutations occur in less than 5% of patients, and few occur in greater than 20% of cases, whilst 20–30 mutations may be present in each case [29]. Agent selection for investigation in a rational subgroup is challenging, and studies may be difficult to power and understand in the context of multiple mutations occurring within each case. Appropriate preclinical guidance and agent-specific biomarkers include those that move beyond the agent: mutation paradigm may be necessary. Precision medicine will rely upon deeper translational characterisation and novel assays relevant to specific therapies (Fig. 18.2).

18.9 Conclusion

At present, clinical decision-making for patients with aggressive lymphomas is limited with respect to the underlying biology. Treatment intensification can be justified for high-risk subtypes, and some novel agents show preferential activity in the context of molecular aberrations or biological subgroups. This knowledge can provide rationale for therapy, whilst an array of agents with differing mechanisms of action against lymphoma are ready for appropriate clinical trials. The complexity of aggressive lymphomas, which increases alongside our growing biological understanding, dictates that this process will be challenging. Basic and translational research will prove crucial in guiding precision medicine, identifying responsive biology and dissecting oncogenic addictions (and their feedback circuits) to develop new therapeutics.

The number of negative first-line studies in DLBCL and the limited response rates of single novel agents are a resounding call for precision medicine (Table 18.1). Detailed molecular characterisation can be incorporated into trials to convert biology to clinical utility and guide future directions; however knowledge of what is pertinent and how to prioritise this are crucial. In addition to genomic and transcriptomic studies elucidating malignant cell characteristics, profiling epigenetic, protein expression or microenvironmental factors may be needed in agent and disease-specific contexts. Predictive biomarkers will rely on mechanism of action of drugs, so a mutation-agent pairing approach may lack the sophistication required to manipulate complex biology. When only a third of patients respond to a novel agent, we should endeavour to explain why, so that future work can be directed. Computational, systems biology techniques are likely needed where disease is complicated and collaborations to amalgamate large datasets are crucial to sufficiently power statistical analyses and appropriately reflect the breadth of the disease.

As we determine that previously homogenous disease entities contain multiple lymphoma endotypes, complex adaptive trial designs may be necessary to investigate agents in terms of the underlying biology most likely to respond. Recruiting only those with highest probability of response to a selected agent or prospective trial design with enrichment through sophisticated statistics could be considered.

As progress builds, how best to incorporate novel agents into optimal regimens, with standard of care or as novel-novel strategies, will require biological as well as clinical understanding. Collaborations between researchers with complementary expertise will be necessary to translate basic science to therapy, design efficient trials, characterise the biology and usher in the next era of improved treatment regimes.

References

1. SEER. National Cancer Institute: Surveillance, Epidemiology, and End Results Program. SEER 2017. https://seer.cancer.gov/statfacts/html/nhl.html. Accessed 2 Apr 2017.
2. https://www.hmrn.org/statistics/incidence. Accessed 25 Jun 2017.
3. Feugier P, et al. Long-term results of the R-CHOP study in the treatment of elderly patients with diffuse large B-cell lymphoma: a study by the Groupe d'Etude des Lymphomes de l'Adulte. J Clin Oncol. 2005;23:4117.
4. Wilson WH, et al. Phase III randomized study of R-CHOP versus DA-EPOCH-R and molecular analysis of untreated diffuse large B-cell lymphoma: CALGB/Alliance 50303. Blood. 2016;128:469.
5. d'Amore F, et al. Up-front autologous stem-cell transplantation in peripheral T-cell lymphoma: NLG-T-01. J Clin Oncol. 2012;30(25):3093–9.
6. Laport GG. Peripheral T-cell lymphoma: autologous hematopoietic cell transplantation as first-line therapy. Curr Opin Oncol. 2010;22(5):409–13.
7. Mounier N, et al. Rituximab plus CHOP (R-CHOP) overcomes bcl-2--associated resistance to chemotherapy in elderly patients with diffuse large B-cell lymphoma (DLBCL). Blood. 2003;101:4279.
8. Cunningham D, et al. Rituximab plus cyclophosphamide, doxorubicin, vincristine, and prednisolone in patients with newly diagnosed diffuse large B-cell non-Hodgkin lymphoma: a phase 3 comparison of dose intensification with 14-day versus 21-day cycles. Lancet. 2013;381(9880):1817–26.
9. Récher C, et al. Intensified chemotherapy with ACVBP plus rituximab versus standard CHOP plus rituximab for the treatment of diffuse large B-cell lymphoma (LNH03-2B): an open-label randomised phase 3 trial. Lancet. 2011;378(9806):1858–67.
10. Jaeger U, et al. Rituximab maintenance for patients with aggressive B-cell lymphoma in first remission: results of the randomized NHL13 trial. Haematologica. 2015;2015:125344.
11. Leppä S, et al. A phase III study of enzastaurin in patients with high-risk diffuse large B cell lymphoma following response to primary treatment: the prelude trial. Am Soc Hematol. 2013.
12. Witzig TE, et al. PILLAR-2: a randomized, double-blind, placebo-controlled, phase III study of adjuvant everolimus (EVE) in patients (pts) with poor-risk diffuse large B-cell lymphoma (DLBCL). Proc Am Soc Clin Oncol. 2016.
13. Vitolo U, et al. Obinutuzumab or rituximab plus CHOP in patients with previously untreated diffuse large B-cell lymphoma: final results from an open-label, randomized phase 3 study (GOYA). Blood. 2016;128:470.
14. Thieblemont C, et al. First analysis of an international double-blind randomized phase III study of lenalidomide maintenance in elderly patients with DLBCL treated with R-CHOP in first line, the REMARC study from Lysa. Blood. 2016;128:471.
15. Davies A, et al. Differential efficacy of bortezomib in subtypes of diffuse large B-cell lymphoma (DLBL): a prospective randomised study stratified by transcriptome profiling: REMODL-B. Hematol Oncol. 2017;35(S2):130–1.
16. Flinn IW, et al. A phase II trial to evaluate the efficacy of fostamatinib in patients with relapsed or refractory diffuse large B-cell lymphoma (DLBCL). Eur J Cancer. 2016;54:11–7.
17. Wilson WH, et al. The Bruton's tyrosine kinase (BTK) inhibitor, ibrutinib (PCI-32765), has preferential activity in the ABC subtype of relapsed/refractory de novo diffuse large B-cell lymphoma (DLBCL): interim results of a multicenter, open-label, phase 2 study. Blood. 2012;120(21):686.
18. Davids MS, et al. Phase I first-in-human study of venetoclax in patients with relapsed or refractory non-Hodgkin lymphoma. J Clin Oncol. 2017;70:4320.
19. Bohl SR, et al. Nivolumab induces remission in high-PD-L1 expressing aggressive B-non Hodgkin lymphoma: a single center experience. Blood. 2016;128:1865.
20. Oki Y, et al. Phase II study of an AKT inhibitor MK2206 in patients with relapsed or refractory lymphoma. Br J Haematol. 2015;171(4):463–70.
21. Horwitz SM, et al. Duvelisib (IPI-145), a phosphoinositide-3-kinase-δ, γ inhibitor, shows activity in patients with relapsed/refractory T-cell lymphoma. Blood. 2014;124:803.
22. Witzig TE, et al. A comprehensive review of lenalidomide therapy for B- cell non-Hodgkin lymphoma. Ann Oncol. 2015;26:1667.
23. Witzig TE, et al. A phase II trial of the oral mTOR inhibitor everolimus in relapsed aggressive lymphoma. Leukemia. 2011;25(2):341–7.
24. Caimi P, et al. A phase 1 study of BET inhibition using RG6146 in relapsed/refractory (R/R) MYC-expressing diffuse large B cell lymphoma (DLBCL). Hematol Oncol. 2017;35(S2):263–5.
25. Morschhauser F, et al. Interim report from a phase 2 multicenter study of TAZEMETOSTAT, an EZH2 inhibitor, in patients with relapsed or refractory B-cell non-Hodgkin lymphomas. Hematol Oncol. 2017;35:24–5.

26. Coiffier B, et al. Romidepsin for the treatment of relapsed/refractory peripheral T-cell lymphoma: pivotal study update demonstrates durable responses. J Hematol Oncol. 2014;7(1):11.
27. Swerdlow SH, et al. The 2016 revision of the World Health Organization classification of lymphoid neoplasms. Blood. 2016;127(20):2375–90.
28. Clozel T, et al. Mechanism-based epigenetic chemosensitization therapy of diffuse large B-cell lymphoma. Cancer Discov. 2013;3:1002.
29. Morin RD, et al. Mutational and structural analysis of diffuse large B-cell lymphoma using whole-genome sequencing. Blood. 2013;122:1256.
30. Park HY, et al. Whole-exome and transcriptome sequencing of refractory diffuse large B-cell lymphoma. Oncotarget. 2016;7(52):86433.
31. Bertier G, Hétu M, Joly Y. Unsolved challenges of clinical whole-exome sequencing: a systematic literature review of end-users' views. BMC Med Genet. 2016;9(1):52.
32. Dubois S, et al. Next generation sequencing in diffuse large B cell lymphoma highlights molecular divergence and therapeutic opportunities: a LYSA study. Clin Cancer Res. 2016;22(12):2919–28.
33. Davies AJ, et al. Differential efficacy of bortezomib in subtypes of diffuse large B-cell lymphoma (dlbl): a prospective randomised study stratified by transcriptome profiling: remodl-B. Hematol Oncol. 2017;35:130–1.
34. Scott DW, et al. Determining cell-of-origin subtypes of diffuse large B-cell lymphoma using gene expression in formalin-fixed paraffin-embedded tissue. Blood. 2014;123(8):1214–7.
35. Alizadeh AA, et al. Distinct types of diffuse large B-cell lymphoma identified by gene expression profiling. Nature. 2000;403:503.
36. Monti S, et al. Molecular profiling of diffuse large B-cell lymphoma identifies robust subtypes including one characterized by host inflammatory response. Blood. 2005;105(5):1851–61.
37. Moffitt AB, Dave SS. Clinical applications of the genomic landscape of aggressive non-Hodgkin lymphoma. J Clin Oncol. 2017;35(9):955–62.
38. Iqbal J, et al. Gene expression signatures delineate biological and prognostic subgroups in peripheral T-cell lymphoma. Blood. 2014;123(19):2915–23.
39. Huang Y, et al. Gene expression profiling identifies emerging oncogenic pathways operating in extranodal NK/T-cell lymphoma, nasal type. Blood. 2010;115(6):1226–37.
40. Manso R, et al. C-MYC is related to GATA3 expression and associated with poor prognosis in nodal peripheral T-cell lymphomas. Haematologica. 2016;101(8):e336.
41. Ennishi D, et al. Genetic profiling of MYC and BCL2 in diffuse large B-cell lymphoma determines cell of origin-specific clinical impact. Blood. 2017;129(20):2760–70.
42. Barrans S, et al. Rearrangement of MYC is associated with poor prognosis in patients with diffuse large B-cell lymphoma treated in the era of rituximab. J Clin Oncol. 2010;28(20):3360–5.
43. Zhang HW, et al. Clinical impact of t (14; 18) in diffuse large B-cell lymphoma. Chin J Cancer Res. 2011;23(2):160–4.
44. Oki Y, et al. Double hit lymphoma: the MD Anderson Cancer Center clinical experience. Br J Haematol. 2014;166(6):891–901.
45. Dunleavy K, et al. Preliminary report of a multicenter prospective phase II study of DA-EPOCH-R in MYC-rearranged aggressive B-cell lymphoma. Blood. 2014;124(21):395.
46. Sehn L, et al. Prognostic impact of BCL2 and MYC expression and translocation in untreated DLBCL: results from the phase III GOYA study. Hematol Oncol. 2017;35(S2):131–3.
47. Lai C, et al. MYC gene rearrangement in diffuse large B-cell lymphoma does not confer a worse prognosis following dose-adjusted EPOCH-R. Leuk Lymphoma. 2018;59:505–8.
48. Kühnl A, et al. Outcome of elderly patients with diffuse large B-cell lymphoma treated with R-CHOP: subgroup analysis from the UK NCRI R-CHOP 14 vs 21 trial. Blood. 2015;126:1516.
49. Roschewski M, et al. Diffuse large B-cell lymphoma-treatment approaches in the molecular era. Nat Rev Clin Oncol. 2014;11:12–23.
50. Staiger AM, et al. Clinical impact of the cell-of-origin classification and the MYC/BCL2 dual expresser status in diffuse large B-cell lymphoma treated within prospective clinical trials of the German High-Grade Non-Hodgkin's Lymphoma Study Group. J Clin Oncol. 2017;35(22):2515–26.
51. Mareschal S, et al. The proportion of activated B-cell like subtype among de novo diffuse large B-cell lymphoma increases with age. Haematologica. 2011;96(12):1888–90.
52. Molina TJ, et al. Young patients with non–germinal center B-cell–like diffuse large B-cell lymphoma benefit from intensified chemotherapy with ACVBP plus rituximab compared with CHOP plus rituximab: analysis of data from the Groupe d'Etudes des Lymphomes de l'Adulte/lymphoma study association phase III trial LNH 03-2B. J Clin Oncol. 2014;32(35):3996–4003.
53. Davis RE, et al. Constitutive nuclear factor κB activity is required for survival of activated B cell-like diffuse large B cell lymphoma cells. J Exp Med. 2001;194(12):1861–74.
54. Gang AO, et al. Cell of origin predicts outcome to treatment with etoposide-containing chemotherapy in young patients with high-risk diffuse large B-cell lymphoma. Leuk Lymphoma. 2015;56(7):2039–46.
55. Byrd JC, et al. Targeting BTK with ibrutinib in relapsed chronic lymphocytic leukemia. N Engl J Med. 2013;369(1):32–42.
56. Wilson WH, et al. Targeting B cell receptor signaling with ibrutinib in diffuse large B cell lymphoma. Nat Med. 2015;21:922.

57. Young RM, et al. CRISPR-CAS9 genetic screens uncover a B cell receptor-MYD88 superpathway in diffuse large B cell lymphoma. Hematol Oncol. 2017;35:25.
58. Phelan JD, et al. A multiprotein supercomplex controlling oncogenic signalling in lymphoma. Nature. 2018;560(7718):387–91.
59. Hernandez-Ilizaliturri FJ, et al. Higher response to lenalidomide in relapsed/refractory diffuse large B-cell lymphoma in nongerminal center B-cell–like than in germinal center B-cell–like phenotype. Cancer. 2011;117(22):5058–66.
60. Davies A, Caddy J, Maishman T, Barrans S, Mamot C, Care M, Pocock C, Stantion L, Hamid D, Pugh K, Mcmillan A, Fields P, Kruger A, Jack A, Johnson P. A prospective randomised trial of targeted therapy for diffuse large B-cell lymphoma (DLBCL) based upon real-time gene expression profiling: the Remodl-B Study of the UK NCRI and SAKK Lymphoma Groups (ISRCTN51837425). ASH Annual Meeting Abstracts. 2015.
61. Thieblemont CC, et al. First analysis of an International Double-Blind Randomized Phase III Study of Lenalidomide maintenance in elderly patients with DLBCL treated with R-CHOP in first line, the Remarc Study from Lysa. American Society of Hematology, San Diego, CA. 2016.
62. Thieblemont C, et al. Lenalidomide maintenance compared with placebo in responding elderly patients with diffuse large B-cell lymphoma treated with first-line rituximab plus cyclophosphamide, doxorubicin, vincristine, and prednisone. J Clin Oncol. 2017;35(22):2473–81.
63. Young RM, et al. B-cell receptor signaling in diffuse large B-cell lymphoma. Semin Hematol. 2015;52(2):77–85.
64. Golay J, et al. Glycoengineered CD20 antibody obinutuzumab activates neutrophils and mediates phagocytosis through CD16B more efficiently than rituximab. Blood. 2013;122(20):3482–91.
65. Chen L, et al. SYK-dependent tonic B-cell receptor signaling is a rational treatment target in diffuse large B-cell lymphoma. Blood. 2008;111(4):2230–7.
66. Paul J, et al. Simultaneous inhibition of PI3Kδ and PI3Kα induces ABC-DLBCL regression by blocking BCR-dependent and-independent activation of NF-κB and AKT. Cancer Cell. 2017;31(1):64–78.
67. Lin T, et al. PILLAR-2: a randomized, double-blind, placebo-controlled, phase III study of adjuvant everolimus in poor-risk diffuse large B-cell lymphoma (DLBCL). Proc Am Soc Clin Oncol. 2012.
68. Carracedo A, Pandolfi P. The PTEN–PI3K pathway: of feedbacks and cross-talks. Oncogene. 2008;27(41):5527–41.
69. Pfeifer M, et al. PTEN loss defines a PI3K/AKT pathway-dependent germinal center subtype of diffuse large B-cell lymphoma. Proc Natl Acad Sci. 2013;110(30):12420–5.
70. Dreyling M, et al. Phase II study of copanlisib, a PI3K inhibitor, in relapsed or refractory, indolent or aggressive lymphoma. Ann Oncol. 2017;28(9):2169–78.
71. Paul J, et al. Simultaneous inhibition of PI3Kδ and PI3Kα induces ABC-DLBCL regression by blocking BCR-dependent and-independent activation of NF-κB and AKT. Cancer Cell. 2017;31(1):64–78.
72. Erdmann T, et al. Sensitivity to PI3K and AKT inhibitors is mediated by divergent molecular mechanisms in subtypes of DLBCL. Blood. 2017;130(3):310–22.
73. Schmitz R, et al. Genetics and pathogenesis of diffuse large B-cell lymphoma. N Engl J Med. 2018;378(15):1396–407.
74. Chapuy B, Stewart C, Dunford AJ, et al. Molecular subtypes of diffuse large B cell lymphoma are associated with distinct pathogenic mechanisms and outcomes. Nat Med. 2018;24:679–90.
75. Cummin TE, Du M, Johnson PW. Genetics of diffuse large B-cell lymphoma. N Engl J Med. 2018;379(5):493–4.
76. Shaw AT, et al. Crizotinib versus chemotherapy in advanced ALK-positive lung cancer. N Engl J Med. 2013;368(25):2385–94.
77. Rimokh R, et al. A translocation involving a specific breakpoint (q35) on chromosome 5 is characteristic of anaplastic large cell lymphoma ('Ki-1 lymphoma'). Br J Haematol. 1989;71(1):31–6.
78. Stein H, et al. CD30+ anaplastic large cell lymphoma: a review of its histopathologic, genetic, and clinical features. Blood. 2000;96(12):3681–95.
79. Passerini CG, et al. Crizotinib in advanced, chemoresistant anaplastic lymphoma kinase–positive lymphoma patients. J Natl Cancer Inst. 2014;106(2):djt378.
80. ALEX. randomised phase III ALEX. 2017. http://www.roche.com/media/store/releases/med-cor-2017-04-10.htm.
81. Béguelin W, et al. EZH2 is required for germinal center formation and somatic EZH2 mutations promote lymphoid transformation. Cancer Cell. 2013;23(5):677–92.
82. McCabe MT, et al. EZH2 inhibition as a therapeutic strategy for lymphoma with EZH2-activating mutations. Nature. 2012;492(7427):108–12.
83. ASH Lymphoma Biology Meeting Report. http://www.epizyme.com/wp-content/uploads/2016/06/EPZM-ASH-L-Data-PR-20160619.pdf.
84. Assouline SE, et al. Phase 2 study of panobinostat with or without rituximab in relapsed diffuse large B-cell lymphoma. Blood. 2016;128(2):185–94.
85. Love C, et al. The genetic landscape of mutations in Burkitt lymphoma. Nat Genet. 2012;44(12):1321–5.
86. Schmitz R, et al. Oncogenic mechanisms in Burkitt lymphoma. Cold Spring Harb Perspect Med. 2014;4(2):a014282.
87. Schmitz R, et al. Burkitt lymphoma pathogenesis and therapeutic targets from structural and functional genomics. Nature. 2012;490(7418):116–20.
88. Spender LC, Inman GJ. Phosphoinositide 3-kinase/AKT/mTORC1/2 signaling determines sensitivity

of Burkitt9s lymphoma cells to BH3 mimetics. Mol Cancer Res. 2012;10:347.
89. Schmitz N, de Leval L. How I manage peripheral T-cell lymphoma, not otherwise specified and angioimmunoblastic T-cell lymphoma: current practice and a glimpse into the future. Br J Haematol. 2017;176(6):851–66.
90. Itzykson R, et al. Impact of TET2 mutations on response rate to azacitidine in myelodysplastic syndromes and low blast count acute myeloid leukemias. Leukemia. 2011;25(7):1147–52.
91. Delarue R, et al. Treatment with hypomethylating agent 5-Azacytidine induces sustained response in angioimmunoblastic T cell lymphomas. Blood. 2016;128:4164.
92. Reddy A, et al. Genetic and functional drivers of diffuse large B cell lymphoma. Cell. 2017;171(2):481–494.e15.
93. Sartorius UA, Krammer PH. Upregulation of bcl-2 is involved in the mediation of chemotherapy resistance in human small cell lung cancer cell lines. Int J Cancer. 2002;97(5):584–92.
94. Michels J, et al. MCL-1 dependency of cisplatin-resistant cancer cells. Biochem Pharmacol. 2014;92(1):55–61.
95. Strasser A. The roles of programmed cell death in tumor development and cancer therapy. Medicographia. 2014;36:311–8.
96. Roberts AW, et al. Targeting BCL2 with venetoclax in relapsed chronic lymphocytic leukemia. N Engl J Med. 2016;374(4):311–22.
97. Choudhary G, et al. MCL-1 and BCL-xL-dependent resistance to the BCL-2 inhibitor ABT-199 can be overcome by preventing PI3K/AKT/mTOR activation in lymphoid malignancies. Cell Death Dis. 2015;6(1):e1593.
98. Certo M, et al. Mitochondria primed by death signals determine cellular addiction to antiapoptotic BCL-2 family members. Cancer Cell. 2006;9(5):351–65.
99. Gregory G, et al. CDK9 inhibition by dinaciclib potently suppresses Mcl-1 to induce durable apoptotic responses in aggressive MYC-driven B-cell lymphoma in vivo. Leukemia. 2015;29(6):1437.
100. Ott PA, Hodi FS, Robert C. CTLA-4 and PD-1/PD-L1 blockade: new immunotherapeutic modalities with durable clinical benefit in melanoma patients. Clin Cancer Res. 2013;19(19): 5300–9.
101. Armand P, et al. Programmed death-1 blockade with pembrolizumab in patients with classical Hodgkin lymphoma after brentuximab vedotin failure. J Clin Oncol. 2016;34(31):3733–9.
102. Ansell SM, et al. PD-1 blockade with nivolumab in relapsed or refractory Hodgkin's lymphoma. N Engl J Med. 2015;372(4):311–9.
103. Green MR, et al. Integrative analysis reveals selective 9p24. 1 amplification, increased PD-1 ligand expression, and further induction via JAK2 in nodular sclerosing Hodgkin lymphoma and primary mediastinal large B-cell lymphoma. Blood. 2010;116(17):3268–77.
104. Shi M, et al. Expression of programmed cell death 1 ligand 2 (PD-L2) is a distinguishing feature of primary mediastinal (thymic) large B-cell lymphoma and associated with PDCD1LG2 copy gain. Am J Surg Pathol. 2014;38(12):1715.
105. Chapuy B, et al. Targetable genetic features of primary testicular and primary central nervous system lymphomas. Blood. 2016;127(7):869–81.
106. Nayak L, et al. PD-1 blockade with nivolumab in relapsed/refractory primary central nervous system and testicular lymphoma. Blood. 2017;129(23):3071–3.
107. Lesokhin AM, et al. Preliminary results of a phase I study of nivolumab (BMS-936558) in patients with relapsed or refractory lymphoid malignancies. Blood. 2014;124(21):291.
108. Gajewski TF, et al. Cancer immunotherapy strategies based on overcoming barriers within the tumor microenvironment. Curr Opin Immunol. 2013;25(2):268–76.
109. Andorsky DJ, et al. Programmed death ligand 1 is expressed by non–Hodgkin lymphomas and inhibits the activity of tumor-associated T cells. Clin Cancer Res. 2011;17(13):4232–44.
110. Rossille D, et al. High level of soluble programmed cell death ligand 1 in blood impacts overall survival in aggressive diffuse large B-cell lymphoma: results from a French multicenter clinical trial. Leukemia. 2014;28(12):2367–75.
111. Shipp MA. Gianni BONADONNA memorial lecture: "genetic signatures and targetable pathways in lymphoid malignancies". Hematol Oncol. 2017;35:23–4.
112. Abu-Eid R, et al. Selective inhibition of regulatory T cells by targeting the PI3K–Akt pathway. Cancer Immunol Res. 2014;2(11):1080–9.
113. Christofides A, et al. Epigenetic regulation of cancer biology and anti-tumor immunity by EZH2. Oncotarget. 2016;7(51):85624–40.
114. Patton DT, et al. Cutting edge: the phosphoinositide 3-kinase p110δ is critical for the function of CD4+ CD25+ Foxp3+ regulatory T cells. J Immunol. 2006;177(10):6598–602.
115. Gunderson AJ, et al. Bruton tyrosine kinase–dependent immune cell cross-talk drives pancreas cancer. Cancer Discov. 2016;6(3):270–85.
116. Turaj AH, et al. Antibody tumor targeting is enhanced by CD27 agonists through myeloid recruitment. Cancer Cell. 2017;32(6):777–91.
117. Roschewski M, et al. Comparative study of circulating tumor DNA and computerized tomography monitoring in untreated diffuse large B-cell lymphoma. Lancet Oncol. 2015;16(5):541.
118. Kurtz DM, et al. Circulating tumor DNA measurements as early outcome predictors in diffuse large B-cell lymphoma. J Clin Oncol. 2018;36(28):2845–53.
119. Scherer F, et al. Distinct biological subtypes and patterns of genome evolution in lymphoma revealed by circulating tumor DNA. Sci Transl Med. 2016;8(364):364ra155.

120. Rossi D, et al. Diffuse large B-cell lymphoma genotyping on the liquid biopsy. Blood. 2017;129(14):1947–57.
121. Thierry A, et al. Clinical utility of circulating DNA analysis for rapid detection of actionable mutations to select metastatic colorectal patients for anti-EGFR treatment. Ann Oncol. 2017;28:2149.
122. Scherer F, et al. Noninvasive molecular subtyping and risk stratification of DLBCL. Proc Am Soc Clin Oncol. 2016.
123. Jin MC, et al. Noninvasive detection of clinically relevant copy number alterations in diffuse large B-cell lymphoma. Proc Am Soc Clin Oncol. 2017.
124. Prasad V. Perspective: the precision-oncology illusion. Nature. 2016;537(7619):S63.
125. Papadimitrakopoulou V, et al. The BATTLE-2 study: a biomarker-integrated targeted therapy study in previously treated patients with advanced non–small-cell lung cancer. J Clin Oncol. 2016;34(30):3638–47.

Correction to: Aggressive Lymphomas

Georg Lenz and Gilles Salles

Correction to:
G. Lenz, G. Salles (eds.), *Aggressive Lymphomas,* Hematologic Malignancies, https://doi.org/10.1007/978-3-030-00362-3

The spelling of book title was incorrect. Book title "Agressive Lymphomas" has been corrected to "Aggressive Lymphomas".

The updated online versions of the book can be found at
https://doi.org/10.1007/978-3-030-00362-3

G. Lenz, G. Salles (eds.), *Aggressive Lymphomas,* Hematologic Malignancies,
https://doi.org/10.1007/978-3-030-00362-3_19

MIX
Papier aus verantwortungsvollen Quellen
Paper from responsible sources
FSC® C105338

If you have any concerns about our products,
you can contact us on
ProductSafety@springernature.com

In case Publisher is established outside the EU,
the EU authorized representative is:
Springer Nature Customer Service Center GmbH
Europaplatz 3, 69115 Heidelberg, Germany

Printed by Libri Plureos GmbH
in Hamburg, Germany